Reshaping Health Promotion and Disease Prevention Through Digital Innovation

Sónia Remondes Costa
https://orcid.org/0000-0003-4282-3964
University of Tras-os-Montes and Alto Douro, Vila Real, Portugal

Jorge Remondes
https://orcid.org/0000-0002-5259-4379
CEOS.PP, ISCAP, Polytechnic of Porto, Portugal

IGI Global
Scientific Publishing
Publishing Tomorrow's Research Today

Published in the United States of America by
IGI Global Scientific Publishing
701 East Chocolate Avenue
Hershey, PA, 17033, USA
Tel: 717-533-8845 | Fax: 717-533-7115
Website: https://www.igi-global.com E-mail: cust@igi-global.com

Library of Congress Cataloging-in-Publication Data

LCCN: 2025024329 (CIP Data Pending)
ISBN13: 9798337335315
Isbn13Softcover: 9798337335322
EISBN13: 9798337335339

British Cataloguing in Publication Data
A Cataloguing in Publication record for this book is available from the British Library.

Table of Contents

Detailed Table of Contents

Over the past twenty years or so, healthcare has been changing in ways we did not see coming. This chapter, Introduction to Digital Health and Prevention, takes a closer look at how things like mobile health apps, eHealth platforms, wearables, telemedicine, big data, blockchain, and AI are now part of public health. These aren't just for treating illnesses—they're helping people stay healthy, spot problems earlier, and take care of themselves day to day. It really began with electronic health records and early telemedicine. Now, AI tools that use machine learning, language processing, and even computer vision can warn about risks and guide better use of resources. Of course, that raises questions—who owns the data, how is it used, and is it fair? Rules like GDPR and HIPAA, plus "data ethics by design," try to keep things in check. In the end, digital health works best when it's fair and open to all.

This chapter examines the economic impact of digital health innovations in disease prevention, focusing on cost-effectiveness, ROI, and policy implications. As health systems face escalating costs and a rising NCD burden, tools like mHealth, telemedicine, wearables, and AI offer scalable, cost-saving preventive solutions. Drawing on global evidence and modeling, the chapter highlights strong ROI, especially in high-risk populations and LMICs. It reviews economic evaluation metrics, showcases real-world case studies, and addresses challenges including the digital divide and policy gaps. Concluding with policy recommendations, it advocates for inclusive design, sustainable investment, and equity-driven evaluation frameworks to guide future innovation.

This chapter examines the transformative evolution of digital health from fragmented technological applications into a comprehensive, multidisciplinary ecosystem that fundamentally redefines healthcare delivery and patient engagement. Driven by rapid advancements in artificial intelligence, wearable devices, the Internet of Things, digital therapeutics, multi-omics integration, and extended reality, digital health shifts care paradigms from reactive, clinician-centered models to proactive, precise, predictive, preventive, and participatory approaches. The COVID-19 pandemic accelerated widespread adoption of digital solutions, demonstrating their capacity for agile crisis response while exposing persistent challenges such as the digital divide, interoperability limitations, and inequities in access. The chapter explores how digital health addresses major systemic pressures—including the rising burden of non-communicable diseases, healthcare workforce shortages, and escalating costs—through scalable, data-driven innovations that support value-based care, real-time monitoring, personalized interventions, lifestyle modification, and improved outcomes that matter to patients. While highlighting the potential to empower individuals as active participants in their health management within everyday contexts, the discussion critically addresses key barriers: ethical concerns, regulatory fragmentation, algorithmic bias, data privacy risks, and the need for inclusive, context-sensitive implementation strategies. Ultimately, this chapter argues that realizing the full promise of digital health requires rigorous evidence generation, participatory design, equitable frameworks, and collaborative governance to ensure that technological progress translates into sustainable, resilient, and human-centered health ecosystems that promote well-being for all populations.

Type 2 diabetes mellitus (T2DM) is rising globally, with low- and middle-income countries, including South Africa, bearing a disproportionate burden. This chapter explores the role of digital health tools such as mobile health (mHealth), wearable technologies, and artificial intelligence in supporting T2DM prevention and management. It critically examines how these innovations promote education, behaviour change, and self-management in under-resourced settings. The chapter highlights that while digital tools offer scalable solutions for diabetes care, their success depends on equitable access, cultural relevance, and integration into primary healthcare. Challenges such as the digital divide, data privacy, and weak system alignment must be addressed. Community engagement enhances trust and long-term use. Looking forward, digital health can transform care if supported by context-specific research, inclusive design, and enabling policies. A hybrid model—blending innovation with person-centred care—is essential for sustainable, accessible diabetes management rooted in local realities.

The rapid digitalisation of healthcare systems has introduced innovative solutions for improved access, efficiency, and patient outcomes. However, without equitable digital competency, these advancements risk exacerbating existing health disparities. This chapter explores the critical role of digital competency in promoting equity within the digital healthcare ecosystem. It examines how varying levels of digital skills among patients, providers, and institutions influence access to and utilisation of digital health services. Through conceptual analysis, global case studies, and policy reflections, the chapter highlights structural barriers, digital divides, and strategies to foster inclusive digital health practices. Emphasising the intersectionality of digital exclusion, the chapter advocates for targeted interventions and capacity-building initiatives that prioritise marginalised populations. Ultimately, it positions digital competency as a foundational pillar for ensuring equity and inclusion in the evolving landscape of digital healthcare.

This chapter introduces the Personalized Health Assistant, an integrated system that combines Internet of Things devices, machine learning, and natural language processing to monitor diabetes and promote proactive, personalized healthcare. For diabetic patients, the system leverages wearable sensors data. For non-diabetic users, physiological parameters are inferred through lifestyle and stress indicators. To support predictive health monitoring, the system incorporates advanced machine learning models: Long Short-Term Memory, Multiple Back-Propagation, and a Convolutional Neural Network. Another component of the system is a clinically aware chatbot, built upon the Falcon-7B large language model and semantically validated using Bio_ClinicalBERT. The chatbot pipeline integrates FAISS-based context retrieval, clinical term detection, and semantic similarity scoring. The validation results underscore the system's reliability for predictive analytics, intelligent interaction, and real-time clinical support, making it a viable solution for scalable and secure chronic disease management.

This chapter examines the dual effects of digital technology on mental health, looking at how AI-powered tools, telepsychiatry, and mobile applications influence modern experiences of psychological identity, emotional regulation, and self-care. With the utility of tools like natural language processing (NLP), cognitive behavioral therapy (CBT) feedback, and predictive risk assessment algorithms, these digital platforms provide scalable and practical interventions. However, they also carry risks, such as over-reliance, a loss of intrinsic motivation, and an inability to recognize deep human nuances. An elaborate discussion of 'surveillance' in the place of 'support' is portrayed in detail through an analysis of the most common underlying technological mechanisms of different digital intervention tools. The chapter ends with an advocation of optimizing digital care by careful planning, moral supervision, and integration with human-centered assistance to guarantee that technology enhances, rather than harms, mental health outcomes.

This chapter is grounded in the results of the ERASMUS+ funded project SmartAgeCare, which investigated active and healthy ageing strategies across eight European countries. The project aims to foster digital inclusion, civic participation, and psychosocial well-being among older adults by exploring innovative models of engagement. This chapter introduces the concept of 'Ikigai Play' as a transdisciplinary framework rooted in a meta-narrative review and inspired by the Japanese philosophy of Ikigai—meaning 'reason for being'. Synthesising evidence from national studies and digital ageing strategies, the chapter identifies regional disparities, psychosocial drivers, and the transformative potential of inclusive technologies. 'Ikigai Play' is proposed as a culturally adaptive model to support autonomy, well-being, and digital health equity.

Digital health technologies are reshaping healthcare by improving disease prevention, early diagnosis, and continuous health monitoring. This chapter delves into the expanding role of digital tools—from e-health and telemedicine to AI and ML—in advancing preventive healthcare. It emphasizes the use of wearable devices and biosensors for real-time monitoring, empowering both patients and providers to detect early health risks. The shift to AI-powered systems enables personalized care, automated diagnostics, and proactive engagement, but also raises concerns around data privacy, ethical use, adoption challenges, and equity in access—especially in underserved regions. Through global case studies, the chapter highlights successful digital health interventions and explores future directions, including digital integration in national health policies, regulation, and literacy. It also examines trends like virtual care, remote monitoring, and AI-linked EHRs, offering insights into how digital health can foster a more inclusive, responsive, and future-ready healthcare system.

This chapter explores the complex relationship between medication adherence, digital health, and patient-centred care (PCC), with a focus on chronic multimorbidity and polypharmacy. It begins by addressing the conceptual evolution of adherence and its determinants, followed by a discussion of how digital technologies can support person-centred approaches to improve therapeutic outcomes. The chapter presents Mobili®, an innovative portable automated dispenser, and outlines the design and implementation of the MobiMAd@PT project in Portugal. Drawing on international evidence and implementation science frameworks, it analyses the usability, effectiveness, and scalability of such interventions. Emphasis is placed on co-design, contextual adaptation, and integrated care models involving community pharmacies. The chapter concludes by outlining best practices for future digital adherence strategies, highlighting the importance of collaborative, user-driven approaches to enhance healthcare quality and sustainability.

The writers of this chapter claim that in surgical nursing, digitalization and technical developments have drastically changed patient care procedures. Digital tools including electronic health records, artificial intelligence-supported decision systems, wearable devices, simulation technologies and augmented reality have helped nurses to make clinical decisions, guarantee patient safety and raise the quality of treatment. Furthermore underlining the need of digital capabilities in professional growth are redefining nurse roles in robotic surgical applications and supporting nursing education with simulations. Although telehealth technologies provide access and flexibility to help surgery patients follow-up, the ethical and legal aspects of digital applications also provide significant topics of conversation. This chapter explores in a multidimensional sense the consequences of digital change on surgical nursing practices.

Preface

In the past two decades, healthcare has undergone a profound transformation driven by the convergence of technology, data science, and public health innovation. What was once the domain of traditional, face-to-face clinical encounters has evolved into a complex ecosystem of digital tools, platforms, and strategies aimed not only at treating disease but also at promoting health and preventing illness. The promise of digital health lies in its potential to empower individuals, enhance system efficiency, and foster equitable access to care, yet this promise comes with challenges, including ethical concerns, data privacy, and the need for inclusive design.

Reshaping Health Promotion and Disease Prevention Through Digital Innovation brings together leading researchers and practitioners from around the globe to explore how digital innovations are transforming health promotion, disease prevention, and patient-centered care. The chapters in this volume address the technological, economic, clinical, and societal dimensions of digital health, offering a comprehensive examination of contemporary challenges and opportunities. By integrating theoretical insights, empirical research, and practical applications, this book aims to inform policymakers, clinicians, educators, and technologists about the evolving landscape of digital healthcare.

CHAPTER OVERVIEW

Chapter 1: Introduction to Digital Health and Prevention

Saha, Singh, and Thakur provide an overview of digital health's evolution, from electronic health records to AI-driven predictive analytics. They discuss the role of telemedicine, wearables, and mobile health apps in prevention, highlighting ethical and regulatory considerations that ensure fair and equitable access.

Chapter 2: The Economic Impact of Digital Health Innovations on Disease Prevention

Abdulwahab et al. examine cost-effectiveness, return on investment, and policy implications of digital health interventions. Case studies from diverse settings demonstrate how innovations such as AI and mHealth can reduce healthcare costs while improving outcomes, with special attention to low- and middle-income countries.

Chapter 3: Code Meets Care: The Digital Shift in Health Promotion

Nogueira, Santos, Pina, and Martins explore the intersection of technology and health promotion, emphasizing how digital tools reshape preventive care strategies through innovative platforms and data-driven approaches.

Chapter 4: App Your Health: Harnessing Digital Tools for Diabetes Prevention and Health Promotion

Mphasha focuses on type 2 diabetes prevention, highlighting mobile apps, wearables, and AI for patient education, self-management, and behavior change. The chapter emphasizes equity, cultural relevance, and integration into primary care.

Chapter 5: Digital Competency's Role in Promoting Equity in the Digital Healthcare Ecosystem

Abubakari and Olamilekan discuss the importance of digital skills in reducing health disparities, exploring global case studies and policy strategies to foster inclusive digital health practices.

Chapter 6: Deep Learning Diabetes Monitoring and Prevention

Ribeiro et al. introduce a Personalized Health Assistant leveraging IoT devices, machine learning, and NLP to support predictive, individualized diabetes care, combining wearable data with advanced AI models for scalable management.

Chapter 7: Digital Cure or Digital Cage? Reassessing Wellness in the Age of Algorithmic Mental Health

Bhaktharam and Tyagi analyze digital mental health tools, weighing their benefits against risks of over-reliance and reduced human nuance. They advocate for ethically guided, human-centered digital interventions.

Chapter 8: Ikigai Play: Towards an Ikigai Paradigm of Healthy and Active Ageing in Europe

Giesteira et al. present 'Ikigai Play,' a framework for promoting active ageing through digital inclusion and psychosocial engagement, synthesizing findings from the ERASMUS+ SmartAgeCare project across Europe.

Chapter 9: Transforming Healthcare Delivery: The Role of Digital Technologies

Kumar and Jain highlight digital tools in disease prevention, real-time monitoring, and AI-powered personalized care, while examining challenges such as equity, data privacy, and integration into healthcare systems.

Chapter 10: From Self-Reports to Sensors in Machine Learning for Chronic Stress Detection

Nag, Vijaya, and Rao review multimodal stress detection, emphasizing wearable sensors, physiological markers, and AI models. They propose a roadmap for privacy-preserving, explainable stress monitoring systems.

Chapter 11: From Virtual Care to Real Satisfaction: Telemedicine Service Quality

Kavipriya and Jesiah evaluate telemedicine service quality using the SERVQUAL framework, linking functional and technical aspects to patient satisfaction, accessibility, and overall care experience.

Chapter 12: Predictive Analytics in Personalized Medical Care

Dehankar and Das discuss AI-driven risk assessment and personalized interventions, exploring ethical frameworks, data privacy, and integration challenges within modern healthcare infrastructures.

Chapter 13: Before the Interface: User Research for ALS Patients with Partial Locked-In Syndrome

Giesteira et al. present tailored user research instruments to inform digital health solutions for neurodegenerative conditions, emphasizing participatory and sensory-based methodologies.

Chapter 14: Digital Technology Supporting Medication Adherence

Gregório et al. analyze the Mobili® automated dose dispenser in Portugal, illustrating how digital solutions can enhance medication adherence, promote person-centered care, and ensure sustainability.

Chapter 15: Digitalization and Technological Innovations in Surgical Nursing

Gümüs explores how digital tools, simulations, AI, and augmented reality transform surgical nursing, supporting clinical decision-making, patient safety, and professional growth.

Chapter 16: Innovating End-of-Life Psychological Care

Leite et al. examine Meaning of Life Therapy via videoconferencing for palliative patients, highlighting digital interventions' potential to promote dignity, purpose, and psychological adjustment in challenging contexts.

This preface situates the book as a global, multidisciplinary exploration of digital health innovations, linking theory, evidence, and practice while emphasizing equity, ethics, and human-centered care.

Chapter 1
Introduction to Digital Health and Prevention

Biswajit Saha
https://orcid.org/0000-0001-8000-6733
JIS University, Kolkata, India & Dr. B.C. Roy Engineering College, Durgapur, India

Dharmpal Singh
JIS University, India

Gour Sundar Mitra Thakur
https://orcid.org/0000-0001-8907-9058
Dr. B.C. Roy Engineering College, Durgapur, India

ABSTRACT

Over the past twenty years or so, healthcare has been changing in ways we did not see coming. This chapter, Introduction to Digital Health and Prevention, takes a closer look at how things like mobile health apps, eHealth platforms, wearables, telemedicine, big data, blockchain, and AI are now part of public health. These aren't just for treating illnesses—they're helping people stay healthy, spot problems earlier, and take care of themselves day to day. It really began with electronic health records and early telemedicine. Now, AI tools that use machine learning, language processing, and even computer vision can warn about risks and guide better use of resources. Of course, that raises questions—who owns the data, how is it used, and is it fair? Rules like GDPR and HIPAA, plus "data ethics by design," try to keep things in check. In the end, digital health works best when it's fair and open to all.

1 INTRODUCTION

Digital technologies and healthcare have drastically revolutionized how societies promote health and prevent sickness in the modern era. As populations increase, age, and more people suffer from chronic diseases, healthcare systems all across the world need to find new, scalable ways to stop them. Digital health includes a lot of different kinds of technology. In line with global definitions, we use the term digital health to describe the safe and effective use of these technologies to strengthen health systems,

DOI: 10.4018/979-8-3373-3531-5.ch001

promote health, and prevent disease across the life course World Health Organization (2019b), Organisation for Economic Co- operation and Development (2019a).

Some examples are mobile health (mHealth), electronic health (eHealth), wearable devices, telemedicine, big data analytics, blockchain technology, and AI (artificial intelligence). Any of these technologies, used alone or combined, might dramatically improve health outcomes by making it easier to keep an eye on diseases, deliver customized treatment, and encourage health. Most of the time, healthcare was reactive, meaning that most therapies were meant to cure problems after they had already happened. Digital health has started a new era of proactive care, where the goal is to find ways to treat people that minimize their risk of getting sick or growing worse. This preventive orientation connects digital health to established traditions in health promotion and population health management, which emphasize early risk detection, behaviour change, and system-level interventions Abernethy et al. (2022), A. Labrique et al. (2013).

Figure 1. Conceptual Framework

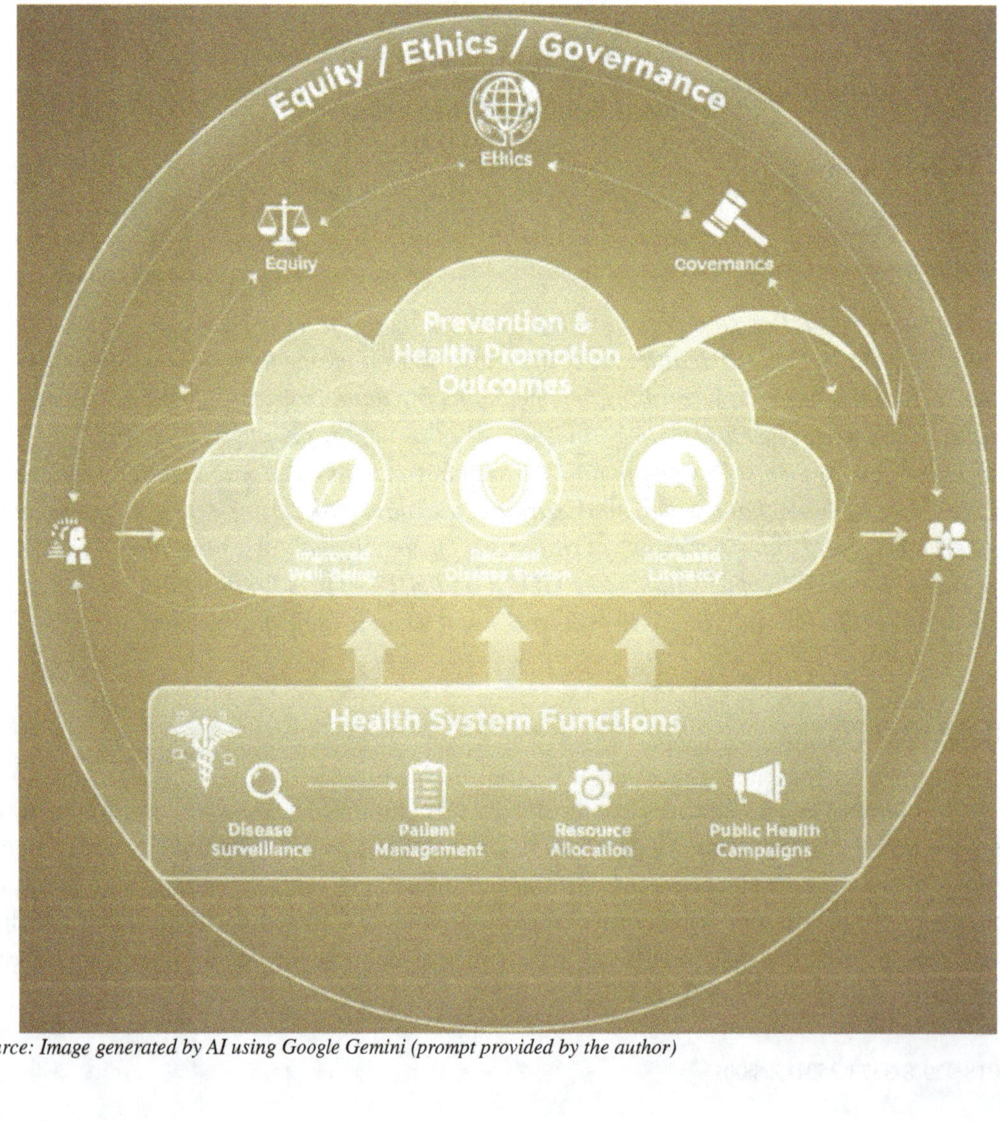

(Source: Image generated by AI using Google Gemini (prompt provided by the author))

Figure 1 shows the link between digital health technologies to health system functions, prevention and health promotion outcomes, under the cross-cutting lens of equity, ethics and governance.

Digital health infrastructure has changed a lot in the last few decades thanks to new technologies. Electronic health records (EHRs) and telemedicine plat- forms were some of the first big changes that made it possible to preserve records digitally and talk to patients from a distance instead of in person. EHRs made it easier to keep and access data, which made clinical environments consider- ably more organized and productive. Telemedicine made it possible for people in rural or poorly developed areas to get medical care. Even though these early technologies were mostly used for writing down information and talking to each other, they were nevertheless quite valuable.

These important technologies are very different from digital health. Now, it is moving towards more complex, smart systems that incorporate computer vision, machine learning, and natural language processing (NLP). These new digital ecosystems not only make it simpler to talk to individuals who are far away, but they also make healthcare better by giving doctors and nurses access to more complex analytical tools. For example, AI-powered predictive analytics can now detect people who are likely to have chronic illnesses before they show symptoms. This lets healthcare providers step in early. Wearable electronics with sensors can always inform you how much activity you have done, your heart rate, and your blood pressure. They give doctors and patients real-time feedback, which helps them stay healthy.

Digital health is particularly important for preventing infections that are not contagious that is which are basically non communicable diseases (NCDs). Heart disease, diabetes, cancer, and chronic lung difficulties are all examples of NCDs that are a big problem all over the world. They cost a lot of money and kill millions of people every year. Digital health solutions help with this problem by helping individuals keep an eye on their health all the time, change their behaviour in ways that work for them, learn about their health from a distance, and instantly get in touch with their doctors and nurses. For example, smartphone apps that encourage people to eat well, work out, or take their med- ications as recommended have been shown to help people make better choices and stay healthy.

Digital health technology could help people on a personal level and also help fill up important gaps in access to healthcare and health information. They offer solutions that can be expanded to serve others who cannot get to them. This helps to fill in the gaps that come from being cut off by location, money, or a lack of healthcare infrastructure. Digital health projects in the community use technology to teach and empower those who are usually left out, giving them more control over their health.

What might seem like a potential assistance from digital health technologies is not always the case. They are not always easy to use when it comes to preventive care. There are technical reasons for this, and one of them is certainly not wanting to share or being unable to share. That is to say, within the preventive care sector, there is a lack of agreement as to what standards are to be used. Now, this is not a direct result of any one law, but certainly, laws like the Health Insurance Portability and Accountability Act (HIPAA) and meaningful use criteria make it difficult for everyone to agree on anything. The effect these laws have is in no way helping facilitate any form of agreement on standards.

One must also consider the moral questions raised by digital health technology. As health information becomes increasingly digital, it creates huge concerns about privacy, safety, and data ownership, along with major questions about informed consent and patients' rights. These developments also raise important ethical questions around privacy, data ownership, consent and algorithmic bias, which are taken up in Section 5 on ethical and regulatory issues.

People across the globe should regard digital health as more than just a tool. It is a crucial part of modern healthcare and MUST be employed in a way that is both USEFUL and ETHICAL, lest we fully squander its potential to link people—and pay a steep price in morality, if not in more tangible ways. At a moment when proffered "solutions" and new healthcare technologies are serving mostly to expand and deepen the fundamental flaws of the system, we must at least figure out ways to use what is at hand more responsibly—if for no other reason than to ensure we do not employ digital health to the manifold ends for which it can be misused.

The chapter is perhaps most relevant to a reader who is an academic (across disciplines), policy-maker, health care practitioner or technology developer. Its main focus is on how digital innovation can enable health promotion and disease prevention for populations and services, not technology for technology's sake. We strive to bridge theoretical considerations with practical applications, so that readers can apply the concepts in this paper toward designing, evaluating and scaling preventative digital health interventions within their own communities. This chapter offers the readers with a narrative, thematically structured overview of how digital health tools support health promotion and disease prevention. We discuss about a socio-technical framework, which recognises digital health as the interplay between people, organizations and technologies Green- halgh et al. (2017), Cresswell et al. (2013). We also consider it from a population health perspective, where the emphasis is on large-scale preventive measures as pointed out by A. Labrique et al. (2013), Abernethy et al. (2022). There are four sections in this chapter: (i) the legacy of digital health technologies; (ii) opportunities for preventing and controlling public health; (iii) challenges and systemic barriers and (iv) ethical, legal concerns.

There is an increasing stream of evidence and review articles which report digital health as offering great potential whilst noting its limitations. For example, Buntin et al. (2011) and Kruse et al. (2018) find largely positive yet idiosyncratic influences of EHR and other HIT on cause-specific causes in the work context. Telemedicine and mHealth were rapidly expanded during COVID-19. At the same time, new research indicates enduring disparities vis-`a-vis equity, human resources preparedness and long-term sustainability Crawford and Serhal (2020), Topol (2019), World Health Organization (2021d). We draw upon these insights in this chapter, in relation to the prevention and health promotion fields.

To facilitate understanding of this wide range, the chapter is structured as follows. First, we describe the trajectory of digital health technology and its use in prevention. We then explore key opportunities and challenges, including ethical considerations, data governance, infrastructure and equity, policy and regulatory landscape, and its influence on the implementation policy We explore further here policy and regulation environment in which EIRBS being adopted came to emergence an enactment. We conclude by spotlighting practical considerations and future directions of digital health in population prevention.

In the following section the evolution of digital health technologies are highlighted starting from EHR and telemedicine to the impact of big data analytics, machine learning, NLP, and computer vision also including the transition from e-Health to advanced AI-driven healthcare.

2 EVOLUTION OF DIGITAL HEALTH TECHNOLOGIES

The digital health transformation continually redefines the manner in which healthcare services are dispensed, administered, and optimized. Although the digital health revolution had its origins in the early 2000s with the develop- ment and implementation of electronic health/medical records, telemedicine, and other health IT solutions, these early e-health initiatives were mainly con- fined to and limited by remote communication solutions, operational efficiencies, and data management with little to no clinical decision-making impacts. From 2010 to 2020, deeper, wider, and more sophisticated forms of AI, driven primarily by big data and the Internet of Things (IoT), started to penetrate the digital health marketplace and supply chain. Collectively, these forms of AI initiated a disruptive, pervasive, and much-anticipated shift in not only the dig- ital health landscape but also in the way healthcare is administrated, delivered, and dispensed. This shift has occurred and is continuing to occur, with pro- found implications for all stakeholders. Clinical, nonclinical, and health plan decision-makers are the primary push/pull stakeholders driving these market- place changes. The next few subsections will provide a more detailed exploration of these critical stages of digital health evolution.

Figure 2. Evolution

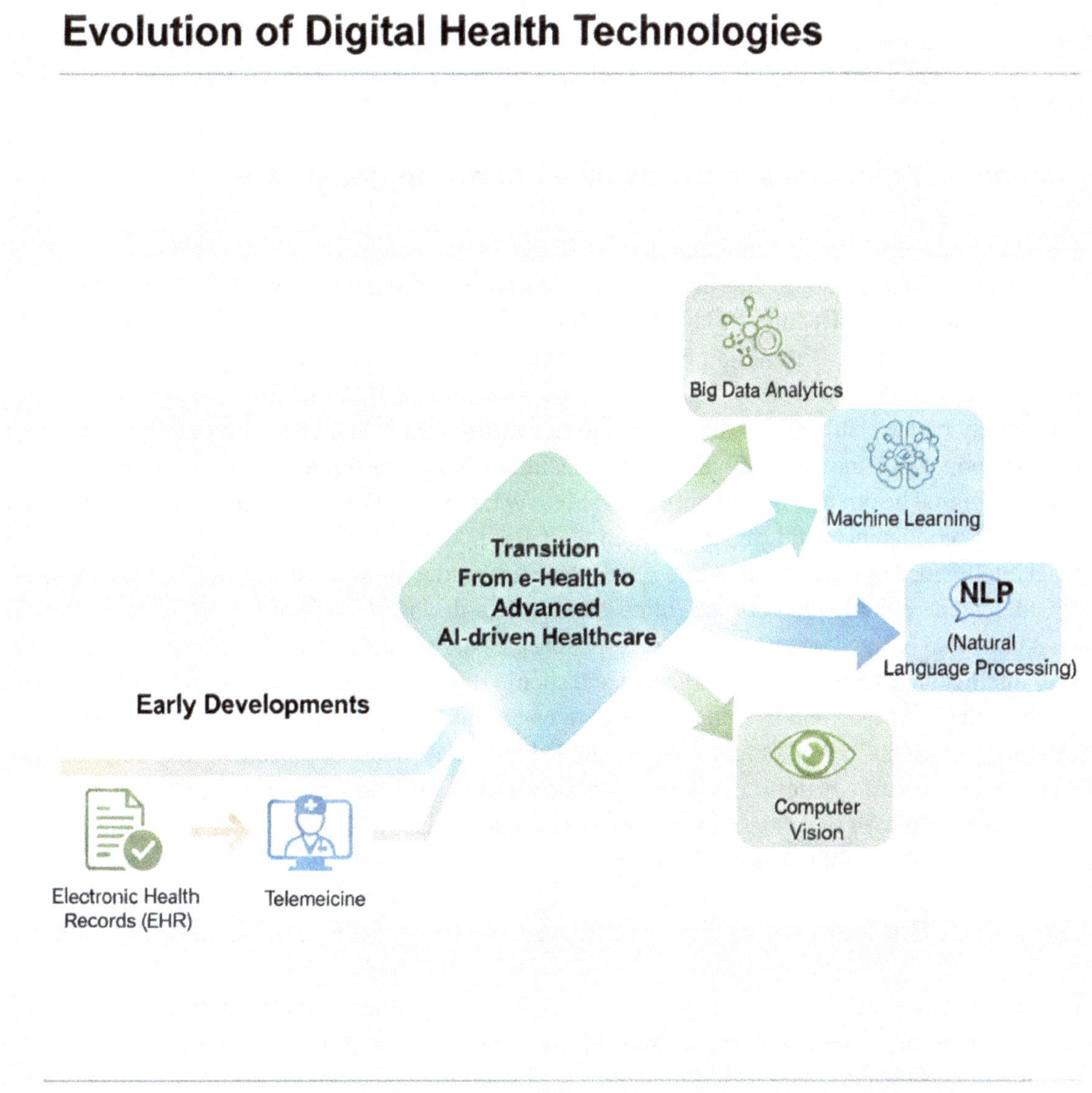

Source: Image generated by AI using Google Gemini (prompt provided by the author).

Figure 2 shows the evolution of digital health technologies.

2.1 Early Developments: Electronic Health Records (EHR) and Telemedicine

The initial stage of digital health innovation was underpinned by two ground- breaking developments: EHR and telemedicine. EHR systems took the traditional, paper-based medical record and transposed it into a digital format. That transition allowed, and in some cases required, healthcare providers to be much more efficient and much more secure in the ways they stored, retrieved, and shared information about patients. EHRs were, and are, a vast improvement over the kinds of record-keeping that had been the norm in healthcare for centuries. EHRs and telemedicine are great 'types' of digital health because they are both so fundamentally important to the way we conceptualize digital health today. They are also domains where the consumer has largely privatized the experience. In other words, one can use an EHR or dial into a telemedicine appointment without ever really understanding what is going on behind the scenes.

2.2 Transition From e-Health to Advanced AI-driven Healthcare

After the first wave of digitization through EHR and telemedicine, the area of digital health started to move in a new direction, one often described as the transition from e-Health to intelligent, AI-driven healthcare ecosystems. E-Health was largely about the documentation of basic healthcare transactions; it was also about the remote provision of health services. In those two primary aspects, e-Health was similar to what had come before it in the history of computing and the internet, mostly just a series of increasingly better platforms for accessing and delivering healthcare. But e-Health also provided a foundation upon which the next edifice of digital health could be constructed. The key moves from that initial, basic digital health platform to the next level (to two next levels, really) were to become not just a better place for conducing healthcare transactions, but also to become something smarter; to incorporate artificial intelligence (AI) and to become a better place for conducing smart healthcare transactions; and finally, to become a cornerstone of the future digital, data-driven smart health ecosystem that would ensue. AI has also been an integral part of this sequence of moves and is rewriting the rule book for the kinds of intelligent systems dig- ital health can and should deploy. In the future, digital health platforms will employ these AI/machine learning (ML) systems to do what they do best: find patterns in digital data, use those patterns to predict future states, and help humans in the loop make nearby decisions that will steer things toward a better state. In the past decade, the computers in our digital health platforms have transformed from passive, static systems into dynamic engines of discovery that are employing AI/ ML methods to influence the next several chapters of digital health history.

2.3 Impact of Big Data Analytics, Machine Learning, NLP, and Computer Vision

The next phase in the evolution of digital health, which is the most transformative so far, is characterized by the integration of large-scale data analytics, ML, natural language processing (NLP), and computer vision into the healthcare sys- tem. The unprecedented volume of health-related information generated from the digital revolution—from EHRs, the Internet of Medical Things (IoMT), genomics, and other patient-generated sources—offers the opportunity to move from deep data storage toward something even more profound: insightful, real- time decision-making that affects the health of populations. Big data affords the opportunity to examine and aggregate diverse, heterogeneous datasets at an unprecedented scale, identifying hidden patterns and correlations not eas- ily discerned by human investigators, that can inform and guide public health interventions, as well as private sector efforts aiming to improve the health of particular populations. Building on this foundation, ML offers the opportunity to continuously (and in near-real time) improve the accuracy of predictive mod- els that inform the kinds of early detection and stratification decisions necessary to anticipate, understand, and address the health of particular individuals in a population. NLP serves the equally important function of understanding and making sense of the enormous volume of unstructured data that health profes- sionals generate. This includes such things as clinical notes, pathology reports, and the medical literature of the last several millennia. A revolution in health- care intelligence is taking place, and it is revolutionizing (again) fields such as radiology, pathology, and dermatology. These advances (in intelligence) involve the use of mostly untrained deep learning neural networks to do what humans have done: look at something and understand it (or not, as in cases of looking at the normal versus the pathologically abnormal).

Even with this fast pace of change, the evidence base within prevention for digital health is mixed. Published work has mostly focused on feasibil- ity and early adoption in high-income contexts, with relatively few rigorous evaluations of long-term health outcomes, cost-effectiveness or equity consequences—particularly in low and middle income countries, as stated in LMICs (Labrique et al., 2018; Crawford & Serhal, 2020; World Health Organization, 2021d). The next section focus not only in technological options but also on ex- isting gaps and frictions in the use of digital health to reinforce prevention. The next section also highlights the opportunities and potential of digital health in- cluding scalable digital interventions for population health management, cost- effectiveness and resource optimization and personalized and precision preven- tive healthcare strategies.

3 OPPORTUNITIES AND POTENTIAL OF DIGITAL HEALTH

In this section, we describe how digital health tools can be employed to particularly bolster health promotion and prevention including detecting risk factors earlier, supporting behaviour change, improving vaccination uptake as well as closely monitoring risk of chronic disease.

Online tools can transform prevention and health promotion — several real- world programs prove it. SMS reminder programs and interactive voice response services have led to increased vaccination uptake, antenatal care attendance and adherence to preventive therapies. Mobile apps and wearables are applied in lifestyle interventions for smoking cessation, physical activity, weight control with or without coaching/ peer support. Telemedicine and remote monitoring services for patients with hypertension or diabetes provide early recognition of poor control, to promptly readjust therapy thus preventing complications. These are examples of the ways in which digital technologies can shift prevention from intermittent, clinic-based counseling to a more continuous and tailored support.

In its initial days digital health technologies were simple electronic tools. Today, they have traversed a long way. We have smart electronic systems that are capable of doing many things. These modern day tools have the capability of suggesting treatments that is proactive, preventive, and tailored to each person. These technologies use real time data, process it to make treatments faster than ever before. These technologies use the available resources more wisely. These combine to give better control over chronic diseases in both individual as well as group settings. The patients have more control over their health. They get tailored counsel, regular feedback and in some cases may also get educational materials that makes them aware of both their diseases that they are suffering from as well as the treatment that are in place to overcome them. This in a way empowers the people to look for their health and themselves. Digital health can improve health outcomes, save costs, and make it easier for people to get good care, especially in areas that do not have a lot of health care options or are hard to get to. This is possible thanks to new technologies like remote monitoring, predictive analytics, and patient interaction platforms.

In terms of emerging trends, predictive analytics, real-time monitoring and AI regulation are especially critical as preventive measures. Predictive ana- lytics applies patterns in clinical data, behavior and sometimes environmental or genomic information to identify people who are at higher risk before their symptoms become severe. Through the use of wearables and connected devices, real-time monitoring can provide continuous monitoring of vital signs and be- haviours to facilitate early feedback for timely intervention. Concurrently, new laws and guidance on AI in healthcare are starting to specify demands for safety, transparency, documentation and human supervision. Combined, these trends will be highly influential on the future of prevention delivery.

3.1 Core Trends in Digital Health and Prevention

Across many health systems, digital health is linked to a wider shift from volume-based to value-based care. Routine digital data, risk scores and dash- boards are used not only to record activity, but also to track outcomes and identify people who might benefit from preventive support earlier. Artificial

intelligence and advanced analytics are increasingly used to move from reactive treatment to predictive and preventive care. Examples include risk prediction models that combine routine clinical data, lifestyle information and sometimes genomic markers to estimate future disease risk, as well as early experimental use of “digital twins” that simulate how an individual patient might respond to different interventions. New delivery models such as digital therapeutics, remote monitoring and hybrid in-person/virtual care are also changing how prevention is delivered. In parallel, some systems are experimenting with more decen- tralised or virtual clinical trials that use apps, wearables and home-based tests to follow participants, which can reduce visit burden and widen participation when designed carefully.

3.2 Scalable Digital Interventions for Population Health Management

According to Abernethy et al. (2022) scalable digital interventions are technolo- gies and program designs that can be used with a small group of people and then with a larger group of people without the cost or complexity going up in a straight line. PHM stands for ”population health management.” Its goal is to find risks ahead of time, provide the right level of intervention (individual, co- hort, community), and keep an eye on outcomes to improve overall health while keeping costs down. When digital tools are designed to be scalable, they can do this. They can reach more people than traditional care settings, automate risk stratification and follow-up, and let people give feedback all the time.

3.3 Cost-Effectiveness and Resource Optimization

Cost-effectiveness and resource optimization are two important reasons to sup- port and justify digital health on a large scale. Digital interventions in popula- tion health management must not only improve outcomes, but they must also do so in a way that gives more value per unit cost than current methods, or they must find better uses for limited resources. Various researches are being carried out across the globe to make digital health cost effective and optimizing the resources required to implement digital health. Thiel et al. (2024) in their research highlights about statistical models based on weather and health data can predict resource utilization and optimize healthcare provision in response to climate impacts. Digital health technology can enhance health promotion campaigns in resource-limited regions, but challenges like internet access and digital literacy must be addressed is emphasized by Pudyastuti et al. (2024).

Kansal et al. (2022) in their research discusses the various ways in which the integration of digital image processing and IoT in healthcare can enable resource optimization and improve care quality while lowering costs while Basu et al. (2021) in their research followed a network slicing approach using 5G tech- nologies which can enable optimized resource provisioning for digital healthcare.

3.4 Personalized and Precision Preventive Healthcare Strate- gies

Gambhir et al. (2018) and Ginsburg and Phillips (2018) states that in recent years, personalized and precision preventive healthcare has shifted from being a futuristic idea to a practical approach in many settings. These strategies draw on digital technologies to create interventions shaped around a person's own health profile—taking into account genetics, lifestyle habits, and even live health data. When paired with tools such as advanced analytics, artificial intelligence, and genomic insights, they make it possible to spot risks early and respond with preventive actions that actually fit the individual. Beyond the tracking, digital platforms that offer practical guidance and self-care ideas put more control in the patient's hands. When this personal touch is combined with early action, better health results are obtained, less pressure are present on hospitals, and, ideally, we get a system that works more smoothly for everyone.

3.5 Case Studies Illustrating Successful Digital Health Im- plementations

The mPower Heart Project in Himachal Pradesh, India, shows how digital tools can strengthen prevention and control of non-communicable diseases in routine primary care. In five community health centres, a nurse care coordinator used a smartphone-based clinical decision support system (CDSS) to screen adults for hypertension and diabetes, enter their clinical data, and generate guideline- based treatment plans, which were then reviewed and approved by a physician. Over 18 months, 6,797 adults were enrolled; more than half of those with hy- pertension and around one-third of those with diabetes were newly detected through this digital screening approach. Mean systolic blood pressure fell by about 15 mmHg and fasting plasma glucose by about 50 mg/dL among partic- ipants, with statistically significant improvements after adjusting for age, sex, and facility. This case not only illustrates how combining task-sharing (nurse- led care) with a simple mobile CDSS can improve detection and risk-factor control for cardiovascular prevention in a resource-constrained setting but also draws attention to practical needs, such as basic digital infrastructure, training for frontline staff, and embedding of digital workflows within under-resourced outpatient departments, Ajay et al. (2016).

MomConnect is a national mHealth program initiated by the South African National Department of Health to support pregnant and post-partum women, which commenced in 2014. It even records pregnancies in public facilities, sends stage-based SMS (and now WhatsApp) messages in all 11 official languages, as well as provides a helpdesk where woman can ask questions or rate services. MomConnect scaled across the public health system to more than 95% of facil- ities and subscriber registrations increased up to 1.5–1.7 million women which is well above half of those attending antenatal care in the public sector, over a period of approximately three years. Evaluations indicate good message de- livery and continued exposure, and narrative reviews report positive impacts on maternal health knowledge, antenatal and postnatal service use and preven- tion of mother-to-child transmission of HIV services. The case study provides an example of how a basic and free messaging service delivering information can be embedded into routine care and provided in local languages to achieve population-wide reach for prevention and health promotion, while generating new questions for consideration, including longer-term sustainability, data gov- ernance and responses to user feedback, Barron et al. (2018).

4 MAJOR CHALLENGES IN DIGITAL HEALTH

The challenges below apply until the point where digital health can be assumed to become a reliable means for enhancing prevention and health promotion, even if better technologies are at hand.

While digital health technologies hold immense promise for reshaping health- care, their integration into existing health systems is accompanied by a complex set of challenges that cannot be overlooked. The transformation from traditional to digital and AI-driven healthcare is not a straightforward process; it is con- strained by a variety of technical, organizational, economic, and social barriers. It is not easy to share information and use required therapy or treatments when the involved digital systems do not work together and there are also lack of enough compatible data formats. Also there are situations when the patient or the doctors and nurses are not well versed in using technology. Purchasing new technology also involves substantial amount of money and some healthcare institutions lack adaptability. Collectively all these obstacles make it challeng- ing for the widespread adoption of these new age technologies. Lack of clear rules that govern the use of telemedicine is also a hindrance considered by many. There are also problems with sharing data across borders. There are apprehen- sions with unfair access to technology, data control and about algorithms that favour some people over others. These problems show that the digital health revolution is more than just new technology. It also requires a change in how things are done and how people think.

Economic and business model questions are also central for digital health and prevention. Every intervention needs a clear plan for who will pay, how costs and savings will be shared, and how services will be reimbursed in public and private health systems. In some settings, digital tools are funded as short-term donor or innovation projects, whereas in others they are incorporated into insurance benefit packages, capitation payments or outcome-based contracts. Technology companies may bundle software, devices and support services into long-term agreements with governments or health organizations. When these financial arrangements are fragile or uncertain, promising preventive initiatives may never move beyond the pilot phase or may collapse once external funding ends. For policy makers and managers, understanding these financing and sustainability models is therefore essential for moving from isolated projects to stable, long- term digital health services that support prevention in an equitable way.

Barriers to implementation are often as critical as the technology. Health workers require training and time to fully embrace new systems, and digital tools must be seamlessly embedded into existing clinical and administrative workflows. Staff tend to resist using processes or views that require them to enter duplicate data, add substantial documentation burden, or be perceived as decreasing professional autonomy. Organizational-level determinants, such as leadership support, incentives and local champions likewise play a major role in determining whether digital-health projects expand beyond the level of pilot and into routine prevention work.

4.1 Technical and Infrastructural Barriers

Kruse et al. (2018) and World Health Organization (2021e) states that people who live in poor or rural places often cannot use telemedicine and other digital services because they cannot connect to the internet properly. it is still hard to keep computers safe, even in places with good internet access. Digital solutions that do not keep patient information safe make people less likely to believe them. A big part of the problem is also how it affects people. A lot of people who work in health care do not have the right tools or know how to use new technology properly. A lot of health care systems are still using old, different tools that do not share data or work well with each other. One of the biggest problems is that things do not work together. For those who are not tech-savvy, it might take longer to get used to new tools, no matter how advanced they are. There is a lot of money that needs to be spent on digital infrastructure, data standardization, strong security, and programs that train trained healthcare workers. No matter where someone is, digital health solutions can only grow in a slow and fair way.

4.1.1 Fragmentation and Interoperability / Legacy Systems

Reisman (2017) and Health Information and Management Systems Society (2021) in their work observes that obsolete systems that fragment and create interop- erability issues hamper use of digital health solutions to their full potential. Most healthcare systems are now of the digital variety, and to some extent re- semble the system structure. This results in data storage that have too many chests and nothing communicates/ exchanges information well. As a result, it significantly becomes a bottleneck for sharing patient information across care sites. Now in case of legacy systems we find that ancient technology is still in use. This complicates matter further because they do not always play well with new digital health platforms or protocols. This leads to more costly and difficult upgrades and integrations. Solving this means working together to set global standards for data and APIs, along with versatile governance frame- works. Similarly so, policymakers and health organizations are encouraged to make intelligent investments in infrastructure improvements, orderly upgrad- ing of legacy systems and adoption of open platforms that promote seamless connectivity across healthcare ecosystems for efficient data sharing.

4.1.2 Connectivity and Digital Infrastructure Gaps

World Health Organization (2021e) and International Telecommunication Union (2022) in their finding states that the absence of both connectivity and digital infrastructure, really hinders any kind of large scale efforts to deploy a digital health solution in an equitable manner. Still, many regions, especially in rural areas where internet access is limited or unreliable, telemedicine access is limited. This includes remote monitoring services and other digital health essen- tials. This disparities continue to manifest with a digital gap, where people are denied quick health access including timely interventions and preventative mea- sures. Lack of broadband infrastructure also hampers the healthcare providers, preventing such cutting-edge technologies to be applied within telemedicine ser- vice. Filling these infrastructure gaps will require specifically targeted public and private investment in expanding broadband access, policies to attract in- vestment for connectivity in poorly served areas, and novel solutions including mobile and satellite-based connectivity. This will require governments, technol- ogy providers and healthcare organizations to work together with their commu- nity stakeholders in order to build resilient, inclusive digital health infrastruc- tures which are foundational to realizing equitable access and universal health coverage.

4.1.3 Data Standards, Integration Complexity, and Semantic Het- erogeneity

Interoperability of digital health systems is impeded by the absence of standard- ized data representation, compounded by interoperability challenges concerning the integration complexity and semantical heterogeneity as pointed by Mandl and Kohane (2016) and Benson and Grieve (2016) in their research. Health- care data come from different sources such as EHRs, wearable devices, imag- ing systems and smartphone apps, each has a different structure, terminology and network protocols. As a result, it makes the semantic heterogeneity an existing problem across different data elements so that when you try to com- bine data from several (distributed) systems, and for same business aspects, they are not understood in the same way. However the catch is that stitch- ing together structured and unstructured data along with legacy and modern platform can be painful, expensive and error prone. This is done using standardized vocabularies eg, Systematized Nomenclature of Medicine – Clinical Terms (SNOMED CT), International Classification of Diseases, 11th Revision (ICD-11), and Logical Observation Identifiers Names and Codes (LOINC) and data exchange protocols eg, Health Level Seven Fast Healthcare Interoperability Resources (HL7 FHIR) for clinical decision support systems, predictive analyt- ics and population-based health management. To overcome these challenges, national and international health authorities need to impose interoperability standards, encourage the adoption of open APIs, semantic harmonization tools and ontologies. Such initiatives will be vital as part of a nuanced digital health ecosystem that allows timely, accurate and patient-oriented care.

4.1.4 Workforce Capacity and Technical Expertise

Topol (2019) and World Health Organization (2021a) in their research opines that however, the penetration of digital health transformation is contingent on the ability, capabilities and skill set(s) of the workforce in deploying, operat- ing and managing new technologies successfully. Nonetheless, we have a long way to go for there is a skills gap in healthcare exposed — Many thousands of healthcare professionals are not taught how to work effectively with digital technologies, data analytics, cybersecurity and importantly the ethics behind AI driven healthcare. The inefficacious adoption and use of innovations like electronic health records, telemedicine platforms as well as predictive decision support systems that can help in filling this gap. This is compounded by already acute shortage of digitally competent health workers in low-resource settings, thus exacerbating equity gaps in their digital health readiness. In the healthcare sector, IT professionals also struggle with deciphering the intricate workflows that clinicians navigate daily and this disconnect hinders alignment between technology solutions and practice-based realities. Addressing these hurdles re- quires initial investments in digital literacy programs, lay education systems and lifelong learning. In this way, partnership across academia, industry, and gov- ernment can contribute to creation of a digitally prepared health care workforce capable of patient-centered use of technology.

4.1.5 Cybersecurity, Privacy, and Trust-Related Infrastructure

Reddy et al. (2019) and European Union Agency for Cybersecurity (ENISA) (2020) in their research emphasizes that secure and trusted digital health input necessarily bet on cyber and privacy protection infrastructures. With healthcare systems increasingly becoming dependent on digital platforms which communi- cate with each other all the time, they are susceptible to cyber attacks that threaten to expose patient data vulnerabilities and disrupt life-saving health services. Instances such as breaches of electron- ic health records, ransomware attacks on hospital systems and tools around the data that touch patient health- care have shown to be disruptive quickly in a time when robust cyber security was needed most. Trust in a solution can be solidified with the implementa- tion of end-to-end encryption, multi-factor authentication, continuous system monitoring and adherence to international standards. Digital health solution development should incorporate privacy-by-design and conform to regulation including GDPR, HIPAA etc. In addition, effective oversight is needed to de- velop trusted digital health spaces, accompa- nied by continuous cyber security training for healthcare professionals, with regular communication to patients. But the stakes for even single use cases are so high that no health system will consistently pick up digital innovation unless it delivers a resilient, secure and ethically responsible digital infrastructure, which retains the trust of its user.

4.1.6 Scalability and Operational Sustainability

According to A. Labrique et al. (2013) and World Health Organization (2021e) the ability to scale and maintain operations are key requirements for digital health innovations, especially in areas with limited resources or an evolving health ecosystem. While digital health pilot programs have shown potential on a small scale, they often fail to maintain effectiveness upon scaling because of deficiencies in infrastructure, funding, workforce capacity and system interoper- ability. So digital solutions need to be scalable — as modular adaptability with cost efficiency allowing them to be tailored for different population needs and health system capacities. For it to be sustainable, it must not be the technologi- cal prowess only but rather an institutional integration, long term financial road map, policy support, soul and commitment from all stakeholders. Introducing user feedback loops, automating updates and hav- ing a cloud based architecture can help in this regard, leading to improved performance and a decrease main- tenance overhead. In addition, public-private partnerships and international collaborations can enable scaling by offering shared infrastructure, Harmonized cross-border regulatory framework and collaborating with innovation ecosys- tems.

4.1.7 Equity and The Digital Divide as Infrastructural Limitations

van Dijk (2020) and Crawford and Serhal (2020) emphasizes that in the digital era, health disparities cannot be addressed without addressing equity and the technology gaps that represent an important part of our critical infrastructure. Digital health technologies (which allow for better access to care and more per- sonalised care) as a whole usually benefit urban, well educated or economically privileged popu- lations. Digital tool accessibility and usability is further com- plicated by the unique challenges faced by marginalized communities, such as those living in rural areas, low-income groups, older adults, or individuals with limited digital literacy. These barriers range from poor internet connectivity, smartphone shortage and language mismatch to limited trust in digital systems. Therefore, the digital divide must lose fuel and people who require medical help need inclusive, prior access to care at any time. Digital health equity must be intentionally pursued, with design and deployment strategies that are inclusive of technology development, cultural competence content on programs, afford- ability measures and en-abling digital literacy. Policy makers need equitable frameworks for them to be focused around investing infrastructure in the most poorly-served areas and have accessibility and inclusivity as design principles. Eliminating the digital divide is not only a moral imperative but also crucial to the performance and public accountability of digital health systems toward universal health coverage.

For instance, a high-income country with a mature health system may con- centrate on embedding digital health tools within existing electronic health records and value-based care programmes while a low-income country could prioritise basic connectivity, SMS reminders or community health worker apps that can work offline. Such variations in infrastructure, funding and workforce capacity are such that implementation strategies and policy decisions should be context specific, rather than simply "rolling out" models developed elsewhere.

4.1.8 Governance Misalignment and Fragmented Investment

World Health Organization (2019a) and Organisation for Economic Co-operation and Development (2019b) states that aligned governance, as well as integrated investing across capital projects in digital health systems remains a substantial barrier to universalization and sustainability. In lots of countries, there is no sin- gle national strategy for digital health that integrates the various initiatives led by differ-ent parts of government, non-governmental organizations (NGOs), the private sector and donor agen-cies. One of the effects of this fragmentation is an overlap in roles and tasks implemented by multiple authorities, reinforcing that sectoral divide and reducing interoperability which maintains a perennial waste in encompassing resources. Without multi-year investment frameworks in place, short-term pilot programs frequently go unfunded or unscaled once they have run their course, resulting in underfunded pilots that either sputter out or are never scaled to system-wide solutions. Moving forward, investment strategies need to move away from short-term project based funding and towards long-term outcomes driven financing models that prioritize integration, capacity-building, and equity. Governance Investment Cohort, a coordinated governance and in- vestment approach is needed to fix fragmented digital health landscapes into resilient, scalable, and patient-centric ecosystems. Governance challenges also arise from unclear roles and responsibilities, weak regulatory enforcement, and limited stakeholder coordination, all of which reduce accountability and strate- gic alignment. To overcome these obstacles, countries must establish robust, centralized digital health governance frameworks that promote inter sectoral coordina-tion, enforce standards, and ensure alignment with broader health sys- tem goals.

4.1.9 Usability and Integration Into Clinical Workflows

While usability and easy integration into clinical workflows are essential factors in the decision to adopt such digital health approaches, these challenges have remained ongoing within healthcare systems as pointed by Ratwani et al. (2019) and Buntin et al. (2011). Digital tools often do not provide opportu-nities for frontline healthcare providers to engage before development, resulting in inter- faces that are difficult to use, take too much time or which depart from existing clinical workflows. Usability issues lead to clinician frustration, workflow disrup- tions, and even medical errors which erode both trust and efficiency. Further, by not integrating digital solutions within these traditional clinical pathways like an

EHR system or care coordination routines it causes fragmentation and excess administrative overhead. To help close these gaps, digital health tools need to be co-developed with clinicians and designed for clear use cases that integrate seamlessly into routine care delivery. This needs to be preceded by usability testing, iterative design and integration with EHR-based decision-support sys- tems. In addition, the embedding of digital interventions within organizational policies as well as clinical training programs and performance metrics (eg, quality indicators) may increase their utility and sustainability. If these issues are addressed through usability and workflow integration, digital health could truly enable high-quality patient centered care rather than feel like an additional burden.

4.1.10 Sustainability in Low-Resource Settings

Mechael and Sloninsky (2008) and A. B. Labrique et al. (2018) states that achieving sustainability of digital health interventions in low-resource settings entails a tradeoff between innovation, affordability and contextual relevance. As such, these environments are plagued with considerable constraints — including limited infrastructure, inadequate resources and funding, unreliable electricity supply, low digital literacy among the population and shortage of trained health professionals. These often rely on expensive high-maintenance complex technol- ogy or frequent internet usage, which are not sustainable in these settings. Cost containment and flexibility can be improved with open-source platforms, modular system designs, and mobile-based interventions. To ensure that solutions are locally relevant and context specific, community engagement and participa- tory design approaches is key. In addition, it helps in forming partnerships with governments, NGOs and private-sectors to ensure continued funding and align- ment with national health strategies. Sustainability in low-resource contexts is not just a technical challenge, but a policy and equity mandate that requires human-centred, resilient, adaptive and context-appropriate digital health solu- tions.

4.2 Interoperability and Standardization Issues

According to Dixon et al. (2013) andHealth Information and Management Sys- tems Society (2021) the lack of interoperability and standardization remains a central challenge in creating cohesive, efficient digital health systems. Digital tools — from electronic health records to remote monitoring devices — are com- monly used in the healthcare space, but tend to work in silos with proprietary formats and lack consistent terminologies or data exchange protocols. Stan- dardization could improve the exchange of data between institutions, systems, and countries. Interoperability is successful only when the globally accepted data standards like HL7 FHIR, LOINC, SNOMED CT are used and the legisla- tion enforces them. Further, the establishment of semantic interoperability (i.e., shared meaning across systems) is also essential for advanced analytics and ef- fective use of health data. Better governance on interoperability combined with the establishment of collective stakeholder platforms can expedite the develop- ment of interoperable digital health ecosystems thereby enabling data liquidity, continuity of care and overall patient outcomes.

4.3 Socioeconomic and Digital Divides

van Dijk (2020) and Golinelli et al. (2020) points out that people from lower socio-economic backgrounds, rural communities and marginalised groups are often among the 10% of households that do not have access to a reliable in- ternet connection in addition to lacking the digital devices and digital literacy required to engage with health technologies effectively. This could include, for example, in-accessibility to telemedicine platforms or app-based self-care tools, if interfaces are too complicated or devices are absent among elderly patients or people with disabilities. Manifestations must include subsidized devices and broadband access, community-based digital literacy efforts, culturally tailored digital content, as well as inclusive technology design. It is imperative that eq- uity be rooted in national digital health frameworks so that no group of people are left unaffected during the transition to digitally empowered first healthcare systems.

4.4 Resistance from Healthcare Professionals and Organi- zations

Greenhalgh et al. (2017) and Cresswell et al. (2013) states that healthcare pro- fessionals and institutions are characterized by a strong resistance to the uptake and implementation of digital health tools. Although digital tools show promise for increasing efficiency, accuracy and patient engagement, many providers worry about additional work, interruption of the current process, and a decline in their relationship with patients. This resistance is typically because of poor training, job fears from automation replacing their work, a lack of input in the design of technology and skepticism about data security and dependability. In- stitutional culture is a significant determinant as well — those with rampant bureaucracy, conservative change management styles, or nebulous top-level sup- port might find digital transformation trickier. There is an inherent resistance to this change but it can be countered if attention is paid from the offset to engage clinicians, providing structured training and proving evidence of clinical effectiveness through implementation science oriented research and establishing feedback pipeline. Enhanced adoption may be achieved by integrating digital tools with contemporary workflows, as opposed to creating parallel systems, and that technology augments, but does not substitute clinical judgment. In addition to driving and communicating a strategic vision of innovation, alter- native reward systems (including those found in open science approaches) and change management strategies such as leadership advocacy or align-ing incen- tives for portions of the provider workforce can support an innovative culture that balances traditionally professional values with new practices.

4.5 Regulatory and Policy-Related Challenges

Regulatory and policy related challenges pose a serious barrier to seamless de- ployment and scale up of even the most promising digital health technology as stated by Cohen et al. (2014) and World Health Organization (2021b). This includes two essential challenges — (i) existing regulations that are not adapted and harmonized to the rapid evolution of innovations such as AI, telemedicine and mobile health applications and (ii) cross border data related issues. Out- dated legal frameworks in most coun-tries are often not adapted to problems such as algorithm accountability, remote diagnostics and data portability. Moreover, there is an inconsistency in regulatory interpretation across regions which makes global collaborations and technology deployment difficult. Additionally, the lack of defined principles for responsible AI operation, as well as data protection in a digital environment and certification require-ments for digital solutions may hamper validation and uptake. To ensure policies are both technologically in- formed and socially grounded, policy frameworks should be co-created with a range of actors who possess perspectives on the issues at stake including tech- nologists, healthcare professionals, legal experts and patient representatives.

Patients and health workers are active agents in the adoption of digital prevention tools. There is a need for people to trust that digital systems are secure, reliable and respect their privacy. Besides they must also have the necessary skills to use those tools with confidence. Human-centered design that puts users at the heart of shaping and testing tools can help make applications more intuitive for users, as well as better linked to local practice and language. From the perspective of a provider, digital solutions must seamlessly integrate within current workflows and professional scopes of work. If it appears to the user that they add time or complexity to documentation, or otherwise interrupt users' clinical routine, they are unlikely to be used in a consistent manner. Creating trust, competences and a common ownership is therefore seen as one essential prerequisite for the success of prevention oriented digital health.

A number of the problems already mentioned are mere symptoms of larger structural problems. Infrastructure deficits frequently reflect chronic underin- vestment in primary care, public health and digital public goods. Algorithmic bias is associated with imbalanced data quality and representation, with some groups missing or underrepresented in training datasets. The coalition believes that interoperability issues stem from siloed procurement, proprietary standards and misaligned incentives between vendors of health technologies and the health organizations that use them. Acknowledging these root causes helps to explain why purely technical "fixes" will not suffice, and solutions must instead incor- porate standards, governance, financing as well as change management.

Table 1. Summary of relatively mature versus still challenging areas in digital health for prevention.

Relatively mature areas	Areas where major challenges remain
Basic digital tools and connectivity in many facilities	Reliable infrastructure in rural and low-resource settings
Simple SMS / IVR reminders for vaccines and antenatal care	Sustained behaviour change and long-term engagement
Telemedicine and virtual visits for selected services	Full integration of telemedicine into routine care and payment
Digitisation of records (EHRs, reg- istries, lab systems)	True interoperability and data shar- ing across providers
Basic dashboards and routine service-coverage analytics	Robust, validated, and fair AI for preventive care
Pilot and donor-funded digital health projects	Sustainable financing, business models, and data governance

In Table 1 we showcase the areas which are mature and the areas still chal- lenging in digital health for prevention.

In the following section we explore ethical considerations and data privacy with respect to digital healthcare.

5 ETHICAL CONSIDERATIONS AND DATA PRIVACY

There are broader ethical considerations when it comes to digital health that extend beyond privacy and confidentiality. The discussion is based on issues of fair play and accountability, transparency, control over data. Patients and their health workers deserve an answer to the question of who is accountable when digital tools make or support decisions, how algorithms arrive at answers and how data are being used in ways that extend far beyond direct care.

5.1 Ethical Implications of Digital Health Technologies

A plethora of ethical concerns arise with digital health technology, which are pivotal for ensuring responsible healthcare reforms. AI, wearables, mobile apps and predictive analytics are growing more significant within health systems due to digitisation. Still, they raise concerns about patient choice, information to be kept as privileged and consented, and algorithmic ethics. The more sensi- tive health information is collected and processed, the more issues arise around how that data is owned and managed. There is, of course, the risk of an al- gorithmic bias — introduced when these non-neutral practices or viewpoints are inducted into AI model training data without accounting for the sufficient and/or representative nature of that training data — which could lead to unfair treatment or oppression towards underprivileged communities as well. While ethical frameworks such as GDPR and HIPAA are offering fundamental protec- tion, the enforcement and application of the same globally remains a challenge. A rising concept, "data ethics by design" proposes that all stages in the develop- ment of digital health solutions — from inception to deployment — are informed by ethical considerations. So, how can we guarantee that the technology is serv- ing" the common good and at the same time not violating our rights, dignity or trust?- well it needs to be opened, with human oversight, there should be an involving stakeholders part. Ultimately, ethical digital health is more than just technical skill and expertise. It also requires the values of equity and inclusion to be baked in from start to finish.

5.2 Issues in Patient Autonomy, Informed Consent, and Data Ownership

The emergence of digital health technologies has radically altered how patient engagement functions, yet numerous concerns regarding patient autonomy, in- formed consent and data ownership remain unaddressed. Since time immemo- rial, healthcare decisions were essentially created in the confines of patient- provider interactions. And although AI-enabled platforms, mobile apps and wearable devices continuously collect data in real-time, patients are typically unaware of how their personal health information is collected, used or shared. True autonomy may be eroded by this asymmetry of information — individuals simply do not understand or control their digital footprints. It represents a fu- sion of informed consent — the legal foundation for ethical practice in medicine — with an algorithmic third-party data processor that has made this far more complicated. In digital platforms, consent mechanisms are usually buried in long, technical terms of service that most users either do not read or do not fully understand. Secondly, the matter of who owns the data itself is also un- clear. They generate the data but often do not store, analyse and monetize them by companies with opaque regulatory and ethic regulations. This creates a disconnect that leads to mistrust, and, ultimately, reduces confidence in dig- ital health ecosystems. Ensuring patient autonomy means improving ways to communicate data practices, streamline consent actions, all while really com- mitting to policies that will guarantee patients enable them to view their data, manage access and even remove the information. Putting patients back into the heart of digital healthcare is therefore critical for trust, ethical alignment and ongoing patient interaction.

5.3 Algorithmic Bias, Fairness, and Equitable Access to Healthcare Technologies

Although this digital evolution has further blurred the lines between mathe- matical and medical models it has also opened up a flood gate of algorithmic bias within inequity in health systems. Algorithms trained on biased, flawed, or incomplete historical datasets can perpetuate ingrained discrimination — often against the most vulnerable populace. For instance, if a model is developed using mainly urban or affluent data and then applied in rural or under served communities the recommendations by that model may not be correct and could cause harm. However, this threatens not only its fairness but in addition con- signs thousands of people to needless lack of life by lacking out on crucial health interventions. Access to healthcare technologies is also an equity issue, as many digital health applications require some degree of baseline digital literacy, inter- net connectivity or socioeconomic status that are not met by all patients.

For example, if a hospital adopts an AI-driven triage or risk prediction tool, it needs to make certain that training data reflect the population served, and that patients know how their data are being used and have a clear mechanism of complaint or override for clinicians as regards algorithmic outputs. Regulations like GDPR and HIPAA, in conjunction with "data ethics by design" methodolo- gies, can offer tangible principles to drive the adoption of such implementations. So, the people who could most benefit from new breakthroughs are often those least likely to have access to them. Ensuring fairness in algorithms to in- volves conscious endeavors to audit, verify and enrich training data as well prac- tice requirement of use ethical frameworks that emphasizes on transparency and stake holders involvement in AI development. Ensuring fairness and equitable access has to involve more than just technical safeguards – it requires wider policy efforts, community engagement, and system designs which contribute to digital ecosystems that are no longer exclusionary in nature.

These ethical and equity questions are not only theoretical. In the Indian case study described earlier, the clinical decision support system depends on ac- curate and up-to-date data for people who may be newly diagnosed and have had limited contact with the health system. This raises practical questions about how consent is taken, how long data are stored, and how patients are informed about any secondary use of their information. In the South African maternal health messaging case, decisions about who gets registered, which languages are supported, and how phone numbers are managed have direct implications for fairness, privacy, and inclusion. These examples show that consent, data pro- tection, and equitable access must be built into the design and governance of digital health tools from the beginning, not treated as afterthoughts.

5.4 Regulatory Frameworks: GDPR, HIPAA, and Na- tional Digital Health Policies

According to European Parliament and Council of the European Union (2016) regulatory frameworks are a key component in determining the ethics of dig- ital health protecting patient privacy, securing data, and enforcing the rights of patients. They include the European Union's GDPR and, in the United States, HIPAA, both of which take different but complementary approaches to safeguard personal health data. The GDPR focuses on transparency, legal ac- countability and end user consent, meaning that any personal data processing must be grounded in a clear specific purpose and not used for additional incom- patible purposes which have not been communicated to the individual before the processing activity. This stems from HIPAA focusing on the confidentiality and integrity of health information by requiring that high-security measures be met along with explicit patient consent when dealing with clinical settings. In addition to these regulatory frameworks, there is an increasing focus on na- tional level Digital Health Policies across the globe to give further shape and reference to digital health practices. In trying to balance the speed of technological progress with societal values and the public interest, these national efforts create guidelines around issues such as interoperability between systems, data ownership, cross-border data transfer and ethical concerns related to AI being leveraged for healthcare.

Diligent, enforcement of these regulations is still dif- ficult because enforcement is complicated and inconsistent across jurisdictions, and technology changes quickly. While digital health innovations are expanding globally, such harmonized regulatory approaches to promote innovation will be essential in protecting the rights of patients while fostering trust and equitable access in view of worldwide burden alleviation through digital health.

Whereas HIPAA has historically been concerned with solely protecting health information within the US healthcare sector, GDPR promulgates cross-sector national level personal data protection throughout the European Union, includ- ing stronger protections for consent, data minimisation and individual rights. Global digital health strategy of WHO, in turn, offers high-level guidance for countries at drastically different points of the digital transformation journey that focuses on governance, equity and capacity-building. Collectively, these frame- works demonstrate how countries reconcile principles of innovation, privacy, and public interest with regard to big data and underscore common challenges despite varied legal traditions.

There are variations in the global standards for regulating digital health technologies and AI. In the European Union we find that laws like the GDPR and new AI rules are particularly concerned with individual rights, data minimi- sation, and transparency. This may slow adoption, but it establishes a strong foundation for privacy and accountability. In the US, HIPAA and FDA guid- ance are more focused on sector-specific health data and a risk-based approach to oversight of digital products, with some open space around commercial apps and non-traditional sources of data. Though many low and middle-income countries are still working to develop robust digital health infrastructure alongside data protection frameworks, they have been adapting much of the global guidelines in environments that do not have adequate capacity for enforcement. These disparities reveal that the scaling up of digital health for prevention is as much a function of technological and human capabilities as it is regulatory philosophy and institutional capacity within each place.

5.5 Data Ethics by Design and Human Oversight in AI- Based Healthcare Systems

Ethics by Design according to Floridi and Taddeo (2016) and World Health Or- ganization (2021c) is the underlying principle of data ethics, which means that we integrate ethical thought process into how products are conceptualized and developed keeping in mind data privacy, fairness in prediction, trans-parency or interpretability and accountability across AI life cycle. stringent standards should be followed from inception to deployment. In healthcare AI, this ap- proach requires to identify and prevent potential biases, protect patient auton- omy, and secure informed consent. At the same time, human interpretation is necessary to assess AI-generated guidance, correct algorithmic errors, and protect patient interests against automated choices that could endanger the safety or rights of a patient.

6 STRATEGIC RECOMMENDATIONS FOR DIGITAL HEALTH ADOPTION

Governments and legislators must provide clear regulatory frameworks that align innovation with pa-tient safety, particularly with telemedicine, AI-driven decision-making, and cross-border data interchange. Investing in capacity build- ing and digital literacy programs for healthcare professionals and patients is essential to ensure the adoption of new technology rather than its rejection. Ethical governance should be included at every stage of adoption through trans- parent algorithms, accountability frameworks, and adherence to principles such as privacy, inclusion, and equity. Public-private partnerships are essential for enhancing digital health initiatives through the integration of technological ex- pertise, legislative support, and financial investment. Companies in the health care field need to plan, prepare, and take the lead to fully use the potential of digital health to change lives of people. To do this, they need to think about both people and technology. A complete plan is needed that involves using technology, educating individuals the way to make use of it, making sure that ethical standards remain in effect, as well as making sure that digital health use is fair and leads to measurable improvements in care and prevention.

The most important thing is to build a strong digital system. To work to- gether well, platforms need to use secure cloud systems, data formats that are the same for everyone, and health information exchanges that are linked to each other. Data on the whole population should be used to plan measures that are specific to each area and help improve health and fairness. It is important to take feedback of healthcare professionals, technologists, policymakers, and pa- tients regularly to make sure that systems are trustworthy and suit demands of users. There should be a complete plan that involves using technology, educat- ing individuals the way to make use of it, making sure that ethical standards remain in effect, as well as making sure that digital health use is fair and leads to measurable improvements in care and prevention.

6.1 Guidelines for Policymakers and Healthcare Organi- zations

Ethical principles should guide administrators and policymakers to establish clear strategies of how digital health technologies should be integrated in the healthcare system. as stated by. As one example, policy makers in Canada and at the regional, national or supra-national level in other jurisdictions should develop strong regulatory regimes for data privacy, informed consent, data in- teroperability and algorithm transparency. Policies should promote digital lit- eracy among both healthcare providers and recipients, with equitable access to technology. We have to bring in systematic evaluations for the assessment of efficiency and equity of digital interventions. Increased public trust, account- ability and sustainable innovation can lead to improved health outcomes and efficiencies in systems World Health Organization (2021d) and Organisation for Economic Co-operation and Development (2019b), as seen through the lens of collaborative governance that involves multi-stakeholder participation.

6.2 Best Practices for Ethical, Transparent, and Inclusive Digital Health Initiatives

World Health Organization (2021d) and Organization for Economic Co-operation and Development (2019b) emphasizes that the ethical, transparent and inclusive conduction of digital health initiatives is nuanced, multifactorial and requires a comprehensive approach that incorporates sound policy development, gover- nance frameworks and broad stakeholder engagement. Transparency in general, healthcare systems and technologists who gather, save, process or transmit pa- tient data should be drama-free — clearly articulating what functions are being conducted. Do you need an explicit expansion of ethical AI-principles in you design and deploy phase? It argues that regular audits and bias assessments are necessary to ensure algorithms benefit all subgroups within the general popula- tion, not just one. Such practices, like inclusive design — where all demographic and socioeconomic ancestries should have patient and community input in the decisions — are necessary to make sure that digital health interventions can be accessed and effective for everyone. In addition, we need continuous training and capacity building for healthcare workers, and patient/user education initiatives to enhance digital literacy among patients/users as well as build confidence and trust. Finally, platforms for feedback and transparent reporting mechanisms open up health systems to patient insights needed to ensure the ongoing trust and authentic engagement with digital health initiatives.

6.3 Strategies for Stakeholder Collaboration and Engage- ment in Digital Health Policy-Making

World Health Organization (2021d) and Organization for Economic Co-operation and Development (2019b) states that effective stakeholder collaboration and engagement is critical for successful digital health policy making — by design- ing policies that are practical, equitable and acceptable. Such processes would also be served well by inclusive participatory approaches, which actively engage across healthcare providers, patients, technology developers and the research community as well as broad-based community representatives in all stages of policy development. The regular consultation workshops with multi stakehold- ers could create for a dialogue, consensus building on multiple interests which would only be of advantage than being seen in different views out there proac- tively. Such groups could serve as formal digital health advisory bodies, with roles and members spanning sectors to ensure alignment and accountability.

Promote transparency by releasing policy drafts regularly, establishing feed- back loops, and clear communication channels through which stakeholders can meaningfully contribute to the process. In addition to this, the setting up of structured training programs to empower stakeholders particularly patient advocacy groups and frontline health care workers helps these stakeholders par- ticipate meaningfully in policy development. Similarly, it is likely that using digital platforms to regularly communicate with key stakeholders, disseminated resources and obtain feedback will further facilitate responsiveness in policy- making processes, which potentially can be more nimble. Thereby conducive for creating a strong foundation of digital health ecosystems grounded on mutual aspirations and trust.

Digital health and prevention do not look the same for everyone around the world. The availability of smartphones, access to internet connectivity, elec- tricity and trained personnel differs largely between as well as within countries, and determines what tools are feasible and acceptable. Cultural beliefs, linguistic and local health priorities can shape reactions to digital interventions too. For example, community health worker platforms or interactive voice response systems might be more appropriate in rural, poor resource environments and patient portals, wearables and mobile apps may be more prevalent among peo- ple with higher income living in urban areas. Awareness of this cross-cultural and global variation can help disrupt that pattern, wherein models are lifted from one culture or setting to another with little accommodation, which in-turn underpins more inclusive and equitable digital health-enabled strategies.

Data governance is a central issue in digital health, especially when AI and large-scale analytics are used. As discussed in Section 5, questions of data ownership, consent, secondary use and accountability need clear stewardship models and oversight mechanisms to sustain trust in preventive digital tools.

7 CONCLUSION

With a focus on preventive digital health numerous scenarios might be envi- sioned for the future of digital healthcare and prevention. In an ideal world, investment in infrastructure, governance and skills of the workforce would enable digital solutions to assist a proactive, equitable prevention that is supported by AI. These should be made transparently and be safe to use to both identify risk and provide direct support. In a more blended and gradual scenario, digital health is still patchy - some of the well-resources organizations and populations benefitting disproportionally from others. In a darker turn, poor governance and powerful commercial pressures result in fragmented, proprietary systems that compound inequalities and further erode trust. Real-world consequences will likely land somewhere in between these two extremes, but it can be helpful for policy-makers and planners to think along the lines of scenarios so they can prepare for risks and select strategies that nudge health systems in a direction toward more desirable futures.

The story of digital health has not been a straight line. What began as a slow transition from paper files to digital records has in just a few short decades evolved into an ecosystem of AI, big data and interconnected systems. This reshaping has recast healthcare from an illness focus after the fact to a risk stratification and preventive approach, and from generic population man- agement to personalized interventions. This might translate in a patient from village X getting advice, monitoring or even diagnostic without the need to ever step into a hospital and on the other side, health systems can be handled in most sustainable way.

Still, this advancement is never uniform. Nevertheless, challenges still persist around the integration of systems which are not interoperable, lack of internet infrastructure and different standards in data. Large portions of the workforce have not been better trained or equipped to adapt with fast developing new technologies and governance frameworks have continued to be piece meal. Built on top of these, practical hurdles are ethical considerations, some of which are: (i) who holds the keys to health data, (ii) whether patients have a clear sense of where their information is going, (iii) how bias can be engineered out of algorithms and (iv) what transparency looks like in decision-making.

Going forward the work to be done on that front is as people-focused as it is technology-focused. Policymakers of tomorrow, healthcare leaders and innova- tors will have to collaborate not only on funding and rolling out new systems, but on building systems that accommodate unique local circumstances, main- tain human oversight of AI decisions, and earn community support in the design phase. Investments in the three categories of Digital Literacy, Fair Governance, and Equitable Infrastructure are a must. In combination, digital health can stop looking like just a toolbox and start to really function in earnest as the architec- tural underpinning for an inclusive, responsive and high performing healthcare system that delivers better health outcomes for all people, in all places.

The narrative of the chapter is centered around the 'digital health' idea, and its central message, is "when digital technology is properly connected to other elements of strong health systems with clear governance" and organized to meet the hidden patients/ professionals needs. For policymakers and implementers, three imperatives are paramount: (i) investing in equitable digital infrastructure and skills, (ii)setting up strong data governance and evaluation systems and (iii) supporting the deployment of digital tools that are part of essential everyday preventive care. Focusing on these areas can propel health systems from stand- alone pilots to long-term, population-level impact.

Conclusively, three general recommendations appear to emerge from a prac- tical perspective for policy and healthcare decision makers who want to leverage digital health to reinforce prevention. First, make equitable digital infrastruc- ture and digital literacy investments so that prevention tools reach a wide

REFERENCES

Abernethy, A. P., Adams, L., Barrett, M., Bechtel, C., Brennan, P., Butte, A., Faulkner, J., Fontaine, E., Friedhoff, S., Halamka, J., Howell, M., Johnson, K., Long, P., McGraw, D., Miller, R., Lee, P., Perlin, J., Rucker, D., Sandy, L., & Valdes, K. (2022). The promise of digital health: Then, now, and the future. *NAM Perspectives, 2022*. Advance online publication. DOI: 10.31478/202206e PMID: 36177208

Ajay, V. S., Jindal, D., Roy, A., Gupta, R., Rastogi, P., & Prabhakaran, D., & mPower Heart Project Investigators. (2016). Development of a smartphone-enabled hypertension and diabetes mellitus management package to facilitate evidence-based care delivery in primary healthcare facilities in India: The mPower Heart Project. *Journal of the American Heart Association, 5*(12), e004343. DOI: 10.1161/JAHA.116.004343 PMID: 28003248

Barron, P., Peter, J., LeFevre, A. E., Sebidi, J., Bekker, M., Allen, R., Parsons, A. N., Benjamin, P., & Pillay, Y. (2018). Mobile health messaging service and helpdesk for South African mothers (MomConnect): History, successes and challenges. *BMJ Global Health, 3*(Suppl 2), e000559. DOI: 10.1136/bmjgh-2017-000559 PMID: 29713503

Basu, D., Krishnakumar, V., Parui, S., Mansoor, W., & Ghosh, U. (2021). Optimum e-health care resource provisioning using network slicing approach for future 5G networks. In *Proceedings of the 4th International Conference on Signal Processing and Information Security (ICSPIS)* (pp. 88–91). IEEE.

Benson, T., & Grieve, G. (2016). *Principles of health interoperability: SNOMED CT, HL7 and FHIR* (3rd ed.). Springer.

Buntin, M. B., Burke, M. F., Hoaglin, M. C., & Blumenthal, D. (2011). The benefits of health information technology: A review of the recent literature shows predominantly positive results. *Health Affairs, 30*(3), 464–471. DOI: 10.1377/hlthaff.2011.0178 PMID: 21383365

Cohen, I. G., Amarasingham, R., Shah, A., Xie, B., & Lo, B. (2014). The legal and ethical concerns that arise from using complex predictive analytics in healthcare. *Health Affairs, 33*(7), 1139–1147. DOI: 10.1377/hlthaff.2014.0048 PMID: 25006139

Crawford, A., & Serhal, E. (2020). Digital health equity and COVID-19: The innovation curve cannot reinforce the social gradient of health. *Journal of Medical Internet Research, 22*(6), e19361. DOI: 10.2196/19361 PMID: 32452816

Cresswell, K., Bates, D. W., & Sheikh, A. (2013). Ten key considerations for the successful implementation and adoption of large-scale health information technology. *Journal of the American Medical Informatics Association : JAMIA, 20*(e1), e9–e13. DOI: 10.1136/amiajnl-2013-001684 PMID: 23599226

Dixon, B. E., Grannis, S. J., & Overhage, J. M. (2013). Measuring the impact of health information technology: A review of the literature. *Journal of Biomedical Informatics, 46*(6), 1181–1190. DOI: 10.1016/j.jbi.2013.08.010

European Parliament & Council of the European Union. (2016). *Regulation (EU) 2016/679 (General Data Protection Regulation)*. Official Journal of the European Union.

European Union Agency for Cybersecurity. (2020). *Cybersecurity in healthcare.* https://www.enisa.europa.eu/publications/cybersecurity-in-healthcare

Floridi, L., & Taddeo, M. (2016). What is data ethics? *Philosophical Transactions of the Royal Society A, 374*(2083), 20160360. DOI: 10.1098/rsta.2016.0360 PMID: 28336805

Gambhir, S. S., Ge, T. J., Vermesh, O., & Spitler, R. (2018). Toward achieving precision health. *Science Translational Medicine, 10*(430), eaao3612. Advance online publication. DOI: 10.1126/scitranslmed.aao3612 PMID: 29491186

Ginsburg, G. S., & Phillips, K. A. (2018). Precision medicine: From science to value. *Health Affairs, 37*(5), 694–701. DOI: 10.1377/hlthaff.2017.1624 PMID: 29733705

Golinelli, D., Boetto, E., Carullo, G., Nuzzolese, A. G., Landini, M. P., & Fantini, M. P. (2020). Adoption of digital technologies in health care during the COVID-19 pandemic: Systematic review of early scientific literature. *Journal of Medical Internet Research, 22*(11), e22280. DOI: 10.2196/22280 PMID: 33079693

Greenhalgh, T., Wherton, J., Papoutsi, C., Lynch, J., & Shaw, S. (2017). Beyond adoption: A new framework for theorizing and evaluating nonadoption, abandonment, and challenges to the scale-up, spread, and sustainability of health and care technologies. *Journal of Medical Internet Research, 19*(11), e367. DOI: 10.2196/jmir.8775 PMID: 29092808

Health Information and Management Systems Society. (2021). *Interoperability in healthcare.* https://www.himss.org/resources/interoperability-healthcare

International Telecommunication Union. (2022). *Connecting humanity: Assessing investment needs of connecting the world.* https://www.itu.int

Kansal, I., Popli, R., Verma, J., Bhardwaj, V., & Bhardwaj, R. (2022). Digital image processing and IoT in smart healthcare: A review. In *Proceedings of the International Conference on Emerging Smart Computing and Informatics (ESCI)* (pp. 1–6). IEEE.

Kruse, C. S., Stein, A., Thomas, H., & Kaur, H. (2018). The use of electronic health records to support population health: A systematic review of the literature. *Journal of Medical Systems, 42*(11), 214. DOI: 10.1007/s10916-018-1075-6 PMID: 30269237

Labrique, A., Vasudevan, L., Kochi, E., Fabricant, R., & Mehl, G. (2013). mHealth innovations as health system strengthening tools: 12 common applications and a visual framework. *Global Health, Science and Practice, 1*(2), 160–171. DOI: 10.9745/GHSP-D-13-00031 PMID: 25276529

Labrique, A. B., Wadhwani, C., Williams, K. A., Lamptey, P., Hesp, C., & Jakubowski, A. (2018). Best practices in scaling digital health in low- and middle-income countries. *Globalization and Health, 14*(1), 103. DOI: 10.1186/s12992-018-0424-z PMID: 30390686

Mandl, K. D., & Kohane, I. S. (2016). Time for a patient-driven health information economy? *The New England Journal of Medicine, 374*(3), 205–208. DOI: 10.1056/NEJMp1512330 PMID: 26789868

Organisation for Economic Co-operation and Development. (2019a). *Health in the 21st century: Putting data to work for stronger health systems.* OECD Publishing.

Organisation for Economic Co-operation and Development. (2019b). *Health in the 21st century: Putting data to work for stronger health systems*. OECD Publishing. https://doi.org/DOI: 10.1787/e3b23f8e-en

Ratwani, R. M., Reider, J., & Singh, H. (2019). A decade of health information technology usability challenges and the path forward. *Journal of the American Medical Association, 321*(8), 743–744. DOI: 10.1001/jama.2019.0161 PMID: 30715133

Reddy, S., Fox, J., & Purohit, M. P. (2019). Artificial intelligence-enabled healthcare delivery. *Journal of the Royal Society of Medicine, 112*(1), 22–28. DOI: 10.1177/0141076818815510 PMID: 30507284

Reisman, M. (2017). EHRs: The challenge of making electronic data usable and interoperable. *P&T : a Peer-Reviewed Journal for Formulary Management, 42*(9), 572–575. https://www.ncbi.nlm.nih.gov/pmc/articles/PMC5565131/ PMID: 28890644

Topol, E. (2019). *Deep medicine: How artificial intelligence can make healthcare human again*. Basic Books.

van Dijk, J. A. G. M. (2020). *The digital divide*. Polity Press.

World Health Organization. (2019). *Recommendations on digital interventions for health system strengthening*. https://www.who.int/publications/i/item/9789241550505

World Health Organization. (2021). *Ethics and governance of artificial intelligence for health*. https://www.who.int/publications/i/item/9789240029200

World Health Organization. (2021). *Global strategy on digital health 2020–2025*. https://www.who.int/publications/i/item/9789240020924

KEY TERMS AND DEFINITIONS

Algorithmic Bias: Systematic errors in AI decision-making caused by bi- ased, incomplete, or unrepresentative training data, which can lead to unfair outcomes for certain patient groups.

Data Ethics by Design: An approach that integrates ethical considera- tions—such as privacy, fairness, transparency, and accountability—into every stage of digital health technology development and deployment.

Digital Health: The use of various digital technologies, including mobile health (mHealth), electronic health (eHealth), wearables, telemedicine, big data, blockchain, and AI, to improve healthcare delivery, prevention, diagnosis, and patient self-care.

Electronic Health Records (EHRs): Digital health records of patients which it easier for healthcare providers to access, share, and update those data.

Interoperability: The ability of different digital health systems and appli- cations to communicate, exchange, and interpret shared data accurately and effectively across various platforms and institutions.

Mobile Health (mHealth): Mobile technologies like smartphones and tablets enhance healthcare practices by allowing things like health monitoring, patient education, and interventions to change behaviour.

Natural Language Processing (NLP): An AI technique that enables com- puters to understand, interpret, and process human language.

Population Health Management (PHM): A strategy that uses data-driven approaches to improve overall population health while keeping costs in control.

Predictive Analytics: The use of statistical algorithms and AI models to analyze health data and predict future health events, such as disease onset or hospitalization risks, enabling early interventions.

Telemedicine: The remote delivery of healthcare services using telecommu- nications technology, enabling consultations, diagnoses, and treatment without the need for in-person visits.

Chapter 2

The Economic Impact of Digital Health Innovations on Disease Prevention: Cost-Effectiveness, ROI, and Policy Implications

Lawal Olamilekan Abdulwahab
https://orcid.org/0000-0003-4955-244X
School of Business and Economics, Universiti Brunei Darussalam, Brunei

Odulusi Daniel
https://orcid.org/0009-0001-3298-8987
Kabale University, Kabale City, Uganda

Akhtar Gul
https://orcid.org/0000-0002-3592-3986
School of Economics and Finance, Xi'an Jiaotong University, China

Hafiz Umar Bubari
https://orcid.org/0000-0003-2093-6570
Federal Polytechnic, Bali, Nigeria

ABSTRACT

This chapter examines the economic impact of digital health innovations in disease prevention, focusing on cost-effectiveness, ROI, and policy implications. As health systems face escalating costs and a rising NCD burden, tools like mHealth, telemedicine, wearables, and AI offer scalable, cost-saving preventive solutions. Drawing on global evidence and modeling, the chapter highlights strong ROI, especially in high-risk populations and LMICs. It reviews economic evaluation metrics, showcases real-world case studies, and addresses challenges including the digital divide and policy gaps. Concluding with policy recommendations, it advocates for inclusive design, sustainable investment, and equity-driven evaluation frameworks to guide future innovation.

DOI: 10.4018/979-8-3373-3531-5.ch002

1. INTRODUCTION

This chapter contributes directly to the overarching theme of Reshaping Health Promotion and Disease Prevention Through Digital Innovation by exploring how economic evaluation can inform the strategic integration of digital technologies into preventive health systems. While digital health is often discussed in clinical or technical terms, its full value for health promotion lies in demonstrating measurable economic returns that sustain and scale innovation. By linking prevention economics with digital transformation, this chapter bridges a critical gap between technology adoption, health behavior change, and evidence-based policy investment. The global surge in chronic and non-communicable diseases (NCDs) such as cardiovascular disease, diabetes, and cancer has created a profound health and economic burden across both developed and developing nations. These preventable conditions account for over 41 million deaths annually, approximately 74% of all global deaths, underscoring the urgent need for effective disease prevention strategies (Pikkarainen et al., 2024). According to WHO and OECD data, global investment in digital health for preventive care has grown from U.S. $4.2 billion in 2016 to more than U.S. $16 billion in 2024, illustrating the scale and momentum of this economic transition.

Despite significant progress in digital health innovation, global health systems remain underprepared to translate these tools into sustainable prevention strategies. The COVID-19 pandemic exposed the fragility of preventive infrastructures and revealed the fiscal strain created by reactive healthcare spending. At the same time, rapid advances in mobile health, telemedicine, and AI created a unique policy moment for re-engineering prevention around digital technologies. However, evidence guiding how to invest efficiently in these tools and how to measure their value beyond clinical outcomes remains fragmented. Addressing this knowledge gap is essential for both policymakers and practitioners seeking to realign prevention financing with 21st-century digital realities. In response to the global rise in chronic and non-communicable diseases (NCDs) such as cardiovascular disease, diabetes, and cancer, digital health innovations have emerged as transformative tools. They offer new pathways for disease prevention, population health management, and system-wide cost containment, inspiring a new wave of innovation and progress in healthcare and instilling a sense of optimism for the future (Leistner & Kowatsch, 2023). Encompassing a broad spectrum of technologies, including mHealth, telemedicine, AI, wearable sensors, and health information systems, digital health enables personalized, data-driven care that supports earlier risk detection and improved patient engagement (Han et al., 2022). These interventions have the potential to significantly reduce hospitalizations and enhance clinical outcomes, offering practical benefits and instilling a sense of optimism and hope for the future of healthcare (Islam & Maddison, 2020). These findings naturally lead into a focused examination of return-on-investment patterns, explored in the following section, which extends the analysis from cost-effectiveness to broader fiscal and social returns.

A deeper analysis of these findings reveals a consistent trend: interventions with simple, behaviorally grounded designs, such as mobile reminders or digital coaching, tend to deliver higher cost-effectiveness ratios than more technologically complex tools like AI-driven analytics or precision prevention platforms. This pattern suggests that economic value often stems from the integration of context and user adoption, rather than from technological sophistication alone. Furthermore, interventions embedded within existing care or community systems show greater scalability and sustained impact, underscoring the importance of system readiness and implementation pathways as key economic determinants.

Empirical evidence demonstrating the measurable economic impact of digital health interventions. The economic case for digital health is increasingly compelling. Studies have shown substantial returns on investment through reduced emergency care utilization, enhanced treatment adherence, and broader societal benefits, including decreased absenteeism and increased productivity (Lawal & Bubari Umar, 2025; Mekniran et al., 2024). ROI patterns across sectors reveal an important distinction between financial and social value. Corporate and insurer-driven digital wellness programs generate rapid monetary returns but primarily benefit already connected or insured populations. By contrast, publicly funded digital prevention programs, such as maternal health or vaccination tracking platforms, offer slower but broader returns, generating benefits that include equity, productivity, and long-term fiscal stability. This comparison highlights the need for multidimensional ROI frameworks that integrate traditional cost recovery with social return on investment (SROI) metrics, encompassing both financial and inclusive value. Econometric analyses from Europe further confirm that digitalization is positively associated with improved life expectancy and lower mortality when aligned with infrastructure and socioeconomic Development (Kuzior et al., 2024). Digital tools have been widely recognized for their potential in addressing inequities and expanding access to essential services in hard-to-reach communities, fostering a sense of empathy and social responsibility among healthcare professionals and policymakers.

While existing research has extensively explored clinical and technological dimensions of digital health, fewer studies have synthesized its economic and preventive implications. Prior reviews have typically focused on isolated interventions such as telehealth, mHealth, or digital therapeutics without evaluating their system-wide fiscal or social returns (De La Torre-Diéz et al., 2015; Santos et al., 2025). Recent contributions (Morris et al., 2023; Ratanawong et al., 2022; Sinha & Schryer-Roy, 2018), emphasize the need to integrate cost-effectiveness, equity, and scalability within a single analytical framework. This chapter addresses that gap by integrating insights from digital innovation studies with the health-economic evidence base to clarify how prevention can be financed, implemented, and justified through measurable economic benefits. Existing frameworks for disease prevention were primarily designed for analogous health systems. Consequently, many economic evaluations focus narrowly on direct healthcare costs and overlook wider social and productivity gains that digital solutions can generate. While there is broad recognition of digital health's potential, consensus is lacking on the economic metrics and policy mechanisms needed to scale these innovations responsibly.

This chapter addresses that gap by integrating economic, policy, and equity perspectives to explain how digital prevention can move from pilot projects to sustainable national strategies. However, despite these challenges, the potential of digital health technologies to revolutionize disease prevention is promising. While evidence supports their effectiveness, digital health technologies are often evaluated through a narrow clinical lens, with limited attention to long-term cost-effectiveness, cross-sectoral ROI, or system-level savings. This underscores the urgent need for strategic investment in promising digital innovations (Xuefei et al., 2018). Evaluations frequently lack methodological consistency and fail to capture broader value dimensions such as improved public health capacity or social return on investment (Weinhold et al., 2019). In low-resource settings, these challenges are further compounded by weak health infrastructure and underdeveloped digital ecosystems, which limit scalability and long-term sustainability (Omotayo et al., 2024). Policymakers and investors are often left without the granular data to make evidence-based decisions on digital health adoption. This chapter addresses these gaps by examining the cost-effectiveness of digital health interventions and the broader ROI and policy implications for disease prevention. A comprehensive understanding of these economic dimensions is crucial for developing more effective, equitable, and scalable digital health strategies globally. These introductory insights establish the problem context and justify the need for a structured analysis of both the conceptual foundations and the empirical evidence that follow.

For healthcare executives, policy planners, and public health managers, this chapter offers an evidence-based roadmap to prioritize, fund, and evaluate digital prevention programs. It demonstrates how economic evaluation tools such as cost-effectiveness and ROI analyses can guide resource allocation, minimize wasteful spending, and scale innovations that yield measurable population-level outcomes. By translating global research into actionable insights, the chapter equips managers to make data-driven decisions that align digital health investment with long-term health system sustainability and equity. To situate this analysis clearly, the following section provides a concise overview of the theoretical and economic foundations that guide cost-effectiveness and ROI assessment in digital prevention. The chapter is organized in a logical progression. Section 1 establishes the global and economic rationale for digital health prevention, and Section 2 presents the theoretical and methodological foundations for evaluating economic value. Sections 4 and 5 synthesize empirical evidence on cost-effectiveness and ROI, translating these insights into policy and managerial guidance. Section 5 examines implementation challenges, Section 6 concludes with forward-looking recommendations, and Sections 7 and 8 provide further insights. This structure ensures clear movement from theory to practice and from evidence to policy.

2. CONCEPTUAL FRAMEWORK

This section clarifies the key theoretical and analytical constructs used throughout the chapter. It defines the main economic evaluation approaches, cost-effectiveness, cost-utility, and cost-benefit analyses, and explains their relevance for digital health. These definitions establish a shared foundation for interpreting the evidence and recommendations that will be presented later.

2.1. Digital Health, Disease Prevention, and Economic Evaluation

Digital health is broadly defined as the use of information and communication technologies (ICT) to improve health outcomes, enhance healthcare delivery, and optimize resource allocation. This includes a spectrum of tools such as mobile health (mHealth), telemedicine, wearable devices, electronic health records, and artificial intelligence-driven diagnostics (Kowatsch & Fleisch, 2021). The World Health Organization further frames digital health as a core component of strengthening health systems through improved access, efficiency, quality, and patient-centeredness (Willis et al., 2021). Disease prevention, particularly in non-communicable diseases (NCDs), focuses on mitigating risk factors, promoting healthier lifestyles, and implementing early detection strategies. When integrated with digital tools, prevention becomes more personalized, proactive, and scalable, targeting individuals and populations with precision interventions that reduce morbidity and health expenditure over time (Bergin et al., 2020). A brief bibliometric review conducted using Scopus and PubMed (search terms: digital health, economic evaluation, disease prevention) identified over 2,300 peer-reviewed studies published between 2015 and 2025, with an average annual growth rate of 18%. The majority (62%) focus on mHealth and telehealth, while only about 12% address ROI or cost-benefit modeling directly. This pattern confirms that economic analyses of digital prevention remain under-represented in the literature, reinforcing the importance of the integrative approach developed in this chapter.

The analysis presented here aligns with the book's focus on digital transformation by emphasizing how economic evaluation frameworks can support health promotion planning, resource allocation, and policy prioritization in digitally enabled prevention systems. Economic healthcare evaluation systematically compares costs and outcomes between competing interventions to inform resource allocation. Core methodologies include cost-effectiveness analysis (CEA), cost-utility analysis (CUA), and cost-benefit analysis (CBA). These approaches aim to quantify the value delivered by interventions, often through metrics like quality-adjusted life years (QALYs), disability-adjusted life years (DALYs), or net monetary benefit (Gils et al., 2011). Traditional economic models in digital health are often insufficient due to the dynamic and complex nature of digital systems. This complexity necessitates the Development of expanded frameworks that incorporate process outcomes, scalability, and long-term system integration. Comparative analyses reveal notable methodological diversity. For example, systematic reviews of digital CVD and diabetes prevention (Buss et al., 2020; Maiga et al., 2021) demonstrate cost-effectiveness across high-income settings, whereas evaluations in LMICs emphasize affordability constraints (Viet et al., 2024). Conversely, modeling studies (Laursen et al., 2023; Watson et al., 2014) argue that standard economic models underestimate productivity gains and equity benefits.

2.2. Categories of Digital Health Tools

Digital health encompasses a broad and evolving ecosystem of technologies designed to support health promotion, disease prevention, and care delivery. These technologies vary widely in their functions, applications, and user interfaces, yet they aim to enhance efficiency, accessibility, and outcomes across healthcare systems (Altibi et al., 2021). One foundational category is mobile health (mHealth), which includes health-related applications on smartphones and tablets. These tools support behavior change through tracking, prompts, educational content, and remote consultations, and have successfully managed cardiometabolic risks, improved medication adherence, and promoted healthier lifestyles (Sharma et al., 2022). Wearable devices, such as fitness trackers and smartwatches, represent another widely used form of mHealth, providing real-time biometric data that enables personalized and preventive health monitoring (Lampreia et al., 2024). Telehealth and telemedicine platforms constitute a second major category, offering synchronous or asynchronous interactions between patients and providers. These systems have been instrumental in expanding access to care, particularly in rural or underserved areas, while reducing travel and intervention delays. Their integration into primary care and preventive screening protocols has become increasingly common, supported by innovations such as AI-enhanced virtual triage systems and real-time diagnostics. This increased accessibility is a significant step towards more equitable healthcare (Sánchez-Castillo et al., 2023). Their integration into primary care and preventive screening protocols has become increasingly common, supported by innovations such as AI-enhanced virtual triage systems and real-time diagnostics (Abbasi, 2024).

Another emerging domain is digital therapeutics (DTx), software-based, evidence-driven interventions that deliver clinical-grade treatments for conditions such as type 2 diabetes, insomnia, or substance use disorders. These tools are often evaluated through regulatory frameworks and can serve as effective supplements or even replacements for pharmacological therapy (Supervia & Lopez-Jimenez, 2018). Artificial intelligence (AI) and machine learning (ML) applications also play a transformative role in prevention by analyzing large datasets to predict disease risk, triage care needs, and guide personalized interventions (Bhatt et al., 2021). This digital health continuum enables more initiative-taking, data-driven, and equitable strategies for disease prevention and management.

2.3. Overview of Economic Evaluation Metrics

Evaluating the economic impact of digital health innovations requires the application of rigorous and standardized economic evaluation metrics. These metrics enable decision-makers to assess whether digital tools provide sufficient value relative to their costs, helping to prioritize investments under resource constraints. The most widely used economic evaluation approaches include cost-effectiveness analysis (CEA), cost-utility analysis (CUA), and cost-benefit analysis (CBA), each providing a different lens for comparing alternatives (Torgerson, 2009). Cost-effectiveness analysis assesses the cost per unit of health outcome achieved, such as the cost per case of disease prevented. It is beneficial to compare interventions with similar health outcomes, but with varying costs and efficiency. In public health, CEA frequently employs natural units such as cases averted or life years gained (Miller & Hendrie, 2012). Cost-utility analysis (CUA), a specialized form of CEA, incorporates both quantity and quality of life into composite indices, typically measured as Quality-Adjusted Life Years (QALYs) or Disability-Adjusted Life Years (DALYs) (Torrance, 1997). Cost-benefit analysis (CBA) translates costs and outcomes into monetary terms to calculate net benefits or benefit-cost ratios, offering a broader societal perspective (Brent, 2023). CBA is particularly well-suited for large-scale digital investments that influence healthcare efficiency, productivity, and social equity (Cohen & Patel, 2009). Complementing these tools, incremental cost-effectiveness ratios (ICERs) express the additional cost per additional unit of benefit gained when comparing interventions, aiding in decisions on adopting digital innovations over standard care (Svensson & Hultkrantz, 2017). Sensitivity analysis is also vital in digital health evaluations, as it tests how variable assumptions (e.g., user retention or implementation costs) impact findings and robustness (Higgins & Harris, 2012). These provide a structured, multidimensional framework for assessing the economic value of digital technologies in disease prevention and guiding data-driven investments across health systems.

Although economic evaluations provide critical evidence, policy translation remains uneven. In many contexts, promising digital interventions fail to achieve scale due to regulatory inertia, misaligned incentives, or fragmented funding structures. To ensure that evidence informs real-world decisions, economic analysis must be integrated into policy design through reimbursement reform, outcome-based Financing, and capacity-building programs that align investment incentives with public health objectives. Despite substantial progress, the literature still reveals three persistent gaps: the limited integration of digital innovation metrics into mainstream cost-effectiveness frameworks, the scarcity of comparative evidence between high-income and low-income contexts, and the underrepresentation of long-term fiscal outcomes, such as productivity, resilience, and social return. Addressing these gaps provides the rationale for the analyses presented in the following sections.

From a managerial perspective, economic evaluation tools can be directly applied to investment decisions in digital prevention. Health system managers can use cost-effectiveness ratios (ICERs) to prioritize interventions that deliver the highest health gain per dollar spent, while cost-utility analyses (QALYs and DALYs) help rank technologies that maximize patient quality of life. For example, a regional health director could compare an mHealth diabetes program and a telecardiology service using ICER values to identify which offers superior long-term value. Similarly, cost-benefit analyses enable ministries of health to demonstrate the fiscal and productivity benefits of prevention programs, thereby strengthening their case for sustained funding. Embedding these tools into annual budgeting cycles helps ensure that digital health investments are not only innovative but also financially responsible.

3. COST-EFFECTIVENESS OF DIGITAL HEALTH IN PREVENTION

3.1. Evidence from Global Sources

The cost-effectiveness of digital health technologies in disease prevention is increasingly supported by empirical evidence from diverse global settings. Digital health interventions, such as mobile applications, telemonitoring platforms, and web-based programs, have demonstrated substantial promise in reducing the burden of chronic disease while offering economic value across both high-income countries and low- and middle-income countries (LMICs). A foundational study reviewed various eHealth applications and found that digital platforms supporting weight loss and mental health management were clinically practical and economically advantageous when integrated into chronic disease prevention strategies (Monzani & Pizzoli, 2019). These interventions typically involved minimal recurring costs and reached large populations, contributing to a favorable cost per health outcome, especially in primary prevention. Similarly, a systematic review study on behavior change interventions found that most digital tools, including SMS, mobile apps, and websites, were cost-effective or cost-saving in chronic disease prevention across high-income settings (Kyaw et al., 2022). A cost-effectiveness analysis in Southeast Asia emphasized that preventive strategies addressing cardiovascular diseases (CVDs), type 2 diabetes, and major NCD risk factors, when supported by digital tools, were either cost-effective or cost-saving across most LMIC contexts (Bertram et al., 2021). Interventions such as sugar-sweetened beverage taxation, mobile-based hypertension monitoring, and digitally enhanced tobacco cessation programs demonstrated high returns per disability-adjusted life year (DALY) averted.

Another similar study found that 80% of evaluated preventive interventions, many of which were digitally supported, fell below the €50,000/QALY threshold, and 60% were below €20,000/QALY, reaffirming the high economic value of digital health (Gils et al., 2011). A 'DALY' measures disease burden, representing the number of healthy years lost due to illness, disability, or early death. Pelletier (1999) evaluated worksite wellness programs in high-income settings and found that embedded digital tools in individualized risk-reduction plans significantly reduced healthcare costs, particularly for high-risk employees. Similarly, other scholars in their study confirmed that integrated prevention campaigns, including digital outreach, yielded cost-effectiveness ratios as low as US$49 per DALY averted in the most favorable LMIC settings (Marseille et al., 2014). These studies reinforce that digital health tools enhance clinical efficiency and patient engagement, offering strong economic justification for their broad-scale implementation in modern disease prevention strategies.

Emerging post-pandemic literature reinforces these findings, highlighting AI-assisted preventive analytics, remote monitoring ecosystems, and hybrid digital-community models as next-generation cost-effective solutions (Bartelheimer et al., 2025; Damera et al., 2025; Gupta et al., 2020; Huang et al., 2025; Khan et al., 2025; Musa et al., 2025). These studies collectively demonstrate that digital innovation now serves as a macroeconomic driver of prevention, rather than an isolated technological enhancement. These global findings underscore that the economic case for digital health extends beyond clinical cost savings to the core goals of health promotion: empowering populations, reducing modifiable risks, and enhancing access to preventive care. In this way, digital tools serve not merely as technological add-ons but as catalysts that reshape the delivery, Financing, and long-term sustainability of health promotion efforts, precisely the transformation this volume seeks to document.

3.2. Case Examples in Disease Prevention

Real-world case studies further reinforce the economic potential of digital health interventions in preventing disease. Across various preventive domains, including vaccination, cardiovascular disease, and diabetes, digital technologies have consistently demonstrated measurable cost-effectiveness in both trial-based and model-based analyses. A systematic review evaluated 35 digital health interventions across high- and middle-income countries. These included text messaging, video consultations, web portals, and mobile applications. The findings revealed that digital tools such as mobile reminders for medication adherence and video-based teleconsultations were clinically effective and showed favorable cost-effectiveness ratios, often below widely accepted willingness-to-pay thresholds (Gentili et al., 2022). In the context of immunization, a systematic review found that digital interventions, including SMS, web-based tools, and automated calls, significantly improved vaccine uptake for influenza, HPV, and childhood immunizations. Most studies concluded that these tools were either cost-effective or cost-saving (Wang et al., 2023). A separate evaluation in Ghana demonstrated that the aerial drone delivery of vaccines using digital logistics systems was highly cost-effective, averting disease cases at a cost of just $41–$58 per DALY (Ospina-Fadul et al., 2024).

Cardiovascular disease (CVD) prevention is another area where digital tools show strong economic viability. A study reviewed over 50 studies and concluded that digital health interventions significantly reduced CVD risk, with a systematic review of cost-effectiveness studies confirming that all evaluated interventions were economically viable (Islam & Maddison, 2020). Additional simulation studies using real-world data, like the one conducted in Liverpool on NHS Health Checks, a comprehensive health check-up program in the UK, demonstrated that combining digital health screening with structural policy changes could deliver thousands of QALYs at low or negative net cost (City, 2023). For type 2 diabetes and hypertension, Nordyke et al. (2019) estimated that digital therapeutics, which are digital tools used to treat medical conditions, could achieve monthly healthcare resource savings of $97–$145 per patient by substituting medication use with behavioral change tools. From a U.S. payer perspective, the treatment proved to be cost-effective over three years. These studies reinforce that digital health interventions are both technologically feasible and economically justified, supporting their broader implementation across public health agendas. Managerial Insights through the Prioritization of Digital Prevention Investments.

i. Health managers can achieve early wins by adopting low-cost, high-impact interventions such as SMS-based behavior change programs or telehealth-supported chronic disease monitoring, both of which demonstrate strong cost-effectiveness and scalability.
ii. National policymakers should prioritize digital tools with a cost per DALY below U.S. $100 or an ROI break-even within three years, ensuring rapid fiscal returns.
iii. In LMIC settings, managers can bundle digital prevention with community programs (e.g., vaccination or nutrition outreach) to leverage existing infrastructure and resources.
iv. Hospital and insurance administrators should consider integrating cost-effectiveness metrics into procurement and reimbursement decisions to align innovation with measurable health and economic outcomes.

3.3. Modeling Approaches and Assumptions

Economic modeling is crucial in evaluating the long-term cost-effectiveness and return on investment (ROI) of digital health interventions for disease prevention. Unlike trial-based evaluations, which are constrained by limited periods and controlled conditions, modeling allows researchers and policymakers to simulate real-world outcomes over extended periods, across diverse populations, and under varying behavior, adherence, and scale assumptions. One of the foundational frameworks for modeling digital health interventions recognizes their inherent complexity. These tools often evolve iteratively, exhibit non-linear usage patterns, and generate multidimensional outcomes, necessitating models that capture these dynamics over time (McNamee et al., 2016). To address this, analysts increasingly apply hybrid models that combine decision trees, Markov chains, and discrete-event simulations to estimate long-term outcomes and cost profiles beyond the scope of clinical trials (Lehnert et al., 2012). These models also adjust for key variables such as technological obsolescence, behavioral fatigue, and varying levels of user engagement.

However, Gomes et al. (2022) have argued that standard health sector models often fail to capture indirect benefits such as productivity gains, social empowerment, or cost avoidance from comorbidity prevention, necessitating a shift toward broader perspectives. Similarly, a study emphasized that simulation-based economic evaluations can extend limited short-term trial data to estimate broader, cumulative health benefits in preventive interventions (Merkur et al., 2013). Pediatric-focused economic models must account for heterogeneity in population coverage, digital literacy, and family engagement to accurately estimate the durability and cost-effectiveness of interventions (Stanić et al., 2023). These provide a flexible and forward-looking toolkit for evaluating digital health interventions in preventive care, delivering methodologically rigorous and policy-relevant insights.

Table 1. High-Value Digital Prevention Tools: Cost and Managerial Considerations

Intervention Type	Estimated Cost per DALY/ QALY	ROI Range	Scalability	Managerial Note
SMS-based tobacco cessation	US $50–70 per DALY	5 – 10: 1	High	Ideal for low-income and rural settings; quick impact
Digital hypertension monitoring	US $41–58 per DALY	8 – 12: 1	Medium	Requires telemedicine infrastructure; strong preventive ROI
AI risk prediction for CVD	< €20 000 per QALY	10 – 15: 1	Moderate	Enhances early detection; ensures data governance readiness
Workplace digital wellness	U.S. $100–300 per team member	1.5 – 2: 1	High	ROI < 3 years; boosts productivity and morale

Source: synthesized by the author from global cost-effectiveness and ROI studies cited.

4. RETURN ON INVESTMENT (ROI) ANALYSIS

Building on the cost-effectiveness results from the previous section, this section expands the scope to include ROI and productivity outcomes. It examines how different sectors, including healthcare, education, and workplaces, translate digital prevention into financial and social value.

4.1. ROI Concepts and Significance

Return on investment (ROI) is a crucial economic metric that measures the financial benefits of an intervention in relation to its cost. In digital health for disease prevention, ROI helps determine whether investing in telehealth platforms, mobile health applications, and predictive analytics tools results in net savings or added value for health systems, employers, or society. Unlike traditional cost-effectiveness analyses, which focus solely on health outcomes, ROI incorporates both direct financial savings and indirect benefits, such as increased productivity and reduced absenteeism. Evidence indicates that well-designed digital health interventions frequently yield a positive ROI within a brief time. Findings from a study that evaluated a digital behavioral counseling program for individuals with prediabetes and cardiovascular risk; their intervention achieved ROI break-even within three years and generated up to $1,565 in savings per participant by year five, primarily through reductions in diabetes incidence and stroke rates. These significant cost savings demonstrate the impressive economic viability of digital health interventions.

At the policy level, the WHO Collaborating Centre for Investment in Health and Wellbeing developed a digital framework to assess preventive interventions' social ROI (SROI). This approach extends beyond fiscal metrics to include environmental, community, and equity outcomes, showcasing how digital tools can support sustainable investment across public health systems (Dyakova et al., 2020). According to Stein & Galea (2020), further research has demonstrated that national public health initiatives, supported by digital interventions, can yield returns of up to $40 for every $1 invested, with exceptionally high returns for remote monitoring, behavioral nudges, and predictive analytics. A related study confirmed a median ROI of 14:1 for public health interventions, with national-level digital programs achieving even higher returns than local implementations. These findings underscore the significant potential for returns on investment in digital health, providing an optimistic outlook for the economic benefits of these interventions. (Mason et al., 2016). This comprehensive approach provides a thorough understanding of the economic implications of digital health interventions, reassuring the audience about the thoroughness of the research.

4.2. Case Studies Across Sectors

Case studies from multiple sectors, including workplaces, schools, public health systems, and Medicaid programs, demonstrate that digital health interventions for disease prevention often yield a substantial return on investment (ROI). These examples demonstrate the financial viability of implementing digital innovations to prevent chronic illness, promote behavioral change, and reduce long-term care costs. A comprehensive systematic review analyzed 138 workplace-based prevention interventions globally and found that 56.5% yielded positive ROI. Digital components such as health tracking apps and remote coaching were among the most effective, particularly in large enterprises with established infrastructure (Stratton et al., 2021; Thonon et al., 2023). Studies in public health found that national-level interventions consistently outperformed local initiatives in ROI, with ratios as high as 28.6:1. Centralized, scalable programs, including digital health campaigns, delivered the most significant returns (Mason et al., 2016). ROI was evaluated across 10 Medicaid managed care organizations, and impressive savings were found: 12.2:1 for adults with chronic conditions and 6.35:1 for children with asthma (Oliveira et al., 2020). Studies in educational settings evaluated school-based prevention programs incorporating digital health platforms, such as activity trackers and nutrition apps, and found ROI exceeding 800% in comprehensive school health models. These tools addressed key NCD risk factors, such as physical inactivity and poor diet (Ekwaru et al., 2021). In clinical pharmacy, a multi-center study in Egypt showed an average ROI of 760% for pharmacist-led digital medication management systems.

These platforms reduced adverse drug events and improved clinical outcomes (Alsetohy et al., 2025). Studies from Mental health interventions also show robust ROI and reported that digital prevention for adolescent anxiety and depression yields a long-term ROI of up to £55:£1. Digital cognitive behavioral therapy (CBT) and online risk assessment tools drove these savings (Fortuna et al., 2019; Jackson-Morris et al., 2024). Furthermore, SROI ratios of up to £28 for every £1 invested in digital mental health interventions have been reported in high-income settings (Kadel et al., 2022). These multi-sector case studies highlight the economic benefits of targeted digital health interventions.

4.3. Long-Term Financial and Productivity Impacts

Beyond immediate cost savings, digital health interventions for disease prevention offer long-term economic and productivity benefits often underestimated in traditional evaluations. These benefits include avoided medical costs resulting from delayed disease onset, enhanced workforce productivity, and reduced absenteeism and presenteeism, particularly relevant for chronic conditions such as diabetes, cardiovascular disease, and mental illness (Huntsman & Bulaj, 2023; Stratton et al., 2021). Moreover, the studies demonstrated how digital interventions that nudge patients with diabetes into regular primary care could significantly reduce long-term costs while generating near-term revenue for health systems. Their economic model, focused on a high-income health system, captured downstream effects such as decreased hospitalization, better disease control, and improved clinical efficiency (Powers & Bucher, 2022). A study highlights how digital prevention strategies, targeting early detection and risk factor reduction, could significantly mitigate vast economic burdens, particularly in low- and middle-income countries (Guerrero-López et al., 2024). These studies reveal that investing in preventive digital health yields immediate fiscal returns and enduring socioeconomic benefits, making it a powerful strategy for sustainable healthcare and workforce development. For decision-makers, the ROI evidence underscores that digital prevention is not a long-term luxury but an immediate fiscal opportunity. Managers should track both direct cost savings (e.g., reduced hospitalizations) and indirect productivity gains (e.g., decreased absenteeism) in their performance dashboards. Embedding ROI metrics into health budgeting, procurement, and performance contracts ensures that digital health interventions deliver sustained economic and social value.

5. POLICY AND SYSTEM-LEVEL IMPLICATIONS

The policy analysis in this section speaks directly to the book's theme of reshaping prevention through digital innovation. Translating cost-effectiveness and ROI data into actionable governance strategies enables policymakers to reposition digital health as a core component of national health promotion policy. This reframing recognizes that financial sustainability and health equity are not competing goals but mutually reinforcing outcomes of well-designed digital innovation systems. Integrating digital health innovations into disease prevention strategies requires a coherent policy framework that aligns technological capabilities with health system priorities. The following discussion connects the economic evidence reviewed earlier to the structural and governance conditions needed for implementation. It explains how cost-effectiveness and ROI data can directly inform national digital health strategy, funding design, and accountability frameworks. Globally, digital health policies have evolved from fragmented pilot programs to more strategic efforts aimed at scaling digital infrastructure, standardizing data governance, and promoting equitable access (Gabrielli et al., 2023; Mburu et al., 2018; Olamilekan & Umar, 2025).

However, the pace and structure of policy development vary significantly across regions, shaped by political will, institutional capacity, and contextual public health needs. Numerous studies emphasize that in low- and middle-income countries (LMICs), policy frameworks must move beyond isolated technology deployments and instead embed multilevel strategies targeting health services, risk factors, environmental determinants, and global influences (Briggs et al., 2019; Owusu et al., 2024). Studies in Ireland describe the national implementation of the "Make Every Contact Count" (MECC) initiative as a digital behavior change policy integrated into chronic disease care that mandates risk factor screening and intervention during routine consultations. These studies underscore the need for adaptive, data-driven, and multilevel policy frameworks that can support the successful deployment of digital health tools in preventive strategies across healthcare systems. Implementation Roadmap for Managers and Policymakers includes the following:

1. Conduct economic screening of existing digital programs to identify those with positive cost-effectiveness or ROI ratios.
2. Develop value-based funding models that reward preventive outcomes rather than service volume.
3. Establish cross-sector partnerships between health, finance, and ICT ministries to align investment and regulation.
4. Integrate equity indicators such as digital inclusion and regional coverage into program evaluation.
5. Create national digital health observatories to monitor implementation costs, returns, and health outcomes over time. Following this roadmap can help managers move from fragmented pilots to scalable, financially sustainable national strategies.

Integrating digital health into national health systems is crucial for realizing the full benefits of disease prevention and control. However, this process demands coordinated policy, sustainable financing models, infrastructure investment, and attention to ethical and equity concerns. Successful integration ensures that digital health is not an external innovation, but a core component of public health strategy (Thomas et al., 2023; Zhang et al., 2023). Emerging technologies, such as 5G-enabled telemedicine, predictive analytics, and virtual care platforms, fundamentally reshape care delivery by enabling more proactive and decentralized prevention strategies. For such systems to succeed nationally, policy and regulatory frameworks must align with digital infrastructure upgrades and cross-sector collaboration (Bhatt et al., 2024; Rukundo, 2024). A study views and argues that integrating digital health into mainstream clinical and preventive services requires a shift from siloed innovation to multidisciplinary system design, highlighting the value of embedding real-time data streams, digital surveillance, and wearable health data into existing infrastructures (Fiordelli, 2024; Kostkova, 2015).

Meanwhile, other studies stress that national health systems must address challenges such as digital literacy, reimbursement policies, and interoperability to facilitate adoption. Their analysis of cardiovascular prevention demonstrates that successful national uptake depends on tailored insurance schemes and user-centric design standards (Komiyama et al., 2025; Tian et al., 2025). These findings show that integrating digital health for disease prevention within national systems demands holistic reforms that bridge policy, practice, people, and technology to deliver equitable and sustainable outcomes.

The reimbursement structure is a powerful determinant of whether digital health technologies for disease prevention are adopted, scaled, and sustained. Traditional reimbursement mechanisms such as fee-for-service (FFS) often fail to incentivize preventive care, including digital interventions, as they reward volume over value. Emerging models increasingly recognize the need to shift toward value-based and population-focused frameworks that promote long-term prevention and improved outcomes (Zwaagstra Salvado et al., 2021). It can be concluded that no single reimbursement scheme works universally across all levels of prevention. While FFS may support short-term interventions, such as immunizations, it often underperforms in preventing chronic diseases.

In contrast, population-based capitation can support broader strategies, such as remote monitoring and lifestyle education, by rewarding outcomes rather than activity volume (Anumudu & Erickson, 2020). The U.S. Institute of Medicine has also supported incentive-based approaches, calling for systems that reward quality and preventive behavior at both provider and patient levels (Heider, 2020). Pay-for-performance (P4P) and bundled payments have emerged as alternatives to FFS, aiming to reduce preventable illness and align financial incentives with patient outcomes. However, studies show that P4P has produced mixed results, with some improvements in process indicators, but these do not always translate into better clinical outcomes, especially when poorly designed or underfunded (Mitchell et al., 2019). Studies in Austria argued that digital therapeutics (DTx) require reimbursement policies grounded in clinical evidence, equity, and digital literacy. Reimbursement should also reflect interoperability and data protection to ensure inclusive adoption (Prodan et al., 2022; Sareban et al., 2025). These findings underscore that aligning reimbursement structures with the preventive goals of digital health is not merely important but essential for achieving sustainable adoption, clinical effectiveness, and equitable access at scale.

As digital health technologies are increasingly adopted for disease prevention, ethical considerations surrounding data governance and health equity have become critically important. These concerns extend beyond data privacy and confidentiality to issues of inclusivity, algorithmic fairness, and the potential for digital interventions to reduce or exacerbate existing health disparities. Studies emphasize that digital health research must be co-designed with racialized and marginalized communities to ensure ethical data collection and governance; their framework supports data self-determination, where communities retain control over how health data are gathered and used (Islam et al., 2024; Voultsos, 2023). A recent framework identifies five key socio-ethical domains essential to equitable digital health development: access and engagement, trial inclusiveness, algorithmic bias, surveillance risks, and trust in data systems. These concerns demand multilevel regulation and design strategies that embed equity from the outset (Paccoud et al., 2024), a call echoed by (Cary et al., 2024), who introduced the BE FAIR framework (Bias Elimination for Fair and Responsible AI), to empower healthcare workers to promote equity in algorithmic tools. A study highlights how historical lessons in medical informatics offer critical guidance on avoiding ethical pitfalls in today's AI-driven systems (Kulikowski, 2022). Ethical digital health implementation requires inclusive design, transparent data practices, and ongoing community engagement to ensure that technologies promote rather than hinder health equity and public trust.

6. CHALLENGES AND BARRIERS

This section critically examines the obstacles that hinder the translation of economic evidence into implementation. By grouping these barriers into infrastructural, regulatory, and socioeconomic categories, the discussion maintains organizational clarity and continuity with preceding sections.

6.1. Digital Divide and Health Disparities

The digital divide, unequal access to and utilization of digital technologies, remains a significant barrier to the equitable deployment of digital health tools for disease prevention. This divide, often driven by socioeconomic status, geography, education, age, and race, can unintentionally reinforce health disparities by limiting access to timely information, remote care, and personalized prevention strategies (Girmay, 2024; Saeed & Masters, 2021). Studies have shown that marginalized groups, including Black, low-income, and rural populations, have disproportionately low telehealth completion rates. While digital health has the potential to expand access to care, structural inequalities in internet availability and device ownership create a gap between technological capability and actual use, ultimately leading to underutilization of preventive services in communities that would benefit most (Bayard et al., 2022; Shaw, 2023). A systematic review found that digital inclusion can be promoted through the application of universal design principles, ongoing evaluation, and targeted interventions, such as digital literacy training and infrastructure expansion (Bhoyar et al., 2024). There is a need for strategic frameworks that propose the Development of telehealth equity dashboards to monitor disparities and guide inclusive service design (Luke et al., 2024). A national survey in China showed that individual and community-level socioeconomic factors significantly influenced digital access, with internet use associated with better self-reported health outcomes (Hong et al., 2017). To ensure the benefits of digital health extend to all populations, closing the digital divide must be prioritized as a foundational component of public health policy and infrastructure development. This includes broadband expansion and coordinated investments in digital literacy, culturally tailored services, and multi-stakeholder engagement.

6.2. Data Security and Patient Privacy

The expansion of digital health technologies for disease prevention has brought patient privacy and data security into sharp focus. As healthcare systems increasingly rely on digital records, mobile applications, and interconnected platforms, ensuring the confidentiality, integrity, and availability of sensitive health information becomes crucial to the ethical and practical implementation of digital health. A study proposed a cybersecurity framework leveraging big data analytics, incorporating encryption, secure authentication, and environmental controls to address common vulnerabilities in EHR systems and promote systemic resilience (Zhu et al., 2020). Furthermore, the importance of HIPAA compliance and adaptive cybersecurity strategies is acknowledged, given the rise of ransomware and phishing as significant threats to digital patient safety (Abbasi & Smith, 2024). The proliferation of connected sensors and mobile devices in healthcare has dramatically increased the volume and granularity of personal health data. While these data enhance prediction and personalization, they also raise serious concerns about privacy. Their analysis supports the use of techniques such as anonymization, differential privacy, and consent protocols (El Ouazzani & El Bakkali, 2020). Protecting health data is not just a technical necessity but foundational to regulatory compliance, public trust, and the equitable expansion of digital health systems.

6.3. Implementation Gaps in LMICs vs. HICs

While digital health technologies have demonstrated effectiveness across various settings, their implementation for disease prevention reveals significant disparities between low- and middle-income countries (LMICs) and high-income countries (HICs). These disparities are shaped by infrastructure, workforce readiness, policy alignment, and sociotechnical complexity, resulting in challenges to scalability, adoption, and long-term sustainability. A study emphasized that LMICs often face systemic barriers, such as fragmented digital systems, weak data governance, and limited workforce capacity, even when digital tools are technically available (Duggal et al., 2023). Studies applying the NASSS (Non-Adoption, Abandonment, Scale-up, Spread, and Sustainability) and ERIC (Expert Recommendations for Implementing Change) frameworks reported improved results, underscoring the need for structured planning and local stakeholder involvement (Seward et al., 2021). In contrast, HICs benefit from more advanced digital ecosystems, policy coherence, and greater provider engagement. However, challenges remain. In the EU, eHealth adoption is hindered by a lack of interoperability and inconsistent clinician engagement (Global Initiative for Children's Surgery et al., 2019). Many HICs still experience socio-technical disconnects during implementation, particularly at later stages of integration into routine care (Hasan et al., 2021).

To bridge these gaps, a set of best practices has been proposed for digital scale-up in LMICs, including aligning digital tools with national priorities, engaging all stakeholders early, and ensuring technical simplicity and policy support (Abdulwahab & Azam, 2026; Fleming et al., 2021). Critical barriers, such as the poor application of diffusion techniques and underinvestment in leadership training, must be addressed through tailored implementation research agendas (Yamey, 2012). These studies reflect complex structural, institutional, and cultural dynamics that require customized strategies, integrated frameworks, and long-term investment in both capacity and context.

7. FUTURE DIRECTIONS AND RECOMMENDATIONS

This section consolidates the chapter's insights into actionable recommendations for health managers, policymakers, and researchers. It outlines strategic directions that can maximize the cost-effectiveness, ROI, and policy relevance of digital prevention initiatives. The future of preventive healthcare lies in embracing digital technologies that are not only clinically effective but also economically smart. Tools like mobile health apps, genomics, electronic health records, and AI-driven platforms are transforming care from reactive treatment to proactive prevention. These innovations enable early disease detection, personalized interventions, and real-time monitoring. One cutting-edge Development is precision prevention using genomics, behavioral data, and mobile tech to tailor strategies to individuals. Technologies such as digital twins and multi-omics data enable accurate risk assessments and early intervention, providing cost-effective methods for managing health before symptoms arise.

However, to fully integrate these tools, governments must realign fiscal priorities. Despite strong evidence supporting the return on investment of digital prevention, funding remains limited. National programs, rather than local initiatives, yield greater economic returns, emphasizing the need for cohesive, high-level policymaking. Strategic investments of around $100 million in digital infrastructure, health literacy, and mobile health are recommended to scale impact. Additionally, Financing must also adapt to challenges like pandemics and climate change. Multisectoral collaboration is crucial through effective partnerships among health, technology, finance, and civil society, which can optimize resource utilization, align goals, and foster trust and confidence. Models like the CDC's 6/18 initiative show how payers, providers, and public health systems can scale evidence-based interventions through joint efforts.

8. CONCLUSION

The conclusion synthesizes the chapter's conceptual, empirical, and policy insights, reaffirming how digital health economics can inform prevention strategies and investment priorities. The conclusion synthesizes the key economic and policy insights presented across the chapter. It reiterates the central argument that digital prevention is both a public health imperative and an economic opportunity and summarizes practical implications for future implementation. Digital health innovations represent a pivotal shift in disease prevention, offering scalable, cost-effective, and personalized approaches to reduce the global burden of non-communicable diseases. Evidence consistently demonstrates their ability to enhance early detection, improve patient engagement, and deliver high returns on investment through reduced healthcare utilization and improved population health outcomes.

However, the full potential of these technologies can only be realized through deliberate policy integration, equitable funding mechanisms, and multisectoral collaboration. Addressing implementation gaps, especially in low- and middle-income countries, requires adaptive infrastructure, inclusive governance, and strategic investment in digital literacy and access. Reimbursement reforms must prioritize value-based care to incentivize long-term preventive strategies, while data governance must safeguard privacy and promote public trust. This chapter advances the book's central argument that digital innovation is transforming prevention from reactive care to proactive, data-driven health promotion. By embedding cost-effectiveness and ROI evidence into digital policy design, health systems can realign incentives toward prevention, ensuring that innovation serves both fiscal prudence and population wellbeing. The analysis presented throughout this chapter highlights that digital health's economic promise lies not in the technology itself, but in how it integrates with human behavior, institutional frameworks, and funding systems. Programs that align technological capacity with user engagement and governance reform consistently achieve superior cost-effectiveness and ROI.

Therefore, successful digital prevention requires analytical attention not only to fiscal metrics but also to the systemic and behavioral contexts that shape their real-world value. The success of digital prevention hinges not only on technological innovation but also on the collective foresight of policymakers, practitioners, and communities to align incentives, bridge disparities, and champion equitable and sustainable health systems. A coordinated global commitment to digital prevention is not only a health imperative, but also an economic and ethical necessity.

Conflict of Interest Statement

The authors declare that there are no known financial, personal, or professional conflicts of interest that could have appeared to influence the content or findings of this chapter.

AI Use Statement

The authors wrote and reviewed this chapter. Artificial intelligence (AI) tools, including Grammarly, Quillbot, and ChatGPT (OpenAI), were utilized solely to support language editing, formatting, and refining sentence clarity. All conceptual ideas, analyses, and contributions remain the original work of the authors. The authors have verified the accuracy and appropriateness of all content.

REFERENCES

Abbasi, N. (2024). Artificial Intelligence in Remote Monitoring and Telemedicine. *Journal of Artificial Intelligence General Science (JAIGS) ISSN:3006-4023*. https://doi.org/DOI: 10.60087/jaigs.v1i1.202

Abbasi, N., & Smith, D. A. (2024). Cybersecurity in Healthcare: Securing Patient Health Information (PHI), HIPPA compliance framework and the responsibilities of healthcare providers. *Journal of Knowledge Learning and Science Technology ISSN: 2959-6386 (Online), 3*(3), 278–287.

Abdulwahab, L. O., & Azam, H. (2026). Platform Work in Europe's Green and Care Economies: Regulatory Pathways for Sustainability, Social Protection, and Fair Work. In *Regulating the Gig Economy in the European Union: Challenges, Innovations, and Global Impacts* (pp. 99–124). IGI Global Scientific Publishing. https://www.igi-global.com/chapter/platform-work-in-europes-green-and-care-economies/395612

Alsetohy, W. M., El-Fass, K. A., El Hadidi, S., Zaitoun, M. F., Badary, O., Ali, K. A., Ezz-Elden, A., Ibrahim, M. R., Makhlouf, B. S., & Hamdy, A. (2025). Economic impact and clinical benefits of clinical pharmacy interventions: A six-year multi-center study using an innovative medication management tool. *PLoS One, 20*(1), e0311707. PMID: 39823444

Altibi, A. M. A., Al'Aref, S., & Khosravi, P. (2021). *Technological advances within digital medicine*. 1–26. https://doi.org/DOI: 10.1016/B978-0-12-820273-9.00001-4

Anumudu, S. J., & Erickson, K. F. (2020). Physician reimbursement for outpatient dialysis care: Past, present, and future. *Seminars in Dialysis, 33*(1), 68–74. DOI: 10.1111/sdi.12853 PMID: 31944418

Bartelheimer, C., Heinz, D., Hönigsberg, S., Siemon, D., Li, M., Strohmann, T., Poeppelbuss, J., & Peters, C. (2025). Conceptualizing hybrid intelligent service ecosystems. *Electronic Markets, 35*. Advance online publication. DOI: 10.1007/s12525-025-00798-4

Bayard, S., Fasano, G., Tamimi, R. M., & Oh, P. S. (2022). Leveraging Electronic Health Records to Address Breast Cancer Disparities. *Current Breast Cancer Reports, 14*(4), 199–204. DOI: 10.1007/s12609-022-00457-z PMID: 36091940

Bergin, A. D., Vallejos, E. P., Davies, E. B., Daley, D., Ford, T., Harold, G., Harold, G., Hetrick, S., Kidner, M., Long, Y., Merry, S., Morriss, R., Sayal, K., Sonuga-Barke, E., Robinson, J. L., Torous, J., & Hollis, C. (2020). Preventive digital mental health interventions for children and young people: A review of the design and reporting of research. *NPJ Digital Medicine, 3*. Advance online publication. DOI: 10.1038/s41746-020-00339-7 PMID: 33083568

Bertram, M., Chisholm, D., Watts, R. D., Waqanivalu, T., Prasad, V., & Varghese, C. (2021). Cost-Effectiveness of Population Level and Individual Level Interventions to Combat Non-communicable Disease in Eastern Sub-Saharan Africa and South East Asia: A WHO-CHOICE Analysis. *International Journal of Health Policy and Management, 10*, 724–733. DOI: 10.34172/ijhpm.2021.37 PMID: 34273918

Bhatt, N., & Bisht, B. G, D. C., Mittal, A., & Garg, N. (2024). Tech-Driven Wellness: Navigating the Confluence of Technology and Digital Health. *2024 2nd International Conference on Artificial Intelligence and Machine Learning Applications Theme: Healthcare and Internet of Things (AIMLA)*, 1–6. https://doi.org/DOI: 10.1109/AIMLA59606.2024.10531325

Bhatt, P., Liu, J., Gong, Y., Wang, J., & Guo, Y. (2021). Emerging Artificial Intelligence–Empowered mHealth: Scoping Review. *JMIR mHealth and uHealth, 10*. Advance online publication. DOI: 10.2196/35053 PMID: 35679107

Bhoyar, A., Vagha, S., Mishra, V., Agrawal, M. S., & Kambala, S. R. (2024). Addressing the Digital Divide in Health Education: A Systematic Review. *Cureus, 16*(9). https://www.cureus.com/articles/257266-addressing-the-digital-divide-in-health-education-a-systematic-review.pdf PMID: 39449933

Brent, R. (2023). Cost-Benefit Analysis versus Cost-Effectiveness Analysis from a Societal Perspective in Healthcare. *International Journal of Environmental Research and Public Health, 20*. Advance online publication. DOI: 10.3390/ijerph20054637 PMID: 36901658

Briggs, A., Persaud, J. G., Deverell, M., Bunzli, S., Tampin, B., Sumi, Y., Amundsen, O., Houlding, E., Cardone, A., Hugosdottir, T., Rogers, S., Pozsgai, M., & Slater, H. (2019). Integrated prevention and management of non-communicable diseases, including musculoskeletal health: A systematic policy analysis among OECD countries. *BMJ Global Health, 4*. Advance online publication. DOI: 10.1136/bmjgh-2019-001806 PMID: 31565419

Buss, V., Leesong, S., Barr, M., Varnfield, M., & Harris, M. (2020). Primary Prevention of Cardiovascular Disease and Type 2 Diabetes Mellitus Using Mobile Health Technology: Systematic Review of the Literature. *Journal of Medical Internet Research, 22*. Advance online publication. DOI: 10.2196/21159 PMID: 33118936

Cary, M. P., De Gagne, J. C., Kauschinger, E. D., & Carter, B. M. (2024). Advancing Health Equity Through Artificial Intelligence: An Educational Framework for Preparing Nurses in Clinical Practice and Research. *Creative Nursing, 30*(2), 154–164. DOI: 10.1177/10784535241249193 PMID: 38689433

City. (2023). *THE COST-EFFECTIVENESS AND EQUITY OF THE NHS HEALTH CHECKS CARDIOVASCULAR DISEASE PREVENTION PROGRAMME: A MICROSIMULATION USING REAL-WORLD DATA FROM A DEPRIVED NORTHERN CITY*. https://consensus.app/papers/the-costeffectiveness-and-equity-of-the-nhs-health-checks-city/41ef207f93b5598bbc073bd3278cee0a/

Cohen, D. R., & Patel, N. (2009). The Potential to Forgo Social Welfare Gains through Overrelianceon Cost Effectiveness/Cost Utility Analyses in the Evidence Base for Public Health. *Journal of Environmental and Public Health, 2009*. Advance online publication. DOI: 10.1155/2009/107927 PMID: 20049165

Damera, V. K., Cheripelli, R., Putta, N., Sirisha, G., & Kalavala, D. (2025). Enhancing remote patient monitoring with AI-driven IoMT and cloud computing technologies. *Scientific Reports, 15*. Advance online publication. DOI: 10.1038/s41598-025-09727-z PMID: 40617852

De La Torre-Diéz, I., López-Coronado, M., Vaca, C., Aguado, J. S., & De Castro, C. (2015). Cost-utility and cost-effectiveness studies of telemedicine, electronic, and mobile health systems in the literature: A systematic review. *Telemedicine Journal and e-Health, 21*(2), 81–85. DOI: 10.1089/tmj.2014.0053 PMID: 25474190

de Oliveira, C., Cho, E., Kavelaars, R., Jamieson, M., Bao, B., & Rehm, J. (2020). Economic analyses of mental health and substance use interventions in the workplace: A systematic literature review and narrative synthesis. *The Lancet. Psychiatry, 7*(10), 893–910. DOI: 10.1016/S2215-0366(20)30145-0 PMID: 32949521

Duggal, M., El Ayadi, A., Duggal, B., Reynolds, N., & Bascaran, C. (2023). Challenges in implementing digital health in public health settings in low and middle income countries. In *Frontiers in public health* (Vol. 10, p. 1090303). Frontiers Media SA. https://www.frontiersin.org/articles/10.3389/fpubh.2022.1090303/full

Dyakova, M., Stielke, A., Ashton-Brown, K., Daniels, P., Kadel, R., & Cotter-Roberts, A. (2020). Evidencing value of public health programmes to enable sustainable investment for health & wellbeing. *European Journal of Public Health, 30*. Advance online publication. DOI: 10.1093/eurpub/ckaa165.103

Ekwaru, J. P., Ohinmaa, A., Dabravolskaj, J., Maximova, K., & Veugelers, P. J. (2021). Cost-effectiveness and return on investment of school based health promotion programmes for chronic disease prevention. *European Journal of Public Health, 31*(6), 1183–1189. PMID: 34355754

El Ouazzani, Z., & El Bakkali, H. (2020). A classification of non-cryptographic anonymization techniques ensuring privacy in big data. *International Journal of Communication Networks and Information Security, 12*(1), 142–152.

Fiordelli, M. (2024). Transitioning Perspectives in Digital Health Through Phenomenology Integration. *Journal of Medical Internet Research, 26*. Advance online publication. DOI: 10.2196/62691 PMID: 39442170

Fleming, K. A., Horton, S., Wilson, M. L., Atun, R., DeStigter, K., Flanigan, J., Sayed, S., Adam, P., Aguilar, B., & Andronikou, S. (2021). The Lancet Commission on diagnostics: Transforming access to diagnostics. *Lancet, 398*(10315), 1997–2050. PMID: 34626542

Fortuna, K. L., Walker, R., Fisher, D., Mois, G., Allan, S., & Deegan, P. (2019). Enhancing Standards and Principles in Digital Mental Health With Recovery-Focused Guidelines for Mobile, Online, and Remote Monitoring Technologies. *Psychiatric Services (Washington, D.C.)*. Advance online publication. DOI: 10.1176/appi.ps.201900166 PMID: 31615369

Gabrielli, S., Ibarra, O. M., & Forti, S. (2023). A Holistic Digital Health Framework to Support Health Prevention Strategies in the First 1000 Days. *JMIR Pediatrics and Parenting, 8*. Advance online publication. DOI: 10.2196/55235 PMID: 39819823

Gentili, A., Failla, G., Melnyk, A., Puleo, V., Tanna, G. L. D., Ricciardi, W., & Cascini, F. (2022). The cost-effectiveness of digital health interventions: A systematic review of the literature. *Frontiers in Public Health, 10*, 787135. PMID: 36033812

Girmay, M. (2024). Digital Health Divide: Opportunities for Reducing Health Disparities and Promoting Equitable Care for Maternal and Child Health Populations. *International Journal of Maternal and Child Health and AIDS, 13*, e026. PMID: 39776789

Guerrero-López, A., Bravo Antón, L., Blázquez-Sánchez, M., Schmidt-Santiago, L., Sevilla-Salcedo, C., Rodríguez-Temporal, D., Rodríguez-Sánchez, B., & Gómez-Verdejo, V. (2024). Overcoming variability challenges for Clostridioides difficile via data augmentation techniques. bioRxiv, 2024–10.

Gupta, D., Bhatt, S., Gupta, M., & Tosun, A. (2020). Future Smart Connected Communities to Fight COVID-19 Outbreak. *Internet of Things : Engineering Cyber Physical Human Systems, 13*, 100342–100342. DOI: 10.1016/j.iot.2020.100342 PMID: 38620326

Han, Y. T., Lyu, J., Yu, C., & Li, L. (2022). [Development and applications of digital public health]. *Zhonghua Liu Xing Bing Xue Za Zhi = Zhonghua Liuxingbingxue Zazhi, 43 6*, 791–797. https://doi.org/ DOI: 10.3760/cma.j.cn112338-20220314-00184

Hasan, B. S., Rasheed, M. A., Wahid, A., Kumar, R. K., & Zuhlke, L. (2021). Generating evidence from contextual clinical research in low-to middle income countries: A roadmap based on theory of change. *Frontiers in Pediatrics, 9*, 764239. PMID: 34956976

Higgins, A., & Harris, A. (2012). Health economic methods: Cost-minimization, cost-effectiveness, cost-utility, and cost-benefit evaluations. *Critical Care Clinics, 28*(1), 11–24. DOI: 10.1016/j.ccc.2011.10.002 PMID: 22123096

Hong, Y. A., Zhou, Z., Fang, Y., & Shi, L. (2017). The digital divide and health disparities in China: Evidence from a national survey and policy implications. *Journal of Medical Internet Research, 19*(9), e317. PMID: 28893724

Huang, G., Chen, X., & Liao, C. (2025). AI-Driven Wearable Bioelectronics in Digital Healthcare. *Biosensors (Basel), 15*. Advance online publication. DOI: 10.3390/bios15070410 PMID: 40710060

Huntsman, J. L., & Bulaj, G. (2023). Health education via "empowerment" digital marketing of consumer products and services: Promoting therapeutic benefits of self-care for depression and chronic pain. *Frontiers in Public Health, 10*. Advance online publication. DOI: 10.3389/fpubh.2022.949518 PMID: 36703812

Islam, M., Valiani, A. A., Datta, R., Chowdhury, M., & Turin, T. C. (2024). Ethical and Equitable Digital Health Research: Ensuring Self-Determination in Data Governance for Racialized Communities. *Cambridge Quarterly of Healthcare Ethics*, •••, 1–11. PMID: 38567458

Islam, S., & Maddison, R. (2020). Digital health approaches for cardiovascular diseases prevention and management: Lessons from preliminary studies. *mHealth, 7*. Advance online publication. DOI: 10.21037/MHEALTH-2020-DHCD-06 PMID: 34345618

Jackson-Morris, A., Meyer, C. L., Morgan, A., Stelmach, R., Jamison, L., & Currie, C. (2024). An investment case analysis for the prevention and treatment of adolescent mental disorders and suicide in England. *European Journal of Public Health, 34*(1), 107–113. PMID: 37997372

Kadel, R., Stielke, A., Ashton, K., Masters, R. B., & Dyakova, M. (2022). Social Return on Investment (SROI) of mental health related interventions—A scoping review. *Frontiers in Public Health, 10.* Advance online publication. DOI: 10.3389/fpubh.2022.965148 PMID: 36568774

Khan, A., Galea, S., & Mendez, I. (2025). Five steps for the deployment of artificial intelligence-driven healthcare delivery for remote and indigenous populations in Canada. *Digital Health, 11.* Advance online publication. DOI: 10.1177/20552076251334422 PMID: 40290270

Komiyama, C., Kuwabara, M., Harima, A., Kanie, T., Yamaguchi, T., & Kodama, T. (2025). Digital Health Interventions for Atherosclerotic Cardiovascular Disease: The Current Impact and Future Directions for Prevention and Management. *Journal of Atherosclerosis and Thrombosis.* Advance online publication. DOI: 10.5551/jat.rv22032 PMID: 39894471

Kostkova, P. (2015). Grand Challenges in Digital Health. *Frontiers in Public Health, 3.* Advance online publication. DOI: 10.3389/fpubh.2015.00134 PMID: 26000272

Kowatsch, T., & Fleisch, E. (2021). *Digital Health Interventions.* Connected Business., DOI: 10.1007/978-3-030-76897-3_4

Kulikowski, C. A. (2022). Ethics in the History of Medical Informatics for Decision-Making: Early Challenges to Digital Health Goals. *Yearbook of Medical Informatics, 31*(01), 317–322. DOI: 10.1055/s-0042-1742491 PMID: 35654428

Kuzior, A., Marszałek-Kotzur, I., Kurovska, Y., & Chvankin, Y. (2024). *The Role of Digital Economy in Transformation of Public Health: Modeling and Analysis.* Health Economics and Management Review., DOI: 10.61093/hem.2024.4-06

Kyaw, T. L., Ng, N., Theocharaki, M., Wennberg, P., & Sahlén, K.-G. (2022). Cost-effectiveness of Digital Tools for Behavior Change Interventions Among People With Chronic Diseases: Systematic Review. *Interactive Journal of Medical Research, 12.* Advance online publication. DOI: 10.2196/42396 PMID: 36795470

Lampreia, F., Madeira, C., & Dores, H. (2024). Digital health technologies and artificial intelligence in cardiovascular clinical trials: A landscape of the European space. *Digital Health, 10.* Advance online publication. DOI: 10.1177/20552076241277703 PMID: 39291150

Laursen, H., Jørgensen, E. P., Vestergaard, P., & Ehlers, L. (2023). A Systematic Review of Cost-Effectiveness Studies of Newer Non-Insulin Antidiabetic Drugs: Trends in Decision-Analytical Models for Modelling of Type 2 Diabetes Mellitus. *PharmacoEconomics, 41,* 1469–1514. DOI: 10.1007/s40273-023-01268-5 PMID: 37410277

Lawal, O. A., & Bubari Umar, H. (2025). Trade, Growth, and Healthcare in ECOWAS: Unlocking Opportunities for Equitable Access. *Trade, Growth, and Healthcare in ECOWAS: Unlocking Opportunities for Equitable Access (January 10, 2025).* https://papers.ssrn.com/sol3/papers.cfm?abstract_id=5206321

Lehnert, T., Sonntag, D., Konnopka, A., Riedel-Heller, S., & König, H. (2012). The long-term cost-effectiveness of obesity prevention interventions: Systematic literature review. *Obesity Reviews, 13.* Advance online publication. DOI: 10.1111/j.1467-789X.2011.00980.x PMID: 22251231

Leistner, T., & Kowatsch, T. (2023). *Digital Therapeutics for Healthy Longevity: A Roadmap*. 616–622. https://doi.org/DOI: 10.5220/0011778500003414

Luke, M. J., Craig, S., Pak-Gorstein, S., Arellano, M., Zhang, J., Wright, S. M., Chuo, J., & Scribano, P. V. (2024). Narrowing the Digital Divide: Framework for Creating Telehealth Equity Dashboards. *Interactive Journal of Medical Research*, *13*(1), e57435. PMID: 39231423

Maiga, B., Bagayoko, C., Ahmed, M. A., Anne, A., Gagnon, M., Traoré, S. A., Landrier, J., & Geissbuhler, A. (2021). Effectiveness of digital health interventions for diabetes: Systematic review of systematic reviews. *African Journal of Diabetes Medicine*. https://doi.org/DOI: 10.21203/rs.3.rs-722330/v1

Marseille, E., Jiwani, A., Raut, A., Verguet, S., Walson, J., & Kahn, J. (2014). Scaling up integrated prevention campaigns for global health: Costs and cost-effectiveness in 70 countries. *BMJ Open*, *4*. Advance online publication. DOI: 10.1136/bmjopen-2013-003987 PMID: 24969782

Mason, R., Anwar, E., Collins, B., Cookson, R., Capewell, S., & Lloyd-Williams, F. (2016). P97 Quantifying the Return on Investment of Public Health Interventions: A systematic review. *Journal of Epidemiology and Community Health*, *70*, 96–96. DOI: 10.1136/jech-2016-208064.195

Mburu, S. N., Kamau, O., & Grace, K. (2018). *Framework for the Development and Implementation of Digital Health Policies to Accelerate the Achievement of Sustainable Development Goals: The Case of Kenya's eHealth Policy (2016-2030)*. https://consensus.app/papers/framework-for-development-and-implementation-of-digital-mburu-kamau/2bdcc225afd55dcaa313beb5a9ebab65/

McNamee, P., Murray, E., Kelly, M., Bojke, L., Chilcott, J., Fischer, A., West, R., & Yardley, L. (2016). Designing and Undertaking a Health Economics Study of Digital Health Interventions. *American Journal of Preventive Medicine*, *51*(5), 852–860. DOI: 10.1016/j.amepre.2016.05.007 PMID: 27745685

Mekniran, W., Kramer, J.-N., & Kowatsch, T. (2024). *Reimagining Preventive Care and Digital Health: A Paradigm Shift in a Health Insurance's Role*. 852–858. https://doi.org/DOI: 10.5220/0012400300003657

Merkur, S., Sassi, F., & McDaid, D. (2013). Promoting health, preventing disease: Is there an economic case? *LSE Research Online Documents on Economics*. https://consensus.app/papers/promoting-health-preventing-disease-is-there-an-economic-merkur-sassi/5359d7352ac75195bc0d8b6822c0f5f3/

Miller, T., & Hendrie, D. (2012). Economic Evaluation of Public Health Laws and Their Enforcement. *Public Health Law & Policy eJournal*. https://consensus.app/papers/economic-evaluation-of-public-health-laws-and-their-miller-hendrie/91510e1dd7c95b04a6e21156a7ba990e/

Mitchell, A. P., Rotter, J. S., Patel, E., Richardson, D., Wheeler, S. B., Basch, E., & Goldstein, D. A. (2019). Association between reimbursement incentives and physician practice in oncology: A systematic review. *JAMA Oncology*, *5*(6), 893–899. PMID: 30605222

Monzani, D., & Pizzoli, S. (2019). The Prevention of Chronic Diseases Through eHealth: A Practical Overview. *P5 eHealth: An Agenda for the Health Technologies of the Future*. https://doi.org/DOI: 10.1007/978-3-030-27994-3_3

Morris, T., Aspinal, F., Ledger, J., Li, K., & Gomes, M. (2023). The Impact of Digital Health Interventions for the Management of Type 2 Diabetes on Health and Social Care Utilisation and Costs: A Systematic Review. *PharmacoEconomics Open*, *7*(2), 163–173. DOI: 10.1007/s41669-022-00377-9 PMID: 36495462

Musa, S., Abubakari, M. S., & Abdulwahab, L. O. (2025). Evaluating the Potential of Adapting Artificial Intelligence (AI) in Small and Medium Enterprises for Competitive Advantage. In *Multi-Industry Digitalization and Technological Governance in the AI Era* (pp. 233–266). IGI Global Scientific Publishing. https://www.igi-global.com/chapter/evaluating-the-potential-of-adapting-artificial-intelligence-ai-in-small-and-medium-enterprises-for-competitive-advantage/372493

Olamilekan, L. A., & Umar, H. B. (2025). *Economic Inequality and Healthcare Access in ECOWAS: The Impact of Government Health Spending*. https://www.preprints.org/manuscript/202504.0605

Omotayo, O., Maduka, C. P., Muonde, M., Olorunsogo, T. O., & Ogugua, J. O. (2024). THE RISE OF NON-COMMUNICABLE DISEASES: A GLOBAL HEALTH REVIEW OF CHALLENGES AND PREVENTION STRATEGIES. *International Medical Science Research Journal*. https://doi.org/DOI: 10.51594/imsrj.v4i1.738

Ospina-Fadul, M. J., Kremer, P., Stevens, S. E., Haruna, F., Okoh-Owusu, M., Sarpong, G., Osei-Kwakye, K., Joshua, B., & Sakyi, O. (2024). Cost-Effectiveness of Aerial Logistics for Immunization: A Model-Based Evaluation of Centralized Storage and Drone Delivery of Vaccines in Ghana Using Empirical Data. *Value in Health Regional Issues*, *46*. Advance online publication. DOI: 10.2139/ssrn.4775458 PMID: 39709942

Owusu, M., Adu, J., Gyamfi, S., Martin-Yeboah, E., & Dortey, B. A. (2024). Tackling the non-communicable disease epidemic: A framework for policy action in low- and middle-income countries. *The Pan African Medical Journal*, *47*. Advance online publication. DOI: 10.11604/pamj.2024.47.82.41089 PMID: 38737222

Paccoud, I., Leist, A. K., Schwaninger, I., Van Kessel, R., & Klucken, J. (2024). Socio-ethical challenges and opportunities for advancing diversity, equity, and inclusion in digital medicine. *Digital Health*, *10*, 20552076241277705. DOI: 10.1177/20552076241277705 PMID: 39372817

Pikkarainen, M., Iivari, M., Gomes, J. F., Kaartinen, J., Xu, Y., He, H., & Gazerani, P. (2024). Identification of required capabilities of digital health ecosystems when preventing and managing non-communicable diseases. *Digital Health*, *10*. Advance online publication. DOI: 10.1177/20552076241271807 PMID: 39281041

Powers, B. M., & Bucher, A. (2022). An Economic Impact Model for Estimating the Value to Health Systems of a Digital Intervention for Diabetes Primary Care: Development and Usefulness Study. *JMIR Formative Research*, *6*. Advance online publication. DOI: 10.2196/37745 PMID: 36155985

Prodan, A., Deimel, L., Ahlqvist, J., Birov, S., Thiel, R., Toivanen, M., Kolitsi, Z., & Kalra, D. (2022). Success factors for scaling up the adoption of digital therapeutics towards the realization of P5 medicine. *Frontiers in Medicine*, *9*, 854665. PMID: 35492346

Ratanawong, J. P., Naslund, J. A., Mikal, J. P., & Grande, S. W. (2022). Achieving the potential of mHealth in medicine requires challenging the ethos of care delivery. *Primary Health Care Research and Development, 23*. Advance online publication. DOI: 10.1017/S1463423622000068 PMID: 35314016

Rukundo, S. K. (2024). *The Role of Digital Health in Preventive Medicine*. RESEARCH INVENTION JOURNAL OF PUBLIC HEALTH AND PHARMACY., DOI: 10.59298/rijpp/2024/323840

Saeed, S. A., & Masters, R. M. (2021). Disparities in Health Care and the Digital Divide. *Current Psychiatry Reports, 23*(9), 61. DOI: 10.1007/s11920-021-01274-4 PMID: 34297202

Sánchez-Castillo, V., Cano, C. A. G., & González-Argote, J. (2023). Telemedicine and mHealth Applications for Health Monitoring in Rural Communities in Colombia: A Systematic Review. *EAI Endorsed Transactions on Pervasive Health and Technology, 9*. Advance online publication. DOI: 10.4108/eetpht.9.3400

Santos, A. R., von Hafe, F., Sampaio, F., Londral, A. R., & Perelman, J. (2025). Mapping Methodologies for Economic Evaluation of Digital Health Technologies: A Scoping Review. *Value in Health*. Advance online publication. DOI: 10.1016/j.jval.2025.09.012 PMID: 41015334

Sareban, M., Treff, G., Smeddinck, J. D., Hussein, R., & Niebauer, J. (2025). Opportunities and barriers for reimbursement of digital therapeutics in Austria: Findings From expert interviews. *Digital Health, 11*, 20552076241299062. DOI: 10.1177/20552076241299062 PMID: 39777062

Seward, N., Hanlon, C., Hinrichs-Kraples, S., Lund, C., Murdoch, J., Salisbury, T. T., Verhey, R., Shidhaye, R., Thornicroft, G., & Araya, R. (2021). A guide to systems-level, participatory, theory-informed implementation research in global health. *BMJ Global Health, 6*(12), e005365. PMID: 34969685

Sharma, S. K., Al-Wanain, M. I., Alowaidi, M. A., & Alsaghier, H. (2022). Mobile healthcare (m-Health) based on artificial intelligence in healthcare 4.0. *Expert Systems: International Journal of Knowledge Engineering and Neural Networks, 41*. Advance online publication. DOI: 10.1111/exsy.13025

Shaw, R. J. (2023). Access to Technology and Digital Literacy as Determinants of Health and Health Care. *Creative Nursing, 29*(3), 258–263. DOI: 10.1177/10784535231211682 PMID: 37909069

Sinha, C., & Schryer-Roy, A.-M. (2018). Digital health, gender and health equity: Invisible imperatives. *Journal of Public Health (United Kingdom), 40*, II1–II5. DOI: 10.1093/pubmed/fdy171 PMID: 30329082

Stanić, T., Avşar, T. S., & Gomes, M. (2023). Economic Evaluations of Digital Health Interventions for Children and Adolescents: Systematic Review. *Journal of Medical Internet Research, 25*. Advance online publication. DOI: 10.2196/45958 PMID: 37921844

Stein, M., & Galea, S. (2020)... *Can We Promote Public Health and Generate Return on Our Investment, 99–102*. Advance online publication. DOI: 10.1093/oso/9780197510384.003.0029

Stratton, E., Jones, N., Peters, S. E., Torous, J., & Glozier, N. (2021). Digital mHealth Interventions for Employees. *Journal of Occupational and Environmental Medicine, 63*, 512–525. DOI: 10.1097/JOM.0000000000002267 PMID: 34050095

Supervia, M., & Lopez-Jimenez, F. (2018). mHealth and cardiovascular diseases self-management: There is still a long way ahead of us. *European Journal of Preventive Cardiology, 25*, 974–975. DOI: 10.1177/2047487318766644 PMID: 29569940

Svensson, M., & Hultkrantz, L. (2017). A Comparison of Cost-Benefit and Cost-Effectiveness Analysis in Practice. *Divergent Policy Practices in Sweden., 5*, 41–53. DOI: 10.5617/NJHE.1592

Thomas, S. A., Browning, C. J., Charchar, F. J., Klein, B., Ory, M. G., Bowden-Jones, H., & Chamberlain, S. R. (2023). Transforming global approaches to chronic disease prevention and management across the lifespan: Integrating genomics, behavior change, and digital health solutions. *Frontiers in Public Health, 11*. Advance online publication. DOI: 10.3389/fpubh.2023.1248254 PMID: 37905238

Thonon, F., Godon-Rensonnet, A.-S., Perozziello, A., Garsi, J., Dab, W., & Emsalem, P. (2023). Return on investment of workplace-based prevention interventions: A systematic review. *European Journal of Public Health, 33*, 612–618. DOI: 10.1093/eurpub/ckad092 PMID: 37290417

Tian, H.-S., Zhang, K., Zhang, J., Shi, J., Qiu, H., Hou, N., Han, F., Kan, C., & Sun, X. (2025). Revolutionizing public health through digital health technology. *Psychology Health and Medicine*, •••, 1–16. DOI: 10.1080/13548506.2025.2458254 PMID: 39864819

Torgerson, D. (2009). Cost-effectiveness analysis and health policy. *Nestle Nutrition Workshop Series. Clinical & Performance Programme, 12*, 95–104. DOI: 10.1159/000235671 PMID: 19858689

Torrance, G. (1997). Preferences for health outcomes and cost-utility analysis. *The American Journal of Managed Care, 3*(Suppl), 8–20. PMID: 10180342

van Gils, P., Tariq, L., Verschuuren, M., & van den Berg, M. (2011). Cost-effectiveness research on preventive interventions: A survey of the publications in 2008. *European Journal of Public Health, 21*(2), 260–264. DOI: 10.1093/eurpub/ckq069 PMID: 20534690

Viet, N. L., Nhi, T. T. Y., Nhi, V. N. Y., Binh, N. T., & Thuy, N. T. T. (2024). Forecasting the cost of diabetes: A systematic review. *T p Chí Khoa H c Trư ng Đ i H c Qu c T H ng Bàng*. https://doi.org/DOI: 10.59294/hiujs.vol.7.2024.689

Voultsos, P. (2023). Ethical considerations surrounding health-related big data research. *Cuadernos de Bioetica: Revista Oficial de La Asociacion Espanola de Bioetica y Etica Medica, 34*(111), 189–218. PMID: 37804492

Wang, Y., Fekadu, G., & You, J. (2023). Cost-Effectiveness Analyses of Digital Health Technology for Improving the Uptake of Vaccination Programs: Systematic Review. *Journal of Medical Internet Research, 25*. Advance online publication. DOI: 10.2196/45493 PMID: 37184916

Watson, P., Preston, L., Squires, H., Chilcott, J., & Brennan, A. (2014). Modelling the Economics of Type 2 Diabetes Mellitus Prevention: A Literature Review of Methods. *Applied Health Economics and Health Policy, 12*, 239–253. DOI: 10.1007/s40258-014-0091-z PMID: 24595522

Weinhold, I., Schindler, C., Kossack, N., Berndt, B., & Häckl, D. (2019). Economic impact of disease prevention in a morbidity-based financing system: Does prevention pay off for a statutory health insurance fund in Germany? *The European Journal of Health Economics*, •••, 1–13. DOI: 10.1007/s10198-019-01086-7 PMID: 31317353

Willis, V., Craig, K. J. T., Yabbarpour, Y., Scheufele, E. L., Arriaga, Y., Ajinkya, M., Rhee, K. B., & Bazemore, A. (2021). Digital Health Interventions to Enhance Prevention in Primary Care: A Scoping Review *(Preprint)*. https://doi.org/DOI: 10.2196/preprints.33518

Xuefei, G., Meili, Z., Xiaoqing, L., Tingting, L., Xiao, H., Chaoqun, W., Nan, X., Guochun, X., Kejun, L., & Runlin, G. (2018). *Strategic Health Economics Study Applied to Policymaking on the Prevention and Control of Chronic Non-Communicable Diseases*. https://consensus.app/papers/strategic-health-economics-study-applied-to-policymaking-xuefei-meili/c0a6b89e41dd54fcb75d2eb0d06798ca/

Yamey, G. (2012). What are the barriers to scaling up health interventions in low and middle income countries? A qualitative study of academic leaders in implementation science. *Globalization and Health*, *8*(1), 11. DOI: 10.1186/1744-8603-8-11 PMID: 22643120

Zhang, J., Gallifant, J., Pierce, R. L., Fordham, A., Teo, J., Celi, L., & Ashrafian, H. (2023). Quantifying digital health inequality across a national healthcare system. *BMJ Health & Care Informatics*, *30*. Advance online publication. DOI: 10.1136/bmjhci-2023-100809 PMID: 38007224

Zhu, S., Saravanan, V., & Muthu, B. (2020). Achieving data security and privacy across healthcare applications using cyber security mechanisms. *The Electronic Library*, *38*(5/6), 979–995.

Zwaagstra Salvado, E., van Elten, H. J., & van Raaij, E. M. (2021a). The linkages between reimbursement and prevention: A mixed-methods approach. *Frontiers in Public Health*, *9*, 750122. PMID: 34778183

Zwaagstra Salvado, E., van Elten, H. J., & van Raaij, E. M. (2021b). The linkages between reimbursement and prevention: A mixed-methods approach. *Frontiers in Public Health*, *9*, 750122. PMID: 34778183

KEY TERMS AND DEFINITIONS

Cost-Effectiveness Analysis (CEA): A method comparing the relative costs and outcomes (effects) of two or more interventions, usually expressed as cost per QALY or DALY averted.

Cost-Utility Analysis (CUA): An evaluation framework using QALYs to measure both quality and quantity of life gained through an intervention.

Digital Divide: The disparity in access to and use of digital technologies across socioeconomic or geographic groups.

Digital Health: The use of information and communication technologies (ICT), such as mobile health (mHealth), telemedicine, wearables, and AI-enabled analytics, to improve health outcomes and system efficiency (WHO, 2021).

Disease Prevention: A set of actions aimed at reducing the occurrence and progression of disease by addressing risk factors and promoting healthy behaviors.

Precision Prevention: The use of personalized data (including genomics, behavior, and environment) to tailor preventive interventions for specific populations.

Return on Investment (ROI): The ratio of net financial gain or benefit to the cost of an intervention is often used by policymakers and managers to assess the fiscal sustainability of an intervention.

Social Return on Investment (SROI): An extension of ROI that incorporates social, health, and equity benefits into the valuation framework.

Chapter 3
Code Meets Care:
The Digital Shift in Health Promotion

Joana Nogueira
https://orcid.org/0009-0001-7139-4460
Future Healthcare Virtual Clinic, Portugal

Teresa Santos
https://orcid.org/0000-0001-9947-6022
Universidade Europeia, Lisbon, Portugal

Ana Pina
https://orcid.org/0000-0001-8135-7420
Future Healthcare Virtual Clinic, Portugal

Sandra S. Martins
https://orcid.org/0000-0001-7217-6273
Universidade Europeia, Lisbon, Portugal

ABSTRACT

This chapter examines the transformative evolution of digital health from fragmented technological applications into a comprehensive, multidisciplinary ecosystem that fundamentally redefines healthcare delivery and patient engagement. Driven by rapid advancements in artificial intelligence, wearable devices, the Internet of Things, digital therapeutics, multi-omics integration, and extended reality, digital health shifts care paradigms from reactive, clinician-centered models to proactive, precise, predictive, preventive, and participatory approaches. The COVID-19 pandemic accelerated widespread adoption of digital solutions, demonstrating their capacity for agile crisis response while exposing persistent challenges such as the digital divide, interoperability limitations, and inequities in access. The chapter explores how digital health addresses major systemic pressures—including the rising burden of non-communicable diseases, healthcare workforce shortages, and escalating costs—through scalable, data-driven innovations that support value-based care, real-time monitoring, personalized interventions, lifestyle modification, and improved outcomes that matter to patients. While highlighting the potential to empower individuals as active participants in their health management within everyday contexts, the discussion critically addresses key barriers: ethical concerns, regulatory fragmentation, algorithmic bias, data privacy risks, and the need for inclusive, context-sensitive implementation strategies. Ultimately,

DOI: 10.4018/979-8-3373-3531-5.ch003

this chapter argues that realizing the full promise of digital health requires rigorous evidence generation, participatory design, equitable frameworks, and collaborative governance to ensure that technological progress translates into sustainable, resilient, and human-centered health ecosystems that promote well-being for all populations.

INTRODUCTION

Figure 1. Evolution of technology-enabled care models

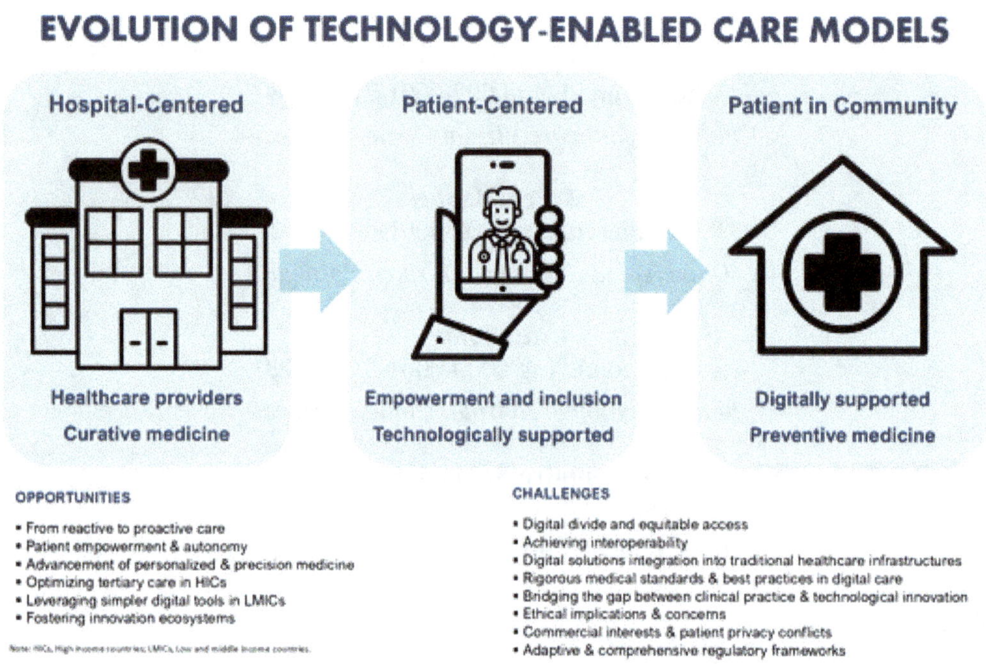

In an age where technology shapes nearly every aspect of our lives, digital health stands at the forefront of a profound transformation - one that promises to reshape healthcare. Far from being a mere extension of traditional clinical care into digital platforms, digital health redefines care, from reactive and episodic care to a vibrant and continuous journey of well-being, catalysed by technological innovation, global health challenges, and shifting societal expectations. It reflects a broader multidisciplinary and rapidly evolving domain that is transforming how health systems operate and how individuals engage with their own health, supporting a more responsive and person-centred care (European Commission, 2020; WHO, 2021). This transformation calls for the reimagination of healthcare journeys in order to promote long-term well-being, enhancing health outcomes and reconfiguring care delivery.

The COVID-19 pandemic served as a global inflection point, accelerating the adoption of digital health solutions and exposing both their potential and limitations. It highlighted the strategic importance of digital infrastructures, the need for interoperability and the value of real-time data in supporting agile, evidence-based responses to health crises (Ganesan & Tong, 2024; OECD, 2023; Ogundiya et al., 2024). At the same time, it underscored persistent gaps in access, digital literacy and system readiness, issues that still remain central to the digital health agenda. Therefore, it becomes essential to critically examine how digital technologies are evolving from niche innovations into integral pillars of contemporary healthcare systems, redefining new paradigms of care and public health engagement.

This chapter, where *"Code meets Care"*, will explore the evolving role of digital technologies in promoting health across populations. The discussion encompasses a broad spectrum of tools and infrastructures, including mobile health applications, wearable devices, artificial intelligence (AI), the Internet of Things (IoT), digital therapeutics (DTx), extended reality (XR), multiomics integration and real-time smart environments, which altogether enable the implementation of precision health strategies. Through these advancements, digital health is transforming traditional care models' by shifting leadership from clinician-centred structures to technology-enabled, patient-empowered systems. In this new paradigm, individuals actively manage their health through autonomous decision-making supported by AI-driven tools, while engaging in everyday life within their communities and participating in collaborative care environments that promote lifestyle changes, early detection and self-care across the continuum of care.

Scalable, data-driven solutions to major health system challenges are being designed, supporting the management of non-communicable diseases, mitigating workforce shortages, enabling value-based healthcare and improving outcomes, including those that matter to patients, through real-time monitoring, interoperability and precision public health strategies. While digital health holds transformative potential, its implementation is shaped by critical challenges, including the digital divide, ethical and regulatory gaps and risks of inequity. Thus, it requires inclusive and context-sensitive strategies that turn innovation into sustainable and equitable opportunities for all.

The current chapter tackles not merely the advancement of digital tools, but the collective challenge of translating their promise into resilient, inclusive and context-aware health ecosystems that can adapt, learn and thrive in the face of evolving global health demands.

Innovation to Integration in Digital Health

Digital health is widespread adopted; however, its designation remains conceptually heterogeneous, with definitions varying across academic, industrial and institutional settings.

Beyond formal definitions, digital health can be interpreted as a broader cultural shift in healthcare, driven by technologies that generate objective digital data and reshape the clinician–patient relationship through shared decision-making and care democratization (Shaffer & Preziosi, 2019). Individuals or patients are seen as active participants, expecting healthcare to reflect the personalization and proactiveness of digital services. Over time, digital health evolves from fragmented technological applications into an integrated ecosystem, encompassing both legacy and emerging tools, and aiming to transform global health systems (Burrell et al., 2022; C, 2022; OECD, 2023; Ogundiya et al., 2024).

Table 1. Digital health definition across different institutions

Institutions	Digital Health Definitions
World Health Organization (WHO, 2021)	Digital health is the field of knowledge and practice associated with the development and use of digital technologies to improve health. This definition encompasses eHealth including digital consumers, with a wider range of smart and connected devices, along with other uses of digital technologies for health such as IoT, advanced computing, big data analytics, artificial intelligence including machine learning, and robotics.
Organisation for Economic Cooperation and Development (OECD, 2023)	Based on the WHO definition, digital health is defined as the field of knowledge and practice associated with the development and use of health data and digital technologies to improve health. Digital health expands the concept of eHealth to include digital consumers, with a wider range of smart devices, connected equipment and digital therapeutics. It also encompasses other uses of data and digital technologies for health, such as the Internet of things, artificial intelligence, big data and robotics, and predictive and prescriptive analytics. Analytics can be for health system improvement, public health preparedness or research and innovation.
European Commission (European Commission, 2020)	Digital health is a set of tools and services that use information and communication technologies to support and improve all stages of healthcare, from prevention and diagnosis to treatment, monitoring and management of health conditions. In the European Union, eHealth is recognised as a vital instrument in advancing healthcare efficiency, enhancing the quality of care, expanding equitable access to services, empowering citizens to take a proactive role in managing their health and supporting healthcare professionals in their daily work. This multidisciplinary field gathers healthcare professionals, researchers, policymakers and technologists, who collaborate to harness innovation for better health outcomes and more sustainable healthcare systems.
U.S. Food and Drug Administration (FDA, 2020)	The broad scope of digital health includes categories such as mobile health (mHealth), health information technology (IT), wearable devices, telehealth and telemedicine and personalized medicine (…). Digital health tools have the vast potential to improve our ability to accurately diagnose and treat diseases and to enhance the delivery of health care for individuals. Digital health technologies use computing platforms, connectivity, software and sensors for health care and related uses. These technologies encompass a broad spectrum of applications, ranging from general wellness tools to regulated medical devices. They include technologies intended for use as a medical product, integrated within medical products, as companion diagnostics or as an adjunct to other medical products (devices, drugs, and biologics). They may also be used to develop or study medical products.
Healthcare Information and Management Systems Society (HIMSS, 2020)	Digital health connects and empowers people and populations to manage health and wellness, augmented by accessible and supportive provider teams working within flexible, integrated, interoperable and digitally-enabled care environments that strategically leverage digital tools, technologies and services to transform care delivery.

The early 2000s marked a shift toward patient empowerment through widespread internet access, which facilitated health information-retrieval behaviours and the formation of online support communities (Ganesan & Tong, 2024). In 2005, the WHO launched the Global Observatory for eHealth, formally recognizing telemedicine as a strategic global healthcare channel (WHO, 2005). Electronic Health Records (EHRs) became standard practice and hospitals began using email and web portals to communicate with patients (Palabindala et al., 2016). From the 2010s onward, digital health entered a phase of integration, grounded by advances in data storage and memory, computing power and high-speed communications - core infrastructures that significantly accelerated development across multiple domains. During this period, the focus shifted towards enabling interoperability and unified data flow across previously disconnected systems, devices and wearables. Concurrently, big data analytics and machine learning (ML), a subfield of AI, are increasingly embedded in digital health platforms to support predictive modelling, disease surveillance and personalized medicine (Ganesan & Tong, 2024). Through multimodal systems, these technologies can integrate heterogeneous complex datasets (such as imaging, text, audio, sensor signals, genomic, structured clinical data and others) to generate a more holistic understanding of patient conditions, enhancing precision care and enabling tailored, real-time interventions. For instance, a multimodal platform might combine EHR data with neuroimaging and voice analysis to more accurately assess cognitive decline (Schouten et al., 2025). The rapid advancement of generative AI, driven by the evolution of Large Language Models (LLMs), such as ChatGPT from openAI, is increasingly explored in clinical contexts. Initially applied in isolated tasks, such as supporting the development of clinical guidelines, LLMs are now being integrated as the brain of autonomous agents (K. Zhang et al., 2025). These agents are designed to collaborate in multi-agent systems, coordinating complex tasks such as continuous patient monitoring, distributed decision support and adaptive care planning. This shift marks a transition from static AI tools to dynamic, reasoning-capable systems that enhance scalability and responsiveness in digital health environments (Yu et al., 2025). Figure 2 depicts this progression over time, presenting a timeline of digital health evolution.

By combining real-time data, including clinical, behavioural and environmental sources, these technologies enable early risk detection, personalized interventions and coordinated care delivery. While LLMs and generative AI support dynamic reasoning and patient engagement by tackling complexity, multimodal and multi-agent systems enhance precision and, thus, scalability. Together, they offer a powerful foundation for predictive, participatory and equitable health systems, as long as they are implemented within ethical, effective, interoperable and inclusive frameworks.

Figure 2. Global timeline of telemedicine and remote healthcare

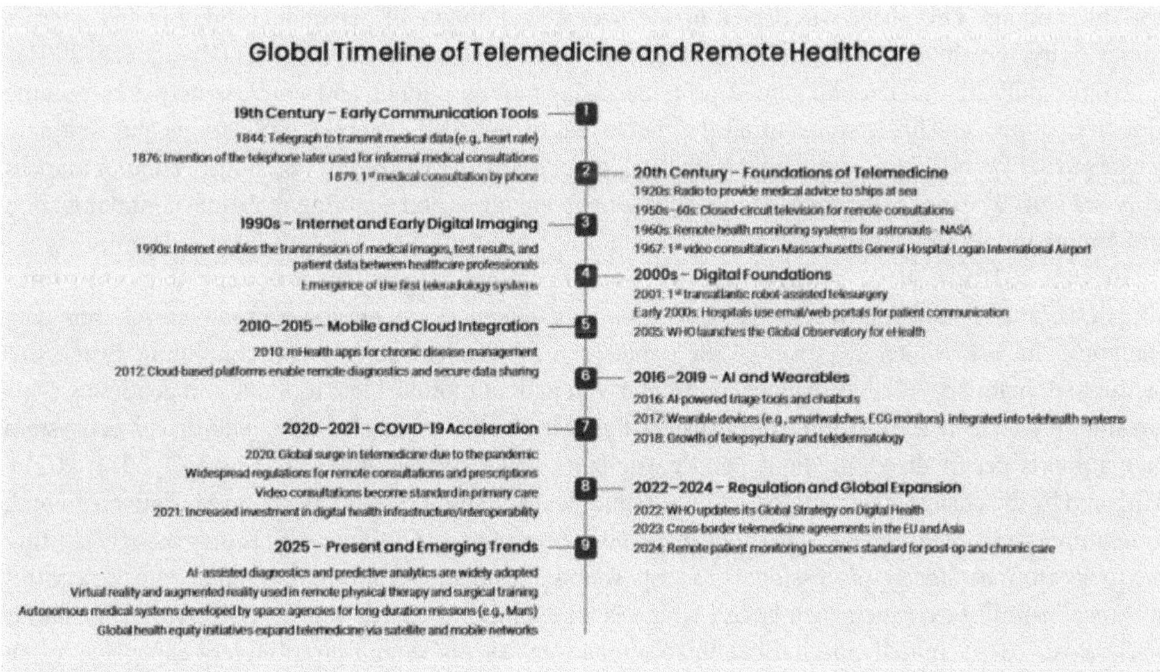

SHIT TO PERSON-CENTRED AND DEMOCRATIZED CARE

As digital health technologies become increasingly embedded in healthcare systems, they are not only driving the transformation of clinical workflows but, more importantly, reshaping the foundational dynamics of care. At the heart of this transformation lies a shift in focus: from healthcare systems and providers to individuals-patients, who increasingly take on an active role in managing their own health, while remaining embedded in their community environments. This reconfiguration is not merely technological but deeply cultural, reflecting evolving expectations regarding autonomy, access and engagement in the digital age.

Evolving Digital Health and Patient Roles

The evolution of digital health terminology - from *eHealth* to *mHealth* and, ultimately, *digital health (dHealth)* - reflects not only technological advancements, but also a fundamental redefinition of the patient's role within health systems. Each term marks a distinct phase in the integration of digital technologies into healthcare, progressively expanding both the scope of intervention and the locus of control.

The term *eHealth* emerged in the late 1990s with the digitization of health records, the development of health information systems and the early adoption of web-based platforms for clinical and administrative functions. This phase was driven by the widespread uptake of personal computing and internet connectivity, which laid the groundwork for digitalizing core healthcare processes (Eysenbach, 2001).

By the mid-2000s, *mHealth* gained prominence as mobile phones and wireless networks became globally pervasive. This term captured the increasing use of SMS, mobile applications and wearable sensors to deliver health services and information, particularly in low-resource settings. *mHealth* marked a pivotal shift by extending care beyond institutional boundaries and enabling real-time communication and remote monitoring (WHO, 2011).

In the 2010s, *digital health* emerged as a broader, integrative concept that subsumes both *eHealth* and *mHealth*, while also encompassing advanced technologies such as AI, big data analytics, the IoT (which has enabled the connection of physical objects and computing systems to facilitate domain-specific intelligence, particularly in patient monitoring), robotics and genomics. This terminology reflects a transition from isolated digital tools to a comprehensive, data-driven ecosystem that supports personalized, predictive and participatory care (Iyamu et al., 2021; WHO, 2011, 2021). Mirrored by the changing terminology, the technological evolution reshaped how care is delivered - and, more importantly, who participates and is involved in providing it. Digital health is increasingly shifting the focus from healthcare professionals to empowered consumers, granting individuals greater control and responsibility over their own health which is an evolution towards self-care (Cuff, 2023; Shaffer & Preziosi, 2019). Initially, digital health solutions were exclusive and prohibitively expensive, often developed for specialized environments such as space missions or military operations. However, relentless innovation, declining hardware costs and the global diffusion of smartphones and broadband have driven *digital health democratization* - the integration of digital tools into the everyday lives of millions (Shaffer & Preziosi, 2019). This transformation aims at reshaping traditional healthcare systems into ecosystems where individuals can self-monitor, self-manage and make informed decisions about their health (HIMSS, 2020). Yet, despite increased accessibility, effective use of digital health technologies still depends on robust digital infrastructure and interoperability, reliable connectivity and sustained investment in system integration. Moreover, many digital health solutions, particularly those involving AI, remote monitoring or personalized therapeutics, remain expensive and are often embedded in business models that impose economic burdens on users. This raises concerns about equity, especially in contexts where digital literacy is low or access to technology is uneven. The digital divide, driven by disparities in infrastructure, affordability and digital skills, risks exacerbating existing health inequities, rather than resolve them. As digital health continues to evolve, addressing these structural barriers will be essential to ensure that its benefits are equitably distributed and that the promise of patient empowerment does not become a new form of exclusion (Butcher & Hussain, 2022; OECD, 2023).

The evolution of digital health is fundamentally reshaping the architecture of healthcare systems, redefining the roles of individuals-patients as active participants in their own health and care. Extending traditionally person-centred care models, individual autonomy is promoted while maintaining everyday living settings, supported by digitally enabled environments. In these emerging configurations, health-care teams are increasingly oriented towards facilitating self-care, where individuals are equipped with digital tools and platforms that support self-monitoring, decision-making and behavioural change. This transformation is sustained by the proliferation of advanced technologies and data infrastructures, which not only enhance access to care, but also enable the deployment of complex algorithms capable of identifying challenges, barriers and opportunities in real time, reshaping interventions to be more adaptive, personalized and responsive. While this transformation offers immense potential to improve health outcomes globally, its successful and equitable implementation requires addressing complex technological, social and ethical challenges.

PRECISION CARE, PERSONALIZED JOURNEYS, AND LIFESTYLE MODIFICATION

Driven by the rapid advancement of AI and digital technologies, the healthcare paradigm is undergoing a profound transformation, steering towards a more personalized, predictive, preventive and participatory model, commonly referred to as precision care (Denysyuk et al., 2024; Wu et al., 2022).

The term precision medicine gained prominence through President Barack Obama's 2015 Precision Medicine Initiative, which emphasized that medicine should be stratified, based on precise biological and contextual characteristics, rather than strictly individualized (Collins & Varmus, 2015). While personalized medicine traditionally refers to individualized care guided by clinical expertise (a concept rooted in Hippocratic practice), precision medicine leverages data-driven technologies, particularly algorithms and machine learning, to analyse multimodal data, including genetic and other clinical data, as well as environmental and lifestyle factors. This enables more targeted and accurate diagnosis and treatment strategies. The application of genetic data is most advanced in monogenic conditions (e.g., tailoring cancer therapies based on tumor genetics), whereas polygenic conditions such as type 2 diabetes or obesity subtypes remain challenging (Bakare, 2025; Barilan, 2022; Collecchia & De Gobbi, 2024). Despite these distinctions, the terms *precision medicine* and *personalized medicine* are often used interchangeably in both academic and clinical discourse (Pandey & Gupta, 2024).

Digital health is evolving from administrative digitization to widespread intelligent clinical decision support systems. Initially, digital health efforts focused primarily on administrative functions, particularly the digitization of clinical documentation through EHR. These systems laid the groundwork for subsequent innovations by enabling functionalities such as laboratory requests and prescription management (Rosenlund et al., 2023; Sharma & Kshetri, 2020). Regarding clinical tasks, digital tools supporting the writing and management of clinical notes are rapidly evolving towards more complex systems capable of assisting, or even automating, elements of diagnosis and treatment.

Traditional Clinical Decision Support Systems (CDSS), often based on static rule sets, have struggled with scalability and adaptability to the complexity of real-world clinical environments. Many early systems failed to meet the nuanced needs of healthcare professionals. The emergence of AI and ML now enables the development of next-generation CDSS that deliver real-time personalized recommendations, improving diagnostic accuracy and optimizing treatment pathways (Mitra & Rehman, 2024).

AI advanced systems can outperform human experts in interpreting medical images, pathology slides, ECGs and even voice recordings - detecting asymptomatic patients or subtle disease markers. These systems integrate diverse data type (genetic, clinical, lifestyle and environmental) into unified diagnostic scores, accelerating early detection and enabling personalized treatment (Davenport & Kalakota, 2019; Meskó, 2022; Tran et al., 2019). Beyond diagnostics, AI supports the development of predictive models that anticipate patient outcomes, detect early signs of deterioration through remote monitoring and recommend timely interventions. These models are already being applied in areas such as chronic kidney disease and oncology, where they inform prognosis and treatment by integrating genomic, histopathological and clinical data (Bouderhem, 2024; Johnson et al., 2021). AI also supports real-time therapy adjustments, such as in closed-loop insulin delivery systems for diabetes management. These technologies identify patient subgroups with atypical drug responses and predict therapeutic efficacy, tailoring interventions to individual profiles (de Jong et al., 2021).

Despite the surge in research and development, the number of licensed and commercially available AI health applications remains limited. Regulatory environments vary in stringency across regions, contributing to a globally heterogeneous landscape in terms of access and implementation (Cancela et al., 2020). Fully automated decision-support tools are classified as medical devices and are therefore subject to stringent regulatory oversight, specifically in Europe and in the USA, which presents implementation challenges (Moberly, 2025). These developments depend heavily on robust digital infrastructure, high-quality interoperable data, computing power and increasingly advanced algorithms. However, data silos and limited data interoperability continue to hinder real-time clinical decision-making and reduce the actionability of digital tools.

Precision health extends beyond the reactive focus of traditional medicine and the gene-centric orientation often associated with precision medicine, adopting a holistic approach that integrates biological, behavioural, environmental and social determinants of health (Wu et al., 2022). Omics sciences - such as genomics, transcriptomics, proteomics, metabolomics, lipidomics and microbiomics - enable comprehensive profiling of biological systems, offering unprecedented insights into disease mechanisms, individual variability and therapeutic response. Their convergence with AI is accelerating the discovery of clinically actionable biomarkers. Moreover, omics-informed digital tools are increasingly influencing public health policy, particularly in areas such as pharmacogenomics, cancer screening and infectious disease surveillance (Hasin et al., 2017; Karczewski & Snyder, 2018; Schüssler-Fiorenza Rose et al., 2019). These advances, however, are not without challenges: omics datasets often reflect the populations from which the training data were derived, limiting their generalizability across diverse groups. Expanding data collection to underrepresented populations is essential, yet the sheer volume of data introduces concerns around quality and accuracy (Huerta-Chagoya et al., 2025).

Given that a significant proportion of the global chronic disease burden is driven by behavioural factors, precision health interventions place strong emphasis on promoting healthier habits and lifestyle changes. The literature underscores that effective interventions require frequent, individualized engagement that reaches people in their daily lives, beyond the confines of traditional clinical settings (Wongvibulsin et al., 2020). Digital technologies are essential enablers of these interventions. Wearable devices, personal health technologies and health apps facilitate the collection of real-time, context-rich data on individuals' behaviours and health states. These include objective metrics, namely physical activity, heart rate, sleep patterns and environmental exposures, such as air quality, data that are often difficult to capture through conventional methods (Riveroll et al., 2018). Continuous data stream is analysed using machine learning, including deep learning algorithms, to identify behavioural patterns, predict health risks or adverse events, and assess the impact of lifestyle and environmental factors on health outcomes (Davenport & Kalakota, 2019; DuBord et al., 2024). For example, data from wearables and sensors can be used to estimate disease severity or predict risks of acute exacerbations of chronic obstructive pulmonary disease (COPD), heart failure, panic disorder or long-term conditions like obesity. Lifestyle and environmental indicators are highly correlated with patient health trajectories and serve as early warning signals for clinical deterioration (Beattie et al., 2020; Wu et al., 2022). Based on predictive insights, precision health offers tailored interventions and feedback (Wongvibulsin et al., 2020). Digital tools provide the right individual with the right information and support, at the right time and in the right context. This may include targeted content, medication or activity reminders, educational resources or behaviour change suggestions based on detected patterns or predicted risks (Denysyuk et al., 2024).

Traditional health interventions have often followed a one-size-fits-all model. Nevertheless, individuals respond differently to the same interventions. This opens new opportunities for personalization and precise care, enabling to discover what works best for people, thereby enhancing motivation and long-term adherence (Bakare, 2025; Riveroll et al., 2018). Digital therapeutics (DTx) are central to personalized behaviour change interventions. For example, DTx for healthy longevity aim to deliver timely preventive care when a vulnerable state is detected or predicted. These include digital programs for conditions such as depression or obesity, which are already being prescribed and reimbursed in some healthcare systems. Such programs integrate behavioural interventions, interactive content and, in some cases, coaching or therapy components delivered digitally. Their goal is to empower individuals to take an active role in managing their health by equipping them with the knowledge, skills and support necessary for self-care and self-management (Leistner & Kowatsch, 2023).

Digital health technologies and AI are increasingly used to complement traditional in person care, enabling continuous and proactive health management (Schwamm et al., 2024). Telemedicine and virtual care platforms facilitate remote consultations and follow-ups, expanding access to care, particularly for individuals with chronic conditions, those in underserved regions or patients with mobility limitations. In such contexts, frequent monitoring and interaction are essential, but often impractical through in-person visits alone (Cancela et al., 2020; Rosenlund et al., 2023). Remote monitoring technologies in everyday environments include digital biomarkers (such as heart rate variability, arrhythmia burden and thoracic impedance from implantable cardioverter defibrillators, glucose variability, sleep patterns, physical activity habits, and others) that have emerged as validated tools using data from devices like smartphones, sensors or wearables. These allow continuous monitoring of physiological and behavioural parameters, providing a more comprehensive view of a patient's health status than sporadic clinical visits, while also empowering them in self-care (Barracca et al., 2023; Kasoju et al., 2023).

AI-assisted platforms integrate clinical records, lifestyle metrics, environmental exposures and patient-reported outcomes into a unified view for healthcare professionals (Wu et al., 2022). These systems support personalized health promotion strategies and enable timely, data-driven clinical decisions (Davenport & Kalakota, 2019). At the same time, digital tools deliver personalized feedback and support to patients, reinforcing positive behaviours and encouraging adherence to treatment or lifestyle plans (Wongvibulsin et al., 2020). Applications may include personalized educational content, symptom tracking, medication reminders and access to peer support communities. Conversational agents (CAs), such as chatbots, offer scalable, personalized education and support, potentially enhancing patient engagement and fostering a "digital therapeutic alliance" (Leistner & Kowatsch, 2023).

The hybrid model of digital and human care recognizes that while technology enhances efficiency and insight, empathy and relational continuity remain indispensable. Clinicians continue to play a central role in diagnosing conditions, interpreting complex data, developing care plans and providing emotional support (Alruwaili et al., 2023; Bitkina et al., 2023). The ideal model integrates digital tools into existing clinical workflows and fosters collaboration among patients, caregivers and healthcare providers. This synergy promotes empowerment, shared decision-making and improved health outcomes (Denysyuk et al., 2024).

However, the integration of certified digital tools into clinical workflows presents regulatory and methodological challenges. Their use in high-stakes domains, such as non-communicable disease management, demands robust validation and multidisciplinary development approaches. For example, patients with type 2 diabetes present highly heterogeneous clinical profiles or subtypes, and while some antidiabetic drugs have shown unexpected cardiovascular benefits, much remains to be discovered (Pina et al., 2023). Digital tools rapid expansion underscores the urgent need for systematic evaluation of their effectiveness and outomes in the real-world (Clements et al., 2023; Shomali et al., 2024).

TRANSITIONING CARE LEADERSHIP AND PROMOTING PATIENT AUTONOMY

While the integration of mobile technologies and AI enables patients to actively participate in their care, healthcare shifts from hierarchical, clinician-led models to collaborative, patient-centred paradigms.

Digital health technologies are reshaping traditional paternalistic models of care, fostering more balanced and collaborative relationships between patients and healthcare professionals (Mesko et al., 2025). As COVID-19 pandemic significantly accelerated the adoption of telemedicine and digital tools, normalizing virtual care across diverse healthcare settings, patients have increasingly embraced these technologies for their convenience, accessibility and ability to maintain continuity of care during periods of disruption (Meskó, 2022; Sust et al., 2020). Digital platforms not only facilitate remote consultations but also provide patients' access to relevant health information and decision-support tools, enhancing their ability to participate in care planning (Topol, 2019).

Effective shared decision-making requires both health literacy - the ability to understand and apply health information - and digital literacy, as patients increasingly interact with technology-mediated care environments (Rosenlund et al., 2023). AI-powered platforms can bridge these gaps by presenting evidence-based content through simplified language and interactive formats (Alfano et al., 2023; Meskó & de Bronkart, 2022). Developing effective digital solutions demands early and sustained collaboration with patients. Co-creation approaches ensure that tools are aligned with real-world needs, patient values and lived experiences (Popa et al., 2024).

Value-Based Healthcare (VBHC) models reinforce a collaborative approach by prioritizing clinical outcomes, as well as the outcomes and experiences that matter most to patients, relative to the costs of care. As new contracting models emerge, linking payment to performance and enhancing transparency in outcome measurement, digital tools play a crucial role in enabling this transformation. By leveraging care pathways' automation and coordination, thus promoting shared decision-making, continuous monitoring and real-time outcome reporting, digital platforms alleviate administrative burdens, and strengthen patient-centred practices (L. Zhang et al., 2025) (refer to point "Addressing Health System Challenges").

Despite all the recent advances, challenges remain. Both patients and clinicians express concerns about data privacy, the potential misuse of AI and overreliance on automated systems. A recent study in the United States found that patients tend to trust physicians less when they use AI in their clinical decision-making (Reis et al., 2025). To build trust, AI must be implemented transparently, with robust safeguards and human oversight. Technology should enhance, not replace, clinical judgment. Ethical integration requires clarity, competence and accountability from all stakeholders involved in the design, deployment and use of digital health systems (Bekbolatova et al., 2024; Bouderhem, 2024; Sagona et al., 2025).

Traditional healthcare models have historically been clinician-centred and professionally led, with patients occupying a largely passive role in managing their health. This hierarchical structure, rooted in centuries of medical practice, assumed that patients lacked the knowledge or capacity to meaningfully participate in care decisions. Treatment decisions were predominantly made by physicians, with patients expected to comply with prescribed plans. Interestingly, the first wave of healthcare digitalization often introduced a computer screen between doctors and patients, unintentionally increasing the distance in clinical encounters (Asgari et al., 2024; Meskó & de Bronkart, 2022; Trzmielak et al., 2024). Digital tools and AI support the transition to patient-centred models by handling technical tasks, allowing clinicians to focus on empathy, communication and trust-building (Schubert et al., 2025). At the core of this transition is the principle of patient autonomy, enabling individuals to make informed decisions about their health. Empowerment rests on three foundational pillars: access to resources (tools, information and assets), individual agency (the capacity and willingness to take control) and a supportive context (cultural and systemic environments that facilitate autonomy) (Mesko et al., 2025).

The democratization of health information retrieval has granted patients access to knowledge once exclusive for professionals. However, they often struggle to interpret this information, preventing it from becoming actionable insight. In response, digital communities have emerged as vital enablers of autonomy and self-management. Platforms like *PatientsLikeMe* illustrate how peer-to-peer networks can enhance health literacy by allowing individuals to share experiences, track their health and learn from others facing similar conditions. These communities foster agency, emotional support and informed participation in care decisions (Wicks et al., 2010). A particularly compelling example of patient-led innovation is the OpenAPS (Open Artificial Pancreas System) project, initiated by patients and caregivers seeking faster and more effective solutions for managing type 1 diabetes. This initiative exemplifies how patients can not only lead technological development, but also drive broader transformation in healthcare. It has given rise to the concept of "patient design", in which patients actively contribute to shaping healthcare strategies and advising organizational decision-making (Mesko et al., 2025; Meskó & de Bronkart, 2022).

AI systems further increase individuals-patients' independence by transforming raw health data into actionable guidance on medication, physical activity, nutrition and symptom management. Some platforms even incorporate virtual health assistants capable of answering questions and scheduling appointments. As a result, people are no longer passive recipients of care, but active participants, often managing their conditions proactively and with reduced reliance on continuous clinical supervision. As awareness grows around the critical role of lifestyle in overall health, the relevance of digital self-management tools becomes increasingly evident. This is reflected in the growing number of applications dedicated to sleep tracking, stress management and other daily behaviours that influence long-term well-being (Alhammad et al., 2024; Johnson Oyeniyi, 2024; Rosenlund et al., 2023). Despite recent advances in technology, there are still significant limitations, such as the "black box" nature of many AI systems, which makes them difficult to interpret and scale. These challenges underscore the importance of transparency, explainability and inclusive design in ensuring that digital health tools genuinely support patient autonomy and equitable care (Hua, 2023; Johnson Oyeniyi, 2024).

The role of healthcare professionals is also evolving. Clinicians are going to be increasingly tasked with interpreting and contextualizing AI outputs, transitioning from sole knowledge providers to facilitators of shared decision-making. They will help patients understand digital feedback, contextualize automated suggestions and make informed choices aligned with their specific health needs. This shift repositions healthcare professionals as educators and navigators within a digitally supported care model, guiding patients through increasingly complex digital health ecosystems. To effectively fulfil this role, clinicians must be equipped with technical literacy to assess AI tools and communicate their implications clearly. Medical education must therefore integrate AI training alongside essential relational competencies such as empathy, active listening and effective communication (Huettemann et al., 2024; Rao, 2023; Schubert et al., 2025).

Transformation in healthcare roles introduces both promising opportunities and new concerns, particularly regarding patient "responsibilization" - the risk of individuals being overburdened with the responsibility for managing their own care. Without adequate support, this shift could overlook structural barriers and exacerbate health inequalities (Meier et al., 2024).

ADDRESSING HEALTH SYSTEM CHALLENGES

Health systems around the world are facing mounting pressures from the growing burden of non-communicable diseases (NCDs), persistent workforce shortages and rising healthcare costs. Digital health has emerged not merely as a technological innovation, but as a strategic response to these systemic challenges. By supporting chronic disease prevention and precise management, improving care coordination, reducing administrative burdens and expanding access to underserved populations, digital tools offer scalable and adaptable solutions. These technologies have the potential to strengthen healthcare systems and foster more sustainable, efficient and patient-centred models of care.

Digital Health for NCD Management

NCDs, including cardiovascular diseases, diabetes, cancer and chronic respiratory conditions, represent one of the most pressing global health challenges. Characterized by a silent onset, slow progression and need for long-term management, NCDs place a substantial burden on patients, healthcare professionals and health systems alike (He et al., 2024; Monzani & Pizzoli, 2020). In the European Union (EU), they account for at least 25% of health spending and contribute to an economic loss of nearly 2% of GDP, underscoring their growing financial impact. Projections indicate a continued rise in NCD-related mortality, compounded by a projected global shortfall of 18 million healthcare workers by 2030 (Bienefeld et al., 2025; Cruz Castañeda & Bertemes Filho, 2023).

NCDs are largely driven by modifiable dysmetabolic risk factors such as hypertension, obesity, dyslipidemia, dysglycemia and insulin resistance. Dysmetabolism is shaped by lifestyle behaviours including poor diet, physical inactivity, smoking and harmful alcohol use, that in turn, are influenced by broader social and environmental determinants (Action Plan for the Prevention and Control of Noncommunicable Diseases in South-East Asia, 2013-2020 SEA-NCD-101 Distribution: General, 2022). Consequently, interventions aimed at any level of this pyramid may produce cascading effects throughout the entire system. For example, emerging evidence indicates that new classes of diabetes medications - initially developed for glycaemic control - also offer benefits in reducing obesity, cardiovascular disease and even certain types of cancer. These findings suggest that well-designed digital health interventions have the potential to achieve similarly broad and transformative impacts, extending benefits beyond their original targets.

Digital health technologies support the full continuum of NCD care, from prevention and early detection to treatment and long-term management (Joshi et al., 2023). In primary prevention, digital health promotion tools such as mobile apps, social media, wearables and chatbots are instrumental in raising awareness, encouraging self-monitoring and promoting healthy behaviour change (Ferretti et al., 2023). A notable example is the WHO's *Be He@lthy Be Mobile* SMS-based initiative in India, which achieved a 19% smoking cessation rate after six months (Gopinathan et al., 2018). Another example is the digital platform developed at Johns Hopkins Hospital that identifies patients with unmet social needs and connects them to community services, demonstrating how EHR-integrated tools can address social determinants of health (Hatef et al., 2025).

Digital technologies also play a critical role in population-based screening and early detection. In India, the *Digital LifeCare* system supports national screening for five major NCDs (cardiovascular diseases, diabetes, oral, breast and cervical cancers) through mobile and web applications tailored for frontline health workers with low digital literacy. The system features intuitive, pictorial interfaces, offline functionality and automated work plans aligned with national protocols (Nadhamuni et al., 2020). AI-powered diagnostic tools further enhance early detection by analysing large volumes of clinical data, including medical images and genetic information, with high precision and speed (Paulchamy, 2024; Pavuluri et al., 2024). Innovations such as AI-based voice analysis for early diabetes detection exemplify the disruptive potential of digital tools in redefining NCD management (Kaufman et al., 2023).

In long-term management, connected health technologies support patient self-management while enhancing provider collaboration. Telemonitoring has demonstrated significant reductions in hospital readmissions and mortality. For example, Partners HealthCare's in the U.S. home monitoring program, managed by a small team of nurses, reduced readmissions by 44% for over 3,000 heart failure patients. Similarly, the U.S. Veterans Health Administration's national home telehealth program achieved nearly $2,000 in annual savings per patient, a 38% reduction in hospital admissions and a 58% drop in inpatient bed days, while maintaining high patient satisfaction (Kvedar et al., 2014). Digital health also enables highly personalized care for NCDs by supporting tailored treatment regimens, customized education and predictive analytics based on individual data (Cruz Castañeda & Bertemes Filho, 2023; Monzani & Pizzoli, 2020). AI algorithms can learn from users' physiological patterns to anticipate fluctuations, such as changes in blood glucose, thus optimizing care delivery over time (Bernardes, 2025; Kanade, 2024). These developments open the door to more precise therapeutic pathways, including improved understanding of patient journeys, diagnostic strategies and optimized drug selection. This aligns with the growing need for precision in prescribing, especially as current clinical guidelines often lack personalization criteria (Garg et al., 2022; Kounatidis et al., 2024).

In low- and middle-income countries (LMICs), digital tools are particularly critical for expanding access to timely, quality care. High mobile phone dissemination enables digital solutions that bridge gaps in human resources and infrastructure. For example, Ghana's *ComHIP* program uses mobile phones for appointment reminders and nutrition education, improving adherence and easing pressure on primary care (Labrique et al., 2018). In Bangladesh, decentralizing hypertension and diabetes management to non-physician health workers via digital platforms has expanded access while reducing dependence on specialist-led clinics (Xie et al., 2023).

Digital health also lays the foundation for *precision public health* (PPH), an emerging model that uses real-time, routinely collected data - including EHRs, wearables, mobile apps and social media - to deliver targeted public health interventions. PPH aims to shift from passive surveillance to proactive action, building agile, data-informed systems capable of managing NCDs at both individual and population levels (Canfell et al., 2022).

Extended reality (XR) technologies, including augmented reality (AR), virtual reality (VR) and mixed reality (MR), are being deployed in medical training, patient education and pain management, and are increasingly integrated into telehealth and therapeutic contexts. Use cases range from immersive learning environments and anatomical visualization to surgical planning. Despite growing adoption, XR still faces barriers related to software maturity, hardware limitations, user experience and cost, which constrain its broader clinical utility (Ganesan & Tong, 2024; Ogundiya et al., 2024; Venkatesan et al., 2021). Nonetheless, its application in medical education and team-based training holds significant promise for enhancing clinical competencies, procedural accuracy and interdisciplinary collaboration. By enabling realistic, risk-free simulations, XR contributes to the development of critical decision-making skills and procedural confidence, ultimately improving the quality of care and the consistency of patient follow-up.

Systems that integrate multiple data sources (such as EHRs, imaging, genomics and wearables) to generate predictive analytics for diagnosis, risk assessment and personalized treatment planning, can improve over time through continuous feedback loops, enhancing their precision and adaptability. The goal is the creation of a Unified Health Platform (UHP) that integrates EHRs, temedicine, IoT devices and AI analytics into a cohesive digital ecosystem. Such platforms would enable performance tracking, strengthen clinical governance and support continuous quality improvement. These capabilities not only contribute to improved patient outcomes and more efficient resource use but also foster a culture of excellence and accountability within healthcare systems (Kanade, 2024; Lebaea et al., 2024).

Mitigating Healthcare Professional Shortages

The global healthcare system is grappling with an intensifying shortage of skilled professionals, compounded by rising levels of clinician burnout and widespread workplace dissatisfaction. Within the next five years, the world is projected to face a healthcare workforce deficit more than twice the current shortfall (Bienefeld et al., 2025). Occupational stressors, administrative overload and the emotional demands inherent to caregiving roles further aggravate the situation. These factors contribute to persistently high attrition rates, with many professionals stepping away from clinical practice due to exhaustion, demotivation or lack of fulfilment (Pavuluri et al., 2024). Ironically, the initial wave of healthcare digitalization, particularly the introduction of electronic health records (EHRs), often intensified clinicians' burdens by increasing documentation requirements and reducing the time available for direct patient care (Keshavarz et al., 2025).

One of AI's most immediate contributions lies in reducing the administrative and cognitive load that contributes to burnout. Currently, healthcare providers spend nearly half their workday on documentation and bureaucrtic tasks. Digital scribes (combining speech recognition with NLP) can transcribe and summarize provider–patient interactions, populate EHRs and generate billing codes. Early studies suggest these tools can improve documentation efficiency by up to 2.7 times (Pavuluri et al., 2024).

However, the use of LLMs introduces important risks. These systems can "hallucinate", generating plausible sounding but factually incorrect information. If used autonomously, without human oversight, they may introduce inaccuracies into clinical records, potentially compromising patient safety. Thus, clinical validation remains essential (Tierney et al., 2024). For example, within the NHS, autonomous voice-based digital scribes are classified as medical devices and require clinician oversight to ensure accuracy and safety (NHS England, 2025). AI helps reduce cognitive fatigue by organizing fragmented health data into cohesive summaries and intuitive visualizations. Generative AI and chatbot tools can also manage high volumes of patient messages by templating responses and triaging inquiries, significantly accelerating communication workflows. By streamlining information retrieval and analysis, AI enables faster, more accurate decision-making and allows clinicians to refocus on patient care. These systems can filter out irrelevant alerts (such as unnecessary medication pop-ups) and surface critical information from remote monitoring devices (Pavuluri et al., 2024; Strika et al., 2024). Additionally, these tools must guarantee data privacy and confidentiality, concerns that are heightened when third-party models are involved. In contrast, open-source models deployed on proprietary infrastructure can offer greater transparency, control and alignment with healthcare data governance requirements (Abrar et al., 2018).

When thoughtfully implemented, AI can also improve work design by redistributing routine or repetitive tasks and augmenting clinical roles. Rather than replicating inefficient workflows, this is an opportunity to redesign care pathways by eliminating outdated processes and creating more effective systems. For instance, AI-enhanced diagnostics can assist physicians in identifying patterns in imaging, lab results or patient histories, thereby improving diagnostic accuracy while supporting ongoing medical education, especially in underserved or resource-limited settings (Strika et al., 2024). In radiology, AI has shown promise in triaging chest X-rays by flagging high-priority cases for earlier review. Prospective clinical studies demonstrate that such systems can help clinicians focus on critical findings more efficiently, potentially improving outcomes (Sridharan et al., 2024). Even in these scenarios, however, AI outputs must be validated by human professionals to ensure diagnostic reliability and clinical accountability. AI can also help nurses reallocate cognitive resources from continuous monitoring to higher-level tasks, such as validating clinical suspicions or contributing to care planning. This human-AI synergy supports skill development, decision-making autonomy and interprofessional collaboration, key factors in professional satisfaction and resilience (Bienefeld et al., 2025).

Ultimately, when integrated through a sociotechnical lens, ensuring alignment between technology, human work and organizational processes, AI not only addresses immediate workforce challenges, but also supports long-term system sustainability by enabling professionals to deliver better care with greater satisfaction and less burnout.

Measuring Success: KPIs and Health Outcomes

Robust measurement through Key Performance Indicators (KPIs) and outcome assessments is essential for evaluating the impact, effectiveness and value of digital health interventions (DHIs). As health systems increasingly adopt VBHC models, standardized and comprehensive evaluation frameworks are critical to guide investment, inform policy and ensure that DHIs achieve their intended health outcomes (McCoy et al., 2025; Wilkinson et al., 2024).

A core component of outcome measurement in VBHC is the use of Patient-Reported Outcome Measures (PROMs). PROMs capture patients' perspectives on symptoms, functional status, treatment goals and overall well-being, offering a more holistic view of health that includes physical, mental and social dimensions (Zhang et al., 2025). PROMs have demonstrated multiple benefits: they enhance communication between patients and clinicians, improve treatment adherence, support shared decision-making and enable more personalized care planning. With the digital transformation of PROMs from paper-based formats to automated platforms, data collection, scoring, analysis and integration with EHRs have become significantly more efficient.

Initiatives such as the International Consortium for Health Outcomes Measurement (ICHOM) and the Patient-Reported Outcomes Measurement Information System (PROMIS) have played a pivotal role in advancing this agenda. These frameworks provide globally recognized standard sets of outcomes that matter the most to patients, facilitating consistent evaluation and international benchmarking (Terwee et al., 2021).

A compelling example comes from a hospital in Brisbane, where a digital PROMs platform was implemented to monitor post-chemotherapy side effects in lung cancer patients. This intervention reduced the average number of follow-up calls per patient from ten to zero, while simultaneously improving clinical efficiency, empowering patients and enhancing treatment outcomes through real-time data and personalized care adjustments (Zhang et al., 2025). Patient feedback plays a critical role in ensuring system sustainability and enhancing performance. Digital platforms that automate the collection of Patient-Reported Outcome Measures (PROMs), Patient-Reported Experience Measures (PREMs) and other patient-generated health data help overcome traditional barriers such as time constraints and limited staff capacity. Additionally, by digitizing data at the point of entry, these platforms support the standardization of outcome measurement, enabling immediate analysis, longitudinal tracking of health status and performance benchmarking across institutions. Collectively, these capabilities contribute to improved patient outcomes and experiences—as captured through PROMs and PREMs—while advancing a more patient-centred, efficient and results-oriented model of care (Ammi et al., 2023; Giger et al., 2025; Zhang et al., 2025).

Beyond PROMs, DHIs support a broader spectrum of outcome evaluations. Clinical outcomes, such as improved blood pressure control, glycaemic regulation, reduced hospitalization rates and lower mortality, are commonly used indicators. While the strength of evidence varies by context, many DHIs have demonstrated positive impacts on these clinical measures. DHIs have also proven effective in improving behavioural outcomes, including medication adherence, increased physical activity and healthier dietary habits, that are critical for disease prevention and self-management (Xiong et al., 2023). Service implementation outcomes represent another key area of value. These include improvements in accessibility, quality and efficiency of healthcare delivery processes. Studies show that DHIs can streamline workflows, enhance user experience and increase the capacity of primary care services (Xiong et al., 2023). From an economic perspective, DHIs contribute to efficiency gains and cost-effectiveness. By reducing reliance on paper-based systems, optimizing resource use and accelerating administrative processes, digital technologies can yield substantial cost savings. Evaluating cost-effectiveness is essential for justifying further investment and ensuring the long-term sustainability of digital health initiatives (Herrick et al., 2024; Willems et al., 2021). In summary, meaningful evaluation of digital health interventions - across clinical, behavioural, experiential and economic dimensions - is key to maximizing their value. These metrics empower stakeholders to identify and scale effective interventions, improve system performance and deliver high-quality, patient-centred care aligned with the principles of VBHC.

Value-Based Digital Health Interventions and ROI

The transition to Value-Based Healthcare represents a significant shift from traditional volume-based models, which emphasize the sheer number of services delivered, towards an approach centred on patient outcomes relative to cost (Porter & Teisberg, 2006). VBHC is designed to improve quality of life, foster functional independence and deliver better health outcomes, while simultaneously reducing inefficiencies and unnecessary time spent in care settings (J. Zhang et al., 2025). Reflecting this broader vision, the European Commission now defines healthcare "value" through four interconnected dimensions:

- **Allocative value:** Ensuring fair and equitable distribution of resources;
- **Technical value:** Maximizing health outcomes with available resources;
- **Personal value:** Aligning care with individual patients' needs and goals;
- **Societal value:** Advancing the well-being of the wider community.

Digital Health Interventions play a crucial role across all these dimensions, helping to build more equitable, efficient, and sustainable health systems (Zhang et al., 2025).

Amidst multidimensional definitions of value, cost-effectiveness remains a central concern. By automating data flows, improving diagnostic precision and enhancing personalization, digital tools have the potential to both improve outcomes and reduce waste, creating value for patients, providers, payers, suppliers and society as a whole (Zhang et al., 2025). However, the real value of digital solutions is not inherent to their digital nature. If these tools simply digitize ineffective processes, their impact will be marginal at best. In today's landscape, where new digital tools proliferate rapidly, robust value-based assessment frameworks are essential. Only with rigorous evaluation can clear benchmarks be established, justifying public or private reimbursement and supporting equitable access to digital solutions that genuinely benefit health management (Herrick et al., 2024).

Accurately quantifying the costs, impacts and overall value of DHIs remains challenging. Many are embedded within broader interventions, making it difficult to isolate their specific effects. Furthermore, while open-source DHIs are often seen as "free", considerable costs can arise from local adaptation, integration and ongoing maintenance – expenses that are frequently excluded from economic analyses. Meanwhile, commercial digital health solutions often depend on subscription or annual licensing models, which may be financially out of reach for many, especially in resource-limited settings (Bostan et al., 2024). To address these limitations, several frameworks have been developed to evaluate DHIs in terms of outcomes and user experience, but also from an economic perspective. One such initiative is *Label2Enable*, a European project that promotes trust and transparency in health and wellness apps by introducing a recognized quality label. It helps users, professionals and systems identify apps that meet high standards for safety, usability and health impact (*Label2Enable*, n.d.). Another approach is the World Bank's five-step economic evaluation framework, designed to guide stakeholders, particularly in low-resource settings, in assessing the value of DHIs (Wilkinson et al., 2024). The framework includes:

- **Determining the context**: understanding system characteristics, user profiles, clinical pathways and digital architecture;
- **Defining the intervention type**: classifying DHIs according to WHO categories and identifying AI functionalities;
- **Establishing complexity**: assessing causal linkages and scope of impact;

- o **Applying analytic principles**: selecting appropriate economic methods that account for scalability, real-time data use and cross-sector impact;
- o **Representing the value proposition**: capturing disaggregated impacts (e.g., user experience, societal benefits, data value) and aggregating findings for decision-makers.

This framework supports the use of Return on Investment (ROI) and Benefit-Cost Analysis (BCA) models to evaluate large-scale DHIs with multisectoral impacts. While traditional BCA methods are useful for estimating general health and system-level benefits, they often fail to capture the unique advantages of digital health, namely predictive capabilities or data generation for future decision-making. To properly evaluate these specific impacts, tailored approaches are needed that go beyond standard economic models (Herrick et al., 2024).

Implementing and evaluating digital health solutions within the framework of VBHC presents a strategic opportunity to advance healthcare delivery. Although technical and methodological challenges in economic evaluation persist, ongoing efforts toward standardization and the development of robust assessment frameworks will better equip decision-makers to identify, prioritize, and scale the most impactful interventions.

Scalling Up Successful Interventions

Digital health is fundamental to expanding the reach of effective health interventions, especially in resource-limited settings (Kvedar et al., 2014). By leveraging technology, it broadens access, increases efficiency and enhances user engagement. Digital tools support care across diverse populations and conditions by connecting clinicians and patients, facilitating collaboration among healthcare professionals and enabling peer-to-peer support. This connectivity underpins remote diagnosis and treatment, continuous monitoring and self-care, significantly improving access to quality healthcare in underserved or remote areas (Chukwudi Cosmos Maha et al., 2024; Strika et al., 2024).

Scaling up successful digital health interventions depends on several interrelated factors that go beyond technological deployment alone. Achieving broad and sustained impact requires attention to user-centred design, effective data integration, interoperability with existing systems, simplicity and adaptability of solutions, and robust mechanisms for training and partnership. Equally important are financial sustainability, multi-channel engagement strategies and fostering strong user motivation – elements that together enable digital initiatives to move from isolated pilots to widespread, transformative healthcare solutions.

User-Centred and Contextual Design: Successful digital health initiatives are grounded in user-centred design, ensuring that solutions are contextually appropriate and aligned with the priorities of all stakeholders. This includes developing localized, culturally sensitive content and conducting user research to address specific needs and preferences (Hazra-Ganju et al., 2023; Labrique et al., 2018). Co-designing AI systems, workflows and responsibilities with clinicians and patients facilitates smoother integration and reduces implementation barriers (Bienefeld et al., 2025). Iterative development, user testing and refinement based on feedback are essential to adapt interventions to local workforce capacities and operational realities (Gadsden et al., 2023).

Multi-Channel Dissemination: An omni-channel approach to content dissemination, utilizing mobile apps, social media, SMS and interactive games, can significantly increase the reach and impact of digital interventions (Hazra-Ganju et al., 2023; He et al., 2024). This diversified strategy supports widespread health communication and encourages sustained behaviour change.

Data and Analytics: Digital platforms enable efficient collection of patient-generated data and automate the generation of insights for clinical and operational decision-making (L. Zhang et al., 2025). These data streams empower users, motivate healthcare workers and support continued investment by enabling performance monitoring and identifying areas for improvement (Labrique et al., 2018). Real-time analytics also help track evolving user needs, informing content updates and outreach strategies to maintain relevance and engagement (Hazra-Ganju et al., 2023).

Integration and Interoperability: Besides data quality, data integration and interoperability are essential for successful scaling. Digital health solutions must be compatible with existing EHR and clinical workflows to reduce administrative burden and support seamless care delivery (Giger et al., 2025; Paulchamy, 2024). Interoperable systems rely on common standards for data exchange, enabling unified, patient-centric communication and analytics (Schlieter et al., 2022). Even with advanced technologies capable of processing unstructured data, ensuring data quality remains critical, particularly when aiming for true interoperability across systems and settings.

Simplicity and Adaptability: Simple solutions, which include SMS-based interventions, are easier to deploy and maintain, especially in low-resource environments. Adaptable and extendable digital tools can be refined based on research findings and user feedback, allowing for continuous improvement (Labrique et al., 2018; Schlieter et al., 2022).

Training and Partnerships: Training and capacity building are essential to ensure adoption and sustained use. Educating healthcare providers and patients on the value, functionality and safety of digital tools, such as telemedicine and remote monitoring, fosters motivation and readiness to engage. Strong partnerships between academia, policymakers, patient groups and private-sector actors are critical for testing, deploying and scaling digital care models. Supportive leadership is equally important to advocate for innovation and enable long-term sustainability (Swartz et al., 2021; Xiong et al., 2023).

Financial Sustainability: Long-term scalability depends on sustainable financial models. While digital health solutions often require significant upfront investment, they can deliver long-term economic benefits through efficiency gains and reduced resource utilization (Bernardes, 2025; Ferretti et al., 2023; Willems et al., 2021). Developing viable financial models, through reimbursement mechanisms, monetization strategies or public-private financing, is essential to maintain impact and ensure equitable access (Giger et al., 2025; Hazra-Ganju et al., 2023).

Engagement and Gamification: Widespread adoption is essential to scaling success. Gamification has emerged as a powerful strategy to enhance user engagement and adherence. Features such as quizzes, leaderboards and real-time feedback encourage sustained participation, motivate behaviour change and can even reduce acquisition costs by promoting user-driven dissemination. Personalized feedback further reinforces user autonomy and supports the effectiveness of interventions (Chukwudi Cosmos Maha et al., 2024; Ferretti et al., 2023; Schlieter et al., 2022).

By systematically applying these strategies, grounded in evidence, user feedback, system integration and value, digital health interventions can move beyond pilot phases and achieve national or global scale. This has the potential to significantly improve population health outcomes and contribute to more sustainable, resilient healthcare systems worldwide (Chukwudi Cosmos Maha et al., 2024; Schlieter et al., 2022).

CHALLENGES AND OPPORTUNITIES

Digital health transformation is neither linear nor uniformly progressive. It occurs within a complex landscape shaped by structural inequalities, fragmented regulations, and sociotechnical tensions that both foster and hinder innovation. The interaction between technological advances and entrenched systemic inertia creates a paradox: digital health can reimagine care delivery, empower individuals, and optimize system performance, yet it also brings to light new and existing vulnerabilities - particularly in areas such as equity, governance, and clinical integrity.

Challenges

The digital transformation of healthcare, while offering significant potential to improve capability, efficiency and access, is accompanied by a complex set of challenges that demand strategic and context-sensitive responses (Martin & Alarcón-Urbistondo, 2024; Pergolizzi Jr. et al., 2023). These challenges span equity, infrastructure, ethics, regulation and clinical standards (Hendl & Shukla, 2024).

Digital Divide and Equitable Access

One of the most urgent concerns is the digital divide and the issue of equitable access. Although digital health technologies are expected to democratize healthcare and reduce costs, they risk reinforcing and amplifying existing health disparities (Hendl & Shukla, 2024; McCoy et al., 2025). This divide is not merely technological, it is deeply rooted in social determinants such as geographic location, poverty, gender discrimination, educational gaps, disability and ethnicity (Kim & Backonja, 2025; WHO, 2025). Vulnerable populations, including those in structurally disadvantaged areas, rural communities, older adults, people with disabilities and ethnic or linguistic minorities, face disproportionate barriers due to limited internet access, poor mobile coverage, lack of digital equipment and low digital literacy (Davis, 2025; Kozlakidis et al., 2024; Rahul A. Lad & Bhawna Sharma Padroo, 2024; WHO, 2025). Evidence shows that many national digital health strategies fail to adequately address these inequalities. They often overlook human rights, fail to remove access barriers and neglect systemic biases or discriminatory practices (Davis, 2025; Sebire et al., 2025). The dominant "technology-first" approach frequently ignores the material realities of healthcare systems, particularly in LMICs, where basic infrastructure is often lacking. As a result, digital health investments in under-resourced contexts risk misallocation and may inadvertently cause harm. They can reinforce technological dependency through reliance on foreign software, limited control over data storage and processing, inadequate local technical capacity and the deployment of solutions misaligned with local needs (McCoy et al., 2025). True democratization of healthcare through digital means requires inclusive, culturally sensitive and community-led strategies (Kozlakidis et al., 2024; Leal Neto & Wyl, 2024). This includes ensuring affordable access to digital tools, designing intuitive user interfaces, providing personal support and developing digital health literacy that incorporates human rights and data governance (Davis, 2025; Fitzpatrick, 2023; WHO, 2025).

Integration Into Traditional Healthcare Infrastructures

Integrating digital solutions into traditional healthcare infrastructures presents another major challenge. The transition from legacy paper-based systems to fully digital environments has been underway for decades and was significantly accelerated by the COVID-19 pandemic, which required widespread adoption of telemedicine and remote monitoring (Dal Mas et al., 2023; Pergolizzi Jr. et al., 2023). However, this transformation is hindered by the substantial financial investment required for development, implementation and maintenance, particularly in lower-income health systems (Bernardes, 2025; Sebire et al., 2025). Many digital health tools still function as standalone applications, resulting in fragmented service delivery rather than cohesive ecosystems (Huettemann et al., 2024; Popa et al., 2024). Achieving interoperability remains difficult due to technological incompatibilities, lack of data standards and divergent stakeholder interests (Kozlakidis et al., 2024; Leal Neto & Wyl, 2024). Resistance to change within healthcare systems accustomed to legacy workflows further complicates integration, creating gaps in data integrity and privacy protection (Pergolizzi Jr. et al., 2023; WHO, 2025). Moreover, the uneven maturity of digital health across countries and institutions means that a universal blueprint is not feasible; implementations must be context-specific and adaptable to local infrastructure, user needs and regulatory environments (Kozlakidis et al., 2024). A unified approach is needed, one that integrates diverse technologies under a common framework and moves beyond isolated silos to a global "puzzle" where each piece addresses local demands (Huettemann et al., 2024). This requires multi-stakeholder collaboration and investment in digital public infrastructure to expand access to essential services (WHO, 2025). A promising example is the European Health Data Space (EHDS), which aims to establish a secure, interoperable framework for health data exchange across EU member states, supporting both individual care and public health while respecting national contexts (Proso, 2024).

Rigorous Medical Standards and Best Practices in Digital Care

Whilst digital health transformation gives the opportunity to reimagine care, maintaining rigorous medical standards and best practices in digital care is essential for patient safety and clinical effectiveness. The rapid proliferation of digital health technologies, including AI-driven diagnostics and self-management apps, raises critical questions about professional judgment, autonomy and clinical competence in an algorithm-influenced environment (Mennella et al., 2024; Natali et al., 2025). While AI and ML offer substantial potential to improve diagnostic accuracy, precise treatments and reduce clinician workload, they also introduce risks (Ammi et al., 2023; Leal Neto & Wyl, 2024; Williamson & Prybutok, 2024). Many digital solutions are developed and marketed without the rigorous regulatory oversight applied to conventional medical interventions, particularly in some regions, and there is often a lack of formal evaluation or standardized validation to confirm their clinical effectiveness (Popa et al., 2024). Moreover, algorithms trained on biased or incomplete datasets may produce inaccurate or inequitable outcomes, particularly for marginalized populations. In both the EU and the US, these technologies are increasingly regulated as medical devices, subject to safety, usability and quality standards, as well as post-market surveillance (Goktas & Grzybowski, 2025; Hendl & Shukla, 2024; Thacharodi et al., 2024).

Ensuring digital health best practices requires a digitally competent health workforce capable of using, managing and maintaining digital health systems effectively (Leal Neto & Wyl, 2024; Rao, 2023; WHO, 2025). This entails comprehensive training, competency frameworks and continuous education to bridge the gap between clinical practice and technological innovation (Garcia et al., 2024). Digital technologies must be designed to solve real-world problems, not simply to showcase technological capabilities (Sebire et al., 2025). Co-creation with patients and rigorous clinical trials are essential to ensure safety and relevance (Popa et al., 2024; Trzmielak et al., 2024). Additionally, AI algorithms must be continuously monitored and updated to detect errors, mitigate bias and maintain public trust (Bouderhem, 2024).

Ethical Implications and Concerns

The integration of AI and digital technologies also raises complex ethical concerns. The sensitive nature of health data, including medical and diagnostic records and treatment plans, intensifies concerns around data security, informed consent, ownership and potential misuse (Fitzpatrick, 2023; Mennella et al., 2024; Williamson & Prybutok, 2024). Patient autonomy may be compromised when data are shared or linked without explicit understanding, especially when consent is obtained through simplified mechanisms such as "I agree" buttons (Mennella et al., 2024; Thacharodi et al., 2024). The use and sharing of extensive patient data in AI development requires robust protection measures, including advanced anonymization, encryption and decentralized data management systems such as Blockchain (Williamson & Prybutok, 2024). Despite these safeguards, re-identification risks persist, and its implementation is still limited by computational overhead and scalability issues, which must be addressed to ensure performance at scale (Ganesan & Tong, 2024; Sabiri et al., 2025; Sharma & Kshetri, 2020).

The involvement of private entities in digital health raises further concerns about conflicts between commercial interests and patient privacy. High-profile cases, such as DeepMind's partnership with the Royal Free London NHS Foundation Trust, highlight the risks of data monetization and third-party sharing (Williamson & Prybutok, 2024). Patients must be clearly informed of their rights to withdraw data and provide renewed consent for new uses (Pergolizzi Jr. et al., 2023). Cultural beliefs, especially in LMICs, also influence attitudes toward digital health and consent, requiring culturally sensitive design and implementation strategies (Kozlakidis et al., 2024).

Comprehensive Regulatory Frameworks

The fast-paced evolution of digital health demands adaptive and comprehensive regulatory frameworks (Fitzpatrick, 2023; Thacharodi et al., 2024). Existing laws such as the General Data Protection Regulation (GDPR) in Europe and the Health Insurance Portability and Accountability Act (HIPAA) in the US are foundational but limited, particularly in governing non-traditional health data collected outside clinical settings, such as from IoT devices, leaving significant gaps in data governance (Goktas & Grzybowski, 2025; Pergolizzi Jr. et al., 2023; Singhal et al., 2024). The EU's AI Act complements GDPR by introducing a framework for the ethical and safe use of high-risk AI systems, including medical devices. It mandates transparency, data quality, human oversight and post-market monitoring, extending responsibilities to both developers and healthcare providers (Vardas et al., 2025). Globally, fragmented regulations hinder cross-border data exchange and limit the scalability of digital health and AI initiatives (Goktas & Grzybowski, 2025; Thacharodi et al., 2024). In many LMICs, regulatory frameworks remain unclear or underdeveloped, undermining trust and adoption (Kozlakidis et al., 2024). Algorithmic bias and discrimination also require urgent attention. AI systems trained on inequitable data risk perpetuating disparities unless dynamic oversight and inclusive design are prioritized (Goktas & Grzybowski, 2025; Leal Neto & Wyl, 2024; McCoy et al., 2025).

Opportunities

While the theoretical potential of digital health is vast, realizing its full benefits requires addressing the persistent disconnect between innovation and impact, a gap that demands rethinking care models and fostering sustained stakeholder commitment (Medical Association, 2022).

From Reactive to Proactive Care

One of the most significant opportunities lies in transitioning from reactive to proactive care. Digital health technologies enable earlier identification of health risks, support preventive interventions and empower individuals to manage their well-being (Maaß et al., 2022). Wearables and mobile applications facilitate continuous self-monitoring of biometric parameters, providing real-time insights that can prompt timely action (Leal Neto & Wyl, 2024; Rukundo, 2024). AI-powered predictive analytics further enhance this shift by identifying individuals at risk of developing specific conditions, enabling earlier diagnosis and more targeted interventions. Shifting from treatment to prevention has the potential to reduce disease burden and improve population health outcomes (Leal Neto & Wyl, 2024). Digital tools also enhance patient engagement and communication in primary care settings, contributing to more efficient and cost-effective service delivery (Kozlakidis et al., 2024).

Patient Empowerment and Autonomy in Everyday Living

Digital health empowers individuals to assume a more active role in managing their health, fostering their confidence and engagement in decision-making processes, all while remaining embedded in the routines of everyday life. Patient-facing applications (PFAs), such as health portals, appointment systems and medication reminders, offer convenient access to personal health data and promote transparency (Kozlakidis et al., 2024). These tools deliver tailored feedback and resources aligned with individual health goals, moving beyond generic public health messaging (Ferretti et al., 2023). This evolution supports the emergence of "consumerized" healthcare, where individuals are more actively involved in managing their own and their families' health. However, careful design is needed to avoid over-monitoring and unintended consequences (Trzmielak et al., 2024).

Advancement of Precision Medicine

By integrating omics data, big data analytics and population health data, digital tools enable data-rich decision-making that supports accurate, proactive and individualized care (Rukundo, 2024). AI plays a transformative role in this context by analysing vast datasets, including demographic, genetic and clinical information, to identify patterns and correlations that may elude human observation. These insights support more accurate diagnoses and highly targeted treatments, particularly in resource-limited settings. The vision of precision medicine, supported by high-quality datasets on diagnoses, treatments and drug effectiveness, promises to deliver tailored therapies and significantly improve health outcomes (Kozlakidis et al., 2024).

Digital Public Health

Beyond individual care, digital health offers immense potential to strengthen public health systems. The field of Digital Public Health has gained visibility, particularly during the COVID-19 pandemic, demonstrating how digital technologies can transform disease prevention, health promotion, surveillance and emergency response. Governments and policymakers are increasingly recognizing the value of leveraging digital health infrastructure for public health benefit. Digital tools support outbreak detection, data exchange, forecasting and evidence generation, enabling more agile and data-informed public health action (*Digital Technologies for Key Public Health Functions : Results of an ECDC Expert Consultation : May/June 2021*, 2021).

Digital tools can reach across geographic, socioeconomic and educational divides, enhancing both health and digital literacy (Fitzpatrick, 2023). Recent advances in LLMs offer new opportunities to deliver tailored, accessible health information at scale. These tools can adapt content to different education levels and cultural contexts, making public health messages more engaging and comprehensible (Leal Neto & Wyl, 2024).

Innovation Ecosystems and Startups

The rapid growth of digital health is also closely tied to innovation ecosystems and the role of startups. Since the COVID-19 pandemic, there has been a surge in digital health entrepreneurship. However, despite significant investment, many longstanding challenges, such as access, quality and equity, remain unresolved, highlighting a persistent "digital health disconnect". To bridge this gap, health technology companies are increasingly expected to develop solutions that reflect the needs of both patients and professionals, emphasizing equity, privacy by design, interoperability and support for integrated care pathways. Solutions that simplify workflows and improve coordination are particularly valuable in publicly funded systems, where efficiency and equitable access are central. Private investment continues to play a key role, especially when aligned with public health priorities and delivered through partnerships with national or regional authorities.

In Europe, the digital health market remains fragmented and sensitive to regulatory and economic shifts. Companies must demonstrate long-term value, sustainability and alignment with public interest to succeed (Medical Association, 2022). European policymakers are uniquely positioned to advance this transformation by streamlining regulatory approval processes, fostering procurement models that incentivize outcome-based care, and reinforcing robust data protection standards under the GDPR. Integrated digital health ecosystems, combining digital and in-person services through unified, citizen-facing platforms, are emerging as a strategic priority. These ecosystems typically involve collaboration among providers, payers, insurers and individuals-patients, coordinated by public institutions to improve system-wide efficiency and population health. Realizing this vision will require not only technical infrastructure, but also new governance models and cultural change across all stakeholders (Huettemann et al., 2024; Trzmielak et al., 2024).

LMICs vs. High-Income Countries (HICs)

Opportunities and challenges differ significantly between high-income countries (HICs) and LMICs. While HICs focus on optimizing tertiary care, LMICs can leverage simpler digital tools, such as SMS and social media, for effective health promotion (Ferretti et al., 2023; Kozlakidis et al., 2024). The COVID-19 pandemic also accelerated digital adoption in LMICs, particularly in the areas of surveillance and diagnostics. However, digitalization pathways in these settings are highly context-dependent and often centred on primary care, in contrast to the hospital-based services more commonly seen in HICs (Kozlakidis et al., 2024). Despite infrastructure barriers, digital health offers transformative potential in LMICs. Telemedicine, digital apps and EHRs can bridge geographic gaps and expand access to care (Kozlakidis et al., 2024). Innovations such as drone delivery of medicines, vaccines and diagnostic tests, as well as for identifying malaria-vector breeding sites, are already making an impact in sub-Saharan

Africa (Leal Neto & Wyl, 2024). Digital tools can also reduce long-term costs by improving efficiency and standardizing information flows. AI can automate administrative tasks, freeing up professionals for more meaningful interactions, while LLMs can enhance public health communication and health literacy (McCoy et al., 2025). To unlock this potential, LMICs require strategic investment in infrastructure, digital literacy, data protection and innovation (Kozlakidis et al., 2024; Rahul A. Lad & Bhawna Sharma Padroo, 2024). Policies must ensure equitable access and provide clear guidance on data governance and ownership (Kozlakidis et al., 2024; Leal Neto & Wyl, 2024). LMICs can also benefit from "reverse innovation", adapting core technologies to local contexts, and from co-creation approaches that build trust and ensure cultural relevance (Kozlakidis et al., 2024; Sebire et al., 2025).

ADVANCING EVIDENCE-BASED DIGITAL HEALTH

Given its inherently broad and interdisciplinary nature, digital health research must reflect its inherent complexity and diversity, encompassing domains such as clinical medicine, public health, biomedical engineering, data science, ethics and health economics (Cuff, 2023). Despite the growing body of work, the high pace of digital health development continues to surpass the generation of robust, generalizable evidence, creating a persistent lag between innovation and validation. This disconnect underscores the urgent need for research frameworks that are both agile and rigorous, capable of keeping pace with technological innovation while ensuring safety, efficacy and contextual relevance. Future research should adopt multidimensional and inclusive approaches that not only address methodological gaps and implementation barriers, but also ensure robust data protection, minimize algorithmic bias and support context-sensitive validation across diverse settings.

Strengthening Methodological Rigor and Participatory Design

The methodological rigor of digital health research must be significantly strengthened to ensure the validity, reproducibility and contextual relevance of findings. This requires the adoption of robust study designs, standardized outcome measures and transparent reporting practices. Moreover, participatory research approaches, where end users, including patients, caregivers and healthcare professionals, are actively involved in the co-design, development and evaluation of interventions, are essential to enhance usability, acceptability and real-world impact (Rauwerdink et al., 2024; Segur-Ferrer et al., 2024).

Bridging the Evidence–Implementation Gap

A persistent gap remains between the generation of evidence and its translation into clinical practice. Bridging this implementation gap is critical to ensure that digital health innovations move beyond pilot studies and academic publications to become integrated components of routine care. Implementation science frameworks should be leveraged to identify barriers and facilitators to adoption, assess fidelity and scalability, and support the adaptation of interventions across diverse healthcare settings (Yao et al., 2025).

Strengthening Validation and Regulatory Science

There is an urgent need to reinforce both scientific and regulatory pathways for the validation and certification of clinical-grade digital devices, especially those incorporating AI, sensors and real-time analytics. This entails not only rigorous academic research but also agile innovation models, often driven by start-ups and Small and medium-sized enterprises (SME), that can accelerate development and testing in real-world environments (Bakker et al., 2025). Regulatory science must evolve in parallel to accommodate the interactive nature of digital innovation while safeguarding patient safety and public trust.

Advancing Data Protection and Trust Frameworks

Safeguarding digital health data must be established as a distinct research priority, given the increasing volume, detail and sensitivity of the information being collected. As these data reflect continuous and richly contextual aspects of individuals' lives, it is essential to establish strong safeguards that ensure privacy, maintain data integrity and preserve user control. Emerging technologies such as blockchain, homomorphic encryption and decentralized identifiers (DIDs) offer promising possibilities for secure, privacy-preserving data exchange. Hybrid blockchain-edge computing architectures, in particular, show potential for enabling secure authentication and anonymization in IoT-based and interoperable environments (Shin et al., 2024; Yaqub et al., 2025).

Addressing Algorithmic Bias and Equity in AI

A critical and often underexplored research gap lies in the detection, mitigation and governance of algorithmic bias. AI systems trained on non-representative datasets risk perpetuating or amplifying health disparities, particularly among marginalized populations. Research should prioritize the development of fairness-aware algorithms, bias auditing tools and inclusive data governance models to ensure that digital health technologies promote equity rather than exacerbate existing inequalities (Alderman et al., 2025; Anderson & Visweswaran, 2025).

Evaluating Human–AI Interaction and Clinical Integration

As AI becomes more embedded in clinical workflows, understanding how healthcare professionals interact with algorithmic outputs is essential. Research should explore how trust is built or eroded, how clinicians interpret and act on AI recommendations, and how these systems influence decision-making, accountability and patient–provider relationships. This includes studying the mental, emotional and organizational impacts of AI integration in real-world settings (Garcia-Rudolph et al., 2025; Padhani & Papanikolaou, 2025).

Investigating Long-Term Impacts and Unintended Consequences

Most digital health studies focus on short-term outcomes, yet the long-term effects, both positive and adverse, remain poorly understood. Research must examine the sustained use of digital tools, their impact on health behaviours, clinical outcomes, system performance and potential unintended consequences such as overdiagnosis, digital fatigue or increased health anxiety (Alanzi et al., 2024; Chauhan et al., 2025; Jacob et al., 2023).

Embracing Multidimensional Outcome Evaluation

Outcome evaluation in digital health must adopt a multidimensional analysis. Beyond clinical efficacy, research must assess economic, technological, organizational, social, cultural, ethical, legal, environmental, political and regulatory dimensions (Yao et al., 2025). This comprehensive perspective is vital to determine not only whether an intervention works, but also for whom, under what conditions and at what cost.

Demonstrating Economic Value and Sustainability

The sustainable adoption of digital health technologies hinges on demonstrating their economic value. Research must apply value-based frameworks that assess cost-effectiveness, resource optimization and long-term impacts on health outcomes and system performance. Without robust economic evidence, even technically sound and clinically effective innovations may struggle to gain traction in policy and practice (Douglas et al., 2025; Khalil et al., 2025; J. Zhang et al., 2025).

Building Capacity for Digital Health Research in Low-Resource Settings

Finally, there is a pressing need to support context-specific research in LMICs, where digital health holds transformative potential but faces unique infrastructural, cultural and regulatory challenges. Research in these settings should prioritize co-creation, local capacity building and the development of scalable, low-cost and culturally appropriate solutions (Craig et al., 2025; Le et al., 2025).

Ensuring that digital health innovations are not only technically robust but also clinically relevant, economically viable and ethically grounded is essential for their long-term integration into health systems. As the field matures, fostering collaborative, interdisciplinary and impact-driven research will be key to translating digital potential into measurable and meaningful health outcomes, through equitable approaches and secure integration into real-world healthcare contexts.

CONCLUSION AND FUTURE DIRECTIONS

The digital transformation of healthcare represents a profound systemic, cultural and epistemological shift that is redefining how health is understood, delivered and experienced. As demonstrated throughout this chapter, digital health is evolving from isolated technological applications into a dynamic, interconnected and multidimensional ecosystem that spans clinical care, public health, biomedical innovation and patient empowerment. The convergence of technologies including artificial intelligence (AI), the Internet of Things (IoT), digital therapeutics (DTx), extended reality (XR) and multi-omics platforms, are enabling precise, predictive, preventive and participatory models of care.

However, healthcare digital transformation is not without its challenges. The digital divide remains a critical barrier, threatening to exacerbate existing health inequities if disparities in access, infrastructure and digital literacy are not addressed. Integrating digital solutions into legacy health systems continues to face structural, financial and interoperability constraints. Moreover, the rapid pace of innovation often outpaces the development of robust evidence, regulatory oversight and ethical safeguards. As the field matures, addressing these multifaceted challenges requires a comprehensive and forward-looking research agenda grounded in a sustained, interdisciplinary and human-centred approach. This includes strengthening methodological rigor, bridging the gap between evidence and implementation, and adopting multidimensional evaluation frameworks that account for clinical, economic, social and ethical dimensions. Regulatory and ethical frameworks must be developed alongside technological innovation, not to hinder progress, but to ensure that advances in digital health enhance data privacy, algorithmic transparency and patient autonomy without imposing unnecessary barriers to innovation. The emergence of AI-driven decision support systems and self-management tools further underscores the need for clear accountability, human oversight and inclusive design that respects diverse user needs and cultural contexts. Ensuring that digital health interventions are clinically validated, ethically grounded, and contextually adapted is essential to avoid unintended harms and to foster trust among users and professionals alike.

Looking ahead, the future of digital health will depend on the ability of stakeholders to co-create inclusive, resilient and ethically grounded digital ecosystems. This will require sustained investment in digital infrastructure, education and governance, the development of interoperable and secure platforms, and the formation of collaborative networks that bridge academia, industry, healthcare systems and civil society. VBHC models, guided by real-world evidence and focused on outcomes rather than volume, must inform the evaluation and adoption of digital interventions to ensure they deliver measurable improvements in health outcomes, system performance and equity.

Ultimately, digital health represents not just a technological revolution, but a human-centred transformation. Its true success lies in its ability to empower individuals, strengthen health systems and promote well-being for people of all backgrounds and in every context, demonstrating that meaningful progress is defined by the positive impact on lives, rather than by technological sophistication alone. Central to this transformation is the shift towards precise health management, where individuals are empowered with digital tools that support autonomous decision-making, self-monitoring and lifestyle modification, meeting them where they are, within their own routines, contexts and communities. This evolution places patients at the center of their health journeys, with intelligent systems that foresee risks, guide prevention and trigger timely responses, calling on healthcare providers when appropriate. As we move forward, the challenge is not simply to innovate, but to do so responsibly, inclusively and with a steadfast commitment to the public good, ensuring that technological progress in healthcare remains aligned with the core principles of human competence, compassion, and fairness.

The time to act decisively and collaboratively is now, ensuring that the digital transformation of healthcare not only advances technological frontiers, but also empowers individuals to take greater ownership of their health, upholds the enduring values of human expertise, empathy and justice, and shapes a future where innovation truly serves the well-being of All.

REFERENCES

Abrar, H., Hussain, S. J., Chaudhry, J., Saleem, K., Orgun, M. A., Al-Muhtadi, J., & Valli, C. (2018). Risk Analysis of Cloud Sourcing in Healthcare and Public Health Industry. *IEEE Access : Practical Innovations, Open Solutions*, *6*, 19140–19150. DOI: 10.1109/ACCESS.2018.2805919

Action plan for the prevention and control of noncommunicable diseases in South-East Asia, 2013-2020 SEA-NCD-101 Distribution: General. (2022). https://apps.who.int/bookorders

Alanzi, T. M., Arif, W., Aljohani, N., Jabali, A., Junainah, M., Aldeen Mohamed, E., Hamdi, T., Mansour, N., Badawood, N., Alghamdi, S., Alanazi, D., Alanzi, N., & Alqurashi, N. (2024). Exploring the Impact of Digital Health Tools in Enhancing Quality of Life and Psychological Adjustment in Long-term Blood Donors: A Cross-Sectional Study. *Cureus*. Advance online publication. DOI: 10.7759/cureus.75123

Alderman, J. E., Palmer, J., Laws, E., McCradden, M. D., Ordish, J., Ghassemi, M., Pfohl, S. R., Rostamzadeh, N., Cole-Lewis, H., Glocker, B., Calvert, M., Pollard, T. J., Gill, J., Gath, J., Adebajo, A., Beng, J., Leung, C. H., Kuku, S., Farmer, L. A., . . . Liu, X. (2025). Tackling algorithmic bias and promoting transparency in health datasets: the STANDING Together consensus recommendations. In *The Lancet Digital Health* (Vol. 7, Issue 1, pp. e64–e88). Elsevier Ltd. DOI: 10.1016/S2589-7500(24)00224-3

Alfano, M., Kellett, J., Lenzitti, B., & Helfert, M. (2023). *Intelligent Provision of Tailored, Easily Understood, and Trusted Health Information for Patient Empowerment*. 384–391. DOI: 10.5220/0011694300003414

Alhammad, N., Alajlani, M., Abd-Alrazaq, A., Epiphaniou, G., & Arvanitis, T. (2024). Patients' Perspectives on the Data Confidentiality, Privacy, and Security of mHealth Apps: Systematic Review. In *Journal of Medical Internet Research* (Vol. 26). JMIR Publications Inc. DOI: 10.2196/50715

Alruwaili, M. M., Shaban, M., & Elsayed Ramadan, O. M. (2023). Digital Health Interventions for Promoting Healthy Aging: A Systematic Review of Adoption Patterns, Efficacy, and User Experience. In *Sustainability (Switzerland)* (Vol. 15, Issue 23). Multidisciplinary Digital Publishing Institute (MDPI). DOI: 10.3390/su152316503

Ammi, C., Kondrateva, G., & Baudier, P. (2023). Healthcare Sustainability: The Role of Artificial Intelligence Acceptance by Medical Staff. *Journal of Innovation Economics & Management. Prépublication*, (0), I159–XXXV. DOI: 10.3917/jie.pr1.0159

Anderson, J. W., & Visweswaran, S. (2025). Algorithmic individual fairness and healthcare: A scoping review. In *JAMIA Open* (Vol. 8, Issue 1). Oxford University Press. DOI: 10.1093/jamiaopen/ooae149

Asgari, E., Kaur, J., Nuredini, G., Balloch, J., Taylor, A. M., Sebire, N., Robinson, R., Peters, C., Sridharan, S., & Pimenta, D. (2024). Impact of Electronic Health Record Use on Cognitive Load and Burnout Among Clinicians: Narrative Review. In *JMIR Medical Informatics* (Vol. 12). JMIR Publications Inc., DOI: 10.2196/55499

Bakare, O. S. (2025). AI-Driven Multi-Omics Integration for Precision Medicine in Complex Disease Diagnosis and Treatment. *International Journal of Research Publication and Reviews*, *6*(6), 5070–5084. DOI: 10.55248/gengpi.6.0125.0650

Bakker, J. P., McClenahan, S. J., Fromy, P., Turner, S., Peterson, B. T., Vandendriessche, B., & Goldsack, J. C. (2025). A Hierarchical Framework for Selecting Reference Measures for the Analytical Validation of Sensor-Based Digital Health Technologies. In *Journal of Medical Internet Research* (Vol. 27). JMIR Publications Inc., DOI: 10.2196/58956

Barilan, Y. M. (2022). Personalization, individuation, and the ethos of precision medicine. In *Can precision medicine be personal; Can personalized medicine be precise?* (pp. 89–106). Oxford University PressOxford., DOI: 10.1093/oso/9780198863465.003.0007

Barracca, A., Ledda, S., Mancosu, G., Pintore, G., Quintaliani, G., Ronco, C., & Kashani, K. B. (2023). Digital Health: A New Frontier. *Journal of Translational Critical Care Medicine*, *5*(2). Advance online publication. DOI: 10.1097/jtccm-d-22-00018

Beattie, Z., Miller, L. M., Almirola, C., Au-Yeung, W.-T. M., Bernard, H., Cosgrove, K. E., Dodge, H. H., Gamboa, C. J., Golonka, O., Gothard, S., Harbison, S., Irish, S., Kornfeld, J., Lee, J., Marcoe, J., Mattek, N. C., Quinn, C., Reynolds, C., Riley, T., & Kaye, J. (2020). The Collaborative Aging Research Using Technology Initiative: An Open, Sharable, Technology-Agnostic Platform for the Research Community. *Digital Biomarkers*, *4*(Suppl. 1), 100–118. DOI: 10.1159/000512208

Bekbolatova, M., Mayer, J., Ong, C. W., & Toma, M. (2024). Transformative Potential of AI in Healthcare: Definitions, Applications, and Navigating the Ethical Landscape and Public Perspectives. In *Healthcare (Switzerland)* (Vol. 12, Issue 2). Multidisciplinary Digital Publishing Institute (MDPI). DOI: 10.3390/healthcare12020125

Bernardes, R. A. (2025). Use of technologies in healthcare: Advances and challenges. *Revista Contexto & Saúde*, *25*(50), e17007. DOI: 10.21527/2176-7114.2025.50.17007

Bienefeld, N., Keller, E., & Grote, G. (2025). AI Interventions to Alleviate Healthcare Shortages and Enhance Work Conditions in Critical Care: Qualitative Analysis. *Journal of Medical Internet Research*, *27*. Advance online publication. DOI: 10.2196/50852

Bitkina, O. V., Park, J., & Kim, H. K. (2023). Application of artificial intelligence in medical technologies: A systematic review of main trends. In *Digital Health* (Vol. 9). SAGE Publications Inc., DOI: 10.1177/20552076231189331

Bostan, S., Johnson, O. A., Jaspersen, L. J., & Randell, R. (2024). Contextual Barriers to Implementing Open-Source Electronic Health Record Systems for Low- and Lower-Middle-Income Countries: Scoping Review. *Journal of Medical Internet Research*, *26*, e45242. DOI: 10.2196/45242

Bouderhem, R. (2024). Shaping the future of AI in healthcare through ethics and governance. *Humanities & Social Sciences Communications*, *11*(1). Advance online publication. DOI: 10.1057/s41599-024-02894-w

Burrell, A., Zrubka, Z., Champion, A., Zah, V., Vinuesa, L., Holtorf, A.-P., Di Bidino, R., Rao Earla, J., Entwistle, J., Tarasovic Boltyenkov, A., Braileanu, G., Kolasa, K., Roydhouse, J., & Asche, C. (2022). How Useful Are Digital Health Terms for Outcomes Research? An ISPOR Special Interest Group Report. *Value in Health*, *25*, 1469–1479. DOI: 10.1016/j.jval.2

Butcher, C. J. T., & Hussain, W. (2022). Digital healthcare: The future. *Future Healthcare Journal*, *9*(2), 113–117. DOI: 10.7861/fhj.2022-0046

C, C. D. (2022). *CDC Global Digital Health Strategy DRAFT Report subtitle Second line if needed.* https://www.cdc.gov/global-health/media/pdfs/GDHS_Strategy2022_REV_508.pdf

Cancela, J., Charlafti, I., Colloud, S., & Wu, C. (2020). Digital health in the era of personalized healthcare: Opportunities and challenges for bringing research and patient care to a new level. In *Digital Health: Mobile and Wearable Devices for Participatory Health Applications* (pp. 7–31). Elsevier. DOI: 10.1016/B978-0-12-820077-3.00002-X

Canfell, O. J., Davidson, K., Woods, L., Sullivan, C., Cocoros, N. M., Klompas, M., Zambarano, B., Eakin, E., Littlewood, R., & Burton-Jones, A. (2022). Precision Public Health for Non-communicable Diseases: An Emerging Strategic Roadmap and Multinational Use Cases. *Frontiers in Public Health, 10.* Advance online publication. DOI: 10.3389/fpubh.2022.854525

Chauhan, G. K., Vavken, P., & Jacob, C. (2025). Mobile Apps and Wearable Devices for Cardiovascular Health: Narrative Review. In *JMIR mHealth and uHealth* (Vol. 13, pp. e65782–e65782). DOI: 10.2196/65782

Clements, M., Kaufman, N., & Mel, E. (2023). Using Digital Health Technology to Prevent and Treat Diabetes. *Diabetes Technology & Therapeutics, 25*(S1), S-90–S-108. DOI: 10.1089/dia.2023.2506

Collecchia, G., & De Gobbi, R. (2024). From personalized medicine to precision medicine. In *AI in Clinical Practice* (pp. 99–103). Elsevier., DOI: 10.1016/B978-0-443-14054-9.00004-1

Collins, F. S., & Varmus, H. (2015). A New Initiative on Precision Medicine. *The New England Journal of Medicine, 372*(9), 793–795. DOI: 10.1056/NEJMp1500523

Craig, A., Lawford, H., Miller, M., Chen-Cao, L., Woods, L., Liaw, S. T., & Godinho, M. A. (2025). Use of Technology to Support Health Care Providers Delivering Care in Low- and Lower-Middle-Income Countries: Systematic Umbrella Review. In *Journal of Medical Internet Research* (Vol. 27). JMIR Publications Inc., DOI: 10.2196/66288

Cruz Castañeda, W. A., & Bertemes Filho, P. (2023). *Towards an Artificial Intelligence Based Chronic Disease Management.* DOI: 10.20944/preprints202304.0491.v1

Cuff, A. (2023). The evolution of digital health and its continuing challenges. *BMC Digital Health, 1*(1). Advance online publication. DOI: 10.1186/s44247-022-00004-x

Dal Mas, F., Massaro, M., Rippa, P., & Secundo, G. (2023). The challenges of digital transformation in healthcare: An interdisciplinary literature review, framework, and future research agenda. *Technovation, 123.* Advance online publication. DOI: 10.1016/j.technovation.2023.102716

Davenport, T., & Kalakota, R. (2019). DIGITAL TECHNOLOGY The potential for artificial intelligence in healthcare. *Future Healthcare Journal, 6*(2), •••.

Davis, S. L. M. (2025). Political determinants of digital health: Beyond the rainbow. *Health Promotion International, 40*(2). Advance online publication. DOI: 10.1093/heapro/daaf014

de Jong, J., Cutcutache, I., Page, M., Elmoufti, S., Dilley, C., Fröhlich, H., & Armstrong, M. (2021). Towards realizing the vision of precision medicine: AI based prediction of clinical drug response. *Brain, 144*(6), 1738–1750. DOI: 10.1093/brain/awab108

Denysyuk, H. V., Pires, I. M., & Garcia, N. M. (2024). A roadmap for empowering cardiovascular disease patients: A 5P-Medicine approach and technological integration. *PeerJ*, *12*(8). Advance online publication. DOI: 10.7717/peerj.17895

Digital technologies for key public health functions : results of an ECDC expert consultation : May/ June 2021. (2021). ECDC.

Douglas, A. O., Senkaiahliyan, S., Bulstra, C. A., Mita, C., Reddy, C. L., & Atun, R. (2025). Global Adoption of Value-Based Health Care Initiatives Within Health Systems: A Scoping Review. In *JAMA Health Forum* (Vol. 6, Issue 5). American Medical Association. DOI: 10.1001/jamahealthforum.2025.0746

DuBord, A. Y., Paolillo, E. W., & Staffaroni, A. M. (2024). Remote Digital Technologies for the Early Detection and Monitoring of Cognitive Decline in Patients With Type 2 Diabetes: Insights From Studies of Neurodegenerative Diseases. *Journal of Diabetes Science and Technology*, *18*(6), 1489–1499. DOI: 10.1177/19322968231171399

European Commission. (2020). Digital health and care. In https://health.ec.europa.eu/ehealth-digital-health-and-care/digital-health-and-care_en. https://health.ec.europa.eu/ehealth-digital-health-and-care/digital-health-and-care_en

Eysenbach, G. (2001). What is e-health? In *Journal of Medical Internet Research* (Vol. 3, Issue 2, pp. 1–5). JMIR Publications Inc. DOI: 10.2196/jmir.3.2.e20

FDA. (2020). What is Digital Health? In https://www.fda.gov/medical-devices/digital-health-center-excellence/what-digital-health

Ferretti, A., Vayena, E., & Blasimme, A. (2023). Unlock digital health promotion in LMICs to benefit the youth. In *PLOS Digital Health* (Vol. 2, Issue 8). Public Library of Science. DOI: 10.1371/journal.pdig.0000315

Fitzpatrick, P. J. (2023). Improving health literacy using the power of digital communications to achieve better health outcomes for patients and practitioners. In *Frontiers in Digital Health* (Vol. 5). Frontiers Media SA. DOI: 10.3389/fdgth.2023.1264780

Gadsden, T., Patel, A., Praveen, D., & Palagyi, A. (2023). Transfer or tailor? Implementing a technology-supported intervention for noncommunicable diseases across contexts. In *Health Care Science* (Vol. 2, Issue 1, pp. 75–78). John Wiley and Sons Inc. DOI: 10.1002/hcs2.26

Ganesan, B., & Tong, R. K. Y. (2024). Historical overview and the evolution of digital health. In *Digital Technology in Public Health and Rehabilitation Care: COVID Era* (pp. 3–18). Elsevier. DOI: 10.1016/B978-0-443-22270-2.00001-0

Garcia, M. B., Arif, Y. M., Khlaif, Z. N., Zhu, M., de Almeida, R. P. P., de Almeida, R. S., & Masters, K. (2024). Effective integration of artificial intelligence in medical education: Practical tips and actionable insights. In *Transformative Approaches to Patient Literacy and Healthcare Innovation* (pp. 1–19). IGI Global., DOI: 10.4018/979-8-3693-3661-8.ch001

Garcia-Rudolph, A., Sánchez-Pinsach, D., Gilabert, A., Sauri, J., Soler, M. D., & Opisso, E. (2025). Building Trust with AI: How Essential is Validating AI Models in the Therapeutic Triad of Therapist, Patient, and Artificial Third? Comment on What is the Current and Future Status of Digital Mental Health Interventions? *The Spanish Journal of Psychology*, *28*, e3–e3. DOI: 10.1017/SJP.2024.32

Garg, S. K., Rodriguez, E., Shah, V. N., & Hirsch, I. B. (2022). New Medications for the Treatment of Diabetes. *Diabetes Technology & Therapeutics*, *24*(S1), S-190–S-208. DOI: 10.1089/dia.2022.2513

Giger, O. F., Fleisch, E., Jovanova, M., & Kowatsch, T. (2025). Barriers and facilitators of implementing value-based care: The case of SwissDiabeter. *Digital Health*, *11*. Advance online publication. DOI: 10.1177/20552076251336322

Goktas, P., & Grzybowski, A. (2025). Shaping the Future of Healthcare: Ethical Clinical Challenges and Pathways to Trustworthy AI. *Journal of Clinical Medicine*, *14*(5). Advance online publication. DOI: 10.3390/jcm14051605

Gopinathan, P., Kaur, J., Joshi, S., Prasad, V. M., Pujari, S., Panda, P., & Murthy, P. (2018). Self-reported quit rates and quit attempts among subscribers of a mobile text messaging-based tobacco cessation programme in India. *BMJ Innovations*, *4*(4), 147–154. DOI: 10.1136/bmjinnov-2018-000285

Hasin, Y., Seldin, M., & Lusis, A. (2017). Multi-omics approaches to disease. In *Genome Biology* (Vol. 18, Issue 1). BioMed Central Ltd. DOI: 10.1186/s13059-017-1215-1

Hatef, E., Richards, T., Hail, S., Zhang, T., Topel, K., Kitchen, C., Shaw, K. C., & Weiner, J. P. (2025). An Electronic Health Record–Based Platform for Social Needs Assessment and Navigation Services: Preliminary Results of an RCT. *AJPM Focus*, *4*(4), 100344. DOI: 10.1016/j.focus.2025.100344

Hazra-Ganju, A., Dlima, S. D., Menezes, S. R., Ganju, A., & Mer, A. (2023). An omni-channel, outcomes-focused approach to scale digital health interventions in resource-limited populations: A case study. *Frontiers in Digital Health*, *5*. Advance online publication. DOI: 10.3389/fdgth.2023.1007687

He, T., Cui, W., Feng, Y., Li, X., & Yu, G. (2024). Digital health integration for noncommunicable diseases: Comprehensive process mapping for full-life-cycle management. *Journal of Evidence-Based Medicine*, *17*(1), 26–36. DOI: 10.1111/jebm.12583

Hendl, T., & Shukla, A. (2024). Can digital health democratize health care? *Bioethics*, *38*(6), 491–502. DOI: 10.1111/bioe.13266

Herrick, T., Digre, P., & Yoden, S. S. (2024). Building the evidence base for the economic value of digital health interventions: Examples of methods and metrics and opportunities for future directions. *Oxford Open Digital Health*, *2*(Supplement_2), ii1–ii3. DOI: 10.1093/oodh/oqae042

HIMSS. (2020). HIMSS Defines Digital Health for the Global Healthcare Industry. In https://legacy.himss.org/news/himss-defines-digital-health-global-healthcare-industry. https://legacy.himss.org/news/himss-defines-digital-health-global-healthcare-industry

Hua, D. (2023). *Understanding the factors influencing acceptability of AI in medical imaging domains among healthcare professionals*.

Huerta-Chagoya, A., Kim, J., Mandla, R., Lu, Y., Suzuki, K., Petty, L. E., Ng, H. K., Choi, J., Lee, S., Rout, M., Lin, K., Adair, L. S., Adeyemo, A., Ahsan, H., Akiyama, M., An, P., Anand, S. S., Becker, D. M., Bertoni, A. G., & Ng, M. C. Y. (2025). *Multi-ancestry polygenic risk scores for the prediction of type 2 diabetes and complications in diverse ancestries*. DOI: 10.1101/2025.07.21.25331778

Huettemann, R., Sevov, B., Meister, S., & Fehring, L. (2024). How to establish digital health ecosystems from the perspective of health service-organizations: A taxonomy developed based on expert interviews conducted as modified Delphi approach. *Digital Health, 10*. Advance online publication. DOI: 10.1177/20552076241271890

Iyamu, I., Xu, A. X. T., Gómez-Ramírez, O., Ablona, A., Chang, H.-J., Mckee, G., & Gilbert, M. (2021). Defining Digital Public Health and the Role of Digitization, Digitalization, and Digital Transformation: Scoping Review. *JMIR Public Health and Surveillance, 11*. Advance online publication. DOI: 10.2196/30399

Jacob, C., Lindeque, J., Klein, A., Ivory, C., Heuss, S., & Peter, M. K. (2023). Assessing the Quality and Impact of eHealth Tools: Systematic Literature Review and Narrative Synthesis. *JMIR Human Factors, 10*. Advance online publication. DOI: 10.2196/45143

Johnson, K. B., Wei, W. Q., Weeraratne, D., Frisse, M. E., Misulis, K., Rhee, K., Zhao, J., & Snowdon, J. L. (2021). Precision Medicine, AI, and the Future of Personalized Health Care. In *Clinical and Translational Science* (Vol. 14, Issue 1, pp. 86–93). Blackwell Publishing Ltd. DOI: 10.1111/cts.12884

Joshi, S., Bagayoko, C. O., Babington-Ashaye, A., & Geissbuhler, A. (2023). Digital technologies for NCD prevention and control. In *Noncommunicable Diseases: A Compendium* (pp. 362–368). Taylor and Francis., DOI: 10.4324/9781003306689-54

Kanade, T. (2024). *Digital Health Innovations to Significantly Improve the Quality of Services in Healthcare Systems.*

Karczewski, K. J., & Snyder, M. P. (2018). Integrative omics for health and disease. *Nature Reviews. Genetics, 19*, 299–310. DOI: 10.1038/nrg.2018.4

Kasoju, N., Remya, N. S., Sasi, R., Sujesh, S., Soman, B., Kesavadas, C., Muraleedharan, C. V., Varma, P. R. H., & Behari, S. (2023). Digital health: Trends, opportunities and challenges in medical devices, pharma and bio-technology. *CSI Transactions on ICT, 11*(1), 11–30. DOI: 10.1007/s40012-023-00380-3

Kaufman, J. M., Thommandram, A., & Fossat, Y. (2023). Acoustic Analysis and Prediction of Type 2 Diabetes Mellitus Using Smartphone-Recorded Voice Segments. *Mayo Clinic Proceedings. Digital Health, 1*(4), 534–544. DOI: 10.1016/j.mcpdig.2023.08.005

Keshavarz, H., Saeidnia, H. R., & Wang, T. (2025). Navigating technostress: A deep dive into health practitioners' technological challenges in hospital settings. *BMC Health Services Research, 25*(1). Advance online publication. DOI: 10.1186/s12913-024-12196-1

Khalil, H., Ameen, M., Davies, C., & Liu, C. (2025). Implementing value-based healthcare: a scoping review of key elements, outcomes, and challenges for sustainable healthcare systems. In *Frontiers in Public Health* (Vol. 13). Frontiers Media SA. DOI: 10.3389/fpubh.2025.1514098

Kim, K. K., & Backonja, U. (2025). Digital health equity frameworks and key concepts: A scoping review. In *Journal of the American Medical Informatics Association* (Vol. 32, Issue 5, pp. 932–944). Oxford University Press. DOI: 10.1093/jamia/ocaf017

Kounatidis, D., Vallianou, N. G., Karampela, I., Rebelos, E., Kouveletsou, M., Dalopoulos, V., Koufopoulos, P., Diakoumopoulou, E., Tentolouris, N., & Dalamaga, M. (2024). Anti-Diabetic Therapies and Cancer: From Bench to Bedside. *Biomolecules*, *14*(11), 1479. DOI: 10.3390/biom14111479

Kozlakidis, Z., Muradyan, A., & Sargsyann, K. (2024). *Digitalization of Medicine in Low- and Middle-Income Countries*.

Kvedar, J., Coye, M. J., & Everett, W. (2014). Connected health: A review of technologies and strategies to improve patient care with telemedicine and telehealth. *Health Affairs*, *33*(2), 194–199. DOI: 10.1377/hlthaff.2013.0992

Label2Enable. (n.d.). Https://Label2enable.Eu/about-the-Project.

Labrique, A. B., Wadhwani, C., Williams, K. A., Lamptey, P., Hesp, C., Luk, R., & Aerts, A. (2018). Best practices in scaling digital health in low and middle income countries. In *Globalization and Health* (Vol. 14, Issue 1). BioMed Central Ltd. DOI: 10.1186/s12992-018-0424-z

Lad, R. A., & Padroo, B. S. (2024). Advancements and challenges in digital health implementation in India: A comprehensive literature review. *World Journal of Biology Pharmacy and Health Sciences*, *18*(1), 205–208. DOI: 10.30574/wjbphs.2024.18.1.0186

Le, H. T., Vu, D. V. T., Nguyen, T. N. A., Thi, H. T., Nguyen, T. V., Tran, T. P., Kekalih, A., Rijal, S., Friska, D., Hamers, R. L., Karkey, A., Chambers, M., Van Nuil, J. I., Lewycka, S., Bhandari, A. R., Bogh, C., Bui, T. H. N., Deokota, D., Dien, S. W. R., . . . Pham, T. Q. (2025). Research Electronic Data Capture (REDCap) for Population-Based Data Collection in Low- and Middle-Income Countries: Opportunities, Challenges, and Solutions. In *Journal of Medical Internet Research* (Vol. 27). JMIR Publications Inc. DOI: 10.2196/65377

Leal Neto, O., & Wyl, V. (2024). *Digital Transformation of Public Health for Noncommunicable Diseases: Narrative Viewpoint of Challenges and Opportunities Rights / license: Creative Commons Attribution 4.0 International*. DOI: 10.3929/ethz-b-000657624

Lebaea, R., Roshe, Y., Ntontela, S., & Thango, B. A. (2024). *The Role of Data Governance in Ensuring System Success and Long-Term IT Performance: A Systematic Review*. DOI: 10.20944/preprints202410.1841.v1

Leistner, T., & Kowatsch, T. (2023). *Digital Therapeutics for Healthy Longevity: A Roadmap*. 616–622. DOI: 10.5220/0011778500003414

Maaß, L., Pan, C. C., & Freye, M. (2022). Mapping Digital Public Health Interventions among Existing Digital Technologies and Internet-Based Interventions to Maintain and Improve Population Health in Practice: Protocol for a Scoping Review. In *JMIR Research Protocols* (Vol. 11, Issue 3). JMIR Publications Inc. DOI: 10.2196/33404

Maha, C. C., Kolawole, T. O., & Abdul, S. (2024). Harnessing data analytics: A new frontier in predicting and preventing non-communicable diseases in the US and Africa. *Computer Science & IT Research Journal*, *5*(6), 1247–1264. DOI: 10.51594/csitrj.v5i6.1196

Martin, M. S., & Alarcón-Urbistondo, P. (2024). *Digital Transformation in Healthcare and Medical Practices.*, DOI: 10.4018/979-8-3693-1214-8.ch009

McCoy, L. G., Bihorac, A., Celi, L. A., Elmore, M., Kewalramani, D., Kwaga, T., Martinez-Martin, N., Prôa, R., Schamroth, J., Shaffer, J. D., Youssef, A., & Fiske, A. (2025). Building health systems capable of leveraging AI: Applying Paul Farmer's 5S framework for equitable global health. *BMC Global and Public Health*, *3*(1), 39. DOI: 10.1186/s44263-025-00158-6

Medical Association. A. (2022). *Future of Health Closing the Digital Health Disconnect: A Blueprint for Optimizing Digitally Enabled Care About the AMA*. https://www.ama-assn.org/terms-use

Meier, E., Rigter, T., Schijven, M. P., van den Hoven, M., & Bak, M. A. R. (2024). The impact of digital health technologies on moral responsibility: a scoping review. In *Medicine, Health Care and Philosophy*. Springer Science and Business Media B.V. DOI: 10.1007/s11019-024-10238-3

Mennella, C., Maniscalco, U., De Pietro, G., & Esposito, M. (2024). Ethical and regulatory challenges of AI technologies in healthcare: A narrative review. In *Heliyon* (Vol. 10, Issue 4). Elsevier Ltd. DOI: 10.1016/j.heliyon.2024.e26297

Meskó, B. (2022). COVID-19's Impact on Digital Health Adoption: The Growing Gap Between a Technological and a Cultural Transformation. *JMIR Human Factors*, *9*(3). Advance online publication. DOI: 10.2196/38926

Meskó, B., & de Bronkart, D. (2022). Patient Design: The Importance of including Patients in Designing Health Care. In *Journal of Medical Internet Research* (Vol. 24, Issue 8). JMIR Publications Inc. DOI: 10.2196/39178

Mesko, B., DeBronkart, D., Dhunnoo, P., Arvai, N., Katonai, G., & Riggare, S. (2025). The Evolution of Patient Empowerment and Its Impact on Health Care's Future. In *Journal of Medical Internet Research* (Vol. 27). JMIR Publications Inc., DOI: 10.2196/60562

Mitra, U., & Rehman, S. U. (2024). *Leveraging AI and Machine Learning for Next-Generation Clinical Decision Support Systems*. CDSS., DOI: 10.4018/979-8-3693-7277-7.ch003

Moberly, T. (2025). Doctors must stop using unregistered AI scribe tools, says NHS England. *BMJ (Clinical Research Ed.)*, *389*, r1302. DOI: 10.1136/bmj.r1302

Monzani, D., & Pizzoli, S. F. M. (2020). The Prevention of Chronic Diseases Through eHealth: A Practical Overview. In *P5 eHealth: An Agenda for the Health Technologies of the Future* (pp. 33–51). Springer International Publishing. DOI: 10.1007/978-3-030-27994-3_3

Nadhamuni, S., Gupta, G., Mullath, R., & Sridhar, S. (2020). Leveraging Technology to Enable Effective Preventive Screening of NCDs at Population Scale: Initial Observations. In *Journal of the Indian Institute of Science* (Vol. 100, Issue 4, pp. 691–700). Springer. DOI: 10.1007/s41745-020-00199-w

Natali, C., Marconi, L., Denisse Dias Duran, L., Miglioretti, M., & Cabitza, F. (2025). *Highlights AI-induced deskilling in medicine: a mixed method literature review for setting a new research agenda AI-induced deskilling in medicine: a mixed method literature review for setting a new research agenda.* https://ssrn.com/abstract=5166364

NHS England. (2025, April). *Guidance on the use of AI-enabled ambient scribing products in health and care settings.* Https://Www.England.Nhs.Uk/Long-Read/Guidance-on-the-Use-of-Ai-Enabled-Ambient-Scribing-Products-in-Health-and-Care-Settings/.

OECD. (2023). *Health at a Glance 2023*. OECD. DOI: 10.1787/7a7afb35-en

Ogundiya, O., Rahman, T. J., Valnarov-Boulter, I., & Young, T. M. (2024). Looking Back on Digital Medical Education Over the Last 25 Years and Looking to the Future: Narrative Review. In *Journal of Medical Internet Research* (Vol. 26). JMIR Publications Inc. DOI: 10.2196/60312

Oyeniyi, J. (2024). The role of AI and mobile apps in patient-centric healthcare delivery. *World Journal of Advanced Research and Reviews*, *22*(1), 1897–1907. DOI: 10.30574/wjarr.2024.22.1.1331

Padhani, A. R., & Papanikolaou, N. (2025). AI and human interactions in prostate cancer diagnosis using MRI. *European Radiology*. Advance online publication. DOI: 10.1007/s00330-025-11498-0

Palabindala, V., Pamarthy, A., & Jonnalagadda, N. R. (2016). Adoption of electronic health records and barriers. *Journal of Community Hospital Internal Medicine Perspectives*, *6*(5), 32643. DOI: 10.3402/jchimp.v6.32643

Pandey, A., & Gupta, S. P. (2024). Personalized Medicine: A Comprehensive Review. *Oriental Journal of Chemistry*, *40*(4), 933–944. DOI: 10.13005/ojc/400403

Paulchamy, B. (2024). *Revolutionizing Healthcare Systems with Advanced Deep Learning Integration for Enhanced Health Information Management.*

Pavuluri, S., Sangal, R., Sather, J., & Taylor, R. A. (2024). Balancing act: The complex role of artificial intelligence in addressing burnout and healthcare workforce dynamics. *BMJ Health & Care Informatics*, *31*(1). Advance online publication. DOI: 10.1136/bmjhci-2024-101120

Pergolizzi, J.Jr, LeQuang, J. A. K., Vasiliu-Feltes, I., Breve, F., & Varrassi, G. (2023). Brave New Healthcare: A Narrative Review of Digital Healthcare in American Medicine. *Cureus*. Advance online publication. DOI: 10.7759/cureus.46489

Pina, A. F., Meneses, M. J., Sousa-Lima, I., Henriques, R., Raposo, J. F., & Macedo, M. P. (2023). Big data and machine learning to tackle diabetes management. *European Journal of Clinical Investigation*, *53*(1). Advance online publication. DOI: 10.1111/eci.13890

Popa, V., Geissler, J., Vermeulen, R., Priest, E., Capperella, K., Susuzlu, G., Terry, S. F., & Brooke, N. (2024). Delivering Digital Health Solutions that Patients Need: A Call to Action. In *Therapeutic Innovation and Regulatory Science* (Vol. 58, Issue 2, pp. 236–241). Springer Science and Business Media Deutschland GmbH. DOI: 10.1007/s43441-023-00592-4

Porter, M. E., & Teisberg, E. O. (2006). Redefining. *Health Care.*

Proso, M. (2024). Digital Transformation of Health: Towards the European Health Data Space. *Medicine. Law & Society, 17*(1). Advance online publication. DOI: 10.18690/mls.17.1.153-170.2024

Rao, D. (2023). The Urgent Need for Healthcare Workforce Upskilling and Ethical Considerations in the Era of AI-Assisted Medicine. *Indian Journal of Otolaryngology and Head and Neck Surgery : Official Publication of the Association of Otolaryngologists of India, 75*(3), 2638–2639. DOI: 10.1007/s12070-023-03755-9

Rauwerdink, A., Spinazze, P., Gijsbers, H., Molendijk, J., Zwolsman, S., Schijven, M. P., Chavannes, N. H., & Kasteleyn, M. J. (2024). Approaches to Evaluating Digital Health Technologies: Scoping Review. In *Journal of Medical Internet Research* (Vol. 26). JMIR Publications Inc. DOI: 10.2196/50251

Reis, M., Reis, F., & Kunde, W. (2025). Public Perception of Physicians Who Use Artificial Intelligence. *JAMA Network Open, 8*(7), e2521643. DOI: 10.1001/jamanetworkopen.2025.21643

Riveroll, A., Murray, S., Thompson, K., Robertson, K., Salijevic, A., & Montelpare, W. (2018). *2018 ACCES23-CMBEC41 Joint Conference PRECISION HEALTH: A PERSONALIZED APPROACH TO ACTIVE HEALTH MANAGEMENT Canadian Partnership Against Cancer, 5 Primary and Integrated Healthcare Innovations Network, 6 Beaconstone.*

Rosenlund, M., Kinnunen, U. M., & Saranto, K. (2023). The Use of Digital Health Services Among Patients and Citizens Living at Home: Scoping Review. In *Journal of Medical Internet Research* (Vol. 25). JMIR Publications Inc., DOI: 10.2196/44711

Rukundo, S. K. (2024). The Role of Digital Health in Preventive Medicine. *RESEARCH INVENTION JOURNAL OF PUBLIC HEALTH AND PHARMACY, 3*(2), 38–40. DOI: 10.59298/RIJPP/2024/323840

Sabiri, K., Sousa, F., & Rocha, T. (2025). A systematic review of privacy-preserving blockchain applications in healthcare. *Multimedia Tools and Applications*. Advance online publication. DOI: 10.1007/s11042-024-20541-z

Sagona, M., Dai, T., Macis, M., & Darden, M. (2025). Trust in AI-assisted health systems and AI's trust in humans. *Npj Health Systems, 2*(1), 10. DOI: 10.1038/s44401-025-00016-5

Schlieter, H., Marsch, L. A., Whitehouse, D., Otto, L., Londral, A. R., Teepe, G. W., Benedict, M., Ollier, J., Ulmer, T., Gasser, N., Ultsch, S., Wollschlaeger, B., & Kowatsch, T. (2022). Scale-up of Digital Innovations in Health Care: Expert Commentary on Enablers and Barriers. In *Journal of Medical Internet Research* (Vol. 24, Issue 3). JMIR Publications Inc. DOI: 10.2196/24582

Schouten, D., Nicoletti, G., Dille, B., Chia, C., Vendittelli, P., Schuurmans, M., Litjens, G., & Khalili, N. (2025). Navigating the landscape of multimodal AI in medicine: A scoping review on technical challenges and clinical applications. In *Medical Image Analysis* (Vol. 105). Elsevier B.V., DOI: 10.1016/j.media.2025.103621

Schubert, T., Oosterlinck, T., Stevens, R. D., Maxwell, P. H., & van der Schaar, M. (2025). AI education for clinicians. In *eClinicalMedicine* (Vol. 79). Elsevier Ltd. DOI: 10.1016/j.eclinm.2024.102968

Schüssler-Fiorenza Rose, S. M., Contrepois, K., Moneghetti, K. J., Zhou, W., Mishra, T., Mataraso, S., Dagan-Rosenfeld, O., Ganz, A. B., Dunn, J., Hornburg, D., Rego, S., Perelman, D., Ahadi, S., Sailani, M. R., Zhou, Y., Leopold, S. R., Chen, J., Ashland, M., & Christle, J. W. Snyder P., M. (2019). A longitudinal big data approach for precision health. *Nature Medicine*, *25*, 792–804. DOI: 10.1038/s41591-019-0414-6

Schwamm, L. H., Pletcher, S., & Erskine, A. (2024). AI and Technology Enabled Clinical Workflow Redesign. *Telemedicine Reports*, *5*(1), 415–420. DOI: 10.1089/tmr.2024.0079

Sebire, N. J., Adams, A., Arpiainen, L., Celi, L., Charlesworth, A., Gorgens, M., Gorsky, M., Magrabi, F., Nagasawa, Y., Onoka, C., & McKee, M. (2025). The Future Hospital in Global Health Systems: The Future Hospital as an Entity. In *International Journal of Health Planning and Management*. John Wiley and Sons Ltd., DOI: 10.1002/hpm.3893

Segur-Ferrer, J., Moltó-Puigmartí, C., Pastells-Peiró, R., & Vivanco-Hidalgo, R. M. (2024). Methodological frameworks and dimensions to be considered in digital health technology assessment: Scoping review and thematic analysis. *Journal of Medical Internet Research*, *26*, e48694–e48694. DOI: 10.2196/48694

Shaffer, F. A., & Preziosi, P. (2019). Digital Health: Join the Movement. *Nursing Administration Quarterly*, *43*(4), 351–353. DOI: 10.1097/NAQ.0000000000000371

Sharma, R., & Kshetri, N. (2020). Digital healthcare: Historical development, applications, and future research directions. In *International Journal of Information Management* (Vol. 53). Elsevier Ltd., DOI: 10.1016/j.ijinfomgt.2020.102105

Shin, H., Ryu, K., Kim, J. Y., & Lee, S. (2024). Application of privacy protection technology to healthcare big data. In *Digital Health* (Vol. 10). SAGE Publications Inc., DOI: 10.1177/20552076241282242

Shomali, M., Mora, P., Aleppo, G., Peeples, M., Kumbara, A., MacLeod, J., & Iyer, A. (2024). The critical elements of digital health in diabetes and cardiometabolic care. *Frontiers in Endocrinology*, *15*. Advance online publication. DOI: 10.3389/fendo.2024.1469471

Singhal, A., Neveditsin, N., Tanveer, H., & Mago, V. (2024). Toward Fairness, Accountability, Transparency, and Ethics in AI for Social Media and Health Care: Scoping Review. In *JMIR Medical Informatics* (Vol. 12). JMIR Publications Inc. DOI: 10.2196/50048

Sridharan, S., Seah Xin Hui, A., Venkataraman, N., Sivanath Tirukonda, P., Pratab Jeyaratnam, R., John, S., Suresh Babu, S., Liew, P., Francis, J., Koh Tzan, T., Kang Min, W., Min Liong, G., & Liew Jin Yee, C. (2024). Real-World evaluation of an AI triaging system for chest X-rays: A prospective clinical study. *European Journal of Radiology*, *181*, 111783. DOI: 10.1016/j.ejrad.2024.111783

Strika, Z., Petkovic, K., Likic, R., & Batenburg, R. (2024). Bridging healthcare gaps: a scoping review on the role of artificial intelligence, deep learning, and large language models in alleviating problems in medical deserts. In *Postgraduate medical journal* (Vol. 101, Issue 1191, pp. 4–16). DOI: 10.1093/postmj/qgae122

Sust, P. P., Solans, O., Fajardo, J. C., Peralta, M. M., Rodenas, P., Gabaldà, J., Eroles, L. G., Comella, A., Muñoz, C. V., Ribes, J. S., Monfa, R. R., & Piera-Jimenez, J. (2020). Turning the crisis into an opportunity: Digital health strategies deployed during the COVID-19 outbreak. In *JMIR Public Health and Surveillance* (Vol. 6, Issue 2). JMIR Publications Inc. DOI: 10.2196/19106

Swartz, A., LeFevre, A. E., Perera, S., Kinney, M. V., & George, A. S. (2021). Multiple pathways to scaling up and sustainability: An exploration of digital health solutions in South Africa. *Globalization and Health*, *17*(1). Advance online publication. DOI: 10.1186/s12992-021-00716-1

Terwee, C. B., Zuidgeest, M., Vonkeman, H. E., Cella, D., Haverman, L., & Roorda, L. D. (2021). Common patient-reported outcomes across ICHOM Standard Sets: The potential contribution of PROMIS®. *BMC Medical Informatics and Decision Making*, *21*(1), 259. DOI: 10.1186/s12911-021-01624-5

Thacharodi, A., Singh, P., Meenatchi, R., Tawfeeq Ahmed, Z. H., Kumar, R. R. S., Neha, V., Kavish, S., Maqbool, M., & Hassan, S. (2024). Revolutionizing healthcare and medicine: The impact of modern technologies for a healthier future—A comprehensive review. In *Health Care Science*. John Wiley and Sons Inc., DOI: 10.1002/hcs2.115

Tierney, A. A., Gayre, G., Hoberman, B., Mattern, B., Ballesca, M., Kipnis, P., Liu, V., & Lee, K. (2024). Ambient Artificial Intelligence Scribes to Alleviate the Burden of Clinical Documentation. *NEJM Catalyst Innovations in Care Delivery*, *5*(3). Advance online publication. DOI: 10.1056/CAT.23.0404

Topol, E. (2019). *Preparing the healthcare workforce to deliver the digital future The Topol Review An independent report on behalf of the Secretary of State for Health and Social Care.*

Tran, V. T., Riveros, C., & Ravaud, P. (2019). Patients' views of wearable devices and AI in healthcare: Findings from the ComPaRe e-cohort. *NPJ Digital Medicine*, *2*(1). Advance online publication. DOI: 10.1038/s41746-019-0132-y

Trzmielak, D. M., Lipka-Matusiak, I., & Oftedal, E. (2024). Responsible Innovation in E-Health Care: Empowering Patients with Emerging Technologies. *Marketing of Scientific and Research Organizations*, *52*(2), 68–87. DOI: 10.2478/minib-2024-0010

Vardas, E. P., Marketou, M., & Vardas, P. E. (2025). Medicine, healthcare and the AI act: Gaps, challenges and future implications. *European Heart Journal. Digital Health*, *6*(4), 833–839. DOI: 10.1093/ehjdh/ztaf041

Venkatesan, M., Mohan, H., Ryan, J. R., Schurch, C. M., Nolan, G. P., Frakes, D. H., & Coskun, A. F. (2021). Virtual_and_augmented_reality_for_biomedical_applications_2021. *Cell Reports Medicine*, *7*. Advance online publication. DOI: 10.1016/j.xcrm.2021.100348

WHO. (2005). *Global Observatory for eHealth*. https://www.who.int/observatories/global-observatory-for-ehealth

WHO. (2011). *mHealth new horizons for health through mobile technologies: based on the findings of the second global survey on eHealth*. World Health Organization. https://iris.who.int/bitstream/handle/10665/44607/9789241564250_eng.pdf?sequence=1&isAllowed=y

WHO. (2021). *Global Strategy on Digital Health 2020-2025*. World Health Organization. https://iris.who.int/bitstream/handle/10665/344249/9789240020924-eng.pdf?sequence=1

WHO. (2025). *Advancing the Responsible Use of Digital Technologies in Global Health.*

Wicks, P., Massagli, M., Frost, J., Brownstein, C., Okun, S., Vaughan, T., Bradley, R., & Heywood, J. (2010). Sharing Health Data for Better Outcomes on PatientsLikeMe. *Journal of Medical Internet Research, 12*(2), e19. DOI: 10.2196/jmir.1549

Wilkinson, T., Wang, M., Friedman, J., Gaye, Y.-E., & Görgens, M. (2024). Knowing when digital adds value to health: A framework for the economic evaluation of digital health interventions. *Oxford Open Digital Health, 2*(Supplement_2), ii75–ii86. DOI: 10.1093/oodh/oqae028

Willems, S. H., Rao, J., Bhambere, S., Patel, D., Biggins, Y., & Guite, J. W. (2021). Digital solutions to alleviate the burden on health systems during a public health care crisis: Covid-19 as an opportunity. In *JMIR mHealth and uHealth* (Vol. 9, Issue 6). JMIR Publications Inc. DOI: 10.2196/25021

Williamson, S. M., & Prybutok, V. (2024). Balancing Privacy and Progress: A Review of Privacy Challenges, Systemic Oversight, and Patient Perceptions in AI-Driven Healthcare. In *Applied Sciences (Switzerland)* (Vol. 14, Issue 2). Multidisciplinary Digital Publishing Institute (MDPI). DOI: 10.3390/app14020675

Wongvibulsin, S., Martin, S. S., Saria, S., Zeger, S. L., & Murphy, S. A. (2020). An Individualized, Data-Driven Digital Approach for Precision Behavior Change. In *American Journal of Lifestyle Medicine* (Vol. 14, Issue 3, pp. 289–293). SAGE Publications Inc. DOI: 10.1177/1559827619843489

Wu, C. T., Wang, S. M., Su, Y. E., Hsieh, T. T., Chen, P. C., Cheng, Y. C., Tseng, T. W., Chang, W. S., Su, C. S., Kuo, L. C., Chien, J. Y., Lai, F., & Wu, C. T. (2022). A Precision Health Service for Chronic Diseases: Development and Cohort Study Using Wearable Device, Machine Learning, and Deep Learning. *IEEE Journal of Translational Engineering in Health and Medicine, 10*. Advance online publication. DOI: 10.1109/JTEHM.2022.3207825

Xie, W., Paul, R. R., Goon, I. Y., Anan, A., Rahim, A., Hossain, M. M., Hersch, F., Oldenburg, B., Chambers, J., & Mridha, M. K. (2023). Enhancing care quality and accessibility through digital technology-supported decentralisation of hypertension and diabetes management: A proof-of-concept study in rural Bangladesh. *BMJ Open, 13*(11). Advance online publication. DOI: 10.1136/bmjopen-2023-073743

Xiong, S., Lu, H., Peoples, N., Duman, E. K., Najarro, A., Ni, Z., Gong, E., Yin, R., Ostbye, T., Palileo-Villanueva, L. M., Doma, R., Kafle, S., Tian, M., & Yan, L. L. (2023). Digital health interventions for non-communicable disease management in primary health care in low-and middle-income countries. In *npj Digital Medicine* (Vol. 6, Issue 1). Nature Research. DOI: 10.1038/s41746-023-00764-4

Yao, L., Liu, Y., Wang, T., Han, C., Li, Q., Li, Q., You, X., Ren, T., & Wang, Y. (2025). Global trends of big data analytics in health research: A bibliometric study. *Frontiers in Medicine, 12*. Advance online publication. DOI: 10.3389/fmed.2025.1456286

Yaqub, N., Zhang, J., Khalid, M. I., Wang, W., Helfert, M., Ahmed, M., & Kim, J. (2025). Blockchain enabled policy-based access controlmechanismto restrict unauthorized access to electronic health records. *PeerJ. Computer Science, 11*. Advance online publication. DOI: 10.7717/PEERJ-CS.2647

Yu, E., Chu, X., Zhang, W., Meng, X., Yang, Y., Ji, X., & Wu, C. (2025). Large Language Models in Medicine: Applications, Challenges, and Future Directions. In *International Journal of Medical Sciences* (Vol. 22, Issue 11, pp. 2792–2801). Ivyspring International Publisher. DOI: 10.7150/ijms.111780

Zhang, Bullen, C., & Chen, J. (2025). Digital Health Innovations to Catalyze the Transition to Value-Based Health Care. *JMIR Medical Informatics, 13*, e57385–e57385. DOI: 10.2196/57385

Zhang, J., Xiang, S., & Li, L. (2025). Economic implications of artificial intelligence-driven recommended systems in healthcare: A focus on neurological disorders. *Frontiers in Public Health, 13*. Advance online publication. DOI: 10.3389/fpubh.2025.1588270

Zhang, K., Meng, X., Yan, X., Ji, J., Liu, J., Xu, H., Zhang, H., Liu, D., Wang, J., Wang, X., Gao, J., Wang, Y. G. S., Shao, C., Wang, W., Li, J., Zheng, M. Q., Yang, Y., & Da Tang, Y. (2025). Revolutionizing Health Care: The Transformative Impact of Large Language Models in Medicine. In *Journal of Medical Internet Research* (Vol. 27). JMIR Publications Inc. DOI: 10.2196/59069

Chapter 4

App Your Health:

Harnessing Digital Tools for Diabetes Prevention and Health Promotion

Mabitsela Mphasha
https://orcid.org/0000-0002-4812-5051
University of Limpopo, South Africa

ABSTRACT

Type 2 diabetes mellitus (T2DM) is rising globally, with low- and middle-income countries, including South Africa, bearing a disproportionate burden. This chapter explores the role of digital health tools such as mobile health (mHealth), wearable technologies, and artificial intelligence in supporting T2DM prevention and management. It critically examines how these innovations promote education, behaviour change, and self-management in under-resourced settings. The chapter highlights that while digital tools offer scalable solutions for diabetes care, their success depends on equitable access, cultural relevance, and integration into primary healthcare. Challenges such as the digital divide, data privacy, and weak system alignment must be addressed. Community engagement enhances trust and long-term use. Looking forward, digital health can transform care if supported by context-specific research, inclusive design, and enabling policies. A hybrid model—blending innovation with person-centred care—is essential for sustainable, accessible diabetes management rooted in local realities.

1. INTRODUCTION

The rapid digitisation of health systems is reshaping how societies approach health promotion, disease prevention, and long-term management of chronic conditions. This shift is especially significant for type 2 diabetes mellitus (T2DM), a condition rising at alarming rates globally and disproportionately burdening low- and middle-income countries (LMICs). Digital health innovations such as mobile applications, wearable sensors, telemedicine platforms, and artificial intelligence present new opportunities to strengthen diabetes prevention, enhance patient engagement, and support sustained self-management. With a particular focus on South Africa, this chapter examines how these technologies can be adapted for resource-limited settings to improve access to care, reinforce health education, encourage behaviour change, and ultimately enhance health outcomes in populations most at risk of developing T2DM.

DOI: 10.4018/979-8-3373-3531-5.ch004

2. BACKGROUND

Diabetes is one of the world's fastest-growing health challenges, affecting an estimated 589 million adults, with projections reaching 853 million by 2050. One in eight adults may be living with diabetes, and over 252 million cases are expected to remain undiagnosed, intensifying the health and economic burden on already strained systems (International Diabetes Federation (IDF), 2025). LMICs face the steepest rise, driven by rapid urbanisation, demographic transitions, and lifestyle shifts that accelerate the emergence of non-communicable diseases (NCDs). The rise of T2DM in LMICs reflects broader societal transformations. Once more prevalent in high-income countries, the burden has shifted toward LMICs due to increased consumption of energy-dense foods, reduced physical activity, higher tobacco and alcohol use, and widespread obesity (Rob et al., 2025; Mphasha, Skaal & Mothiba, 2022; Ford, Patel, & Narayan, 2017). These risk factors: intensified by globalisation, socioeconomic inequality, and food system changes (Gong et al., 2025; Fox, Feng & Asal, 2019; Ruel et al., 2017) result in earlier disease onset, more severe complications, and poorer long-term outcomes.

T2DM remains largely preventable, as it is strongly associated with modifiable lifestyle factors such as unhealthy diets, physical inactivity, and excess body weight (IDF,2021). Yet prevalence continues to grow, revealing weaknesses in prevention efforts, early detection systems, and continuous self-management support. Digital health interventions offer scalable, cost-effective solutions that can address these gaps. They provide personalised coaching, real-time glucose tracking, lifestyle guidance, and remote consultations, empowering individuals to adopt healthier behaviours and maintain long-term disease control (Giansanti, 2025; Chatterjee et al., 2021; Rollo et al., 2016). When integrated effectively, these tools can complement overburdened healthcare systems and expand access to care in resource-constrained LMIC environments.

2.1. Description and Diagnosis

Type 2 diabetes mellitus is a chronic metabolic condition characterised by insulin resistance, progressive β-cell dysfunction, and sustained hyperglycaemia (IDF, 2025). In LMICs, its pathophysiology reflects complex interactions between genetic, lifestyle, and environmental factors (Pledger & Ahmadizar, 2023). Insulin resistance reduces glucose uptake in muscle and adipose tissue, while impaired hepatic insulin signalling increases glucose production (DaSilva et al., 2020). Chronic inflammation and prolonged hyperinsulinaemia eventually exhaust β-cells, worsening glycaemic control (Thouvenot et al., 2022). Emerging evidence from African populations suggests that reduced insulin clearance, not only resistance, may represent an early metabolic defect preceding β-cell deterioration (Kunyiha et al., 2025).

The rising prevalence of T2DM in LMICs is further linked to sedentary lifestyles, rapid urbanisation, and increased consumption of ultra-processed, high-calorie foods (Popkin & Ng,, 2022). Central obesity, alcohol and tobacco use, and newer risk contributors such as air pollution compound vulnerability (Bell et al., 2011). Socioeconomic barriers such as low income, limited health literacy, poor access to care, and under-resourced health systems delay diagnosis and hinder long-term management (Woodward et al., 2024). In many LMIC contexts, individuals develop T2DM at younger ages and sometimes at lower BMI thresholds, increasing lifetime complications (Ford, Patel, & Narayan, 2017). Diagnosis follows standard WHO/ADA criteria:

- Fasting plasma glucose ≥7.0 mmol/L

- 2-hour OGTT ≥11.1 mmol/L
- HbA1c ≥6.5%
- Random glucose ≥11.1 mmol/L in symptomatic individuals (Colagiuri, 2021).

Underdiagnosis remains widespread and millions of South Africans live with undetected diabetes (IDF, 2021). Barriers include limited laboratory capacity, financial constraints, and weak screening programmes.

Conventional management combines lifestyle modification (diet quality, physical activity, weight control, tobacco/alcohol reduction) with pharmacotherapy. Metformin remains first-line therapy, followed by sulfonylureas, SGLT2 inhibitors, GLP-1 receptor agonists, or insulin, depending on glycaemic needs (Esayed et al., 2024). Long-term monitoring includes HbA1c evaluations, lipid profiles, blood pressure control, and screening for complications such as nephropathy, retinopathy, and neuropathy. However, many LMIC systems face medication shortages, inadequate diagnostics, clinic overcrowding, and poor adherence challenges that significantly limit effective diabetes control (Ntinginya et al., 2021).

3. MAIN FOCUS OF THE CHAPTER

This chapter examines the transformative potential of digital health interventions in enhancing diabetes prevention and care in LMICs, with a particular focus on South Africa. It explores how digital tools can strengthen health literacy, support behaviour change, and close longstanding gaps in healthcare service delivery. Drawing on emerging evidence, the chapter emphasises the importance of integrating digital innovation into mainstream public health strategies to reduce inequities, improve early detection, and promote sustained community engagement.

3.1. Issues, Controversies, and Problems

Digital health technologies offer significant promise for chronic disease management, yet their implementation encounters complex challenges, especially in LMICs. Persistent digital divides, poor connectivity, limited smartphone access, and low digital literacy restrict uptake among vulnerable populations. Weak regulatory frameworks, insufficient data protection laws, and concerns about privacy and algorithmic bias further complicate adoption. Moreover, many digital tools are not culturally adapted, resulting in poor user engagement and low adherence. A lack of user-centred design, limited integration with public health systems, and inadequate long-term evaluation create uncertainty about sustainability and impact. These issues highlight the urgent need for inclusive, context-sensitive, and ethically grounded digital strategies that complement rather than replace person-centred care.

3.2. Digital Gaps and Opportunities in LMICs

Digital tools are increasingly recognised as essential for addressing persistent gaps in diabetes care in LMICs, where workforce shortages, geographical barriers, and weak primary healthcare disrupt routine management (Maita et al., 2024). Mobile apps and SMS platforms expand access to culturally tailored information on diet, physical activity, and medication adherence (Materia et al., 2023). Unlike in-person counselling, digital tools offer continuous reinforcement via reminders, personalised feedback, and behaviour tracking, strengthening self-management (Li et al., 2025). Remote monitoring through glucose-logging apps, wearables, and telemedicine reduces reliance on clinics, which is especially critical where transport barriers and long waiting times impede care (Materia et al., 2023). At a system level, digital infrastructure such as appointment scheduling, supply-chain alerts, and clinical decision-support tools helps mitigate workforce shortages and strengthens continuity of care (Suganthi & Kalaiselvi, 2024). Consequently, digital solutions offer scalable, cost-effective strategies that complement weak health systems and extend services to underserved communities (Abernethy et al., 2022).

Digital tools also align with all levels of diabetes prevention. For primary prevention, apps supporting physical activity, nutrition, weight control, and smoking cessation help reduce behavioural risks, particularly among rapidly urbanising youth (Schoeppe et al., 2017). Secondary prevention benefits from digital risk calculators, screening reminders, and teleconsultations that improve early detection of prediabetes and early T2DM stages commonly missed in LMICs (Kengne & Ramachandran, 2024). Tertiary prevention is strengthened through connected glucose monitors, medication-adherence tools, foot-care education and remote follow-up, improving glycaemic control and reducing severe complications (Najafi & Mishra, 2021).

4. MOBILE HEALTH (MHEALTH) TECHNOLOGIES IN PUBLIC HEALTH AND DIABETES PREVENTION

4.1. Overview and Global Uptake of mHealth Technologies

Mobile health refers to the use of mobile and wireless technologies including smartphones, feature phones, tablets, and wearable sensors to support public health functions, clinical decision-making, and patient self-management (Abaza, & Marschollek, 2017). As a central component of the wider digital-health ecosystem, mHealth has become a transformative force in expanding healthcare access beyond traditional clinic-based settings. Its capabilities includes remote monitoring, behaviour change support, continuous patient education, and enhanced communication are particularly valuable for chronic diseases such as T2DM, where ongoing lifestyle adjustments and long-term self-management are fundamental for effective care (Holl et al., 2024).

4.1.1. Global trends and specific innovations

The global uptake of mHealth has accelerated rapidly, propelled by near-universal mobile network penetration and the demand for flexible care models during the COVID-19 pandemic. Over 70% of the world's population now has access to mobile networks, and smartphone ownership continues to rise even among lower-income and remote populations (Intelligence, 2018). However, beyond these global statistics, several specific innovations illustrate how mHealth is reshaping care delivery:

- India's mDiabetes Programme (Rani et al., 2025): A text-based intervention reaching more than one million people with personalised lifestyle messages significantly improved dietary behaviour and self-care among participants.
- mySugr, BlueStar, and Dario: These are advanced digital diabetes-management applications that combine carbohydrate counting, medication and glucose logging, and personalised coaching.

Using AI-driven feedback, trend analysis, and goal-setting tools, these platforms enhance daily self-management, support behavioural change, and strengthen patient–provider communication, ultimately improving glycaemic control and long-term diabetes outcomes (Lee & Lee, 2023; Fitzpatrick, 2023; Schroeder, Haug & Gewald, 2022; Sanz, Acha, & García, 2021; World Health Organization (WHO). 2021).

This case illustrate that while mHealth is global in scope, impact is maximised when tools respond to specific local health priorities and are embedded in existing healthcare structures.

4.1.2. South African Context and Illustrative Success Stories

South Africa has increasingly integrated mHealth into national health strategies, particularly for maternal and child health, HIV management, and the growing burden of non-communicable diseases. The country hosts several successful and widely recognised mHealth innovations:

- MomConnect: A flagship national programme delivering stage-based pregnancy information via SMS to over 3 million women. It also includes a helpdesk that strengthens accountability and patient feedback within the health system (Barron et al., 2018; Seebregts et al., 2018).
- Vula Mobile: A referral and teleconsultation app used by clinicians across the country, allowing healthcare workers to connect instantly with specialist teams. This has improved referral efficiency for diabetic complications such as retinopathy, foot ulcers, and hypertension (Gloster, Mash, & Swartz, 2021).
- B-Wise: This is a youth-focused digital health platform delivered through WhatsApp and web-based channels, offering accessible, culturally relevant, and visually engaging information on sexual, reproductive, and general health. Designed for South African adolescents, it provides interactive content, advice, and motivational messaging, helping young people make informed decisions and access trustworthy health guidance in real time (Barron et al., 2018; LeFevre et al., 2018).

These examples demonstrate that South Africa offers not only widespread adoption but also concrete success stories that show how digital innovation can address real systemic gaps.

4.1.3. Issues, problems, and trends: A more critical analysis

Persistent Structural Inequities: Digital literacy disparities, inadequate network coverage, and the high cost of data continue to limit mHealth use in rural and resource-poor communities. These inequities risk widening existing health disparities if not deliberately mitigated.

Fragmentation of Digital Health Systems: South Africa, like many LMICs, faces challenges related to parallel, unintegrated mHealth platforms. Lack of interoperability results in duplicated data, inefficiencies, and limited continuity of care—problems recognised across the global digital-health landscape.

Cultural and Linguistic Misalignment: Many mHealth apps remain poorly localised, offering English-only content or failing to reflect local cultural norms, dietary patterns, and health beliefs. This reduces relevance and long-term user engagement, particularly in multilingual contexts.

Heightened Data-Privacy Concerns: As digital platforms collect sensitive health information, questions around consent, security, data ownership, and ethical use have intensified. These concerns have prompted calls for stronger national governance frameworks.

Variable Evidence of Effectiveness: While pilot projects are widespread, few have undergone rigorous evaluation. This limits the ability of health systems to scale up interventions confidently and sustainably.

The Value of Locally Adaptive and Participatory Approaches: Growing evidence shows that mHealth interventions are most effective when they adopt participatory co-design methodologies, engaging community members, clinicians, and software developers from the outset (Fitzpatrick, 2023; Schroeder, Haug & Gewald, 2022; Sanz, Acha, & García, 2021). Successful tools in diverse South African settings incorporate:

- Multilingual features aligned to local languages
- Food and lifestyle guidance that reflects local diets
- Culturally sensitive graphics and simplified user interfaces
- Community health-worker integration
- Iterative design processes informed by user feedback

Such approaches improve trust, usability, and long-term adoption, especially for chronic conditions requiring sustained behaviour change such as T2DM.

5. DIGITAL TOOLS FOR DIABETES PREVENTION

Digital tools, which includes mHealth applications, SMS messaging services, social media platforms, and virtual assistants are playing an increasingly central role in health promotion. These technologies help raise public awareness, support healthy behaviour changes, and improve access to preventive care, especially in the context of NCDs like T2DM (WHO, 2021; Rinaldi, Hijazi, & Haghparast-Bidgoli, 2020). Their interactive and widely accessible nature makes them effective for influencing individual and community-level behaviours.

Table 1. Key Features of Effective Diabetes Health Promotion Apps

Feature	Purpose	Behavioural Impact
Goal setting	Enables users to define personalised health targets	Enhances motivation, focus, and accountability
Reminders & notifications	Sends prompts for medication, exercise, or meals	Supports routine adherence and timely health actions
Gamification (e.g., points, badges)	Introduces game-like elements to user tasks	Increases engagement and sustains long-term participation
Personalisation	Tailors content and feedback to individual user data	Improves relevance and user satisfaction
Educational content	Delivers culturally appropriate and accessible information	Boosts health literacy and informed self-management

5.1. Mobile Applications (Apps)

mHealth applications have become increasingly practical, affordable, and scalable tools for preventing and managing T2DM. These apps enable users to monitor a wide range of health behaviours and clinical indicators, including dietary intake, physical activity, blood glucose levels, weight, medication adherence, and emotional wellbeing (Debon et al., 2019). Beyond basic tracking, many advanced platforms integrate personalised feedback, health education, behavioural nudges, and virtual coaching to support sustained lifestyle modification.

- Several applications are also linked to electronic health records (EHRs), enhancing clinical oversight and promoting continuity of care. For example, the mDiab study in India evaluated a mobile-based lifestyle intervention targeting high-risk adults. The app delivered video lessons and remote coaching via smartphones, aiming to improve weight management, clinical markers, and health-related behaviours. If validated further, mDiab may serve as a scalable mHealth model for chronic disease prevention in low-resource settings (Muralidharan et al., 2017). Other evidence-based platforms such as mySugr, BlueStar, and Dario include features like carbohydrate counting, goal setting, personalised coaching, and educational modules. Many incorporate artificial intelligence (AI) to adapt to user needs over time, offering tailored support that enhances glycaemic control, medication adherence, and overall self-management (Lee & Lee, 2023; Fitzpatrick, 2023; Schroeder, Haug & Gewald, 2022; Sanz, Acha, & García, 2021; WHO, 2021).

5.2. SMS and USSD-Based Messaging Systems

In LMICs, where access to smartphones and reliable internet connectivity may be limited, text-based communication platforms have demonstrated significant potential in delivering health interventions. These systems commonly provide reminders for medication adherence, upcoming clinic visits, and motivational health messages. Prominent examples include South Africa's MomConnect and B-Wise programmes, which utilise SMS and WhatsApp to deliver targeted health education and behavioural support (LeFevre et al., 2018; Barron et al., 2018). MomConnect, for instance, sends regular SMS messages in local languages to guide pregnant women through the stages of antenatal care, while B-Wise engages youth with culturally relevant sexual and reproductive health information, using accessible language and visual icons (Barron et al., 2018). These models demonstrate how simple, low-cost messaging systems can be adapted to meet the specific needs of diverse populations. A similar approach could be tailored for diabetes prevention and management, offering regular prompts, self-care tips, and lifestyle guidance to individuals in resource-limited settings.

5.3. Telemedicine Platforms

Telemedicine platforms enable real-time audio or video consultations between patients and healthcare providers, significantly improving access in regions with limited infrastructure or specialist availability. These platforms are particularly valuable for the ongoing monitoring, management, and education of patients with chronic conditions such as diabetes and hypertension (Haleem et al., 2021). With an ageing population and a global shortage of specialists, home-based care through telemedicine shows strong potential, especially for cardiovascular and respiratory diseases. It reduces the need for hospitalisation, preserves bed capacity, and supports patient comfort by allowing vital signs and video communications to be transmitted directly from home to care providers (Habukawa et al., 2021). This approach can also be adapted for diabetes management, enabling remote monitoring of patients' adherence to treatment and lifestyle modifications.

5.4. Wearable Devices

Devices such as fitness trackers, smartwatches, and continuous glucose monitors (CGMs) are capable of real-time biometric tracking. These devices often integrate with digital health platforms, providing immediate feedback to users and facilitating more responsive, data-driven clinical decision-making. In the context of diabetes care, CGMs are particularly valuable, as they allow users to monitor glucose fluctuations continuously and adjust dietary intake, physical activity, or insulin dosage accordingly (Vijayan et al., 2021). Beyond individual monitoring, these technologies offer healthcare providers a more comprehensive view of patient trends, enabling early intervention and personalised treatment adjustments. Evidence from a systematic review confirms that wearable devices significantly contribute to effective diabetes management and the prevention of related complications. Their use has also been associated with better glycaemic control, increased adherence to treatment plans, and overall improvements in quality of life for people living with diabetes (Makroum et al., 2022)

5.5. AI-powered Chatbots and Virtual Health Assistants (VHAs)

They are becoming integral components of digital health systems, offering enhanced patient support and engagement. These technologies deliver customised health information, assist users in managing self-care routines, and triage symptoms using real-time data inputs. Available around the clock, they offer instant responses to patient queries—an essential feature in settings where access to healthcare providers may be limited or delayed. VHAs hold significant promise for advancing lifestyle medicine by delivering ongoing, personalised guidance through adaptive conversations that help users sustain healthy behaviours. When thoughtfully designed, these AI tools can contribute to improved health outcomes while preserving the human connection vital to effective and compassionate care (Maher et al., 2024). By streamlining routine tasks and providing consistent, evidence-based information, they ease pressure on strained healthcare systems while ensuring continuity of care. Additionally, they play a pivotal role in patient education, treatment adherence, and promoting behaviour change, particularly among individuals managing long-term conditions like diabetes (Clark & Bailey, 2024).

5.6. Social Media Platforms

The social media platforms includes Facebook, WhatsApp, Instagram, and YouTube have become powerful tools for disseminating health information, offering formats that are visually engaging, culturally relevant, and easily shareable. These platforms are particularly effective in promoting health communication that encourages user interaction, peer support, and message retention features that are often lacking in more traditional forms of health education (Sepulveda-Escobar & Morrison, 2020). Social media enables real-time, personalised health education through videos, infographics, live sessions, and user stories. Platforms like Facebook support peer interaction and motivation, while WhatsApp groups deliver targeted messages in local languages, building trust and promoting sustained behaviour change.

Their interactive nature allows two-way communication with peers and health workers, enhancing empowerment and self-efficacy, key to lasting health improvements, especially in low-resource and multilingual settings.

Table 2. Comparison of common digital tools used in diabetes prevention and management

Tool Type	Description	Strengths	Limitations
Mobile Apps	Apps for tracking diet, activity, glucose levels	Accessible, scalable, user-friendly	Requires smartphone, digital literacy
SMS Reminders	Text messages for medication/dietary reminders	Works on basic phones, low cost	Limited personalisation, no visual content
Wearable Devices	Fitness trackers, CGMs	Real-time feedback, behaviour reinforcement	Costly, requires maintenance and connectivity
AI-powered Chatbots	Conversational support tools	24/7 support, adaptive learning	Limited in handling complex queries
Social Media Campaigns	Platforms for health education	Broad reach, social engagement	Risk of misinformation

6. PATIENT ENGAGEMENT AND HEALTH LITERACY IN DIGITAL HEALTH INTERVENTIONS

Patient engagement and digital health literacy are central to the effectiveness of digital health interventions, particularly within underserved and marginalised populations. Digital health literacy is more than just the ability to read—it involves the skills needed to search for, understand, evaluate, and apply health information delivered through digital platforms (Van Der Vaart & Drossaert, 2017). However, in many low-income and rural contexts, individuals often struggle with limited exposure to digital tools, language barriers, and unfamiliarity with clinical terminology (Badr, Motulsky, & Denis, 2024). To improve uptake and sustained use, digital health solutions must be developed with user-centred design in mind. Interfaces should be easy to navigate, and information should be communicated using clear, culturally appropriate language. Visual and interactive features such as voice prompts, videos, quizzes, and pictorial guides can support better comprehension and increase engagement, particularly among users with limited literacy. Tailoring content to align with local customs, language preferences, and daily routines enhances the relevance of the intervention and encourages ongoing participation.

Moreover, the involvement of family members and peers plays a critical role in promoting engagement and improving outcomes. Peer-led models offer emotional encouragement, shared learning opportunities, and collective motivation, which can be particularly powerful in community settings (Sherman et al.,2023). Family support is equally important, as it can shape health-related decision-making, especially for users with limited confidence in using digital tools. When families adopt these tools together, they help normalise their use within the home and promote consistent engagement (Mphasha, Mothiba & Skaal, 2022).

Strengthening these social and support networks not only increases participation but also ensures that digital health interventions are inclusive, locally grounded, and sustainable. In doing so, they contribute meaningfully to reducing health disparities and ensuring that digital innovation benefits all regardless of literacy level, digital experience, or geographic location.

7. CHALLENGES AND CONCERNS IN DIGITAL HEALTH IMPLEMENTATION

Digital health technologies are increasingly seen as transformative in improving healthcare access, reducing delivery costs, and enhancing system efficiency particularly in low-resource and remote areas. Tools such as mobile apps, telemedicine platforms, wearable devices, and AI-driven diagnostics support remote consultations, real-time monitoring, and personalised care. These innovations are especially valuable in managing chronic conditions like type 2 diabetes. However, their equitable and sustainable implementation is challenged by technical, social, ethical, and systemic barriers that must be addressed (Jerjes & Harding, 2024).

7.1. Digital Divide

One of the most persistent barriers to achieving equity in digital health is the digital divide. This term refers to the stark inequalities in access to digital technologies such as smartphones, reliable internet, and supporting infrastructure. While mobile phone penetration has increased across sub-Saharan Africa, access to smartphones and consistent, affordable internet remains a challenge particularly in rural and economically disadvantaged areas. In many of these contexts, high data costs and patchy network coverage severely limit meaningful engagement with digital health platforms (Badr, Motulsky, & Denis, 2024; Okano et al., 2022).

Yet access alone is not enough. The digital divide also includes significant gaps in digital literacy—the confidence and skills required to use technology effectively. Many individuals are unfamiliar with navigating mobile applications, interpreting health content, or using online platforms for self-care or monitoring. These limitations reduce the reach and impact of digital interventions and risk leaving behind groups who are already vulnerable, including the elderly, persons with disabilities, and low-income populations (Statti & Torres, 2020).

Bridging this divide calls for a dual approach. On one hand, investments are needed in infrastructure expanding network coverage, lowering data costs, and improving access to digital devices. On the other, efforts must focus on building users' capacity to engage with these technologies. Community-based training, user-friendly platform design, and culturally relevant content delivered in local languages can make a significant difference in building trust and usability. These measures ensure that digital tools are not only available but genuinely accessible and inclusive (Wierda et al., 2020)

7.2. Privacy and Ethical Considerations

The success of digital health interventions depends not only on access but also on trust particularly when sensitive personal health data are involved. Many digital platforms require users to share private health information, which raises concerns about privacy, informed consent, and data security. In countries where legal frameworks for data protection are still evolving or poorly enforced, individuals may face serious risks, including data breaches, misuse of information, or discrimination based on their health status (Brall, Schröder-Bäck & Maeckelberghe, 2019).

These concerns are particularly acute in contexts involving stigmatised conditions such as HIV, diabetes, or mental illness. Without clarity on how data will be used or stored, people may be reluctant to use digital tools, fearing that unauthorised sharing could result in social stigma, rejection, or even reduced access to care. Ethical implementation must therefore prioritise user autonomy, transparency, and protection from harm (McGraw & Mandl, 2021).

Best practices in this space begin with clear and accessible information about data collection and use. Users should be offered genuine choices such as opt-in or opt-out features and be able to control what information they share. From a technical standpoint, strong encryption, secure data transmission, and strict access controls are essential to protect confidentiality (Scheibner et al.,2020) Digital health systems should also comply with national and global standards, such as the General Data Protection Regulation (GDPR), and be subject to routine oversight by independent ethical review bodies (Clifford, 2016). Beyond technical safeguards, ethical responsibility includes designing for inclusion. Developers and implementers must be aware of power imbalances and actively involve underrepresented groups in the creation of digital health interventions. Engaging communities in co-design processes not only improves relevance and usability but also helps ensure that digital health technologies serve all users fairly and respectfully.

7.3. Cultural and User-Centred Design Limitations

One of the key obstacles to the success of digital health interventions in LMICs is the lack of cultural and contextual relevance in their design. Many digital health tools are developed in high-income settings and are shaped by Western biomedical models, which often fail to consider the diverse sociocultural realities of users in LMICs (Al Shamsi et al.,2020). This disconnect can reduce user engagement, lead to misinterpretation of content, and ultimately result in poor retention or outright rejection of the intervention.

Language is a critical factor in this equation. In multilingual contexts such as South Africa, the absence of language diversity in digital platforms marginalises non-English speakers or those with limited literacy. Digital content that relies heavily on clinical or technical jargon, without local translation or simplification, risks alienating the very populations it aims to empower. Furthermore, differing health beliefs including reliance on traditional remedies or community-based care can shape how digital messages are received and acted upon (Kirk et al., 2021). Applying user-centred design principles, especially participatory co-design, is essential to address these issues. Engaging local users, healthcare workers, and community leaders in the development process ensures that interventions are culturally relevant, contextually grounded, and reflective of real-life experiences (Gillett-Swan et al.,2024; Nguyen, Chib & Mahalingam, 2017). Co-design fosters trust, increases local ownership, and enhances the credibility and usability of digital tools.

Social and household dynamics also influence the uptake of digital technologies. In some communities, gender roles and family hierarchies may restrict women's access to mobile devices or require male approval to engage with digital tools (Ortiz-Escobar et al., 2023). These structural inequalities must be recognised and addressed through inclusive design, targeted training, and supportive policies. Usability is another vital component of user-centred design. Platforms should include intuitive interfaces, visual cues, and voice prompts for users with limited literacy or visual impairments (Kim, Coiera & Magrabi, 2017). Content must reflect culturally familiar dietary patterns, idiomatic expressions, and locally accepted imagery. Overlooking these elements risks reinforcing digital exclusion and exacerbating existing health disparities.

7.4. Integration into Health Systems

Digital health technologies offer great potential, but their full value can only be realised when integrated into the wider health system rather than implemented as standalone or parallel solutions. Fragmented digital initiatives often lead to duplicated efforts, confusion among providers, and resistance from health workers who may find them burdensome or misaligned with existing workflows (Junaid et al.,2022). A major barrier to integration is the lack of interoperability between digital platforms and national health information systems. For example, mobile applications designed for diabetes management or maternal health tracking must sync with electronic medical records to ensure continuity of care. Without such integration, providers may be left without essential patient information, resulting in fragmented service delivery and missed opportunities for early intervention (Zakaria et al., 2024).

Effective integration also depends on aligning digital health tools with offline services. Systems for referrals, medication tracking, and appointment scheduling should be linked with facility-based care to ensure consistency and avoid service disruption. Evidence suggests that hybrid models where digital solutions supplement face-to-face care are particularly effective in chronic disease management, offering a balance between convenience and personal connection (South African National Department of Health, 2019). Health system integration requires more than technical alignment; it also demands capacity-building and supportive policy environments. Frontline health workers need adequate training in digital literacy, data use, and change management to promote digital adoption. At the same time, national health strategies must include digital health within formal frameworks—governance, budgeting, standards, and monitoring to ensure long-term sustainability (Miller, Cafazzo & Seto, 2016).

Integrated systems also allow for improved measurement of outcomes and better scalability across regions. Embedding digital health into routine care delivery and linking it to national health budgets and monitoring systems helps secure longevity beyond donor-driven or pilot-phase projects. Despite the progress made, digital health implementation continues to face structural hurdles such as digital literacy gaps, cultural barriers, fragmented systems, and unreliable connectivity, particularly in rural areas. In parallel, rising concerns about privacy, informed consent, and secure data management further complicate widespread adoption (Lee & Lee, 2023).

Table 3. Barriers to digital health adoption in rural South African communities

Barrier Category	Specific Challenge	Proposed Solutions
Infrastructure	Unreliable internet and mobile network coverage	Expand connectivity via satellite networks or community Wi-Fi hubs
Economic	High cost of smartphones, data, and maintenance	Government subsidies or donor-funded device/data packages
Cultural & Linguistic	Lack of translation and contextual relevance	Localise content, co-design with communities, multilingual platforms
Digital Literacy	Low familiarity with digital tools and apps	Digital skills training via PHC facilities and peer education

continued on following page

Table 3. Continued

Barrier Category	Specific Challenge	Proposed Solutions
Social Norms	Gender-based access disparities; male-dominated device ownership	Women-focused programmes, shared household tech access, inclusive design
System Integration	Tools not aligned with clinic workflows or health records	Ensure interoperability with national EHR systems and clinic tools
Privacy & Ethics	Fear of data misuse, lack of consent clarity	Transparent data policies, localised privacy education, GDPR-aligned systems

8. OPPORTUNITIES AND INNOVATIONS IN DIGITAL HEALTH

The rapid evolution of digital technology presents unprecedented opportunities to enhance the prevention, management, and promotion of health in relation to T2DM. Innovations such as AI, gamification, wearable technologies, and integrated data systems are increasingly being leveraged to improve service delivery and patient outcomes, especially in low-resource and remote contexts (Iftikhar et al., 2024). These advancements are helping to close gaps in access, support behavioural change, and strengthen the responsiveness of health systems.

8.1. AI and Personalised Care

Artificial intelligence is playing a transformative role in the evolution of digital health, offering greater precision, responsiveness, and personalisation in healthcare delivery. By leveraging machine learning, natural language processing, and predictive analytics, AI enables the processing of large, complex datasets to generate tailored health interventions in real time. This functionality is particularly relevant in the management of T2DM, where successful care relies on continuous monitoring, behavioural adjustment, and timely clinical responses. A key application of AI in diabetes care is predictive analytics. Using data drawn from CGMs, electronic health records, dietary logs, and physical activity trackers, AI algorithms can anticipate fluctuations in glucose levels and detect early signs of hyperglycaemia or hypoglycaemia. These predictive capabilities allow for timely intervention and support proactive treatment planning, reducing the risk of complications and enhancing disease control (Lee et al., 2025).

AI also plays a crucial role in providing real-time personalised guidance. Learning from individual behavioural patterns and physiological responses, AI systems can offer context-specific suggestions such as dietary adjustments, exercise recommendations, or medication reminders. For example, if a user logs a high-carbohydrate meal, the system may propose a brief walk or advise an insulin adjustment based on previous data trends. This type of feedback empowers patients to make informed daily decisions, improving both engagement and adherence to treatment plans (Ortiz-Escobar et al., 2023).

Beyond data interpretation, AI enables the development of intelligent chatbots and virtual health assistants that offer round-the-clock support. These tools simulate natural conversation, answering queries related to symptoms, medication schedules, and lifestyle advice. Unlike conventional digital resources, AI-powered assistants can adapt their responses based on user input, respond in local languages, and provide culturally relevant suggestions—broadening accessibility for diverse user groups (Mauroner, 2019). This is particularly valuable in low-resource settings, where direct access to healthcare professionals may be limited. Additionally, AI enhances remote monitoring and clinical decision-making for healthcare providers. When integrated with EHRs, AI systems can flag patients at risk, track glycaemic trends, and suggest evidence-based adjustments to care plans. This not only improves the timeliness of clinical interventions but also helps reduce provider burden and prevent avoidable hospitalisations (Sanz, Acha, & García, 2021).

However, as the integration of AI in personalised diabetes care expands, it also raises important ethical and practical concerns. Issues such as data privacy, algorithmic bias, and unequal access to digital technologies must be addressed to ensure responsible and equitable implementation. Inclusive data sets, transparent algorithms, and robust data governance are critical for building user trust and ensuring that AI enhances, rather than exacerbates, disparities in healthcare.

8.2. Gamification and Behaviour Change

Gamification refers to the use of game-design elements such as points, rewards, progress bars, badges, levels, challenges, and leaderboards in non-game settings to enhance user engagement and motivation (Riar et al., 2022). Within digital health, it has emerged as an effective strategy to encourage patient adherence to self-care behaviours, especially in the prevention and management of chronic conditions like T2DM (Miller, Cafazzo & Seto, 2016).

Gamification transforms routine health tasks into engaging experiences by adding interactive and motivating elements, making them feel less monotonous and more enjoyable. For example, users may earn virtual points or badges for completing daily exercise goals, recording meals, or consistently monitoring their blood glucose levels. Some platforms introduce friendly competition through leaderboards or peer challenges, while others present health tasks as 'missions' or 'quests' that must be completed to unlock additional features or progress to a higher level (Nour, Rouf & Allman-Farinelli, 2018). These elements tap into intrinsic motivation, reinforcing desired behaviours through recognition and progression (Miller, Cafazzo & Seto, 2016).

Evidence suggests that gamification is particularly effective among adolescents and young adults, who are more responsive to digital interaction and social reinforcement (Behl et al.,2022; Schmidt-Kraepelin et al., 2020). A In this demographic, the appeal of challenges, competition, and virtual rewards can help overcome resistance to behaviour change. Gamified tools can support goal-setting, promote self-monitoring, and foster longer-term engagement with health interventions. For instance, fitness-tracking apps that offer real-time feedback and achievements have been shown to promote more active lifestyles among youth at risk of developing T2DM.

In addition to enhancing engagement, gamification supports behaviour change by incorporating principles from established behavioural theories such as the Transtheoretical Model (TTM) and Self-Determination Theory (SDT) (Schmidt-Kraepelin et al., 2020). These theories emphasise the importance of goal-setting, perceived competence, and timely feedback in facilitating long-term behavioural shifts. Gamified features can help users build self-efficacy by setting manageable goals, tracking progress, and receiving positive reinforcement, for example, earning a badge for a week of consistent healthy eating or stable blood sugar levels.

Social components further strengthen the impact of gamification. Many platforms allow users to share achievements, support one another, and participate in team-based challenges. These features promote accountability and create a sense of community, which can be particularly beneficial in rural or underserved areas where in-person peer support may be limited but digital connectivity is available

(Nour, Rouf & Allman-Farinelli, 2018). However, the success of gamification depends heavily on thoughtful and culturally sensitive design. Rewards and challenges must be meaningful and relevant to users' experiences. The interface should be intuitive, and feedback should be timely and supportive. If poorly designed, gamified elements may seem superficial, lose their appeal over time, or fail to engage users with limited digital literacy. Care must also be taken to avoid trivialising serious health issues or excluding users from low-resource settings.

8.3. Wearable Technology and Real-Time Monitoring

Wearable technology has become an increasingly important tool in digital health, particularly for the management and prevention of non-communicable diseases such as T2DM (Jafleh et al., 2024). Devices such as fitness trackers, smartwatches, and CGMs enable users to monitor a range of health indicators in real time, including physical activity, heart rate, sleep quality, and blood glucose levels. One of the most significant innovations in diabetes care is the CGM, which provides continuous, non-invasive glucose monitoring throughout the day and night (Liu & Zhang, 2024). Unlike traditional finger-prick tests, CGMs offer real-time insights into glucose fluctuations, allowing users to respond quickly to risks of hyperglycaemia or hypoglycaemia (Ghosh & Verma, 2024). This dynamic feedback supports better glycaemic control, reduces anxiety, and increases users' confidence in managing their condition (Franceschi et al., 2021). Fitness wearables such as Fitbit, Apple Watch, and Garmin devices further support diabetes prevention by tracking daily steps, calorie expenditure, and sleep patterns. These metrics encourage healthier lifestyles such as regular physical activity which are essential for improving insulin sensitivity and maintaining a healthy weight (Shei et al., 2022).

When integrated with mHealth applications, wearable devices form part of a seamless digital health ecosystem. They allow users to visualise long-term trends, receive personalised recommendations, and set behaviour-related goals. Remote data sharing also enables healthcare providers to offer timely, informed guidance. As Cohen et al. (2016) note, access to patient-generated data enhances clinical decision-making, facilitates early intervention, and promotes adherence to treatment. Wearables also empower individuals by making health management more interactive. Real-time data helps users understand how their behaviours such as dietary choices or sleep habits affect their health (Jafleh et al., 2024). For instance, noticing a spike in glucose after a high-carbohydrate meal can prompt immediate dietary adjustments. Some wearable platforms include gamification elements or social features, allowing users to participate in challenges, celebrate milestones, and gain support from peers (Girginov et al., 2020). These features improve motivation and help sustain engagement over time.

8.4. Data Analytics and Population Health Insights

The integration of data analytics into digital health systems is transforming how population health is monitored, evaluated, and improved particularly in the prevention and management of chronic diseases such as T2DM (Avoke et al., 2024). Digital platforms, including mobile apps, wearable technologies, and telemedicine services, generate substantial volumes of user data, ranging from behavioural and physiological metrics to treatment adherence and user engagement patterns. When aggregated and analysed systematically, these data provide valuable insights at both individual and population levels. Data analytics plays a pivotal role in identifying high-risk groups, uncovering behavioural patterns, and highlighting unmet healthcare needs across diverse population segments. For example, patterns in glucose fluctuations, physical inactivity, or poor dietary habits derived from app data can be used to tailor targeted interventions. These may include personalised SMS reminders, culturally adapted nutrition content, or community-based education initiatives (Chatterjee et al., 2021).

In low-resource settings, digital health data offers a vital alternative to traditional surveillance, enabling real-time tracking of outcomes. This supports evidence-based planning, helping ensure interventions are effective, context-specific, and equitable. Machine learning and predictive analytics further enhance the value of health data. Algorithms can forecast disease progression, predict non-adherence, or identify individuals at risk of hospital readmission (Kataria & Ravindran, 2019). For instance, a user showing declining engagement and rising glucose levels might be flagged automatically for follow-up, allowing for early intervention and proactive chronic disease management.

In addition, real-time dashboards are being used to visualise and summarise key performance indicators such as app usage trends, biometric outcomes, and progress against behaviour change goals (Helminski et al., 2022). These tools allow healthcare teams and programme managers to monitor the effectiveness and reach of digital interventions. Public health campaigns, for example, can track engagement rates by age, gender, or geographic region, and adjust strategies accordingly to maximise impact.

Beyond clinical application, data analytics also informs health policy and programme evaluation. Trends in glycaemic control, physical activity, and treatment adherence provide evidence for shaping national strategies on diabetes prevention and informing broader health system investments (Avoke et al., 2024). Data analytics also facilitates cross-sector collaboration, enabling coordination between government agencies, non-governmental organisations, and private sector partners engaged in digital health implementation. Nevertheless, the benefits of data-driven insights must be balanced with strong governance and ethical safeguards. Key concerns around data privacy, informed consent, and digital equity must be addressed to avoid perpetuating or deepening existing disparities (Adeniyi et al.,2024). Ensuring data are disaggregated by gender, socioeconomic status, and geography is vital for revealing hidden inequities and designing responsive, inclusive interventions.

8.5. Linking Digital Tools to Primary Health Care and Peer Support

The integration of digital health tools into primary health care (PHC) systems is pivotal for the delivery of sustainable, equitable, and person-centred care particularly in the management of chronic conditions such as T2DM. When appropriately embedded within formal health infrastructure, digital technologies can improve service efficiency, enhance patient monitoring, and strengthen the responsiveness of health systems (Sanz, Acha, & García, 2021). Mobile applications, wearable devices, and remote monitoring tools must not operate in silos but rather complement existing PHC models to ensure continuity of care, trust, and accessibility.

A central component of this integration is the linkage of digital tools to EHRs, allowing clinicians access to real-time, comprehensive patient data (WHO, 2021). Information collected from personal devices such as glucose readings, dietary logs, and physical activity levels can be used to inform clinical decision-making and guide personalised treatment adjustments (Lim et al., 2016). Integrating these tools with EHR systems also facilitates referral coordination, streamlines follow-up appointments, and supports timely prescription renewals, ultimately reducing administrative burden and enhancing care quality.

Moreover, digital tools that enable secure communication such as appointment booking systems, messaging functions, and medication reminders contribute to reducing missed appointments and enabling early intervention. These features are especially valuable in resource-constrained or geographically remote settings, where physical access to care may be limited (Rinaldi, Hijazi & Haghparast-Bidgoli, 2020). They allow for remote management, reducing unnecessary clinic visits and supporting patients in maintaining continuity of care under challenging circumstances.

Beyond the clinical interface, peer support represents a vital but often underutilised resource in digital health. Peer-led interventions where individuals living with diabetes offer support to others managing the same condition have demonstrated improved outcomes in terms of self-management, emotional wellbeing, and adherence to care plans (Fortuna et al., 2019). Digital platforms such as WhatsApp, Telegram, and SMS offer flexible and accessible means to facilitate these connections, allowing participants to share experiences, ask questions, and provide mutual encouragement. Community health workers (CHWs) can also play a significant role by using mobile platforms to deliver health education, track patient progress, and provide culturally sensitive guidance. Research shows that hybrid models, combining digital tools with interpersonal or community-based support, are more effective than purely digital or face-to-face interventions (Mulenga & Shilongo, 2025). These integrated models harness the benefits of both technology and human connection, addressing the motivational, emotional, and social dimensions of diabetes care that digital tools alone may overlook.

Importantly, linking digital health tools to community-based health systems can increase reach and relevance. CHWs may act as digital intermediaries, supporting users with limited literacy or unfamiliarity with mobile technology. This is particularly important in rural, older, or low-income populations, where smartphone ownership and digital proficiency may be lower. These efforts ensure that digital innovation promotes inclusion rather than exacerbating existing disparities. At a systemic level, robust policy frameworks and institutional backing are essential to support integration and scale. Ministries of health and digital health strategies must incorporate these tools into PHC policies, training curricula, and clinical guidelines. This should include clear protocols for data privacy, role definitions for task-sharing, and mechanisms for accountability and quality assurance (Stevens, 2018).

8.6. Localising Digital Health Solutions for Greater Relevance and Impact

Localising digital health interventions is crucial to ensure their relevance, accessibility, and effectiveness especially in diverse, resource-constrained settings such as rural South Africa. This process involves tailoring digital content and platforms to reflect the cultural, linguistic, and social realities of the target population, thereby fostering user engagement and improving health outcomes. A key element of localisation is cultural and linguistic adaptation. Effective digital health solutions must go beyond mere technical functionality to resonate with the lived experiences, cultural identities, and everyday practices of users (Brewer et al., 2020). In multilingual, socio-economically varied environments like many parts of South Africa and other low- and middle-income countries, neglecting localisation risks poor uptake, misunderstanding, and ultimately limited impact.

Language adaptation is foundational. Delivering health messages in local languages such as isiZulu, Xitsonga, Sepedi, or Setswana enhances comprehension and builds trust. Language not only aids understanding but also signals respect for users' identities and contexts. Research demonstrates that people engage more deeply and respond better when health information is communicated in their mother tongue (Clayman et al., 2010). Moreover, some health concepts lack direct translations or may carry different connotations across languages, necessitating careful adaptation with community input to prevent confusion or stigma. Localising dietary guidance is particularly important in diabetes prevention and management, where nutrition is central. Recommending Western foods like quinoa or kale can be irrelevant, unaffordable, or inaccessible to many rural or low-income users. Instead, guidance should emphasise familiar local staples such as pap (maize meal porridge), *morogo (*traditional leafy greens), samp (crushed maize), beans, and traditional meats or legumes. Incorporating culturally accepted cooking methods and typical portion sizes ensures advice is practical and respects household routines and economic realities (Domosławska-Żylińska et al., 2023).

Cultural beliefs about illness and treatment also shape how digital health messages are perceived. For example, some communities may attribute chronic diseases like diabetes to spiritual causes or traditional imbalances rather than biomedical factors (Clayman et al., 2010). Ignoring these perspectives can alienate users. Instead, digital content should seek to bridge biomedical knowledge with cultural understandings of health, potentially integrating respectful references to traditional healing or involving traditional leaders in design. Visual and audio aids further enhance accessibility, particularly for populations with limited literacy or digital skills. Illustrations, diagrams, and animations can effectively demonstrate procedures such as glucose testing or foot care. Audio messages in local dialects, disseminated via WhatsApp or pre-recorded calls, can reach users less comfortable with reading text. Such multimedia formats improve inclusivity and retention, especially among older adults, women, and rural residents with limited formal education (Tomczyk et al., 2023).

Participatory content development is vital for cultural alignment. Involving community members, healthcare workers, and peer educators in co-design workshops ensures that digital health content is both accurate and relatable [74]. [45]. (Gillett-Swan et al., 2024). These engagements help identify local idioms, taboos, and preferences that influence message reception, while end-user testing fine-tunes tone, format, and delivery channels. Finally, gender and social norms must be accounted for in localisation efforts. In some households, women may require permission to use mobile phones, while men might be less willing to discuss health matters openly. Gender-sensitive content design such as incorporating role models, couple-based messaging, or discreet message delivery can help overcome these barriers (Chace Dwyer et al., 2022).

Figure 1. Ecosystem of Digital Health Tools for Diabetes Management

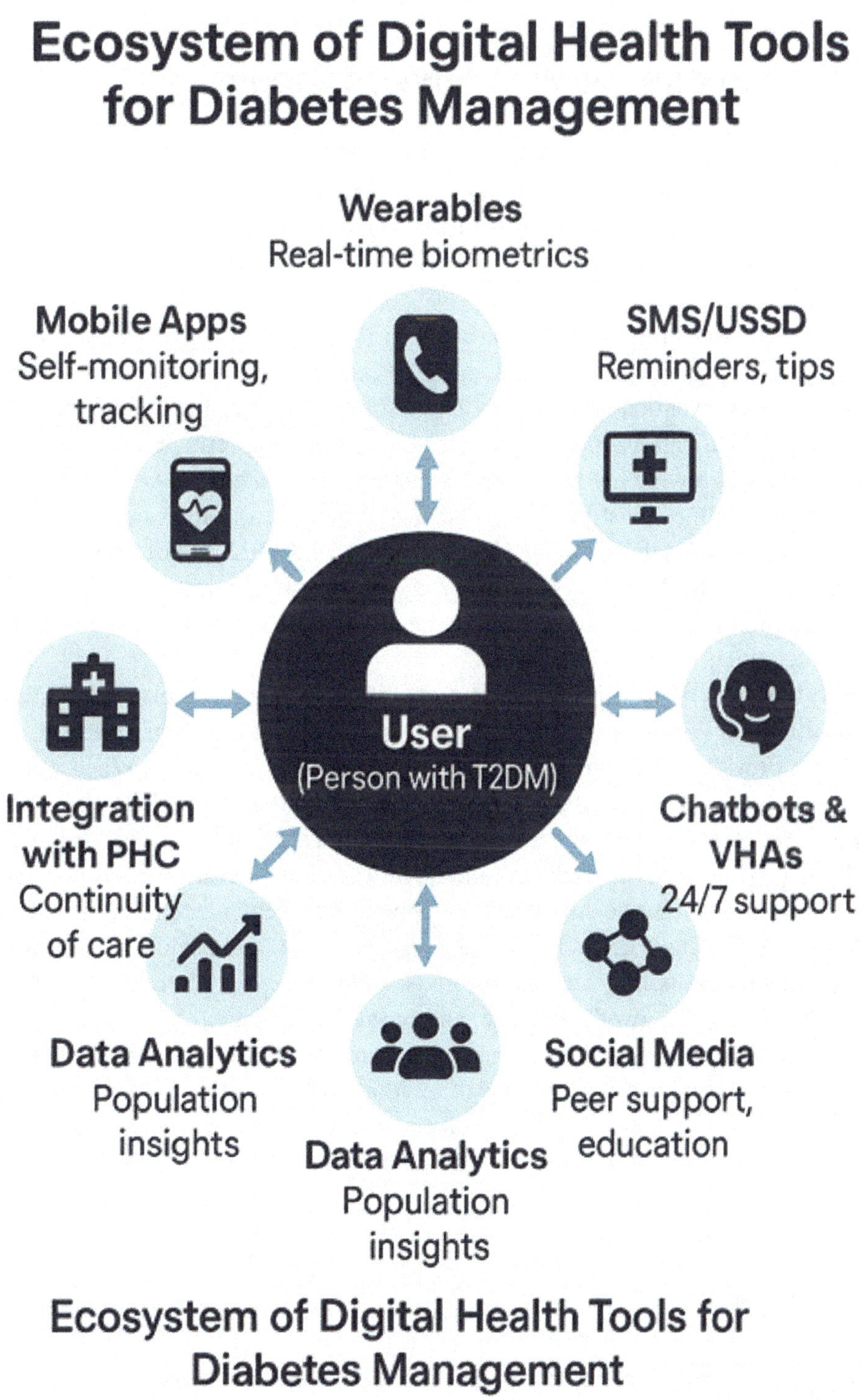

This diagram illustrates the user-centred digital health ecosystem for managing T2DM. The central figure represents the person with T2DM, surrounded by various digital tools that support different aspects of care.

9. FUTURE DIRECTIONS AND POLICY IMPLICATIONS

Harnessing digital health for diabetes prevention and UHC: As digital health tools continue to demonstrate their effectiveness in preventing and managing diabetes, there is increasing impetus to integrate them into national health systems. In LMICs such as South Africa, this integration must be supported by deliberate policy frameworks that promote accessibility, scalability, and alignment with broader health priorities.

Integrating digital tools into national diabetes strategies: Digital solutions including mobile applications, SMS messaging, wearable devices, and EHRs should be formally incorporated into national strategies for diabetes prevention and control. These tools support critical components such as early diagnosis, lifestyle modification, medication adherence, and long-term monitoring. Their effective use can help reduce the growing burden of type 2 diabetes and related NCDs. To facilitate meaningful adoption, national guidelines must prioritise evidence-based, locally relevant digital platforms. The World Health Organization's Global Digital Health Strategy 2020–2025 advocates for integrating digital innovations into primary healthcare systems to promote equity and person-centred care. Ministries of Health can leverage this framework to establish national standards for interoperability, data privacy, and health service integration.

Public-private partnerships (PPPs) as catalysts for scale: The PPPs play a crucial role in scaling digital health initiatives. While the private sector offers innovation, technical expertise, and infrastructure, governments provide regulation, policy direction, and public legitimacy. When well-aligned, such partnerships can enable sustainable digital transformation that protects public health interests.

Advancing UHC through digital innovation: Digital health can be a powerful enabler of UHC, particularly by improving access, efficiency, and quality of care for marginalised populations. Mobile technologies allow for low-cost health education, appointment reminders, teleconsultations, and peer support, helping to overcome barriers related to geography, cost, and healthcare workforce shortages. To ensure digital inclusion, policy interventions must address the digital divide through investment in infrastructure, expansion of network coverage, and promotion of digital literacy. Localisation of content linguistically and culturally is also essential to ensure that digital tools are relevant and engaging for diverse user groups. Embedding digital health within UHC frameworks will require multisectoral collaboration and strong political will. Policy-makers must commit to inclusive, ethical, and evidence-informed digital innovation that prioritises the health needs of all citizens, particularly those most at risk of being left behind.

10. CONCLUSION

Digital health tools are reshaping approaches to diabetes prevention and management, particularly in LMICs such as South Africa. This chapter has underscored the value of mHealth apps, SMS messaging, wearable technologies, AI, and user-centred digital interventions in raising awareness, promoting healthy behaviours, and supporting T2DM management. While digital innovations offer scalable and cost-effective solutions, their impact depends on equitable access, cultural relevance, and integration into primary healthcare. Addressing challenges such as the digital divide, data privacy, and weak health system alignment is essential. Engagement with users, families, and communities further enhances trust, usability, and long-term adherence.

Looking ahead, digital tools hold strong potential to transform diabetes care, but this requires coordinated action. Researchers must produce context-specific evidence; developers should prioritise inclusive, localised design; and policymakers must foster enabling environments through investment, integration, and capacity building. The future of diabetes care lies in hybrid models that combine technological innovation with person-centred, accessible care firmly grounded in the realities of those most affected.

11. LIMITATIONS

While this chapter provides valuable insights into the role of digital health in diabetes prevention and management, several limitations must be acknowledged. The geographic and contextual focus is largely centred on LMICs, with a particular emphasis on South Africa. However, the significant diversity within LMICs ranging from variations in infrastructure and health systems to differing cultural norms and policy environments means the findings may not be universally applicable across all settings. A further limitation lies in the chapter's technology-centric perspective. While digital tools are foregrounded as transformative, there is a risk of underplaying the continued importance of in-person, community-based, and traditional care models. In many under-resourced environments, these conventional systems remain the backbone of healthcare provision. Therefore, digital interventions should be seen as complementary, rather than substitutive.

Moreover, the chapter draws upon emerging literature and programme evaluations, yet there is still a scarcity of large-scale, longitudinal evidence to fully assess the effectiveness, cost-efficiency, and long-term sustainability of digital health interventions in LMICs. This limits the ability to draw definitive conclusions about their broader impact. Equity and inclusion, though addressed, require deeper exploration. The experiences of marginalised groups such as individuals with disabilities, rural youth, or gender-diverse populations are not examined in sufficient detail. These communities often face unique barriers to accessing digital health services, and greater attention is needed to ensure their needs are adequately represented in both design and implementation. Finally, while the chapter outlines general policy implications, it does not delve into the specific political, economic, and institutional obstacles that often hinder the successful scale-up of digital health initiatives. Challenges such as limited funding, bureaucratic resistance, and poor inter-sectoral coordination are common and must be considered in any future strategic planning.

These limitations underscore the need for further context-specific research, participatory and inclusive design processes, and proactive policy engagement to ensure digital health tools can truly meet the needs of those most affected by the diabetes epidemic in LMICs.

ABBREVIATIONS

AI - Artificial Intelligence
CGM - Continuous glucose monitor
EHR - Electronic Health Records
GDPR -General Data Protection Regulation
LMICs Low- and Middle-Income Countries
mDiab - Mobile Diabetes Prevention App
mHealth - Mobile Health
NCDs - Non-Communicable Diseases
NGO - Non-Governmental Organisation
PHC - Primary Health Care
PPP - Public-Private Partnership
SDT - Self-Determination Theory
SMS - Short message service
T2DM - Type 2 Diabetes Mellitus
TTM - Transtheoretical Model
UHC - Universal Health Coverage
USSD - Unstructured Supplementary Service Data
VHA - Virtual Health Assistant
WHO - World Health Organization

REFERENCES

Abaza, H., & Marschollek, M. (2017). mHealth application areas and technology combinations. *Methods of information in medicine, 56*(S 01), e105-e122.

Abernethy, A., Adams, L., Barrett, M., Bechtel, C., Brennan, P., Butte, A., & Valdes, K. (2022). The promise of digital health: Then, now, and the future. *NAM Perspectives, 2022*, 10–31478.

Adeniyi, A. O., Arowoogun, J. O., Okolo, C. A., Chidi, R., & Babawarun, O. (2024). Ethical considerations in healthcare IT: A review of data privacy and patient consent issues. *World Journal of Advanced Research and Reviews, 21*(2), 1660–1668.

Al Shamsi, H., Almutairi, A. G., Al Mashrafi, S., & Al Kalbani, T. (2020). Implications of language barriers for healthcare: A systematic review. *Oman Medical Journal, 35*(2), e122.

Avoke, D., Elshafeey, A., Weinstein, R., Kim, C. H., & Martin, S. S. (2024). Digital health in diabetes and cardiovascular disease. *Endocrine Research, 49*(3), 124–136.

Badr, J., Motulsky, A., & Denis, J. L. (2024). Digital health technologies and inequalities: A scoping review of potential impacts and policy recommendations. *Health Policy (Amsterdam)*, •••, 105122.

Barron, P., Peter, J., LeFevre, A. E., Sebidi, J., Bekker, M., Allen, R., & Pillay, Y. (2018). Mobile health messaging service and helpdesk for South African mothers (MomConnect): History, successes and challenges. *BMJ Global Health, 3*(Suppl 2), e000559.

Behl, A., Jayawardena, N., Pereira, V., Islam, N., Del Giudice, M., & Choudrie, J. (2022). Gamification and e-learning for young learners: A systematic literature review, bibliometric analysis, and future research agenda. *Technological Forecasting and Social Change, 176*, 121445.

Bell, K., Salmon, A., & McNaughton, D. (2011). Alcohol, tobacco, obesity and the new public health. *Critical Public Health, 21*(1), 1–8.

Brall, C., Schröder-Bäck, P., & Maeckelberghe, E. (2019). Ethical aspects of digital health from a justice point of view. *European Journal of Public Health, 29*(Supplement_3), 18–22.

Brewer, L. C., Fortuna, K. L., Jones, C., Walker, R., Hayes, S. N., Patten, C. A., & Cooper, L. A. (2020). Back to the future: Achieving health equity through health informatics and digital health. *JMIR mHealth and uHealth, 8*(1), e14512.

Chace Dwyer, S., Mathur, S., Kirk, K., Dadi, C., & Dougherty, L. (2022). "When you live in good health with your husband, then your children are in good health…." A qualitative exploration of how households make healthcare decisions in Maradi and Zinder Regions, Niger. *BMC Public Health, 22*(1), 1350.

Chatterjee, A., Prinz, A., Gerdes, M., & Martinez, S. (2021). Digital interventions on healthy lifestyle management: Systematic review. *Journal of Medical Internet Research, 23*(11), e26931.

Clark, M., & Bailey, S. (2024). Chatbots in health care: Connecting patients to information. *Canadian Journal of Health Technologies, 4*(1).

Clayman, M. L., Manganello, J. A., Viswanath, K., Hesse, B. W., & Arora, N. K. (2010). Providing health messages to Hispanics/Latinos: understanding the importance of language, trust in health information sources, and media use. Journal of health communication, 15(sup3), 252-263.

Clifford, G. D. (2016). E-health in low to middle income countries. *Journal of Medical Engineering & Technology*, *40*(7-8), 336–341.

Cohen, D. J., Keller, S. R., Hayes, G. R., Dorr, D. A., Ash, J. S., & Sittig, D. F. (2016). Integrating patient-generated health data into clinical care settings or clinical decision-making: Lessons learned from project healthdesign. *JMIR Human Factors*, *3*(2), e5919.

Colagiuri, S. (2021). Definition and classification of diabetes and prediabetes and emerging data on phenotypes. *Endocrinology and Metabolism Clinics*, *50*(3), 319–336.

da Silva Rosa, S. C., Nayak, N., Caymo, A. M., & Gordon, J. W. (2020). Mechanisms of muscle insulin resistance and the cross-talk with liver and adipose tissue. *Physiological Reports*, *8*(19), e14607.

Debon, R., Coleone, J. D., Bellei, E. A., & De Marchi, A. C. B. (2019). Mobile health applications for chronic diseases: A systematic review of features for lifestyle improvement. *Diabetes & Metabolic Syndrome*, *13*(4), 2507–2512.

Domosławska-Żylińska, K., Łopatek, M., Krysińska-Pisarek, M., & Sugay, L. (2023). Barriers to adherence to healthy diet and recommended physical activity perceived by the polish population. *Journal of Clinical Medicine*, *13*(1), 22.

Fitzpatrick, P. J. (2023). Improving health literacy using the power of digital communications to achieve better health outcomes for patients and practitioners. *Frontiers in Digital Health*, *5*, 1264780.

Ford, N. D., Patel, S. A., & Narayan, K. V. (2017). Obesity in low-and middle-income countries: Burden, drivers, and emerging challenges. *Annual Review of Public Health*, *38*(1), 145–164.

Fortuna, K. L., Brooks, J. M., Umucu, E., Walker, R., & Chow, P. I. (2019). Peer support: A human factor to enhance engagement in digital health behavior change interventions. *Journal of Technology in Behavioral Science*, *4*, 152–161.

Fox, A., Feng, W., & Asal, V. (2019). What is driving global obesity trends? Globalization or "modernization"? *Globalization and Health*, *15*(1), 32.

Franceschi, R., Micheli, F., Mozzillo, E., Cauvin, V., Liguori, A., Soffiati, M., & Giani, E. (2021). Intermittently scanned and continuous glucose monitor systems: A systematic review on psychological outcomes in pediatric patients. *Frontiers in Pediatrics*, *9*, 660173.

Ghosh, N., & Verma, S. (2024). Technological advancements in glucose monitoring and artificial pancreas systems for shaping diabetes care. *Current Medical Research and Opinion*, *40*(12), 2095–2107.

Giansanti, D. (2025, April). The Future of Healthcare Is Digital: Unlocking the Potential of Mobile Health and E-Health Solutions. In Healthcare (Vol. 13, No. 7, p. 802). MDPI.

Gillett-Swan, J., Kerr, J., Winter, A., & Callard, N. (2024). Co-designing place-based co-located health and wellbeing infrastructure and services with high school students, educators, and health service providers. *Children and Youth Services Review*, *166*, 107971.

Girginov, V., Moore, P., Olsen, N., Godfrey, T., & Cooke, F. (2020). Wearable technology-stimulated social interaction for promoting physical activity: A systematic review. *Cogent Social Sciences*, *6*(1), 1742517.

Gloster, P., Mash, R., & Swartz, S. (2021). Investigating the effect of the Vula Mobile app on coordination of care and capacity building in district health services, Cape Town: Convergent mixed methods study. *South African Family Practice*, *63*(4).

Gong, J. Y., Sajjadi, S. F., Motala, A. A., Shaw, J. E., & Magliano, D. J. (2025). Variation in type 2 diabetes prevalence across different populations: The key drivers. *Diabetologia*, •••, 1–13.

Habukawa, C., Ohgami, N., Arai, T., Makata, H., Tomikawa, M., Fujino, T., & Murakami, K. (2021). Wheeze recognition algorithm for remote medical care device in children: Validation study. *JMIR Pediatrics and Parenting*, *4*(2), e28865.

Haleem, A., Javaid, M., Singh, R. P., & Suman, R. (2021). Telemedicine for healthcare: Capabilities, features, barriers, and applications. *Sensors International*, *2*, 100117.

Helminski, D., Kurlander, J. E., Renji, A. D., Sussman, J. B., Pfeiffer, P. N., Conte, M. L., & Landis-Lewis, Z. (2022). Dashboards in health care settings: Protocol for a scoping review. *JMIR Research Protocols*, *11*(3), e34894.

Holl, F., Kircher, J., Hertelendy, A. J., Sukums, F., & Swoboda, W. (2024). Tanzania's and Germany's digital health strategies and their consistency with the World Health Organization's global strategy on digital health 2020-2025: Comparative policy analysis. *Journal of Medical Internet Research*, *26*, e52150.

Iftikhar, M., Saqib, M., Qayyum, S. N., Asmat, R., Mumtaz, H., Rehan, M., & Ejaz, Z. (2024). Artificial intelligence-driven transformations in diabetes care: A comprehensive literature review. *Annals of Medicine and Surgery (London)*, *86*(9), 5334–5342.

Intelligence, G. S. M. A. (2018). The mobile economy sub-saharan Africa.

International Diabetes Federation. 2021. IDF Diabetes Atlas. 10th ed. Brussel Belgium: IDF, 2019. 1-169. https://www. diabetesatlas.org

International Diabetes Federation (IDF). 2025. Diabetes Atlas. 11th Edition. (Accessed 20 April, 2025). https://diabetesatlas.org/resources/idf-diabetes-atlas-2025/?mc_cid=b5d31665df&mc_eid=672aa4d27c

Jafleh, E. A., Alnaqbi, F. A., Almaeeni, H. A., Faqeeh, S., Alzaabi, M. A., Al Zaman, K., & Alzaabi, M. (2024). The role of wearable devices in chronic disease monitoring and patient care: A comprehensive review. *Cureus*, *16*(9).

Jerjes, W., & Harding, D. (2024). Telemedicine in the post-COVID era: Balancing accessibility, equity, and sustainability in primary healthcare. *Frontiers in Digital Health*, *6*, 1432871.

Junaid, S. B., Imam, A. A., Balogun, A. O., De Silva, L. C., Surakat, Y. A., Kumar, G., . . . Mahamad, S. (2022, October). Recent advancements in emerging technologies for healthcare management systems: a survey. In Healthcare (Vol. 10, No. 10, p. 1940). MDPI.

Kataria, S., & Ravindran, V. (2019). Emerging role of ehealth in the identification of very early inflammatory rheumatic diseases. *Best Practice & Research. Clinical Rheumatology*, *33*(4), 101429.

Kengne, A. P., & Ramachandran, A. (2024). Feasibility of prevention of type 2 diabetes in low-and middle-income countries. *Diabetologia*, *67*(5), 763–772.

Kim, M. O., Coiera, E., & Magrabi, F. (2017). Problems with health information technology and their effects on care delivery and patient outcomes: A systematic review. *Journal of the American Medical Informatics Association : JAMIA*, *24*(2), 246–250.

Kirk, J., Bandholm, T., Andersen, O., Husted, R. S., Tjørnhøj-Thomsen, T., Nilsen, P., & Pedersen, M. M. (2021). Challenges in co-designing an intervention to increase mobility in older patients: A qualitative study. *Journal of Health Organization and Management*, *35*(9), 140–162.

Kunyiha, N., Adan, R., Ngugi, R., Odhiambo, J., & Sokwalla, S. M. (2025). The unique ethnicity-specific aspects of burden, pathogenesis and management of prediabetes: Insights from Africa. *Current Diabetes Reports*, *25*(1), 25.

Lee, E. Y. F., & Lee, E. L. S. (2023). *Trends and Issues of Promoting Digital Learning in High-Digital-Competitiveness Countries: Country Reports and International Comparison*. Online Submission.

Lee, S., Choi, D., Truong, L., Sawhney, N., & Paakki, H. (2025, April). Into the Unknown: Leveraging Conversational AI in Supporting Young Migrants' Journeys Towards Cultural Adaptation. In *Proceedings of the 2025 CHI Conference on Human Factors in Computing Systems* (pp. 1-19).

LeFevre, A. E., Dane, P., Copley, C. J., Pienaar, C., Parsons, A. N., Engelhard, M., & Mohan, D. (2018). Unpacking the performance of a mobile health information messaging program for mothers (MomConnect) in South Africa: Evidence on program reach and messaging exposure. *BMJ Global Health*, *3*(Suppl 2), e000583.

Li, L. C., Xie, H., Feehan, L. M., Shaw, C., Lu, N., Ramachandran, S., & Lacaille, D. (2025). Effect of digital monitoring and counselling on self-management ability in patients with rheumatoid arthritis: A randomised controlled trial. *Rheumatology*, *64*(1), 310–320.

Lim, S., Kang, S. M., Kim, K. M., Moon, J. H., Choi, S. H., Hwang, H., & Jang, H. C. (2016). Multifactorial intervention in diabetes care using real-time monitoring and tailored feedback in type 2 diabetes. *Acta Diabetologica*, *53*, 189–198.

Liu, X., & Zhang, J. (2024). Continuous Glucose Monitoring: A Transformative Approach to the Detection of Prediabetes. *Journal of Multidisciplinary Healthcare*, •••, 5513–5519.

Maher, C., Singh, B., Wylde, A., & Chastin, S. (2024). Virtual health assistants: A grand challenge in health communications and behavior change. *Frontiers in Digital Health*, *6*, 1418695.

Maita, K. C., Maniaci, M. J., Haider, C. R., Avila, F. R., Torres-Guzman, R. A., Borna, S., & Forte, A. J. (2024). The impact of digital health solutions on bridging the health care gap in rural areas: A scoping review. *The Permanente Journal, 28*(3), 130.

Makroum, M. A., Adda, M., Bouzouane, A., & Ibrahim, H. (2022). Machine learning and smart devices for diabetes management: Systematic review. *Sensors (Basel), 22*(5), 1843.

Materia, F. T., Smyth, J. M., Puoane, T., Tsolekile, L., Goggin, K., Kodish, S. R., & Catley, D. (2023). Implementing text-messaging to support and enhance delivery of health behavior change interventions in low-to middle-income countries: Case study of the Lifestyle Africa intervention. *BMC Public Health, 23*(1), 1526.

Mauroner, O. (2019). Gamification in management and other non-game contexts—Understanding game elements, motivation, reward systems, and user types. *Open Journal of Business and Management, 7*(4), 1815–1830.

McGraw, D., & Mandl, K. D. (2021). Privacy protections to encourage use of health-relevant digital data in a learning health system. *NPJ Digital Medicine, 4*(1), 2.

Miller, A. S., Cafazzo, J. A., & Seto, E. (2016). A game plan: Gamification design principles in mHealth applications for chronic disease management. *Health Informatics Journal, 22*(2), 184–193.

Mphasha, M. H., Mothiba, T. M., & Skaal, L. (2022). Family support in the management of diabetes patients' perspectives from Limpopo province in South Africa. *BMC Public Health, 22*(1), 2421.

Mphasha, M. H. P., Skaal, L., & Mothiba, T. M. (2022). Prevalence of overweight and obesity amongst patients with diabetes and their non-diabetic family members in Senwabarwana, Limpopo province, South Africa. *South African Family Practice, 64*(2).

Mulenga, R., & Shilongo, H. (2025). Hybrid and blended learning models: Innovations, challenges, and future directions in education. *Acta Pedagogia Asiana, 4*(1), 1–13.

Muralidharan, S., Mohan, V., Anjana, R. M., Jena, S., Tandon, N., Allender, S., & Ranjani, H. (2017). Mobile health technology (mDiab) for the prevention of type 2 diabetes: Protocol for a randomized controlled trial. *JMIR Research Protocols, 6*(12), e8644.

Najafi, B., & Mishra, R. (2021). Harnessing digital health technologies to remotely manage diabetic foot syndrome: A narrative review. *Medicina, 57*(4), 377.

Nguyen, H., Chib, A., & Mahalingam, R. (2017). Mobile phones and gender empowerment: Negotiating the essentialist-aspirational dialectic. *Information Technologies and International Development, 13*, 181–185.

Nour, M. M., Rouf, A. S., & Allman-Farinelli, M. (2018). Exploring young adult perspectives on the use of gamification and social media in a smartphone platform for improving vegetable intake. *Appetite, 120*, 547–556.

Ntinginya, N. E., Kuchaka, D., Orina, F., Mwebaza, I., Liyoyo, A., Miheso, B., & Sabiiti, W. (2021). Unlocking the health system barriers to maximise the uptake and utilisation of molecular diagnostics in low-income and middle-income country setting. *BMJ Global Health, 6*(8), e005357.

Okano, J. T., Ponce, J., Krönke, M., & Blower, S. (2022). Lack of ownership of mobile phones could hinder the rollout of mHealth interventions in Africa. *eLife*, *11*, e79615.

Ortiz-Escobar, L. M., Chavarria, M. A., Schönenberger, K., Hurst, S., Stein, M. A., Mugeere, A., & Rivas Velarde, M. (2023). Assessing the implementation of user-centred design standards on assistive technology for persons with visual impairments: A systematic review. *Frontiers in Rehabilitation Sciences*, *4*, 1238158.

Pledger, S. L., & Ahmadizar, F. (2023). Gene-environment interactions and the effect on obesity risk in low and middle-income countries: A scoping review. *Frontiers in Endocrinology*, *14*, 1230445.

Popkin, B. M., & Ng, S. W. (2022). The nutrition transition to a stage of high obesity and noncommunicable disease prevalence dominated by ultra-processed foods is not inevitable. *Obesity Reviews*, *23*(1), e13366.

Rani, P. K., Williams, J. D., Jaswal, N., Yandluri, V., Sangani, P., Sanagavarapu, K., & Khanna, R. C. (2025). Effectiveness of mDiabetes intervention in enhancing diabetes awareness and promoting healthy lifestyle changes among the general population in rural India. *Frontiers in Public Health*, *12*, 1470615.

Riar, M., Morschheuser, B., Zarnekow, R., & Hamari, J. (2022). Gamification of cooperation: A framework, literature review and future research agenda. *International Journal of Information Management*, *67*, 102549.

Rinaldi, G., Hijazi, A., & Haghparast-Bidgoli, H. (2020). Cost and cost-effectiveness of mHealth interventions for the prevention and control of type 2 diabetes mellitus: A systematic review. *Diabetes Research and Clinical Practice*, *162*, 108084.

Rob, A., Hoque, A., Asaduzzaman, M. M., Khatoon, M. A. A., Khalil, R., Thomas, D., & Chowdhury, T. A. (2025). The Global Challenges of Type 2 Diabetes. *Bangladesh Journal of Medicine*, *36*(2), 92–98.

Rollo, M. E., Aguiar, E. J., Williams, R. L., Wynne, K., Kriss, M., Callister, R., & Collins, C. E. (2016). eHealth technologies to support nutrition and physical activity behaviors in diabetes self-management. *Diabetes, Metabolic Syndrome and Obesity*, •••, 381–390.

Ruel, M. T., Garrett, J., Yosef, S., & Olivier, M. (2017). Urbanization, food security and nutrition. *Nutrition and health in a developing world*, 705-735.

Sanz, M. F., Acha, B. V., & García, M. F. (2021). Co-design for people-centred care digital solutions: A literature review. *International Journal of Integrated Care*, *21*(2), 16.

Scheibner, J., Ienca, M., Kechagia, S., Troncoso-Pastoriza, J. R., Raisaro, J. L., Hubaux, J. P., & Vayena, E. (2020). Data protection and ethics requirements for multisite research with health data: A comparative examination of legislative governance frameworks and the role of data protection technologies. *Journal of Law and the Biosciences*, *7*(1), lsaa010.

Schmidt-Kraepelin, M., Warsinsky, S., Thiebes, S., & Sunyaev, A. (2020). The role of gamification in health behavior change: a review of theory-driven studies.

Schoeppe, S., Alley, S., Rebar, A. L., Hayman, M., Bray, N. A., Van Lippevelde, W., & Vandelanotte, C. (2017). Apps to improve diet, physical activity and sedentary behaviour in children and adolescents: A review of quality, features and behaviour change techniques. *The International Journal of Behavioral Nutrition and Physical Activity*, *14*(1), 83.

Schroeder, T., Haug, M., & Gewald, H. (2022). Data privacy concerns using mHealth apps and smart speakers: Comparative interview study among mature adults. *JMIR Formative Research*, *6*(6), e28025.

Seebregts, C., Dane, P., Parsons, A. N., Fogwill, T., Rogers, D., Bekker, M., ... & Barron, P. (2018). Designing for scale: optimising the health information system architecture for mobile maternal health messaging in South Africa (MomConnect). *BMJ global health, 3*(Suppl 2).

Sepulveda-Escobar, P., & Morrison, A. (2020). Online teaching placement during the COVID-19 pandemic in Chile: Challenges and opportunities. *European Journal of Teacher Education*, *43*(4), 587–607.

Shei, R. J., Holder, I. G., Oumsang, A. S., Paris, B. A., & Paris, H. L. (2022). Wearable activity trackers–advanced technology or advanced marketing? *European Journal of Applied Physiology*, *122*(9), 1975–1990.

Sherman, A. D., Balthazar, M., Kim, S., Carroll, L., Casseus, K., & Febres-Cordero, S. (2023). Peer Facilitation: Accelerating Individual, Community, and Societal Change. *Advances in Peer-Led Learning*, *3*, 18.

South African National Department of Health. (2019). National digital health strategy for South Africa 2019–2024. Pretoria, South Africa.

Statti, A., & Torres, K. M. (2020). Digital literacy: The need for technology integration and its impact on learning and engagement in community school environments. *Peabody Journal of Education*, *95*(1), 90–100.

Stevens, C. (2018). Scales of integration for sustainable development governance. *International Journal of Sustainable Development and World Ecology*, *25*(1), 1–8.

Suganthi, V., & Kalaiselvi, K. (2024). Decision Support System in Healthcare Monitoring. *Artificial Intelligence-Based System Models in Healthcare*, 55-78.

Thouvenot, K., Turpin, T., Taïlé, J., Clément, K., Meilhac, O., & Gonthier, M. P. (2022). Links between insulin resistance and periodontal bacteria: Insights on molecular players and therapeutic potential of polyphenols. *Biomolecules*, *12*(3), 378.

Tomczyk, Ł., Mascia, M. L., Gierszewski, D., & Walker, C. (2023). Barriers to digital inclusion among older people: a intergenerational reflection on the need to develop digital competences for the group with the highest level of digital exclusion.

Van Der Vaart, R., & Drossaert, C. (2017). Development of the digital health literacy instrument: Measuring a broad spectrum of health 1.0 and health 2.0 skills. *Journal of Medical Internet Research*, *19*(1), e27.

Vijayan, V., Connolly, J. P., Condell, J., McKelvey, N., & Gardiner, P. (2021). Review of wearable devices and data collection considerations for connected health. *Sensors (Basel)*, *21*(16), 5589.

Wierda, E., Blok, S., Somsen, G. A., van der Velde, E. T., Tulevski, I. I., Stavrov, B., & Winter, M. M. (2020). Protecting patient privacy in digital health technology: The Dutch m-Health infrastructure of Hartwacht as a learning case. *BMJ Innovations*, *6*(4).

Woodward, A., Walters, K., Davies, N., Nimmons, D., Protheroe, J., Chew-Graham, C. A., & Armstrong, M. (2024). Barriers and facilitators of self-management of diabetes amongst people experiencing socio-economic deprivation: A systematic review and qualitative synthesis. *Health Expectations*, *27*(3), e14070.

World Health Organization (WHO). (2021). Global strategy on digital health 2020-2025. Geneva: World Health Organization; 2021. Licence: CC BY-NC-SA 3.0 IGO.

Zakaria, H., Said, Y., Aleabova, S., Bangayan, J., Dandan, M., Debs, J., & Almarzooqi, I. (2024). Measuring the effectiveness of hybrid diabetes care over 90 days through continuous data monitoring in type 2 diabetic patients. *Frontiers in Endocrinology*, *15*, 1355792.

KEY TERMS AND DEFINITIONS

Digital health: is defined as any use of mobile apps, teleconsultation platforms, or wearable devices by patients for diabetes-related care, self-monitoring, or health education purposes.

Gamification: refers to the use of game-like elements such as achievement badges, progress tracking, and health challenges within health applications to increase patient motivation, engagement, and adherence to daily diabetes management routines.

Health literacy: is the patients' ability to interpret health messages delivered via digital platforms and respond appropriately for example, following treatment instructions, seeking help, or adopting recommended behaviours.

Mobile Health (mHealth): refers to the use of mobile phones or related devices by patients to receive health messages, use health tracking applications, or participate in remote consultations, particularly in the context of diabetes management.

Type 2 Diabetes Mellitus (T2DM): refers to individuals who have been diagnosed by a healthcare professional and are currently managing the condition through the use of glucose-lowering medication or lifestyle modifications.

Universal health coverage(UHC): refers to patients' ability to access diabetes-related services such as education, medication, and digital tools without experiencing significant financial hardship, along with their perceptions of healthcare accessibility, availability, and equity.

User-centred design: is the inclusion of end-user feedback specifically from patients with diabetes in the development, adaptation, or use of digital health tools or mobile applications aimed at supporting their care and self-management.

Chapter 5
Digital Competency's Role in Promoting Equity in the Digital Healthcare Ecosystem:
An Overview

Mussa Saidi Abubakari
https://orcid.org/0000-0003-3782-281X
Universiti Brunei Darussalam, Brunei & Dig Connectivity Research Laboratory (DCRLab), Uganda

Lawal Abdulwahab Olamilekan
https://orcid.org/0000-0003-4955-244X
Accord University, Mogadishu, Somalia

ABSTRACT

The rapid digitalisation of healthcare systems has introduced innovative solutions for improved access, efficiency, and patient outcomes. However, without equitable digital competency, these advancements risk exacerbating existing health disparities. This chapter explores the critical role of digital competency in promoting equity within the digital healthcare ecosystem. It examines how varying levels of digital skills among patients, providers, and institutions influence access to and utilisation of digital health services. Through conceptual analysis, global case studies, and policy reflections, the chapter highlights structural barriers, digital divides, and strategies to foster inclusive digital health practices. Emphasising the intersectionality of digital exclusion, the chapter advocates for targeted interventions and capacity-building initiatives that prioritise marginalised populations. Ultimately, it positions digital competency as a foundational pillar for ensuring equity and inclusion in the evolving landscape of digital healthcare.

1. INTRODUCTION

Digital Transformation in Healthcare and the Importance of Digital Competency

The accelerated integration of digital technologies into healthcare delivery has transformed the landscape of global health services. From electronic health records and telemedicine to mobile health

DOI: 10.4018/979-8-3373-3531-5.ch005

applications and artificial intelligence-driven diagnostics, the digital healthcare ecosystem is rapidly expanding (K. K. Kim & Backonja, 2025; Mukhtar et al., 2025). While these innovations promise improved healthcare accessibility, efficiency, and patient outcomes, they also pose a significant risk: deepening existing inequalities for populations with limited digital access or low digital competency (Badr et al., 2024). The mission of this chapter is to critically examine the role of digital competency in promoting equity within this evolving ecosystem and to highlight how targeted interventions in digital literacy and skill-building can foster inclusive digital healthcare systems.

While digital health solutions are often framed as inherently progressive and inclusive, the chapter interrogates this assumption. A key concern addressed is that many digital health initiatives assume a baseline level of digital access and capability that does not reflect reality for a significant portion of the global population (Girmay, 2024; Whitehead et al., 2023). Populations such as older adults, people with disabilities, ethnic minorities, low-income communities, and residents of rural or underserved areas are disproportionately affected by low digital competency (Ausserhofer et al., 2024; Tso et al., 2022). This limits their ability to navigate patient portals, participate in virtual consultations, understand digital health information, or engage with wearable health technologies, leading to missed diagnoses, delayed treatments, and poorer health outcomes.

Another concern is that healthcare professionals themselves are often insufficiently trained in digital tools and platforms. Without adequate digital skills and understanding, providers may fail to deliver patient-centred digital care or to recognise the digital literacy needs of their patients. This digital competency gap among providers not only undermines the quality of digital service delivery but also further disenfranchises already marginalised patient populations (Girmay, 2024; Mukhtar et al., 2025). Finally, the chapter is concerned with policy and system-level oversights. Current digital health policies and strategies may not fully account for the disparities in digital competency across populations or incorporate digital inclusion as a core principle. As such, they risk perpetuating structural inequalities by designing and implementing digital health interventions that are out of reach for many of the people they are intended to serve.

Therefore, at the heart of this chapter lies a central concern: digital technologies, if not implemented thoughtfully and inclusively, can exacerbate health disparities rather than resolve them. Equity in healthcare is fundamentally about ensuring that all individuals, regardless of their socioeconomic status, age, gender, disability, or geographic location, can access and benefit from quality healthcare services (Girmay, 2024; Lyles et al., 2022). However, the digital divide—the gap between those with access to digital technologies and those without—mirrors, and in some cases intensifies, existing health inequalities (Girmay, 2024). This divide is not merely technological but deeply intertwined with individual and systemic levels of digital competency. The chapter, therefore, positions digital competency as a critical enabler—or barrier (if lacking)—to equitable health outcomes in digitally mediated healthcare environments.

By drawing from interdisciplinary literature in public health, digital literacy, education, and health informatics, this chapter synthesises theoretical and empirical insights to develop a comprehensive framework that situates digital competency as a linchpin of equitable digital healthcare systems. It examines how gaps in digital skills manifest among patients and healthcare providers alike and how these gaps can systematically exclude vulnerable groups from the benefits of digital health innovations.

Chapter Objectives, Methodology, and Organisation

The overarching aim of this chapter is threefold:

1. To conceptualise digital competency and its relevance within digital healthcare settings.
2. To explore the intersection between digital competency and equity in access, utilisation, and outcomes within digital healthcare ecosystems and
3. To propose evidence-informed strategies and policy recommendations that leverage digital competency development as a mechanism to promote health equity across diverse populations.

As for the methodology, this chapter employed a narrative review approach, drawing on interdisciplinary, peer-reviewed literature published recently (especially prioritising between 2020 and 2025 from Scopus- and Web of Science–indexed journals). A systematic search was conducted using key terms such as "digital competency," "digital health equity," "health literacy," "telemedicine," and "digital divide in healthcare" across major academic databases. The selection of sources prioritised empirical studies, systematic reviews, and policy reports relevant to digital health ecosystems. Illustrative global and regional case studies complemented the review to provide contextual depth and practical relevance. This approach enabled a comprehensive synthesis of theoretical perspectives, policy frameworks, and real-world interventions, offering insights into the role of digital competency in promoting equity across diverse healthcare contexts.

This chapter is organised thematically to provide a coherent and progressive exploration of digital competency's role in fostering equity within digital healthcare ecosystems. It begins by introducing the core concepts and framing the relevance of digital skills in the context of healthcare digitalisation. The chapter then defines digital competency and maps the structure of digital healthcare systems, followed by an in-depth discussion on health equity and its intersection with digital inclusion. Subsequent sections examine the barriers to digital competency, highlight successful global case studies, and propose evidence-based strategies and policy recommendations. The chapter concludes with reflections on the implications for research, practice, and policy, reinforcing digital competency as a foundational element of equitable healthcare.

2. CONCEPTUALISING DIGITAL COMPETENCY IN HEALTHCARE SYSTEMS

Defining Digital Health Literacy and Competency

Digital competency in health care is a multi-dimensional concept that builds on general digital literacy and health literacy. Digital literacy is commonly defined as the ability to use information and communication technologies to find, evaluate, create, and communicate information, requiring both cognitive and technical skills (van Kessel et al., 2022). It is now considered a fundamental prerequisite for participating in modern society. Health literacy refers to the ability to obtain, understand, and use health information to make appropriate decisions. Digital health literacy emerges at the convergence of these two domains. In simple terms, digital health literacy is the capacity to seek, find, understand, and apply health information from digital sources (Girmay, 2024). It enables patients and the public to effectively navigate telehealth services and other eHealth tools, making informed health decisions in a digital context. Importantly, these literacies overlap and interact – for example, age, education, income, and other social determinants influence both digital and health literacy, which in turn shape one's digital health literacy (van Kessel et al., 2022).

Digital competency in the healthcare sector is increasingly recognised as a multidimensional construct that requires a blend of technical skills and an understanding of the broader implications of digital health tools on health equity (Lawrence & Levine, 2024). Practitioners, patients, and other health stakeholders must stay current with digital tools and innovations, which are transforming public health practices, by engaging in continuous learning and adaptation to new technologies (Iyamu et al., 2025). This engagement is not solely about acquiring technical skills but also involves understanding the implications of digitisation for personalised precision medicine, which is an emerging field in the healthcare sector (Martin-Sanchez et al., 2023). Furthermore, public health practitioners are encouraged to inform interdisciplinary and transdisciplinary teams about the opportunities presented by digital technologies, thereby fostering collaborative environments that enhance the integration of these tools into practice (Iyamu et al., 2025). Such integration requires competencies that are adaptable to the diverse needs of public health practitioners, emphasising the necessity for both specialised and generalised competencies. Hence, effective digital competency should not only focus on the technical aspect but also prioritise the understanding of its implications for health equity, ensuring that digital health tools are used to address, rather than exacerbate, existing health disparities (Lawrence & Levine, 2024). This holistic approach to digital competency development is essential to drive forward the digital transformation in healthcare, leading to more equitable and efficient health outcomes.

Competency Frameworks: Key Components of Digital Health Competency

Both health literacy and digital literacy are often described through competency frameworks that break down the necessary skills and attitudes. A seminal European framework (DigComp) outlines five key domains of general digital competence: (1) information and data literacy, (2) communication and collaboration, (3) digital content creation, (4) safety (including privacy and cybersecurity awareness), and (5) problem-solving (Abubakari et al., 2025; Abubakari & Kalinaki, 2024; van Kessel et al., 2022; Vuorikari et al., 2022). These domains each include sub-competencies ranging from basic technical know-how to critical evaluation of online information. In healthcare, a complementary model is the *eHealth Literacy-Transactional Model*, which describes four progressive levels of digital health competence (Paige et al., 2018; van Kessel et al., 2022):

- **Functional literacy:** Ability to read and type (write) about health using digital devices. This literacy helps in location and understanding digital health-related information.
- **Communicative literacy:** Ability to adapt and collaborate via online communication about health.
- **Critical literacy:** Ability to evaluate the relevance and trustworthiness of digital health information.
- **Translational literacy:** Ability to apply digital health information to real-life health contexts.

Cultural and Linguistic Dimensions

An often underappreciated aspect of digital health competency is cultural and linguistic appropriateness. Competence includes being able to engage with digital health tools in one's own language and culturally relevant ways. A recent qualitative systematic review of culturally and linguistically diverse populations identified language proficiency and cultural relevance as pivotal factors in digital health engagement (Whitehead et al., 2023). Many patients strongly prefer health apps and websites in their native language; for example, refugee women in one study praised a mental health app delivered in the local Arabic dialect instead of formal medical language. Likewise, seeing one's culture accurately represented (through images, narratives, or having providers of a similar background) can greatly increase trust and willingness to use digital tools (Whitehead et al., 2023). Thus, digital competency extends beyond technical skill to include cultural competency – the ability of digital health interventions to meet users' cultural and linguistic needs, and the capacity of users to effectively use those tools given their cultural context.

Privacy and Cybersecurity Awareness

In the digital health competency spectrum, safety is a core domain that covers privacy, data security, and ethical use of technology (van Kessel et al., 2022). Both healthcare providers and consumers need a basic awareness of cybersecurity practices – for instance, knowing how to protect personal health information, recognise phishing attempts, or use secure communication channels. Studies indicate that the health sector has low awareness of cyber risks among staff and often insufficient training on security best practices. In one review, health workers were found to have poor awareness of how their behaviours (like weak passwords or improper data sharing) could compromise data security (He et al., 2021). Digital competency frameworks, therefore, include knowledge of privacy regulations, data protection strategies, and the ethical implications of digital health data use. This awareness is essential for fostering trust: patients who understand how their data is protected (or conversely, those who fear it is not) will differ in their willingness to engage with telehealth or mobile health apps.

Together, these frameworks, therefore, illustrate that digital competency in healthcare is not a single skill but a spectrum of abilities – from technical skills (using devices and apps) to cognitive skills (critical thinking, information management) and social skills (communication, cultural competence) (Abubakari, 2025a; van Kessel et al., 2022). For instance, navigating a patient portal might require technical ability (logging in, clicking through results), health knowledge to interpret information, and communication skills to discuss findings with providers. In summary, digital competency in healthcare can be conceptualised as a combination of literacies and skills – technical, informational, cultural, and ethical. It is the toolbox that all stakeholders need to use digital health innovations safely and effectively. A lack in any one dimension (be it internet skills, health knowledge, or language proficiency) can become a barrier to equitable participation in the digital health ecosystem (Abubakari et al., 2023; van Kessel et al., 2022). This conceptual foundation informs the discussion of specific equity challenges and stakeholder groups in the sections that follow.

Digital Skills and Competency Among Healthcare Providers

Healthcare providers are central to the digital health ecosystem – they must be able to use electronic health records, telemedicine platforms, data analytics, and more. Several studies between 2020 and 2025 highlight gaps in digital competencies among healthcare professionals, as well as efforts to define and improve the skills needed for modern practice. In many settings, especially low- and middle-income countries, providers' basic digital skills remain limited. For example, a cross-sectional survey of 167 frontline healthcare providers in public clinics in North-West Ethiopia found that overall digital competency levels were relatively low (Shiferaw et al., 2020). Using a questionnaire based on the EU digital competency framework, the study revealed that providers struggled the most with tasks in the problem-solving, safety, and communication domains. In other words, many could perform simple digital tasks but had difficulty troubleshooting technology issues, protecting data security, or communicating with patients via digital tools. Factors such as younger age, higher educational level, and higher income were associated with better digital competency in this study (Shiferaw et al., 2020). The authors conclude that there is an urgent need to address these skill gaps through targeted training, as even basic eHealth implementations (like electronic medical record systems) depend on a digitally literate workforce. Notably, they emphasised that digital literacy is not a one-time achievement – given the pace of change, health professionals must continually update their skills as new technologies emerge.

Even in high-income countries, variability in providers' digital skills is evident. A large study in Finland profiled the digital health competences of over 800 healthcare professionals and found several distinct competence profiles, suggesting that some clinicians are "power users" of digital health, while others lag behind (Jarva, 2024; Jarva et al., 2024). Key competency areas identified for providers included: ability to conduct human-centred remote consultations, positive attitudes towards integrating digital solutions in daily work, general ICT proficiency, ability to evaluate and effectively use digital health solutions, and ethical competence regarding digital data use. Importantly, the study found that organizational factors heavily influence these competencies. Providers who reported strong management support and an organizational culture of digital innovation had significantly higher competence levels (Jarva et al., 2024). Peer influence was also a factor – having colleagues who adopt new technologies encourages others to learn. This suggests that building provider competencies is not just about individual training but also about creating a supportive environment (through leadership, policies, and teamwork) that promotes digital skill development.

Patient-Centred Digital Literacy and Access

An important thread in recent literature is the idea that digital health can either empower patients or exclude them, depending on their competency and support. On one hand, those who have or gain adequate digital skills often become more empowered in managing their health. They can access their medical information through portals, communicate with providers via email or messaging, and use wearable data to make lifestyle changes. Studies on chronic disease self-management show that patients who use digital tracking tools often report greater understanding and control over their condition (Bober et al., 2024). On the other hand, patients who lack digital literacy or access can feel even more disenfranchised. For example, if appointment scheduling moves primarily online, a patient who cannot navigate the online system may find it harder to get care than before. This creates a risk of a new kind of health disparity: digital exclusion leading to worse health outcomes. As one review succinctly put it, improving digital health literacy is crucial for addressing health disparities in the modern era, because those with low digital skills might otherwise struggle to obtain vital health information and services (Girmay, 2024). The consensus in the literature is that patient-focused interventions – such as digital literacy classes at community centres, library programs to teach health app usage, or one-on-one tech support in clinics – are needed to raise the floor for everyone (Bober et al., 2024; Mukhtar et al., 2025). Some healthcare organizations have begun deploying "digital navigators" or patient tech support lines specifically to assist those having trouble with patient portals or telehealth apps (Bober et al., 2024; Wisniewski & Torous, 2020). These efforts, while still nascent, are promising practices to make digital health more inclusive.

In conclusion, patient-centred digital competency is a linchpin of equitable digital health. The studies reviewed indicate that while many patients are adapting to and even thriving with digital health tools, significant segments – especially older adults, the less educated, and culturally diverse groups – face barriers in digital literacy and access. Bridging this gap will require multifaceted approaches: education and training to improve eHealth literacy, designing technologies with simplicity and cultural relevance in mind, and providing alternative support for those who cannot easily go digital (Abubakari, 2025b; Abubakari et al., 2024, 2025; Mizzi et al., 2023; Whitehead et al., 2023). The goal is to ensure that digital health empowers all patients to take charge of their health, rather than creating a new divide between the digitally literate healthy and the digitally disconnected sick.

3. EQUITY IN DIGITAL HEALTHCARE ECOSYSTEM

Understanding Digital Equity in Healthcare Contexts

Equity in healthcare refers to the principle of ensuring that all individuals have fair and just access to health services, regardless of their social, economic, or demographic background. In the context of digital healthcare, this principle extends to encompass equal opportunities to access, understand, and benefit from digital health technologies (K. K. Kim & Backonja, 2025). As healthcare systems increasingly incorporate digital tools— from telemedicine and electronic health records to AI-driven diagnostics and wearable health devices— understanding how equity operates in these digital domains becomes paramount. Equity in digital healthcare does not imply uniformity in service provision but recognises that different groups may require different types and levels of support to achieve comparable health outcomes.

The notion of equity in digital healthcare is deeply influenced by the digital divide, which refers to disparities in access to digital technologies and the skills required to use them effectively. This divide manifests in multiple dimensions: access to infrastructure (e.g., devices, internet connectivity), digital literacy and skills, and the ability to engage meaningfully with digital health platforms (Fisher & Magin, 2022). In high-income countries, the divide often relates to skills and usage gaps, while in many low- and middle-income contexts, access remains a primary barrier. However, both access and competency gaps can co-exist, and each plays a significant role in shaping who benefits from digital health services.

Digital health equity further encompasses the availability, accessibility, acceptability, and quality of digital services for all segments of the population. It requires not only that services exist but that they are designed to be culturally appropriate, linguistically accessible, and responsive to users' needs. For example, digital health interfaces available only in dominant languages or requiring high levels of health literacy can alienate significant user groups. Thus, the design and delivery of digital healthcare must account for diverse patient profiles and contexts to avoid reinforcing systemic health inequities.

Addressing equity in digital healthcare also requires attention to the institutional and systemic structures that influence health service delivery. Health policies must embed principles of digital inclusion and proactively identify at-risk populations for targeted interventions. Moreover, equity must be integrated into procurement processes, funding decisions, and evaluation metrics for digital health programmes. Digital health equity cannot be achieved through isolated interventions; it must be institutionalised within broader health system reforms.

In summary, equity in digital healthcare goes beyond mere access to technologies; it demands thoughtful design, inclusive policies, and culturally responsive implementation. It recognises that digital tools, when deployed without attention to social disparities, can replicate or even deepen existing inequities. Promoting digital health equity, therefore, involves acknowledging the complex interplay between digital competency, social determinants of health, and systemic healthcare inequalities. By centring equity in digital health initiatives, healthcare systems can ensure that digital innovation contributes to rather than detracts from universal health coverage and inclusive health outcomes.

Current Equity Challenges Faced in Digital Healthcare

The current equity challenges in digital healthcare are multifaceted and deeply entrenched, largely exacerbated by the digital divide, which is affected by diverse socioeconomic and political factors (Shaw & Glover, 2024). Economically marginalised communities bear the brunt of this divide, facing significant obstacles in accessing essential technologies and services that are crucial for equitable healthcare delivery. Moreover, the lack of coherent investment in digital health literacy exacerbates these challenges, as individuals struggle to effectively utilise digital tools for health management (Shaw & Glover, 2024). This literacy gap is critical, as digital health literacy, defined as the ability to use emerging information and communications technologies to improve health, is a linchpin in addressing these equity challenges. The interconnections between these issues highlight a pressing need for culturally appropriate and patient-centred design strategies that can specifically address the needs of diverse populations and facilitate better communication between patients, caregivers, and healthcare providers (Ha et al., 2023). To combat these disparities, interventions should focus on improving access to affordable technologies and infrastructure, while fostering digital health literacy to ensure all communities can benefit from digital healthcare advancements. Addressing these core aspects collectively is essential to developing a more equitable digital healthcare landscape, requiring targeted actions and interventions at multiple levels within the healthcare system.

4. THE INTERLINK BETWEEN DIGITAL COMPETENCY AND EQUITY

Digital Competency as a Tool for Promoting Equity

Digital competency (DC) holds immense potential in reducing disparities in healthcare access by leveraging technological advancements to bridge gaps between patients and providers (Shiferaw et al., 2020). The proliferation of health information online and the ability to schedule appointments digitally empower individuals to access healthcare services more efficiently, breaking down barriers traditionally posed by geographical and physical limitations (Arias López et al., 2023). Furthermore, digital technologies, such as health tracking wearables and self-monitoring devices, enable individuals to actively participate in managing their health, fostering a sense of self-efficacy and potentially diminishing disparities in healthcare access. These devices not only provide real-time data to users but also facilitate continuous interactions with healthcare providers, ensuring that individuals receive timely and personalised care. Moreover, digital health innovations, including virtual visits and asynchronous messaging, revolutionise care delivery by allowing simultaneous consultations, reducing the necessity for travel, and thus significantly benefiting underserved populations in rural or remote areas (Arias López et al.,

2023). However, the effective governance of digital transformations, which include promoting DC of individuals, is critical. Without it, efforts to enhance digital competency could inadvertently exacerbate health inequities, as those lacking access to or skills in using technology may be left behind. Therefore, it is imperative to implement inclusive digital strategies that prioritise equitable access and ensure all individuals can benefit from these technological advancements.

Impact of Improved Digital Competency on Equitable Patient Outcomes

Enhancing digital competency among patients is pivotal for improving patient outcomes, particularly in terms of equity, as it directly influences patients' ability to engage effectively with digital health services. This is especially crucial for marginalised and vulnerable populations who may otherwise be disadvantaged due to the digital divide (H. Kim et al., 2024). Addressing digital competency involves not only improving access to technology but also ensuring that individuals possess the necessary digital literacy and skills to utilise these resources effectively. This requires a comprehensive approach that includes assessing digital readiness through customised assessment tools, which provide a validated framework for understanding patients' digital capabilities (H. Kim et al., 2024). By focusing on digital inclusion, healthcare systems can bridge existing gaps in service provision, allowing for equitable access to digital health services and ultimately leading to improved health outcomes for all patient groups. To achieve this, healthcare policymakers and providers need to integrate digital health resources with community-based healthcare services, ensuring that advancements in digital health do not leave behind those who are most in need of care (Crawford & Serhal, 2020).

5. CHALLENGES AND BARRIERS

Beyond the individual-level factors (such as skills and competencies) discussed previously, systemic and infrastructural factors play a decisive role in enabling or hindering equitable digital health. These include the availability of technology infrastructure, institutional policies, funding mechanisms, and broader socioeconomic conditions. Research often points to these macro-level barriers that must be addressed to create a supportive ecosystem for digital competency and equity.

Technology Infrastructure and Access

The most fundamental infrastructure for digital health is access to the internet and devices. As highlighted earlier, large parts of the world still lack reliable broadband. Even within wealthy countries, rural areas may have poor connectivity (for instance, parts of rural Australia or Appalachia in the U.S. have spotty internet, limiting telehealth uptake). The ITU's 2024 report noted that while around 93% of the global population had at least some mobile broadband coverage, nearly half the population remained offline due to cost, lack of devices, or other barriers (Fisher & Magin, 2022; ITU, 2024). Infrastructure inequities are thus a root cause of digital health inequities. Studies emphasize that national and regional investments in broadband expansion, 5G networks, and public internet access (e.g., free Wi-Fi in community centres) are prerequisites for digital health inclusion. In healthcare contexts, infrastructure also means having the necessary hardware and software in clinics and hospitals. In some low-resource settings, clinics may not have enough computers or a stable power supply to maintain electronic systems – an issue observed in parts of Africa and South Asia in various case reports. Thus, digital health readiness at a system level involves upgrading physical infrastructure alongside human skills. A concept called 'digital health readiness' has emerged to assess not just individuals but also how prepared health systems are to implement digital solutions (Bober et al., 2024). This encompasses infrastructure, staff training, workflow integration, and data systems.

Policy and Funding Environments

The policy landscape can significantly influence digital health equity. For example, during COVID-19, many countries introduced temporary policies to reimburse telehealth or to provide free data packages for tele-education and telemedicine (Abubakari & Mashoedah, 2021; Torous et al., 2020). These policies greatly facilitated access. However, if such support is withdrawn without alternatives, it can widen disparities. In Australia, researchers warned that ending public funding for telehealth after the pandemic would disproportionately hurt rural and low-income patients who came to rely on it (Fisher & Magin, 2022). Similarly, in the U.S., telehealth reimbursement and licensing flexibilities are policy choices that will affect long-term equity (Hinkley & Briskin, 2020). Funding for digital literacy initiatives is another policy lever – some countries have begun to fund community-based digital skills training for seniors or marginalized groups as part of their digital inclusion strategies. Cybersecurity and privacy regulations also play a role; if regulations are too onerous, small clinics might avoid adopting digital tools, but if too lax, patients may lose trust after data breaches. Achieving the right balance is important so that safety concerns do not become a barrier to innovation or a cause of distrust. The need for clear guidelines on privacy, informed consent for telehealth, and equitable data governance has been noted in multiple commentaries.

Organizational Barriers

Within healthcare organizations, leadership and culture can either promote or impede digital equity efforts. An international survey via the Global Digital Health Partnership (GDHP) in 2023 found that lack of organizational structure and leadership was one of the most-cited barriers to implementing digital health, with 7 out of 10 respondent countries highlighting it (Cascini et al., 2023). If hospital leaders do not prioritize digital training or if no one is accountable for digital inclusion, these issues may fall by the wayside. Another related barrier is clinician scepticism or resistance (Cascini et al., 2023; Girmay, 2024). If a significant number of providers in a system are reluctant to use new digital tools, patients will have fewer opportunities to engage with those tools. Overcoming this may require change management strategies and demonstrating that digital tools can actually reduce workload or improve care, rather than adding burdens. The GDHP survey also underscored population accessibility as a barrier – essentially the difficulty of ensuring the general population can access digital health – reinforcing that organizations and governments are aware of the challenge but may not yet have solved it (Cascini et al., 2023). To address these issues, some health systems have created dedicated roles such as Chief Digital Inclusion Officers or committees focused on health equity in IT deployments.

Cybersecurity and Trust Infrastructure

As health systems digitalise, cybersecurity challenges have increasingly become a systemic concern. Hospitals and clinics have been targets of ransomware attacks, and data breaches expose patient information. A 2021 scoping review summarised that healthcare organisations often suffer from inadequate cybersecurity practices – common issues include insufficient endpoint protection, outdated software, and, critically, human factors like a lack of staff training in security (He et al., 2021). The review noted a lack of security awareness across the health sector and that most organizations react to breaches by adding staff training after the fact. This reactive approach suggests that initiative-taking integration of cybersecurity competence is still lacking. From an equity perspective, high-profile security failures can erode public trust in digital health, particularly among communities already cautious about technology. For instance, if a telehealth platform leaks sensitive data, patients who are on the fence about using such services may firmly opt out, and these may often be those from marginalized communities with historical reasons to mistrust institutions. Therefore, building robust security infrastructure and cultivating a culture of privacy protection is part of ensuring equitable uptake – everyone needs confidence that their data is safe. Some proposed solutions include requiring cybersecurity literacy as part of medical staff competencies and educating patients about how their data is used and protected. Indeed, making cybersecurity a 'team effort from board members to front-line employees' is recommended (He et al., 2021), implying that governance structures must treat digital security as an organisational priority.

Cost and Economic Barriers

Affordability of technology is a non-negligible systemic barrier. The cost of smartphones, data plans, or broadband subscriptions can be prohibitive for low-income families (McDonald et al., 2024). Digital health interventions that assume patient-owned devices can inadvertently exclude those who cannot afford them. Some health economics studies suggest subsidising devices for patients with chronic diseases might actually be cost-effective by improving disease management and reducing hospitalisations (Nouri et al., 2020) – but such programs are not yet widespread. On the provider side, small clinics or solo practitioners may find the cost of health IT systems (and maintaining them) too high, leading to a digital divide between well-resourced health facilities and under-resourced ones. Policymakers are grappling with how to include digital health in insurance coverage and national health benefits (Bejarano, 2022). For instance, should internet access be considered a social determinant worth addressing through healthcare policy? These systemic questions go beyond traditional healthcare but have real impacts on equity.

In summary, system-level barriers – infrastructure, policy, organizational culture, security, and cost – critically shape the landscape in which individual digital competencies are exercised. The literature suggests that to achieve digital health equity, efforts like improving literacy or training providers must be accompanied by parallel improvements in infrastructure and supportive policy. As one global survey concluded, effective communication strategies and improved digital health literacy for both clinicians and citizens are key system priorities for the future of digital health (Cascini et al., 2023). Health systems need to invest not only in technologies themselves but in the surrounding ecosystem – from broadband and cybersecurity to policies that ensure no population is left behind in the digital transition. Tackling these systemic barriers is challenging and often requires multi-sector collaboration (health, technology, education, telecom, etc.), but it is essential for equitably scaling digital health innovations.

6. STRATEGIES FOR PROMOTING DIGITAL HEALTH COMPETENCY AND HEALTHCARE EQUITY

Enhancing Digital Competency Among Healthcare Providers

To enhance digital competency among healthcare providers, a multifaceted approach is necessary, focusing on both individual proficiency and systemic integration. Organisations must prioritise empowering healthcare providers to effectively harness digital technology in their daily operations, which is vital for advancing overall healthcare delivery. By involving healthcare professionals as end-users in the development of digital systems, these solutions can be tailored to fit their specific needs, ensuring that they are practical and beneficial in real-world applications (Alotaibi et al., 2025). Furthermore, investment in professional development is crucial; healthcare organisations should offer continuous learning opportunities that focus on building digital skills and competencies. Such initiatives not only address the immediate need for technological proficiency but also contribute to long-term improvements in patient outcomes by equipping providers with the necessary tools to integrate digital health solutions seamlessly into their practice (Alotaibi et al., 2025). Additionally, addressing concerns related to the use of technology at the point of care is essential for fostering an environment where digital interventions are effectively integrated, thereby enhancing the overall quality of care provided (Mukhtar et al., 2025). Collectively, these strategies underscore the importance of a comprehensive framework to elevate digital competency, ultimately leading to more efficient healthcare delivery and improved patient experiences.

Emerging Frameworks and Policy Models

In recent years, awareness of the challenges outlined above has led to the development of various frameworks, strategies, and policy models aiming to guide the integration of digital competency and equity considerations into health systems. Between 2020 and 2025, researchers, professional bodies, and international organisations have proposed several notable frameworks to ensure that digital health advances are inclusive. This section highlights some of these emerging models and how they address equity.

Global and National Digital Health Strategies

The World Health Organization (WHO) launched a Global Strategy on Digital Health 2020–2025, which explicitly frames digital health as a means to advance health for all and emphasises appropriate, accessible, affordable, scalable digital solutions (World Health Organization, 2021). A key principle of the WHO strategy is 'leave no one behind,' which translates into promoting digital health literacy and user-centred design globally. The strategy calls on member states to strengthen health workforce digital capacities and to invest in infrastructure so that rural and underserved areas are connected. Many countries have aligned their national policies with this strategy: for example, countries in the European Union, as well as Australia, India, and others, have published national digital health blueprints that include components on building digital skills among both providers and the public, and on monitoring equity outcomes of digital health initiatives. The formation of the Global Digital Health Partnership (GDHP) in 2019 (with over thirty country members) further facilitated policy exchange. As reported by Cascini *et al.* (2023) from the GDHP survey, member countries identified common obstacles and are sharing best practices on issues like expanding telehealth in primary care and ensuring accessibility. This kind of international collaboration is itself a new model – treating digital health equity as a global public good that benefits from collective action.

Digital Health Equity Frameworks

Researchers have been working to conceptualise what digital health equity entails in a structured way. A 2025 scoping review by Kim *et al.* examined existing frameworks and concepts in the literature related to digital health equity (K. K. Kim & Backonja, 2025). They found forty-two frameworks across different studies, each shedding light on parts of the "ecosystem" of digital health equity, though none were entirely comprehensive. Common elements across these frameworks included individual characteristics (like age, race, literacy), community and societal factors (like infrastructure, culture, policy), and the design and implementation of the digital intervention itself. The authors grouped 243 unique concepts into 43 categories that spanned micro to macro levels – from personal digital skills and trust, to organisational readiness, to broader issues of access to services and data governance (K. K. Kim & Backonja, 2025). The review highlighted the need for a consolidated definition of digital health equity and a more unified framework to guide both intervention development and evaluation. In response, they suggested a working definition: digital health equity is the opportunity for all to engage with digital health tools to achieve good health outcomes, and they pointed to key domains that any comprehensive framework should cover (technology access, digital literacy, usability, usefulness, cost, etc., intersecting with social determinants). This work is expected to inform future policymakers and communities seeking to improve digital inclusion in health.

One example of a proposed comprehensive framework is the Framework for Digital Health Equity, published in 2022. This framework introduces the concept of Digital Determinants of Health (DDoH), analogous to social determinants of health (Richardson et al., 2022). It details how factors like broadband availability, device access, digital literacy education, inclusive design, and data privacy are all DDoHs that influence health outcomes in the digital age. By delineating these determinants, the framework provides a checklist for developers and policymakers (Lawrence & Levine, 2024; Richardson et al., 2022): e.g., *Accessibility* (do intended users have the required tech?), *Literacy* (do they have skills to use it?), *Design* (was it co-created with diverse users?), *Legislation* (are there policies to support its equitable implementation?), and *Ethics* (are algorithms bias-free and fair?). Others have also advocated a similar view, stating digital health services are not second-tier but first-tier of a different nature, and calling for building public demand and trust in digital health as part of future health systems (van Kessel et al., 2022). These frameworks serve as north stars to ensure that, as digital health expands, it does so with equity front and centre rather than as an afterthought.

Competency Frameworks in Professional Training

Earlier, the DECODE framework for medical education was mentioned. This is an example of an institutional policy model that embeds digital competencies (and implicitly equity considerations) into the training of future providers (Car et al., 2025). By specifying learning outcomes like understanding telehealth barriers for vulnerable populations or using health information systems in a patient-centred way, such frameworks ensure new graduates are aware of equity issues. Another example is the incorporation of digital ethics in curricula, as recommended by multiple authors (Wong et al., 2021). Training clinicians in data ethics and awareness of biases in digital tools can help safeguard against technologies inadvertently worsening disparities (for instance, if an AI risk score performs poorly on minority patients, a digitally literate and ethically aware clinician can recognize and mitigate this). This kind of education reform is essentially a policy intervention at the academic level, aiming to produce a workforce that can operationalize equity-focused digital health.

Community Engagement and Co-design Models

An emerging best practice to promote equity is involving end-users in the design of digital health interventions. This goes beyond frameworks into methodology, but is worth noting as a model: Participatory design or community co-design has been used in projects to develop digital health apps for Indigenous communities, refugee populations, or patients with low literacy. Studies document that when such users are included from the outset – helping determine features, language, and interface design – the end product is more accessible and acceptable to the target group (Whitehead et al., 2023). Some health systems are formalizing this by setting up patient advisory panels for digital health or partnering with community organizations (for example, a barbershop-based program to teach digital blood pressure tracking to Black male patrons). These are more grassroots models, but they complement high-level frameworks by putting principles into practice.

Monitoring and Evaluation Models

Another important development is the push to better measure digital health equity outcomes. A few papers propose equity-focused evaluation frameworks – for instance, by always disaggregating digital health usage data by age, gender, race/ethnicity, etc., to spot disparities (Hatef et al., 2024). In the U.S., some health systems have created 'telehealth equity dashboards' to track which patient groups are using telehealth versus who is not, allowing targeted interventions (Luke et al., 2024). This data-driven approach is crucial for accountability. If a new patient portal is rolled out and only 20% of patients in low-income ZIP codes use it, that signals a need for corrective action (such as outreach or alternative modalities). Policymakers are increasingly calling for equity impact assessments when approving digital health programs – similar to environmental impact assessments for new projects. All these represent a shift to systematically include equity metrics in digital health governance.

In sum, the period 2020–2025 has seen a maturation in our collective approach to digital health equity. From high-level international strategies (WHO's call to action) to granular frameworks (digital determinants and competency models) to on-the-ground co-design initiatives, there is a convergence towards structured, principle-driven integration of equity in digital health efforts. While these frameworks are relatively new and still being tested, they provide a roadmap for stakeholders. The challenge ahead will be in the implementation – turning framework boxes and arrows into real-world changes. Nonetheless, the existence of these models is a positive sign that the health community is proactively addressing what used to be unintended consequences of tech innovation. The next section will look at some concrete case studies across different regions, illustrating how digital competency and equity issues manifest in various contexts and what lessons have been learned.

7. CASE STUDIES ON DIGITAL HEALTH SKILLS AND COMPETENCY

Digital Competency in Improving Equity in Healthcare

Baseline health literacy varies widely across populations, and this translates into uneven *eHealth literacy*. Recent works have noted that digital health literacy has become "increasingly essential" for consumers in managing their health (Girmay, 2024). Individuals with strong digital skills can more easily use telehealth, patient portals, and online education resources, often leading to improved health knowledge and outcomes (Mukhtar et al., 2025). For example, a study found that pregnant women with high digital literacy could locate quality information about prenatal care and thus feel more empowered in decision-making (Perestelo-Perez et al., 2020). On the other hand, those with lower digital skills may struggle to even find or access such resources, widening outcome gaps (Arias López et al., 2023; Perestelo-Perez et al., 2020). Importantly, some interventions have shown success in boosting patients' eHealth literacy. One randomized trial provided patients with an online decision aid for hypertension and observed a significant increase in participants' ability to understand, appraise, and apply health information compared to controls (Wehkamp et al., 2021). Notably, the improvement was seen across different education levels, suggesting that well-designed digital tools can benefit even those with less formal education. This indicates that patient-facing digital interventions, if carefully tailored, can enhance specific competencies and not just cater to the already health-literate.

Furthermore, another successful example of digital competency improving equity in healthcare is the Digital Opportunities for Outcomes in Recovery Services (DOORS) program. This initiative is specifically tailored to enhance digital literacy among individuals with serious mental illness, a group often marginalised in accessing healthcare resources (Hoffman et al., 2020). The DOORS program offered 6-8 weeks of group sessions aimed at developing smartphone skills and competencies, which are crucial for navigating digital health services. By focusing on digital literacy rather than on more technologically advanced solutions like artificial intelligence, the program addresses the fundamental barriers that prevent vulnerable populations from accessing equitable healthcare. Moreover, the positive reception of the DOORS program by its participants underscores its effectiveness in bridging the digital divide, thereby enabling these individuals to better manage their health through digital platforms (Hoffman et al., 2020). This approach not only empowers participants but also contributes to a more inclusive healthcare system where digital health services are accessible to all, regardless of their initial level of digital competence. Thus, enhancing digital literacy through targeted interventions like DOORS is a critical step towards achieving equity in healthcare.

Lessons Learned from Successful Implementations

Building upon the digital competence framework for healthcare professionals, successful implementations of guidelines in this domain highlight the necessity of a multifaceted approach. Implementers must employ a variety of strategies to address the complexities inherent in guideline implementation, emphasising the role of organisational and change management characteristics. This comprehensive approach ensures that the implementation is not merely reliant on individual clinicians or the guidelines themselves, but rather on a broader organisational context. The success of such implementations often hinges on the adoption of multiple strategies, as focusing on a single approach can limit effectiveness (Solberg et al., 2000). Furthermore, the external environment and organisational contexts are critical, as they significantly influence the implementation process and its outcomes. To ensure that these efforts are sustained and achieve their intended impact, it is crucial to integrate continuous performance measurement and data sharing, which are vital components of quality improvement initiatives (Solberg et al., 2000). Thus, by recognising these interconnected elements, healthcare organisations can better strategise and implement guidelines, thereby enhancing both the adoption and effectiveness of digital competence frameworks in practice.

8. IMPLICATIONS FOR POLICY, PRACTICE, AND RESEARCH

The findings and analyses presented in this chapter have significant implications for policy development, clinical practice, and future research. As digital technologies become increasingly central to health service delivery, strategies to enhance digital competency must be embedded within broader efforts to promote equity in healthcare access and outcomes. Addressing digital health inequities through a competency lens requires a shift in how policymakers, practitioners, and researchers conceptualise, design, and evaluate digital health initiatives.

Practical Implications

In terms of clinical practice, healthcare professionals must be equipped with the digital competencies required to deliver effective and inclusive care. This calls for the integration of digital health literacy and technology training into the professional development curricula of doctors, nurses, allied health workers, and community health personnel. Beyond technical proficiency, practitioners must also develop cultural competence and communication skills that enable them to support patients with varying levels of digital literacy. Clinical workflows should include processes for assessing patients' digital competency and offering tailored support, such as step-by-step guidance, accessible resources, and helplines. Thus, in practical terms, the following can be suggested and summarised:

- Integrate digital health training into professional development for healthcare providers.
- Train health workers in cultural competence and patient support for digital tool usage.
- Implement digital navigators in clinical settings to assist patients with low digital skills.
- Routinely assess patients' digital competency and provide tailored support.
- Ensure digital systems are intuitive, multilingual, and inclusive for people with disabilities or low literacy.

Healthcare institutions should also invest in digital navigators or trained support staff who can assist patients in accessing and using digital health services, particularly in telemedicine settings (Bober et al., 2024; Wisniewski & Torous, 2020). In addition, institutions must critically evaluate the design and usability of their digital health platforms to ensure they are intuitive and accessible for all users, including those with low literacy or disabilities. Embedding equity-focused digital practices into clinical routines will not only improve patient outcomes but also enhance the overall effectiveness of digital health integration.

Policy Implications and Directions

From a policy perspective, digital competency should be formally recognised as a public health priority and an essential component of digital health strategies. Governments and health ministries must adopt inclusive digital health frameworks that explicitly address the digital divide and prioritise digital literacy as a social determinant of health. This includes integrating digital skills training into national health education policies, primary care outreach programmes, and digital health infrastructure planning. Funding mechanisms should support not only technological infrastructure but also the development of human capital through community-based digital literacy programmes and culturally responsive training initiatives. Policies must also ensure that digital health tools comply with universal accessibility standards and are developed with input from diverse user groups, particularly those who are historically underserved. The following can be summarised for policymakers:

- Recognise digital competency as a public health priority and core component of national digital health strategies.
- Embed digital literacy training in health education, community outreach, and public health campaigns.
- Allocate funding not only for infrastructure but also for human capacity-building in digital skills.
- Ensure accessibility, inclusivity, and user-centred design in digital health platforms.
- Establish monitoring systems with disaggregated data to identify digital equity gaps (e.g., by age, gender, geography).
- Promote international cooperation to support digital health equity in low- and middle-income countries.

Moreover, policies should incorporate monitoring and evaluation mechanisms to track digital competency levels across different population groups, using disaggregated data by age, gender, ethnicity, disability status, and geography. This will enable health systems to identify gaps and respond with targeted interventions. International agencies and donors also have a role to play in supporting low- and middle-income countries in building digital health capacities that are equitable and sustainable, particularly through South-South collaborations, technical assistance, and knowledge-sharing platforms.

Future Research Directions

The research implications of this chapter highlight several important directions. First, there is a need for longitudinal and large-scale studies that measure the impact of digital competency interventions on health equity outcomes, especially across diverse settings. While there is growing recognition of digital competency as a determinant of healthcare access, more empirical evidence is needed to establish causal relationships and the cost-effectiveness of training programmes and inclusive design practices. Second, research should explore how intersectionality affects digital health engagement— examining how overlapping factors such as race, gender, income, and disability intersect to create unique barriers and opportunities for different populations. Participatory action research involving end-users— particularly marginalised communities— can offer rich insights into the lived experiences of digital exclusion and inform the co-creation of more inclusive solutions.

Third, there is a pressing need for the development and validation of context-sensitive digital health competency assessment tools. Many existing frameworks, such as DigComp or the Digital Health Literacy Instrument (DHLI), have been developed in high-income settings and may not adequately capture the realities of users in low-resource environments. Adapting or creating new tools that reflect local languages, cultural norms, and usage contexts will enhance the relevance and effectiveness of digital competency research. Finally, interdisciplinary collaboration among researchers in health informatics, public health, education, behavioural science, and technology studies is essential to capture the complexity of digital health equity. Future studies should also investigate the role of emerging technologies, such as AI, wearable devices, and blockchain, in reshaping digital competencies and access, ensuring that ethical and inclusive principles guide innovation. In sum, advancing digital competency for equitable healthcare is not a task confined to one sector or discipline. It requires coordinated and sustained action across policy, practice, and research domains. By recognising digital skills as foundational to participation in contemporary health systems, stakeholders can co-create inclusive digital health ecosystems that truly serve the needs of all. Thus, in summary, the following can be suggested as future directions in digital health research:

- Conduct longitudinal studies to evaluate how digital competency affects health equity outcomes.
- Apply intersectionality frameworks to understand multi-dimensional barriers to digital engagement.
- Involve marginalised populations in participatory research and co-design of digital solutions.
- Develop context-sensitive assessment tools for digital health literacy in diverse regions.
- Explore emerging technologies (e.g., AI, blockchain, wearables, IoT) and their impact on digital health skills and inclusion (Abubakari & Mashoedah, 2021).
- Promote interdisciplinary research across public health, education, tech, and behavioural science.

9. CONCLUSION

The digital transformation of healthcare holds immense promise for enhancing the accessibility, quality, and efficiency of health services. However, as this chapter has demonstrated, the potential of digital health technologies to promote inclusive and equitable healthcare can only be fully realised if digital competency is recognised and addressed as one of the critical enablers. Without the necessary skills and confidence to navigate digital tools, large segments of the population— especially those already marginalised by social, economic, or geographical factors— face the risk of further exclusion in the digital healthcare landscape. Throughout the chapter, we have highlighted how digital competency is more than a technical skillset; it is a multidimensional construct encompassing information literacy, communication, content creation, problem-solving, and digital safety, all of which are vital for meaningful engagement in modern healthcare systems. For patients, digital competency determines the ability to access telemedicine services, interpret electronic health records, use mobile health apps, and make informed health decisions. For healthcare professionals, it is essential to deliver patient-centred care in increasingly digital environments and to ensure that the shift towards e-health does not widen disparities in care delivery.

By critically examining the digital healthcare ecosystem, this chapter has shed light on the ways in which digital inequities mirror— and at times intensify— existing health disparities. These inequities are not only technological but also social and structural, influenced by factors such as age, education, income, disability, and geographic location. Addressing digital health equity, therefore, requires more than deploying infrastructure or designing new technologies. It demands an ecosystemic approach that integrates digital competency development into public health strategies, clinical practice, education systems, and technology design. The chapter has further explored a range of barriers to digital competency, including individual-level challenges (such as low digital literacy or confidence), institutional limitations (such as inadequate training or digital support), and systemic issues (such as exclusionary design or limited connectivity in remote areas). In response, we have proposed a set of strategies rooted in evidence and inclusivity. These include multi-stakeholder collaboration, targeted digital skill-building initiatives, culturally and linguistically appropriate digital content, and participatory design methods that engage end-users in the creation of health technologies.

Global and regional case studies were presented to demonstrate how countries and communities are confronting digital exclusion and innovating to improve digital health outcomes. These examples underscore the value of context-sensitive approaches that account for local realities while advancing global goals such as the Sustainable Development Goals (SDG 3 on good health and well-being and SDG 10 on reducing inequalities).

In conclusion, if digital healthcare is to be a tool for equity rather than exclusion, digital competency must be treated as a public health imperative. Health systems must invest not only in technological innovation but also in human capacity— equipping individuals and institutions with the skills and confidence to participate meaningfully in digital health ecosystems. Ensuring that no one is left behind in the digital era requires deliberate, inclusive, and sustained efforts to close the digital skills gap across all sectors of society. Ultimately, fostering digital competency is not merely a technological challenge but a social justice endeavour— one that is essential to building equitable, inclusive, and resilient healthcare systems for the future.

REFERENCES

Abubakari, M. S., & Mashoedah. (2021). The Internet of Things (IoT) as an Emerging Technological Solution for the Covid-19 Pandemic Mitigation: An Overview. *Journal of Physics: Conference Series*, *1737*(1), 012003. DOI: 10.1088/1742-6596/1737/1/012003

Abubakari, M. S. (2025a). Digital Competence for Enhancing Financial Inclusion in FinTech Adoption: Addressing the Digital Divide. In Masri, M., Sait, M. A., & Anshari, M. (Eds.), *Promoting Inclusivity and Accessibility With FinTech* (pp. 65–102). IGI Global Scientific Publishing., DOI: 10.4018/979-8-3373-1112-8.ch003

Abubakari, M. S. (2025b). Digital Technologies Adoption in Islamic Education for Fostering Lifelong Learning Culture: Pilot Survey Preliminary Insights. In Anshari, M., Almunawar, M. N., & Ordóñez de Pablos, P. (Eds.), *Multi-Industry Digitalization and Technological Governance in the AI Era* (pp. 103–126). IGI Global., DOI: 10.4018/979-8-3373-1681-9.ch005

Abubakari, M. S., & Kalinaki, K. (2024). Digital Competence in Islamic Education for Lifelong Learning: Preliminary Analysis Using DigComp 2.1 Framework. In Hawamdeh, M. M. K., & Abdelhafid, F. (Eds.), *Embracing Technological Advancements for Lifelong Learning* (pp. 1–31). IGI Global., DOI: 10.4018/979-8-3693-1410-4.ch001

Abubakari, M. S., Zakaria, G. A. N., & Musa, J. (2024). Perceived compatibility and students' intention to adopt digital technologies in Islamic education institutions. *Cogent Education*, *11*(1), 2430869. DOI: 10.1080/2331186X.2024.2430869

Abubakari, M. S., Zakaria, G. A. N., & Musa, J. (2025). Validating the DigComp framework among university students across different educational systems. *Discover Education*, *4*(1), 200. DOI: 10.1007/s44217-025-00652-x

Abubakari, M. S., Zakaria, G. A. N., Musa, J., & Kalinaki, K. (2023). Assessing Digital Competence in Higher Education: A Gender Analysis of DigComp 2.1 Framework in Uganda. *SAGA: Journal of Technology and Information System*, *1*(4), 114–120. DOI: 10.58905/saga.v1i4.210

Alotaibi, N., Wilson, C. B., & Traynor, M. (2025). Enhancing digital readiness and capability in healthcare: A systematic review of interventions, barriers, and facilitators. *BMC Health Services Research*, *25*(1), 500. DOI: 10.1186/s12913-025-12663-3 PMID: 40186200

Arias López, M. del P., Ong, B. A., Borrat Frigola, X., Fernández, A. L., Hicklent, R. S., Obeles, A. J. T., Rocimo, A. M., & Celi, L. A. (2023). Digital literacy as a new determinant of health: A scoping review. *PLOS Digital Health*, *2*(10), e0000279. DOI: 10.1371/journal.pdig.0000279 PMID: 37824584

Ausserhofer, D., Piccoliori, G., Engl, A., Mahlknecht, A., Plagg, B., Barbieri, V., Colletti, N., Lombardo, S., Gärtner, T., Tappeiner, W., Wieser, H., & Wiedermann, C. J. (2024). Community-Dwelling Older Adults' Readiness for Adopting Digital Health Technologies: Cross-Sectional Survey Study. *JMIR Formative Research*, *8*, e54120. DOI: 10.2196/54120 PMID: 38687989

Badr, J., Motulsky, A., & Denis, J. L. (2024). Digital health technologies and inequalities: A scoping review of potential impacts and policy recommendations. *Health Policy (Amsterdam)*, *146*(June), 105122. DOI: 10.1016/j.healthpol.2024.105122 PMID: 38986333

Bejarano, G. (2022). Digital Literacy, Health Inequities, and the COVID-19 Pandemic. *American Journal of Public Health*, *112*(4), 588–589. DOI: 10.2105/AJPH.2021.306661 PMID: 35319941

Bober, T., Rollman, B. L., Handler, S., Watson, A., Nelson, L. A., Faieta, J., & Rosland, A.-M. (2024). Digital Health Readiness: Making Digital Health Care More Inclusive. *JMIR mHealth and uHealth*, *12*, e58035. DOI: 10.2196/58035 PMID: 39383524

Car, J., Ong, Q. C., Erlikh Fox, T., Leightley, D., Kemp, S. J., Švab, I., Tsoi, K. K. F., Sam, A. H., Kent, F. M., Hertelendy, A. J., Longhurst, C. A., Powell, J., Hamdy, H., Nguyen, H. V. Q., Aoun Bahous, S., Wang, M., Baumgartner, M., Mahendradhata, Y., Popovic, N., & Obadiel, Y. A. (2025). The Digital Health Competencies in Medical Education Framework: An International Consensus Statement Based on a Delphi Study. *JAMA Network Open*, *8*(1), e2453131. DOI: 10.1001/jamanetworkopen.2024.53131 PMID: 39888625

Cascini, F., Gentili, A., Causio, F. A., Altamura, G., Melnyk, A., Beccia, F., Pappalardo, C., Lontano, A., & Ricciardi, W. (2023). Strengthening and promoting digital health practice: Results from a Global Digital Health Partnership's survey. *Frontiers in Public Health*, *11*, 1147210. DOI: 10.3389/fpubh.2023.1147210 PMID: 37404277

Crawford, A., & Serhal, E. (2020). Digital Health Equity and COVID-19: The Innovation Curve Cannot Reinforce the Social Gradient of Health. *Journal of Medical Internet Research*, *22*(6), e19361. DOI: 10.2196/19361 PMID: 32452816

Fisher, K., & Magin, P. (2022). The telehealth divide: Health inequity during the COVID-19 pandemic. *Family Practice*, *39*(3), 547–549. DOI: 10.1093/fampra/cmab173 PMID: 34964886

Girmay, M. (2024). Digital Health Divide: Opportunities for Reducing Health Disparities and Promoting Equitable Care for Maternal and Child Health Populations. *International Journal of Maternal and Child Health and AIDS*, *13*, e026. DOI: 10.25259/IJMA_41_2024 PMID: 39776789

Ha, S., Ho, S. H., Bae, Y.-H., Lee, M., Kim, J. H., Kim, J. H., & Lee, J. (2023). Digital Health Equity and Tailored Health Care Service for People With Disability: User-Centered Design and Usability Study. *Journal of Medical Internet Research*, *25*, e50029. DOI: 10.2196/50029 PMID: 38015589

Hatef, E., Hudson Scholle, S., Buckley, B., Weiner, J. P., & Austin, J. M. (2024). Development of an evidence- and consensus-based Digital Healthcare Equity Framework. *JAMIA Open*, *7*(4), ooae136. Advance online publication. DOI: 10.1093/jamiaopen/ooae136 PMID: 39553827

He, Y., Aliyu, A., Evans, M., & Luo, C. (2021). Health Care Cybersecurity Challenges and Solutions Under the Climate of COVID-19: Scoping Review. *Journal of Medical Internet Research*, *23*(4), e21747. DOI: 10.2196/21747 PMID: 33764885

Hinkley, G., & Briskin, A. (2020). *U.S. Waives Medicare and HIPAA Rules to Promote Telehealth.* https://www.pillsburylaw.com/en/news-and-insights/us-waives-medicare-and-hipaa-rules-to-promote-telehealth.html

Hoffman, L., Wisniewski, H., Hays, R., Henson, P., Vaidyam, A., Hendel, V., Keshavan, M., & Torous, J. (2020). Digital Opportunities for Outcomes in Recovery Services (DOORS): A Pragmatic Hands-On Group Approach Toward Increasing Digital Health and Smartphone Competencies, Autonomy, Relatedness, and Alliance for Those With Serious Mental Illness. *Journal of Psychiatric Practice*, *26*(2), 80–88. DOI: 10.1097/PRA.0000000000000450 PMID: 32134881

ITU. (2024). *Measuring digital development – Facts and Figures 2024*. International Telecommunication Union (ITU).

Iyamu, I., Ramachandran, S., Chang, H.-J., Kushniruk, A., Ibáñez-Carrasco, F., Worthington, C., Davies, H., McKee, G., Brown, A., & Gilbert, M. (2025). Considerations for adapting digital competencies and training approaches to the public health workforce: An interpretive description of practitioners' perspectives in Canada. *BMC Public Health*, *25*(1), 122. DOI: 10.1186/s12889-024-21089-1 PMID: 39794767

Jarva, E. (2024). *Digital Health Competence of Healthcare Professionals in Healthcare Settings*. University of Oulu.

Jarva, E., Oikarinen, A., Andersson, J., Pramila-Savukoski, S., Hammarén, M., & Mikkonen, K. (2024). Healthcare professionals' digital health competence profiles and associated factors: A cross-sectional study. *Journal of Advanced Nursing*, *80*(8), 3236–3252. DOI: 10.1111/jan.16096 PMID: 38323687

Kim, H., Schnall, R., Yoon, N., Koh, S.-J., Lee, J., & Cheon, J. H. (2024). Development and Validation of a Mobile-Centered Digital Health Readiness Scale (mDiHERS): Health Literacy and Equity Scale. *Journal of Medical Internet Research*, *26*, e58497. DOI: 10.2196/58497 PMID: 39137409

Kim, K. K., & Backonja, U. (2025). Digital health equity frameworks and key concepts: A scoping review. *Journal of the American Medical Informatics Association : JAMIA*, *00*(0), 1–13. DOI: 10.1093/jamia/ocaf017 PMID: 39936843

Lawrence, K., & Levine, D. L. (2024). The Digital Determinants of Health: A Guide for Competency Development in Digital Care Delivery for Health Professions Trainees. *JMIR Medical Education*, *10*, e54173. DOI: 10.2196/54173 PMID: 39207389

Luke, M. J., Craig, S., Pak-Gorstein, S., Arellano, M., Zhang, J., Wright, S. M., Chuo, J., & Scribano, P. V. (2024). Narrowing the Digital Divide: Framework for Creating Telehealth Equity Dashboards. *Interactive Journal of Medical Research*, *13*, e57435. DOI: 10.2196/57435 PMID: 39231423

Lyles, C. R., Sharma, A. E., Fields, J. D., Getachew, Y., Sarkar, U., & Zephyrin, L. (2022). Centering Health Equity in Telemedicine. *Annals of Family Medicine*, *20*(4), 362–367. DOI: 10.1370/afm.2823 PMID: 35879077

Martin-Sanchez, F., Lázaro, M., López-Otín, C., Andreu, A. L., Cigudosa, J. C., & Garcia-Barbero, M. (2023). Personalized Precision Medicine for Health Care Professionals: Development of a Competency Framework. *JMIR Medical Education*, *9*, e43656. DOI: 10.2196/43656 PMID: 36749626

McDonald, N., Stamato, L., & Hamidi, F. (2024). Connecting in Crisis: Investigating Equitable Community Internet Access in the US During the COVID-19 Pandemic. *ACM Journal on Computing and Sustainable Societies*, *2*(3), 1–20. DOI: 10.1145/3677326

Mizzi, R. C., Hawley, J. D., Rocco, T. S., Smith, M. C., & Merriweather, L. R. (2023). *The Handbook of Adult and Continuing Education*. Routledge., DOI: 10.4324/9781003447849

Mukhtar, T., Babur, M. N., Abbas, R., Irshad, A., & Kiran, Q. (2025). Digital Health Literacy: A systematic review of interventions and their influence on healthcare access and sustainable development Goal-3 (SDG-3). *Pakistan Journal of Medical Sciences*, *41*(3), 910–918. DOI: 10.12669/pjms.41.3.10639 PMID: 40103887

Nouri, S., Khoong, E. C., Lyles, C. R., & Karliner, L. (2020). Addressing Equity in Telemedicine for Chronic Disease Management During the Covid-19 Pandemic. *NEJM Catalyst Innovations in Care Delivery*, *1*(3), 1–13. DOI: 10.1056/CAT.20.0123

Paige, S. R., Stellefson, M., Krieger, J. L., Anderson-Lewis, C., Cheong, J., & Stopka, C. (2018). Proposing a Transactional Model of eHealth Literacy: Concept Analysis. *Journal of Medical Internet Research*, *20*(10), e10175. DOI: 10.2196/10175 PMID: 30279155

Perestelo-Perez, L., Torres-Castaño, A., González-González, C., Alvarez-Perez, Y., Toledo-Chavarri, A., Wagner, A., Perello, M., Van Der Broucke, S., Díaz-Meneses, G., Piccini, B., Rivero-Santana, A., & Serrano-Aguilar, P. (2020). IC-Health Project: Development of MOOCs to Promote Digital Health Literacy: First Results and Future Challenges. *Sustainability*, *12*(16), 6642. DOI: 10.3390/su12166642

Richardson, S., Lawrence, K., Schoenthaler, A. M., & Mann, D. (2022). A framework for digital health equity. *NPJ Digital Medicine*, *5*(1), 119. DOI: 10.1038/s41746-022-00663-0 PMID: 35982146

Shaw, J., & Glover, W. (2024). The Political Economy of Digital Health Equity: Structural Analysis. *Journal of Medical Internet Research*, *26*, e46971. DOI: 10.2196/46971 PMID: 38530341

Shiferaw, K. B., Tilahun, B. C., & Endehabtu, B. F. (2020). Healthcare providers' digital competency: A cross-sectional survey in a low-income country setting. *BMC Health Services Research*, *20*(1), 1021. DOI: 10.1186/s12913-020-05848-5 PMID: 33168002

Solberg, L. I., Brekke, M. L., Fazio, C. J., Fowles, J., Jacobsen, D. N., Kottke, T. E., Mosser, G., O'Connor, P. J., Ohnsorg, K. A., & Rolnick, S. J. (2000). Lessons from Experienced Guideline Implementers: Attend to Many Factors and Use Multiple Strategies. *The Joint Commission Journal on Quality Improvement*, *26*(4), 171–188. DOI: 10.1016/S1070-3241(00)26013-6 PMID: 10749003

Torous, J., Jän Myrick, K., Rauseo-Ricupero, N., & Firth, J. (2020). Digital Mental Health and COVID-19: Using Technology Today to Accelerate the Curve on Access and Quality Tomorrow. *JMIR Mental Health*, *7*(3), e18848. DOI: 10.2196/18848 PMID: 32213476

Tso, W. W. Y., Reichert, F., Law, N., Fu, K. W., de la Torre, J., Rao, N., Leung, L. K., Wang, Y.-L., Wong, W. H. S., & Ip, P. (2022). Digital competence as a protective factor against gaming addiction in children and adolescents: A cross-sectional study in Hong Kong. *The Lancet Regional Health. Western Pacific*, *20*, 100382. DOI: 10.1016/j.lanwpc.2022.100382 PMID: 35967602

van Kessel, R., Wong, B. L. H., Clemens, T., & Brand, H. (2022). Digital health literacy as a super determinant of health: More than simply the sum of its parts. *Internet Interventions : the Application of Information Technology in Mental and Behavioural Health*, *27*, 100500. DOI: 10.1016/j.invent.2022.100500 PMID: 35242586

Vuorikari, R., Kluzer, S., & Punie, Y. (2022). *DigComp 2.2, The Digital Competence Framework for Citizens - with new examples of knowledge, skills and attitudes*. Publications Office of the European Union., DOI: 10.2760/115376

Wehkamp, K., Kiefer, F. B., Geiger, F., Scheibler, F., Rueffer, J. U., Donner-Banzhoff, N., & Betsch, C. (2021). Enhancing Specific Health Literacy with a Digital Evidence-Based Patient Decision Aid for Hypertension: A Randomized Controlled Trial. *Patient Preference and Adherence, 15*, 1269–1279. DOI: 10.2147/PPA.S311470 PMID: 34163144

Whitehead, L., Talevski, J., Fatehi, F., & Beauchamp, A. (2023). Barriers to and Facilitators of Digital Health Among Culturally and Linguistically Diverse Populations: Qualitative Systematic Review. *Journal of Medical Internet Research, 25*, e42719. DOI: 10.2196/42719 PMID: 36853742

Wisniewski, H., & Torous, J. (2020). Digital navigators to implement smartphone and digital tools in care. *Acta Psychiatrica Scandinavica, 141*(4), 350–355. DOI: 10.1111/acps.13149 PMID: 31930477

Wong, B. L. H., Khurana, M. P., Smith, R. D., El-Omrani, O., Pold, A., Lotfi, A., O'Leary, C. A., & Saminarsih, D. S. (2021). Harnessing the digital potential of the next generation of health professionals. *Human Resources for Health, 19*(1), 50. DOI: 10.1186/s12960-021-00591-2 PMID: 33853625

World Health Organization. (2021). Global strategy on digital health 2020-2025. In *World Health Organization*. World Health Organization. https://iris.who.int/handle/10665/344249

KEY TERMS AND DEFINITIONS

Digital Competency: The knowledge, skills, and attitudes required to effectively use digital technologies to access, evaluate, create, and communicate information within healthcare environments.

Digital Divide: The disparities in access to, use of, and benefit from digital technologies resulting from socioeconomic, geographic, educational, or infrastructural inequalities.

Digital Health Equity: The attainment of the highest level of health through fair and just access to digital health resources, services, and technologies for all populations.

Digital Healthcare Ecosystem: An integrated system of digital technologies, stakeholders, data infrastructures, and services that collectively support healthcare delivery and management.

Health Informatics: The application of information science and digital technologies to collect, manage, and analyse health data for improving healthcare services and outcomes.

Health Literacy: The degree to which individuals can obtain, process, and understand basic health information and services needed to make informed health decisions.

Inclusive Healthcare: Healthcare practices and systems designed to ensure equitable access, participation, and outcomes for diverse and marginalised populations.

Telemedicine Access: The availability and usability of remote healthcare services enabled through digital communication tools, including video consultations and mobile health platforms.

Chapter 6

Deep Learning Diabetes Monitoring and Prevention: Personalized Health Assistant Contribution

Diogo Ribeiro
Polytechnic Institute of Guarda, Portugal

Celestino Gonçalves
https://orcid.org/0000-0001-6144-0980
Polytechnic Institute of Guarda, Portugal

Clara Silveira
https://orcid.org/0000-0003-2809-4208
Polytechnic Institute of Guarda, Portugal

Filipe Caetano
https://orcid.org/0000-0001-6857-7971
Polytechnic Institute of Guarda, Portugal

Paulo Vieira
https://orcid.org/0000-0003-4692-5546
Polytechnic Institute of Guarda, Portugal

ABSTRACT

This chapter introduces the Personalized Health Assistant, an integrated system that combines Internet of Things devices, machine learning, and natural language processing to monitor diabetes and promote proactive, personalized healthcare. For diabetic patients, the system leverages wearable sensors data. For non-diabetic users, physiological parameters are inferred through lifestyle and stress indicators. To support predictive health monitoring, the system incorporates advanced machine learning models: Long Short-Term Memory, Multiple Back-Propagation, and a Convolutional Neural Network. Another component of the system is a clinically aware chatbot, built upon the Falcon-7B large language model and semantically validated using Bio_ClinicalBERT. The chatbot pipeline integrates FAISS-based context

DOI: 10.4018/979-8-3373-3531-5.ch006

retrieval, clinical term detection, and semantic similarity scoring. The validation results underscore the system's reliability for predictive analytics, intelligent interaction, and real-time clinical support, making it a viable solution for scalable and secure chronic disease management.

INTRODUCTION

Diabetes mellitus is one of the most prevalent chronic diseases globally, leading to severe complications that significantly impact patients' quality of life and generate substantial pressure on healthcare systems (Naveed, Kaleem, Keshavjee, & Guergachi, 2023). Recent advances in digital health - namely, the Internet of Things (IoT) (Rodríguez-Rodríguez, Campo-Valera, Rodríguez, & Frisa-Rubio, 2023), machine learning (ML), and conversational agents - have enabled the development of innovative, patient-centered approaches for chronic disease monitoring and management (Fagherazzi & Ravaud, 2019). These technologies offer the potential to personalize care, improve disease control, and empower patients through real-time feedback and data-driven decision support.

The Personalized Health Assistant (PHA) system (Ribeiro, Gonçalves, & Silveira, 2025) was designed to address this challenge by integrating a modular and scalable architecture that continuously monitors health parameters using IoT devices such as the Fitbit Charge 4 and Dexcom G6. These devices can collect vital metrics including heart rate, physical activity, sleep quality, glucose levels, and calorie expenditure. Data is transmitted securely using OAuth 2.0 and stored in Firebase Firestore, forming the system's Online Transaction Processing (OLTP) layer. A Python-based ETL (Extract, Transform, Load) pipeline transforms the data into structured analytical tables and loads it into Google BigQuery, enabling advanced Online Analytical Processing (OLAP) and visual exploration through interactive dashboards in Power BI.

To ensure regulatory compliance and user trust, the system adopts a privacy-by-design strategy, aligned with the General Data Protection Regulation (GDPR) and ISO/IEC 27001:2022. Measures such as pseudonymization, encryption, role-based access control, incident logging, and risk assessments are implemented across all stages of data collection and processing.

From an analytical standpoint, the system integrates multiple artificial intelligence models tailored to different user profiles. In the hospital triage phase, initial clinical parameters - such as blood glucose, blood pressure, and other vital signs - are collected and entered via a chatbot interface. The data is analyzed using the K-Means algorithm (Hartigan & Wong, 1979) to segment patients into risk clusters, with dimensionality reduction applied to improve clustering quality. For diabetic patients, a Long Short-Term Memory (LSTM) model (Hochreiter & Schmidhuber, 1997) predicts critical fluctuations in glucose levels with high temporal resolution. For non-diabetic patients, a neural network with Multiple Back-Propagation (MBP) algorithm (Lopes & Ribeiro, 2009) and the LightGBM model (Ke, et al., 2017) are used to predict glucose and blood pressure values based on indirect variables, leveraging parallel computing to improve performance. Additionally, dietary habits are assessed using a Convolutional Neural Network (CNN) (LeCun, Bottou, Bengio, & Haffner, 2002) trained to classify food images and estimate nutritional balance.

An intelligent and clinically aware chatbot was also developed to improve patient engagement and automate the collection of lifestyle and clinical data. The chatbot leverages a pipeline of FAISS-based (Douze, et al., 2025) context retrieval, Falcon-7B (Almazrouei, et al., 2023) for response generation, and

Bio_ClinicalBERT (Alsentzer, et al., 2019) for semantic validation, ensuring that clinical interactions are contextually relevant and medically sound.

All collected data is encrypted, securely stored, and analyzed to ensure a less intrusive, continuous monitoring process that adapts to individual patient needs. The integration of IoT, Big Data, Artificial Intelligence (AI), and privacy-preserving strategies positions PHA system as a comprehensive and intelligent solution for the management and prevention of diabetes.

This chapter is structured as follows: next section reviews related work and presents a comparative analysis with the proposed system; Follows a section that outlines the proposed methodology; Next two sections describe the system's design, implementation, and evaluation; Follows a section that discusses the results obtained; And finally, a section that concludes with final remarks and future perspectives.

STATE OF THE ART

The use of IoT devices and artificial intelligence algorithms has transformed healthcare monitoring, offering advanced solutions for chronic diseases such as diabetes mellitus. These advances enable real-time data collection and analysis, providing valuable insights for early risk factor detection and predicting critical metabolic events. Recent studies demonstrate that deep learning models, such as LSTM and CNN, are highly effective in predicting glycemic events and identifying metabolic risk factors (Toledo-Marín, Ali, van Rooij, Görges, & Wasserman, 2023). Studies on the genetic epidemiology of type 2 diabetes highlight how hereditary and environmental factors interact, offering opportunities for personalized prevention and new treatment strategies (Meigs, 2019). The interrelationship between metabolic syndrome, diabetes, and cardiovascular risk has been explored, emphasizing the importance of the management of these factors to reduce complications and improve clinical outcomes (Mottillo, et al., 2010).

LSTM-based temporal models have demonstrated greater accuracy in diabetes-related predictions by using longitudinal blood glucose data. This approach has outperformed traditional methods in recent studies (Naveed, Kaleem, Keshavjee, & Guergachi, 2023). An example is the study (Rajalakshmi, Sivakumar, Kumari, & Selvi, 2024), where the authors propose a Bidirectional Long Short-Term Memory (BLSTM) with an accuracy of 98,26%. Another study used deep learning models to predict type 2 diabetes with over 91% accuracy by integrating blood glucose data and other risk factors over time (American Diabetes Association, 2014). The application demonstrated reduced predictive errors and advancements in personalized medicine. In the study (Rodríguez-Rodríguez, Campo-Valera, Rodríguez, & Frisa-Rubio, 2023), IoT devices and lightweight algorithms, such as Random Forest (RF) and Support Vector Regression (SVR), were used to predict blood glucose levels with high real-time accuracy, highlighting the feasibility of cost-effective solutions for continuous monitoring. CNN-based models have been successfully used for diabetes prediction in specific populations, such as industrial workers, enabling risk identification in highly vulnerable populations (Wu, et al., 2020). The authors of (Zhao, et al., 2024) also considered a CNN, proposing an attention-oriented convolutional neural network (SECNN), with which have achieved an accuracy of 94,12%. CNN were also used to identify dietary patterns associated with glycemic spikes, providing an additional tool for personalized metabolic risk analysis (Rajalakshmi, Sivakumar, Kumari, & Selvi, 2024).

In (Nassar, Dunlea, Montero, Tweedt, & Magee, 2025) an educational chatbot demonstrated effectiveness in improving patient engagement and reducing Hemoglobin A1C (HbA1c) levels, suggesting a promising role in diabetes management. In (Lokman, Zain, Komputer, & Perisian, 2009) an architectural design of a chatbot is proposed, to function as a virtual diabetes doctor. In (Nawabi, Tolgyesi, Bianchi, Toffanin, & Dondi, 2025) a Large Language Model (LLM)-based chatbot assistant for diabetes patients, D-Care, is proposed and validated through a user study. Intelligent chatbots, by interacting directly with patients, help educate them on diabetes management, offering real-time tips and information, thus enhancing self-management of the condition.

Based on the highlighted studies, the integration of IoT devices with artificial intelligence algorithms demonstrates an effective approach to continuous monitoring and personalized follow-up for diabetes patients. In this context, some relevant studies from the literature were selected for comparative analysis, considering their contributions and limitations. The studies used reveals that the proposed monitoring system goes beyond the limitations observed in the analyzed studies by integrating different components. This integration results in a robust system capable of addressing the demands of continuous monitoring, glucose prediction, and personalized support. The comparative study (Table 1) illustrates the differences and advancements of PHA, the proposed system, compared to the selected studies.

The integration of AI and ML techniques into medical systems and healthcare is not done without great concern for legal, ethical and trust issues (Kumar, Chauhan, & Awasthi, 2023), and its intense debate has allowed some recent solutions to be reached (Iniesta, 2025).

Table 1. Comparison of Models and Technologies for Glucose Management and Prediction with the Proposed Solution, Source: Own Elaboration

Project	Use of IoT	Chatbot Assistant	Prediction Model	Glucose Management and Prediction	Computational Efficiency
(Rajalakshmi, Sivakumar, Kumari, & Selvi, 2024)	Yes	No	BLSTM	Partial. Accuracy: 98,26%	High
(Rodríguez-Rodríguez, Campo-Valera, Rodríguez, & Frisa-Rubio, 2023)	Yes	No	RF, SVR	Short-term monitoring	High. For low-resource devices
(Wu, et al., 2020)	No	No	CNN	Yes. Accuracy: 89,00%	Moderate
(Zhao, et al., 2024)	No	No	SECNN	Yes. Accuracy: 94,12%	High
(Nassar, Dunlea, Montero, Tweedt, & Magee, 2025)	No	Yes, deterministic	Not Applicable	Yes, focused only on self-management	Not Applicable
(Lokman, Zain, Komputer, & Perisian, 2009)	No	Yes, deterministic	Not Applicable	Yes, focused only on self-management	Not Applicable
D-Care (Nawabi, Tolgyesi, Bianchi, Toffanin, & Dondi, 2025)	No	Yes, generative	Not Applicable	Yes, focused only on self-management	Not Applicable
PHA	Yes	Yes, generative Focused on personalized alerts	K-Means, LSTM, MBP, CNN	Continuous prediction. Accuracy: 94,56%	High. Support for mobile devices

METHODOLOGY

The SCRUM methodology (Schwaber & Sutherland, 2020) was adopted for the development of the project, enabling an agile and iterative approach. The project was structured into sprints with incremental deliveries and continuous validation. In the initial phase, the focus was on creating the visual identity of the application, defining its name, designing the logo, and establishing a consistent branding. The next phases involved the implementation and validation of the machine learning models.

The project utilized an innovative approach for requirements elicitation by leveraging the GPT-4 language model to create interview scripts. The technique was based on the study (Görer & Aydemir, 2024), which proposes the use of prompt chaining to create detailed and realistic interviews for requirements engineering. This method was applied to overcome common challenges in requirements elicitation, such as interview complexity and the difficulty of involving real stakeholders in the early stages of the project. GPT-4 was configured with a specific knowledge base and personalized instructions, enabling the creation of scripts that simulate interactions with stakeholders.

Functional Requirements

The functional requirements of the PHA system are the following (User Story format):

1. As a patient, I want to view real-time blood glucose levels through my IoT device to monitor my health condition and be alerted about abnormal values. Acceptance Criteria: The system displays updated glucose levels every 5 minutes; the patient can view detailed graphs of the last 24 hours; notifications are sent when levels exceed defined thresholds.
2. As a patient, I want to receive automatic alerts when abnormal glucose values are detected, allowing immediate action. Acceptance Criteria: Real-time notifications provide guidance for actions such as consulting a doctor or taking medication.
3. As a doctor, I want to classify patients into risk categories using the K-Means model to prioritize critical cases and make informed decisions. Acceptance Criteria: The system classifies patients into five risk categories; the algorithm automatically recalculates categories when new data is added.
4. As a patient, I want to monitor glucose, heart rate, blood pressure, and physical activity integrated with my IoT device. Acceptance Criteria: The device collects data continuously and transmits it to the system at regular intervals; the system centralizes information on a dashboard accessible to the doctor.
5. As a patient, I want to interact with a chatbot to report my symptoms and receive guidance based on the provided data. Acceptance Criteria: The chatbot requests additional clinical information in a structured manner; recommendations provided by the chatbot are accurate and tailored to the patient's history.
6. As a doctor, I want detailed reports with graphical data to facilitate clinical evaluation. Acceptance Criteria: Reports include graphs of glucose and other parameters; the system suggests automatic recommendations based on the data.
7. As a patient, I want my data to be stored in an encrypted manner to ensure privacy. Acceptance Criteria: All data is encrypted during storage and transmission; the system complies with GDPR.

8. As a patient, I want to input information such as medical history, symptoms, and medication to complement automatic data. Acceptance Criteria: The patient can manually add relevant data; the data is integrated into the system's overall analysis.

Non-Functional Requirements

The non-functional requirements of the system are fundamental to ensuring a high-quality, secure, and user-centered experience. These include:

1. Performance – The system must support fast and efficient processing of large volumes of real-time physiological and clinical data. All components, from data collection through Fitbit API to visualization in Power BI, must operate with low latency to allow timely alerts, continuous monitoring, and accurate health predictions.
2. Security – Sensitive medical and personal data must be fully encrypted in transit and at rest. The platform adheres to GDPR and ISO/IEC 27001:2022 standards, ensuring access control, pseudonymization, secure API authentication (OAuth 2.0), and a privacy-by-design approach in all layers of the system.
3. Usability – The interface must be accessible, intuitive, and adapted for both patients and healthcare professionals. Dashboards must present clear graphs, meaningful summaries, and personalized recommendations in natural language. The chatbot must be user-friendly, supporting proactive conversations and memory-based responses.
4. Scalability and Modularity – The system architecture must allow new components (e.g., additional devices, models, or visualizations) to be integrated with minimal changes to the overall structure. All services (data ingestion, processing, analysis, and presentation) are designed to function independently but collaboratively.
5. Reliability – The application must ensure high availability and robust fault tolerance in data synchronization, prediction models, and real-time communication modules. Backup mechanisms and logging systems should be in place to monitor system status and recover from failures.

These requirements guarantee that the PHA system meets the demands of a clinical-grade monitoring platform while offering a smooth and secure experience for users.

The proposed PHA system is presented in the section that follows.

PROPOSED SOLUTION: PERSONALIZED HEALTH ASSISTANT

The proposed solution for diabetes monitoring and management integrates advanced technologies and machine learning algorithms to provide real-time monitoring, accurate predictions, and personalized support for patients. The PHA system, whose architecture is illustrated in Figure 1, is composed of four main components.

The first component is intended to involve IoT devices, specifically the Dexcom G6, Fitbit Sense 2, and Fitbit Charge 4, to collect biometric data continuously. The Dexcom G6 monitors real-time glucose levels, while the Fitbit Sense 2 and Charge 4 record vital parameters such as heart rate, blood pressure, sleep quality, and physical activity (Rajalakshmi, Sivakumar, Kumari, & Selvi, 2024).

For diabetic patients, glucose levels are measured in real time. In contrast, non-diabetic patients do not have access to continuous glucose monitoring. Instead, glucose levels are predicted using machine learning models based on variables including heart rate, oxygen saturation, physical activity, and sleep patterns. All data are synchronized in real time with Firebase Firestore, where they are structured and visualized through interactive dashboards, allowing both patients and healthcare professionals to monitor health status continuously and receive timely alerts or recommendations.

The second component focuses on machine learning models. Various algorithms were implemented for data analysis and prediction. The LSTM model is used to predict fluctuations in glucose levels based on historical data. A neural network with the MBP algorithm is applied to predict variables in non-diabetic patients, ensuring greater accuracy in complex scenarios. Additionally, the CNN model was trained to analyze images sent by patients, such as diet photos, correlating food intake with metabolic changes. These models were trained using multimodal datasets (Dubosson, et al., 2018), (Ulianova, 2018), (Fazeli, 2018), (Rachakonda, 2022), (Tharmalingam, 2023), (Koldijk, Sappelli, Verberne, Neerincx, & Kraaij, 2014), (Darabi, 2023), (UCI Machine Learning, 2016) and (Rashid, 2020), including glucose measurements, ECG, heart rate, and food images. Those datasets are usually highly imbalanced, therefore it becomes necessary to apply data balancing methods so that it does not negatively affect the classification results (Aymaz, 2025).

To support the data ingestion pipeline, a Python-based script collects data via the Fitbit API using OAuth 2.0 authentication. This script stores physiological signals such as heart rate, sleep patterns, steps, and calories into Firestore, establishing the OLTP layer. A second script performs ETL operations: it cleans and normalizes the raw data, creates time-indexed features, and loads it into BigQuery as structured analytical tables for longitudinal analysis and clustering. For continuous monitoring and clinical feedback, an additional service connects to BigQuery, extracts key patient metrics via SQL queries, and routes this information to the chatbot module.

Figure 1. PHA system architecture integrating IoT, machine learning, chatbot, database, medical reports and personalized notifications, Source: Own Elaboration

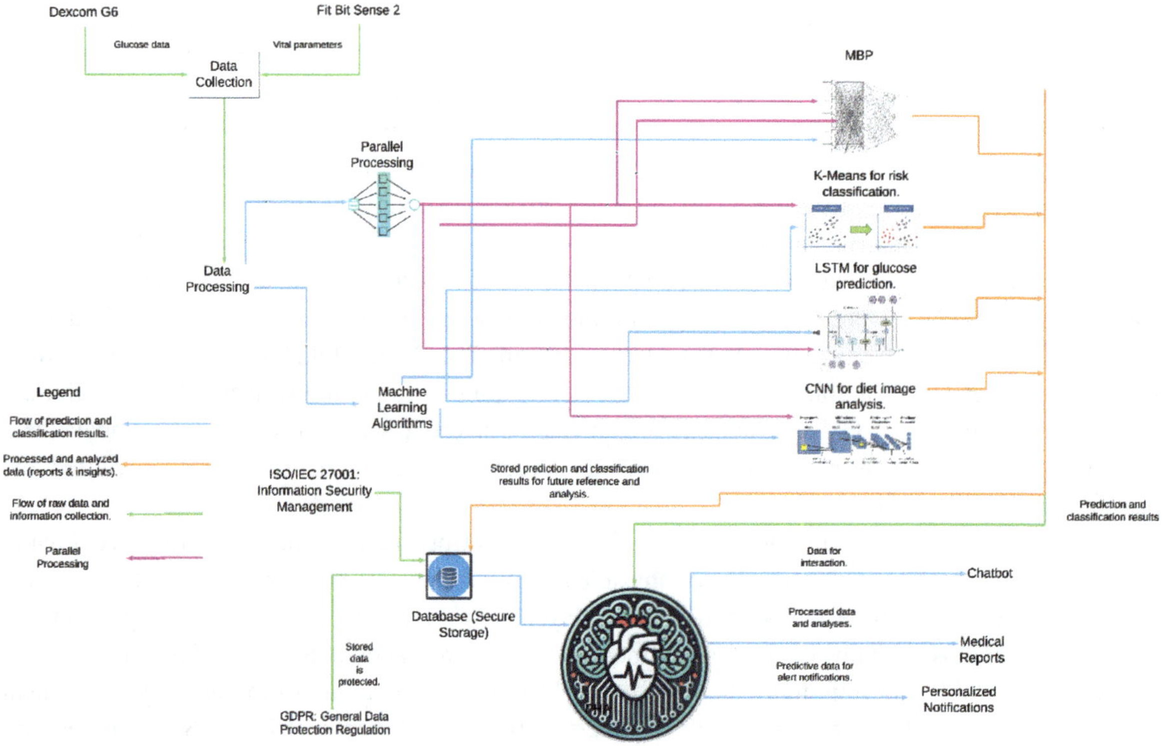

The third component is the intelligent chatbot, integrated with NLP (Natural Language Processing) and LLM, providing direct support to patients through personalized interactions based on collected data and issuing real-time alerts. Leveraging parallel thread processing, the chatbot can simultaneously monitor multiple patient conditions and accelerate the collection of supplementary patient data, such as symptoms and dietary habits, optimizing system responsiveness and efficiency.

The fourth component encompasses automated medical reports and personalized notifications. Based on processed data and predictive insights from the machine learning models, the system generates clinical summaries and delivers real-time alerts to patients. This functionality supports continuous monitoring and facilitates communication between patients and healthcare professionals, ensuring a closed-loop feedback mechanism for improved diabetes management. Figure 2 illustrates the PHA system activity diagram to manage alerts and corrective actions.

Figure 2. Activity diagram that will manage alerts and corrective actions, Source: Own Elaboration

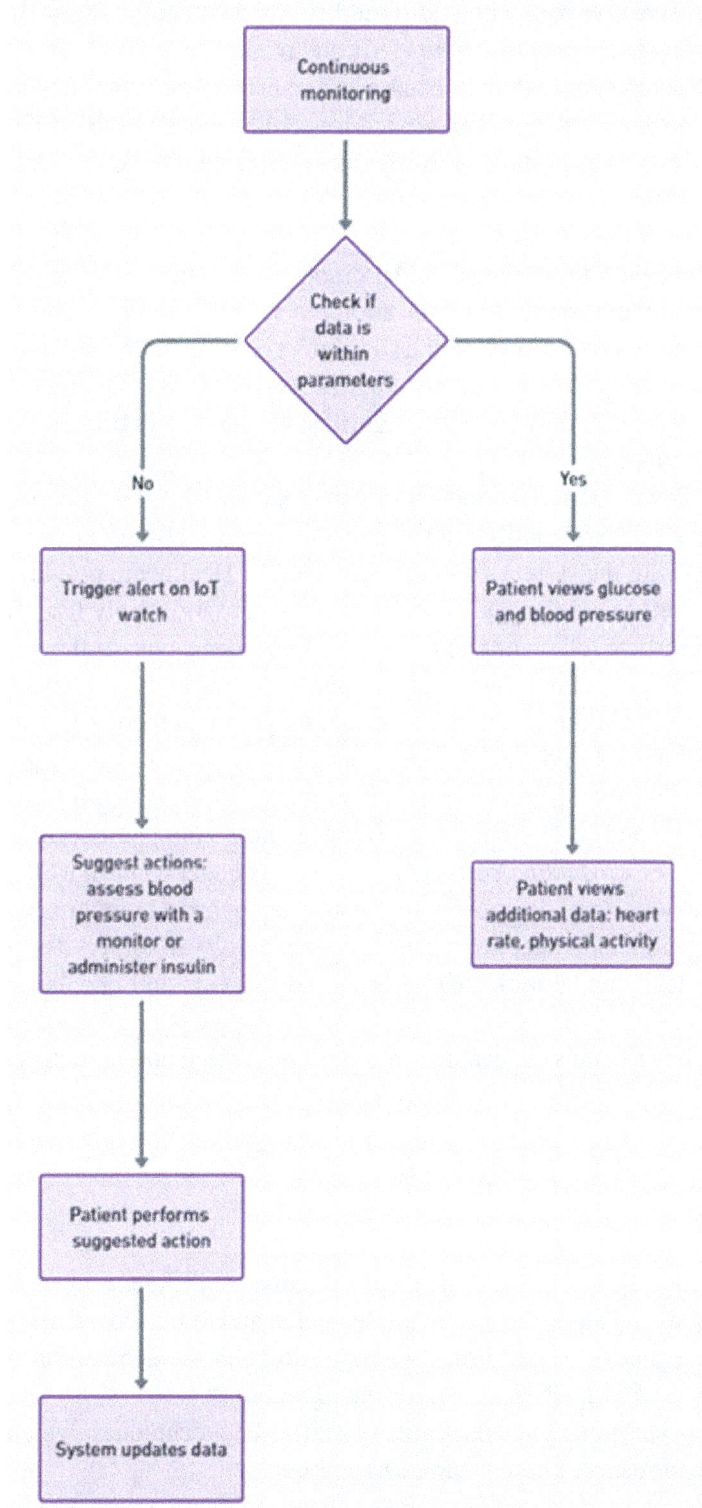

The system leverages Firebase to ensure:

- Secure storage of sensitive data with end-to-end encryption, complying with GDPR;
- Fast data processing to support real-time alerts and medical queries;
- ETL pipelines developed in Python to extract and transform Firestore data into BigQuery;
- BigQuery serves as the OLAP system, while Firestore operates as the OLTP layer;
- Power BI dashboards connect directly to BigQuery, offering interactive visualizations for doctors and patients.

Beyond GDPR compliance, the design should promote patient autonomy and data ownership through granular consent, clear sharing controls, and the ability to access, download, and revoke data use at any time. Role-based access, encryption, and audit trails protect confidentiality without undermining usability. To reduce alert fatigue, systems should personalize thresholds, bundle and rate-limit notifications, respect quiet hours, and escalate only clinically significant events - with brief, actionable rationales and an easy path to human support.

For visualization, Power BI is integrated through a native BigQuery connector. Dashboards are configured with temporal filters, multi-variable indicators, and real-time updates, enabling clinicians and patients to interact with the system's outputs dynamically. Healthcare providers would thus use the dashboards to track trends (e.g., glucose, heart rate, sleep, activity), apply time filters, and view real-time alerts that help prioritize follow-ups and support clinical decisions. At the patient side, the chatbot gathers symptoms and context, offers plain-language guidance, and nudges adherence to care plans. Most patients respond positively to timely, actionable messages, provided there is transparency, the option to opt out or snooze notifications, and short explanations for why an alert was triggered.

The PHA system architecture is modular and cloud-ready, allowing teams to start small (data ingestion + basic dashboards) and scale components (models, notifications, reporting) as value is proven. Parallelization and batched processing keep latency and costs under control, while commodity Android phones and simple gateways (e.g., Raspberry Pi) enable deployment in low-resource settings. Key implementation challenges include data governance, connectivity variability, device heterogeneity, and staff training, all of which can be mitigated with phased roll-outs and open-source tooling to reduce total cost of ownership.

The section that follows details the evaluation procedure carried out on each component of the PHA system.

EVALUATION

The evaluation section aims to present the results obtained at different stages and approaches of the project. Various methods and algorithms were implemented and tested, covering everything from initial patient screening via a chatbot to risk group classification and the application of advanced machine learning models such as LSTM, CNN, and MBP-based methods.

A special focus was placed on the use of parallel processing techniques, which played a key role in optimizing system performance. These techniques enabled:

- Faster data collection;

- Efficient statistical analysis;
- Simultaneous execution of tasks such as alert notifications and scenario simulations for health monitoring.

Each subsection details the results obtained, highlighting:

- The evaluated metrics;
- The relevance of the proposed models in the context of health monitoring and diagnosis;
- The benefits of parallel processing approaches for performance optimization.

Security, Privacy and Data Governance

The PHA system was developed with a strong commitment to data protection, ethical responsibility, and regulatory compliance, recognizing the high sensitivity of health-related information. Its backend infrastructure employs secure OAuth 2.0 authentication for data transmission and stores all patient data in a GDPR-compliant Firebase Firestore environment, ensuring pseudonymization, multi-factor authentication, and fine-grained access control.

A comprehensive Data Protection Impact Assessment (DPIA) was carried out in accordance with ISO/IEC 27005:2022 guidelines, and the implemented technical and organizational safeguards align with the principles established in ISO/IEC 27001:2022. The platform enforces data minimization, explicit user consent, and role-based access control, in full compliance with Articles 5, 6, 9, and 25 of the GDPR.

Beyond technical protections, PHA system adopts a privacy-by-design strategy embedded throughout the system's lifecycle. This includes:

- Continuous logging and monitoring of access events;
- Regular audit procedures and dynamic risk re evaluation;
- Transparent, user-friendly privacy policies inspired by industry leaders such as Apple Health and Fitbit.

These measures ensure that the PHA system is not only technologically advanced and clinically reliable but also ethically aligned and legally sustainable.

As illustrated in Figure 3, the privacy and data protection pipeline follows a structured flow designed to enforce GDPR compliance from initial user input to ongoing monitoring and risk reassessment.

Figure 3. Privacy and data protection pipeline in the PHA system, Source: Own Elaboration

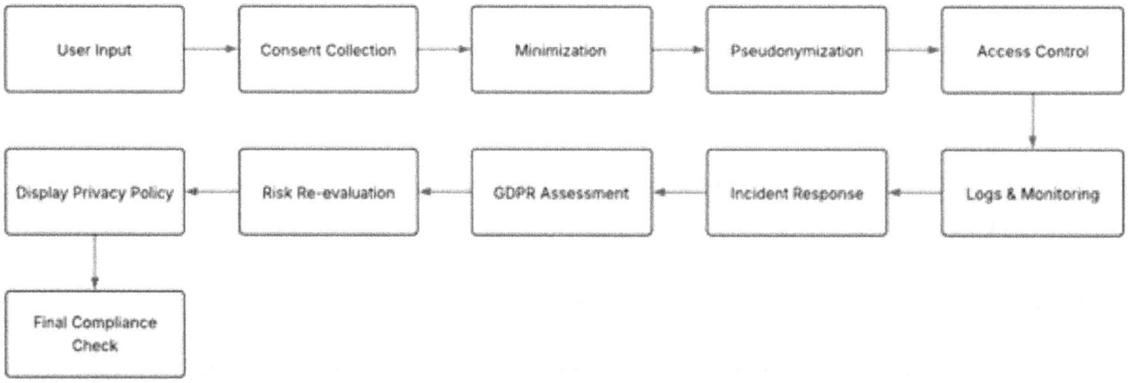

The flowchart of Figure 3 illustrates the sequential steps implemented to guarantee full adherence to GDPR data protection principles. The process begins with user input and advances through consent collection, data minimization, pseudonymization, and access control. Continuous monitoring and logging are used to trigger incident response protocols and support GDPR compliance assessments. Based on these evaluations, risks are re-assessed, privacy policies are updated and displayed to users, and a final compliance check is conducted to ensure the security and privacy of all stored health data.

Key Achievements and Compliance Results

The effectiveness of the privacy and security measures was assessed through dedicated metrics and compliance indicators, as summarized in Table 2.

Table 2. Summary of Privacy Compliance Metrics and Outcomes in the PHA System, Source: Own Elaboration

Privacy Dimension	Metric / Result
Audit Frequency	Internal audits conducted every 6 months, with corrective action plans created
Incident Response Time GDPR Request Compliance	Mean response time to incidents: < 48 hours 92% of GDPR-related requests were resolved in under 30 days
Team Awareness	100% participation in mandatory privacy training and sensitization sessions
Privacy Reviews	Privacy policies reviewed quarterly, aligned with evolving app modules
High-Risk Scenarios (DPIA)	No uncontrolled risks; all HIGH/MEDIUM risks have documented mitigations
Automated Decision Monitoring	LSTM and MBP models undergo monthly clinical validation
GDPR Request Compliance	All endpoints protected via RBAC, MFA, and encryption protocols
Export and Log Monitoring	Verified access logs and export permissions regularly via Firestore

The DPIA identified specific risk scenarios that were subsequently mitigated through technical and procedural controls, as summarized in Table 3. This ensures that both preventive and corrective measures are systematically applied across the system lifecycle. Between Tables 2 and 3, it is important to highlight that while compliance metrics validate the robustness of the implemented framework, a thorough risk-based perspective remains crucial.

Table 3. Main Privacy Risks and Mitigations (From DPIA), Source: Own Elaboration

Risk	Residual Risk	Mitigation Implemented
Unauthorized access to health data	High → Low	RBAC, MFA, encryption
AI prediction error (e.g., glucose)	Medium	Monthly review by medical staff
Credential theft (phishing)	High → Medium	Secure login, user education
System/data failure	Medium	Automated backups, monthly testing
Inappropriate third-party use	Medium	Legal contracts, pseudonymization, access logs

Big Data Architecture and Analytics

The PHA system integrates a scalable Big Data architecture to manage and process high-frequency data streams collected from IoT devices such as continuous glucose monitors, smartwatches, and mobile applications. This architecture is based on real-time data ingestion into a NoSQL database (Firebase Firestore), with scheduled ETL pipelines exporting weekly snapshots to Google BigQuery for OLAP analysis. The conceived Big Data pipeline is illustrated in Figure 4.

To ensure efficient storage and fast querying of longitudinal health data, the system employs a schema optimized for medical time series and risk clustering. The processed data is used to:

- Monitor temporal trends of glucose and vital signs;
- Segment patients using clustering algorithms (e.g., K-Means);
- Feed predictive models such as LSTM and MBP;
- Enable data visualization via dashboards (e.g., Looker Studio);
- Support clinical decisions through aggregated pattern recognition.

This architecture allows healthcare providers to scale their analysis and gain valuable insights from multivariate health data, while ensuring compliance with privacy regulations.

Figure 4. Big Data pipeline used in the Personalized Health Assistant system, Source: Own Elaboration

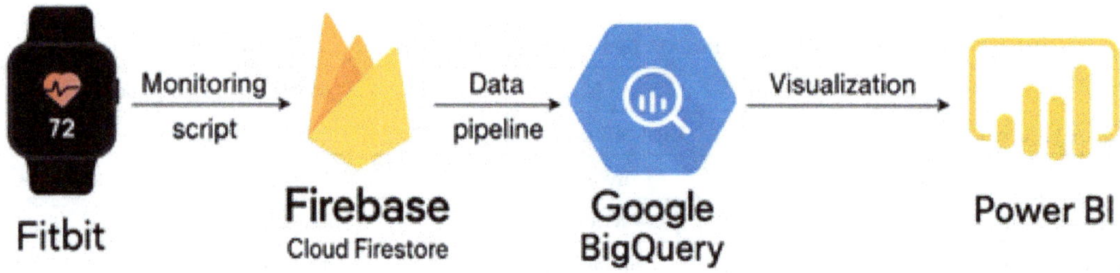

Real-time monitoring data from Fitbit is collected via scripts and stored in Firebase Cloud Firestore. Periodic ETL processes send the data to Google BigQuery for advanced analysis and visualization through Power BI dashboards.

To demonstrate how clinical data is structured for OLAP analysis, Figure 5 shows an example of a partitioned fact table in BigQuery. This table consolidates timestamped cardiac zone readings, including fat burn and out-of-range glucose intervals, organized by patient ID. The data used in this demonstration was collected using a Fitbit Charge 4, ensuring realistic and personalized time-series patterns for testing and validation. Such a structure allows for efficient querying and aggregation of cardiovascular and metabolic metrics over time.

Figure 5. Structure of clinical data of an example for OLAP analysis, Source: Own Elaboration

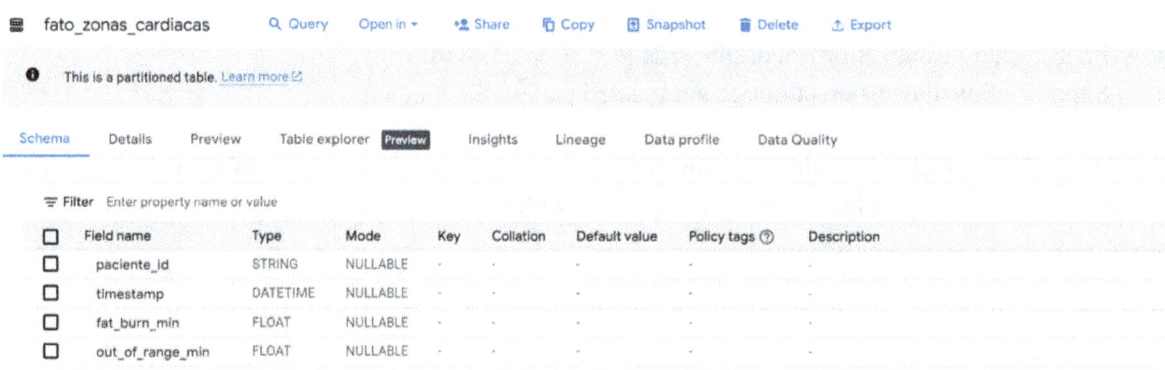

Additionally, to illustrate how physiological parameters are linked, Figure 6 uses the same Fitbit Charge 4 dataset to analyze the relationship between total sleep time and the total minutes of physical activity, stratified by time out of range (minutes of glucose outside the healthy range). The results show that patients with less sleep generally engage in less physical activity and exhibit greater variability in glucose regulation, indicating a potential correlation between poor sleep and metabolic imbalance.

Figure 6. Analysis Example - Relationship between sleep time and physical activity, Source: Own Elaboration

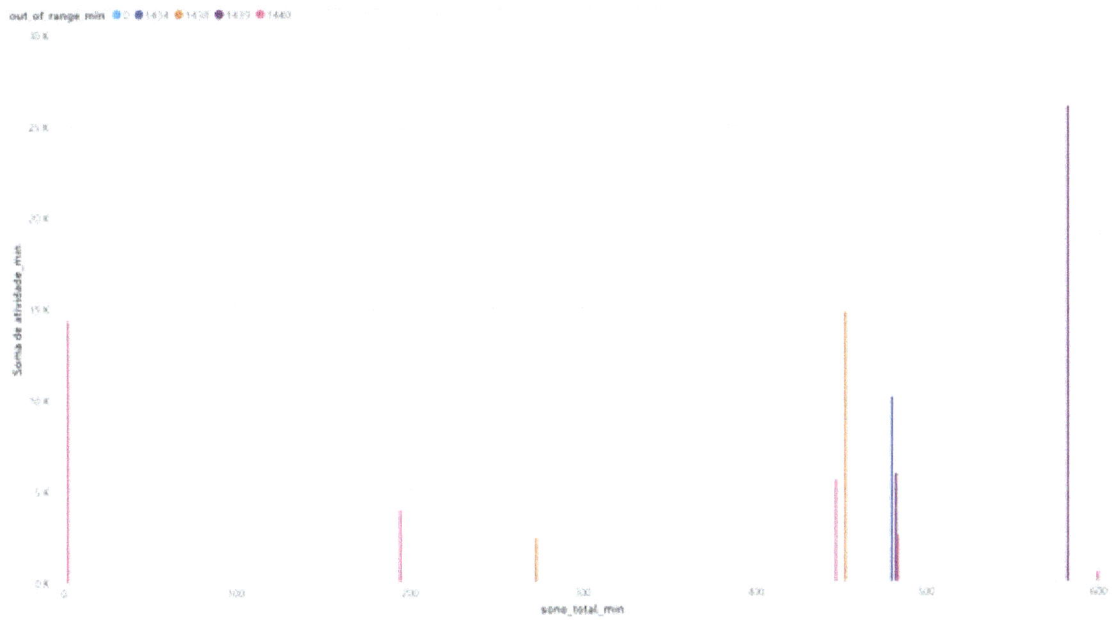

Furthermore, Figure 7 presents how different heart rate indicators (minimum, average, and maximum bpm) vary across physical activity levels, also derived from the Fitbit Charge 4 dataset. The analysis shows strong consistency between bpm metrics, particularly at lower activity levels, with greater dispersion occurring in highly active individuals. This supports the hypothesis that increased physical effort induces wider cardiovascular response variability, a factor that should be monitored for early signs of autonomic imbalance.

Figure 7. Analysis Example - Heart rate and physical activity levels, Source: Own Elaboration

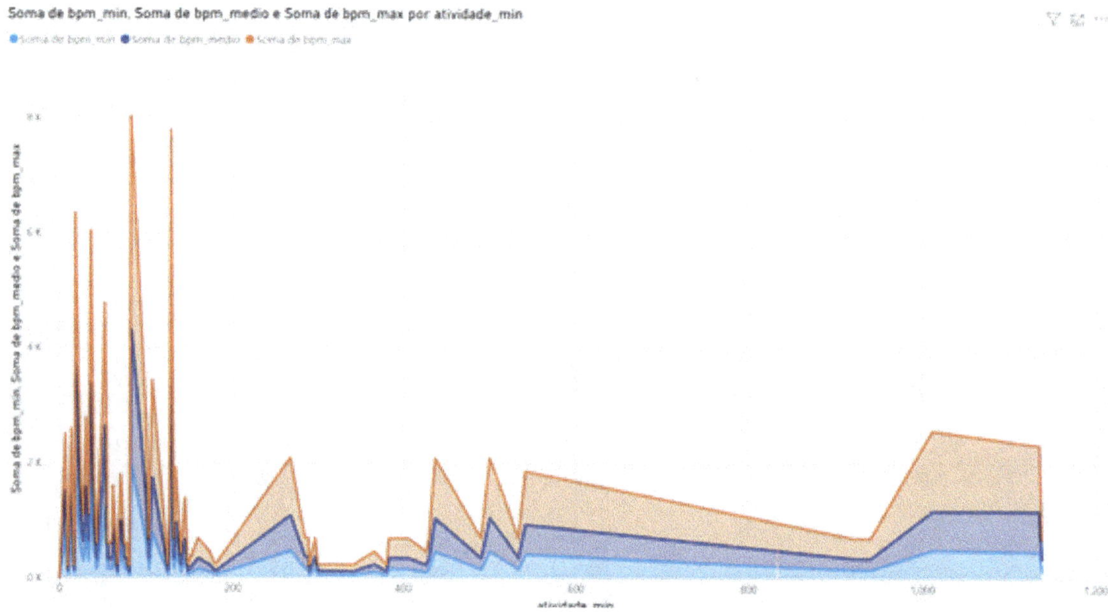

Chatbot Functionality

The initial version of the chatbot was based on a rule-based model capable of classifying patients into predefined risk categories and storing clinical inputs using deterministic logic. While functional, this early version lacked the flexibility to handle free-form questions and provide context-aware feedback. To address these limitations, an intelligent and clinically aware conversational system was developed.

The enhanced chatbot integrates state-of-the-art large language models with clinical validation techniques, ensuring that responses are both semantically accurate and medically sound. The new architecture combines:

- Falcon-7B Instruct for generating medically relevant natural language responses;
- Bio_ClinicalBERT for semantic validation, ensuring alignment with clinical terminology and guidelines.

Intelligent Clinical Pipeline

To achieve this, a robust multi-stage pipeline was implemented:

- Context Retrieval using FAISS for fetching semantically similar examples;
- Response Generation with Falcon-7B based on user input and retrieved context;
- Semantic Validation using embeddings from Bio_ClinicalBERT to measure similarity;
- Clinical Term Detection, quantifying the number of relevant medical terms in each output;
- Scoring and Classification, assigning each response a specificity score and type label.

Evaluation Context and Key Results

To evaluate the chatbot, a test set of 50 clinically relevant questions was compiled, covering diabetes symptoms, treatment recommendations, lifestyle habits, and preventive care. Each response was assessed in terms of semantic similarity (using Bio_ClinicalBERT embeddings), the number of clinical terms detected, and its classification as "specific" (medically precise and targeted) or "generic" (general advice or non-specific).

Figure 8 presents the distribution of clinical terms detected per response during this evaluation. The majority of answers classified as "specific" contained three or more clinically relevant terms, demonstrating the model's ability to embed appropriate medical terminology and context into its outputs. This reflects the chatbot's improved clinical precision compared to generic LLM responses.

This visualization illustrates the correlation between the classification of answers ("specific" vs. "generic") and the number of medical terms present. Higher counts are associated with clinically focused outputs, confirming that the semantic validation pipeline effectively filters non-specific or unsafe answers.

Figure 8. Chatbot Evaluation - Number of Clinical Terms Detected in Each Response, Source: Own Elaboration

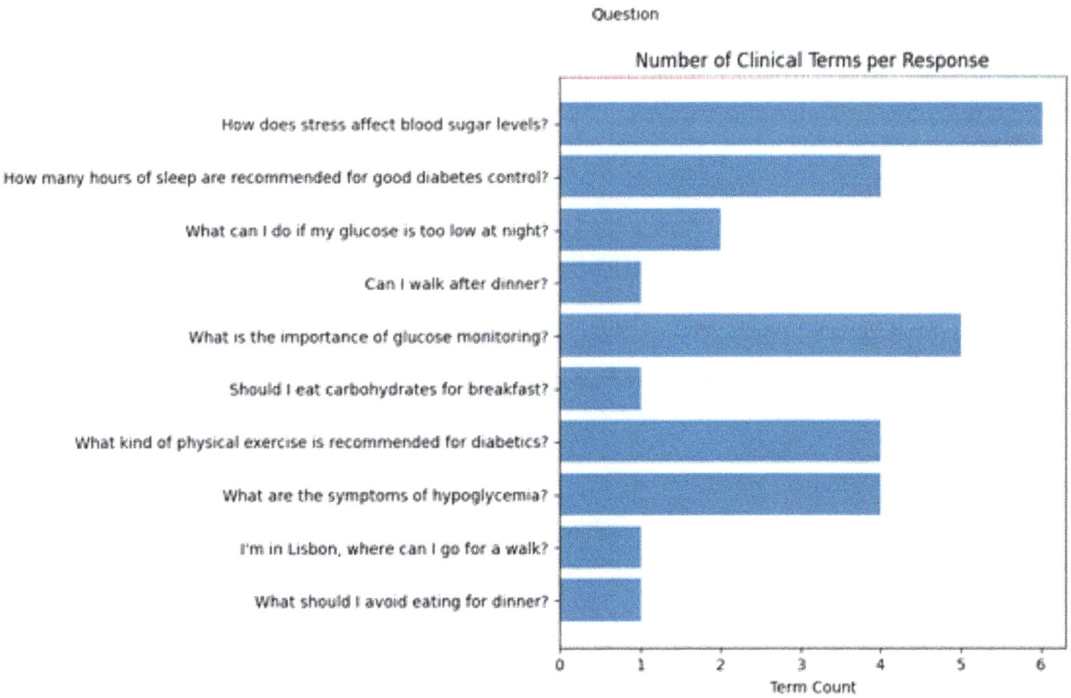

In addition, Table 4 provides examples from the evaluation dataset, showcasing typical user questions, their similarity scores, clinical term counts, classification, and overall response quality scores. This table highlights how the chatbot balances domain-specific rigor with conversational naturalness. For instance, questions like "What are the symptoms of hypoglycemia?" achieved both high similarity (0.91) and high clinical term density (5), resulting in precise and actionable answers. Conversely, lifestyle-oriented questions such as "Can I walk after dinner?" received lower clinical term counts, aligning with their generic, non-clinical nature.

Table 4. Chatbot Evaluation - Examples of Questions and Metrics Collected, Source: Own Elaboration

Question	Similarity	Clinical Terms	Type	Score
What are the symptoms of hypoglycemia?	0.91	5	Specific	0.94
What to do if glucose is low at night?	0.89	5	Specific	0.92
Can I walk after dinner?	0.86	1	Generic	0.66
What to avoid at dinner?	0.86	1	Generic	0.66

In conclusion, this upgraded chatbot framework successfully merges generative AI with domain-specific validation, enabling:

- Personalized and clinically coherent interactions, grounded in real patient data;
- Real-time triage and lifestyle coaching, supporting both diabetic and non-diabetic users;
- Scalable deployment, suitable for integration with remote monitoring platforms and mobile applications.

Future work will focus on optimizing fluency and inference speed, refining prompt design, and deploying lighter LLM variants (e.g., quantized or distilled models) to enable edge computing and real-time responsiveness in mobile environments.

Grouping Patients into Risk Groups (K-Means Model)

The K-Means model was trained using 1,768 samples, which were preprocessed to correct missing values and normalize the data. The number of clusters was set to five, based on exploratory analysis and the use of the elbow method.

The evaluated metrics include:

- Inertia: Measures the sum of squared distances between each point and the center of its cluster;
- Silhouette Coefficient: Assesses the separation and compactness of clusters. Higher values indicate better clustering quality.

The graph in Figure 9 shows a sharp decrease in inertia up to three clusters, with a gradual reduction thereafter, stabilizing around five clusters.

Figure 9. K-Means Model - Inertia and Number of Clusters, Source: Own Elaboration

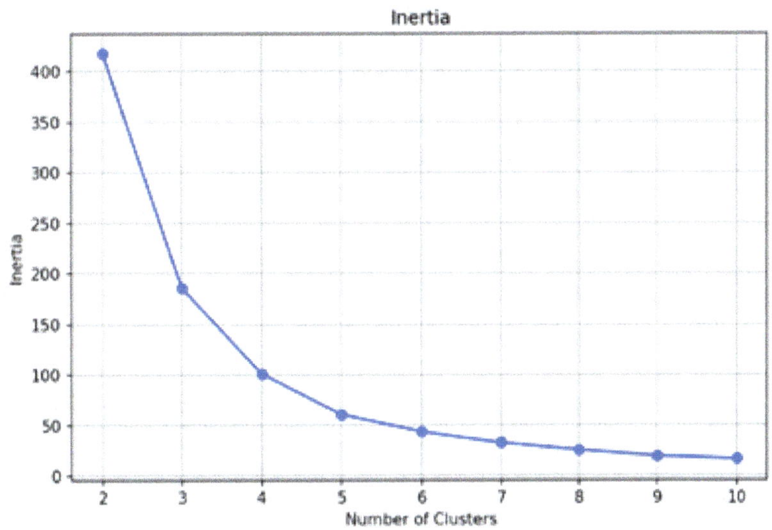

In Figure 10 the silhouette coefficient reaches its highest value at five clusters, indicating the most appropriate clustering structure despite some local peaks at three and nine clusters.

Figure 10. K-Means Model - Silhouette Coefficient and Number of Clusters, Source: Own Elaboration

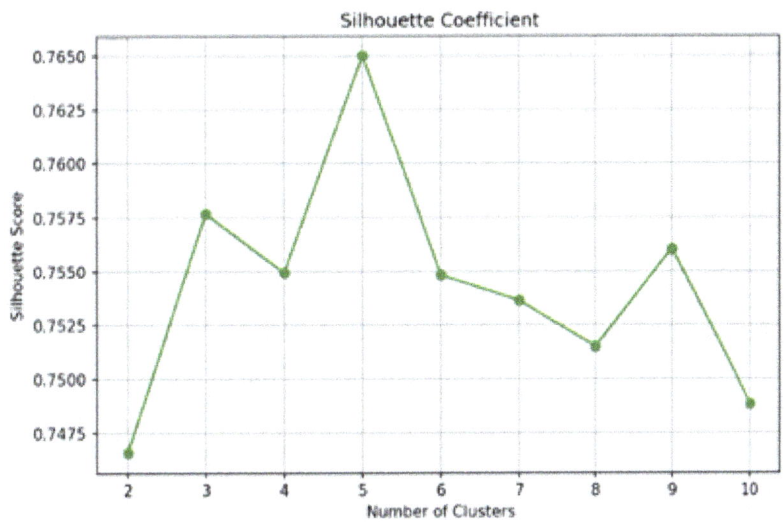

Critical Analysis of Patient Clustering

The K-Means results, illustrated in Figure 11, proved useful in categorizing patients into five distinct clusters, considering weighted clinical variables. The choice of the number of clusters was based on the analysis of inertia and the silhouette coefficient, ensuring a reasonable balance between separation and compactness.

However, the algorithm has intrinsic limitations, such as the assumption of spherical cluster shapes, which may not accurately reflect the complexity of clinical data. Additionally, the weights assigned to the variables were defined based on pre-established criteria, which may reduce flexibility and limit the model's applicability to other scenarios.

Finally, the visual analysis provides a good understanding, but incorporating more robust cross-validation methods and additional metrics could strengthen the conclusions and enhance the interpretation of results.

Figure 11. K-Means Model - The clusters categorize patients based on the calculated diabetes risk, Source: Own Elaboration

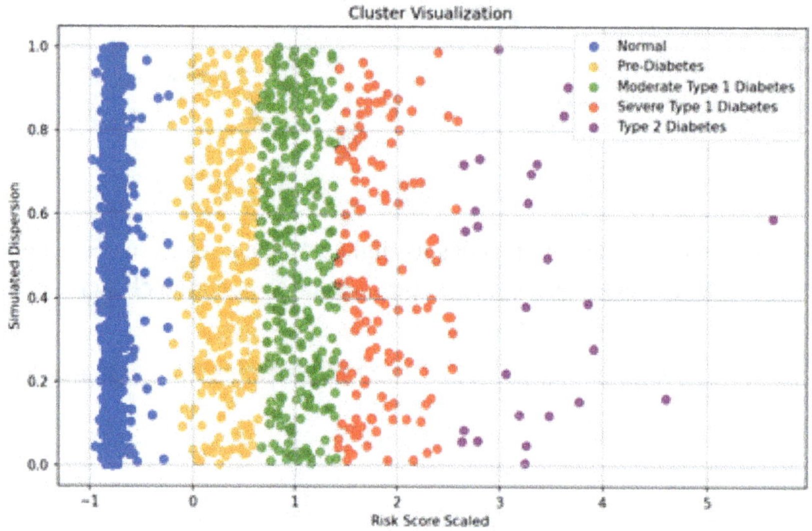

LSTM Model Evaluation

The LSTM model was developed to estimate blood glucose values based on previous temporal data. It is composed of two stacked LSTM layers with 64 units each, both using ReLU activation, followed by dropout layers with a 30% rate to reduce overfitting, and a final dense layer for regression output. The model was compiled using Adam optimizer, with Mean Squared Error (MSE) as the loss function and Mean Absolute Error (MAE) as the evaluation metric. Training was configured for a maximum of 100 epochs with a batch size of 32, and included an EarlyStopping mechanism with a patience of 10 epochs. This strategy automatically stopped training when validation loss ceased to improve, restoring the best-performing model weights. In practice, the training stopped after 43 epochs.

To assess the model's performance, multiple metrics and visualizations were used. A detailed breakdown of precision, sensitivity, and specificity for each blood glucose risk class is presented in Table 5, highlighting the model's strong performance across all categories. The highest precision was observed in the Hyper Severe class, while all average metric values remained above 0.94, confirming the model's reliability in accurately distinguishing between clinically relevant states. The results demonstrate that the LSTM model maintains high predictive accuracy, especially in detecting severe hyperglycemia and hypoglycemia cases. The balanced metrics indicate robust classification capabilities across all clinical risk levels.

Table 5. LSTM Model - Evaluation Metrics, Source: Own Elaboration

Class	Precision	Sensitivity	Specificity
0 – Hypo	0,954545	0,849515	0,996711
1 – Normal	0,943065	0,940907	0,973375
2 – Hyper Mild	0,906027	0,943456	0,967452
3 – Hyper Severe	0,977366	0,973776	0,987530
Average	**0,945251**	**0,926914**	**0,981267**

Figure 12 illustrates the evolution of the training and validation loss over the epochs, where a consistent decrease in both curves can be observed, indicating proper convergence of the model.

Figure 12. LSTM Model - Training and Validation Loss, Source: Own Elaboration

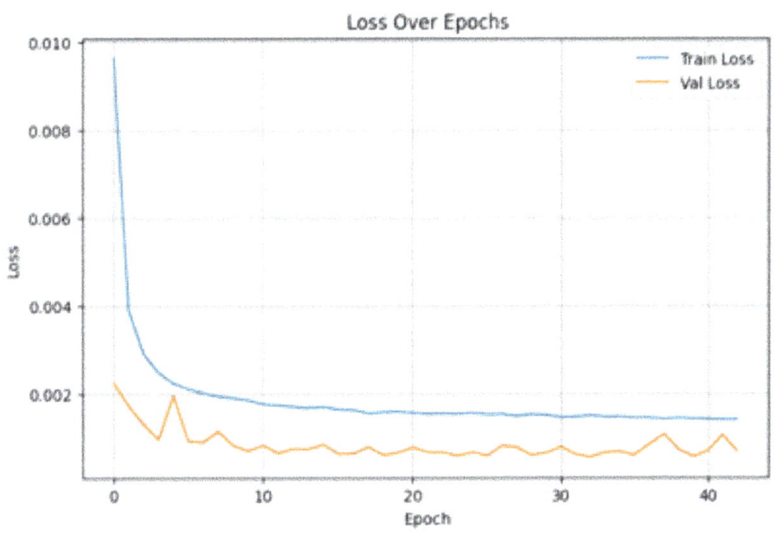

Figure 13 shows the values of MAE per epoch. The validation MAE fluctuates but remains low, reinforcing the generalization capability of the LSTM model.

Figure 13. LSTM Model - Mean Absolute Error, Source: Own Elaboration

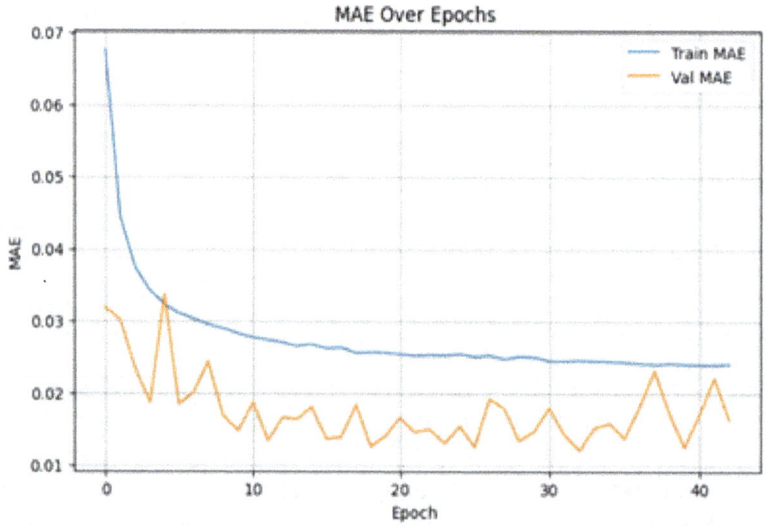

In Figure 14, the validation accuracy remains consistently high throughout the training, maintaining values above 90% after epoch 10 and stabilizing near the peak performance range.

Figure 14. LSTM Model - Validation Accuracy, Source: Own Elaboration

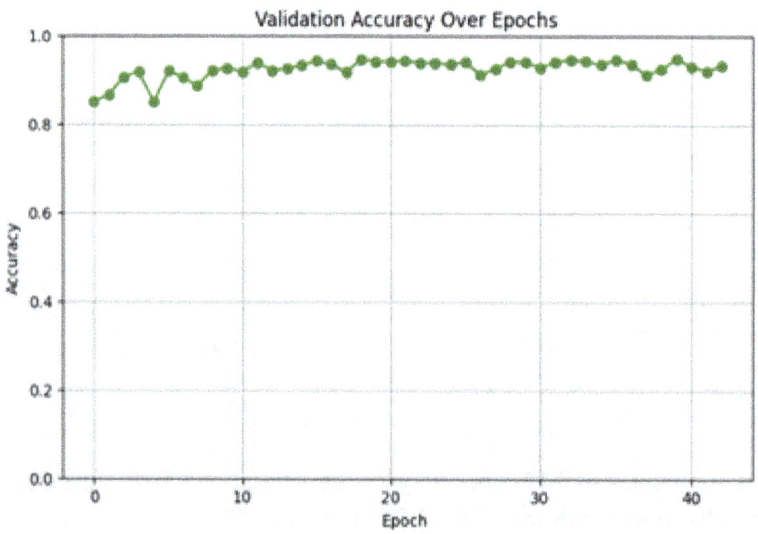

To further validate the classification performance, Figure 15 presents the confusion matrix using the predicted risk classes (Hypoglycemia, Normal, Hyper Mild, and Hyper Severe). The model demonstrates high accuracy in distinguishing between these categories, with the most confusion occurring between adjacent classes, which is expected in clinical contexts.

In terms of metrics, the model achieved the following results:

- MSE: 0.0006
- MAE: 0.0122
- RMSE: 0.0243
- R^2: 0.9867
- Classification Accuracy: 94.64%

Figure 15. LSTM Model - Confusion Matrix, Source: Own Elaboration

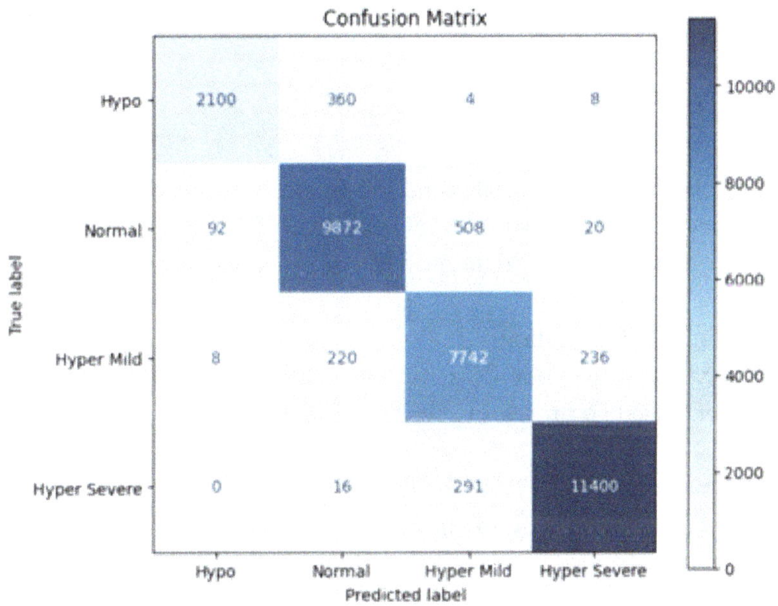


```
✅ MSE: 0.0006 | MAE: 0.0122 | RMSE: 0.0243 | R²: 0.9867 | Accuracy:
0.9464
📌 Epochs used: 43
```

These results highlight the model's strong performance not only in predicting continuous glucose values but also in effectively classifying them into clinically relevant risk levels. This dual capability is essential for real-time monitoring systems aiming to provide both predictive analytics and immediate alerts. Figure 16 illustrates an example.

Figure 16. Alerts generated by the LSTM model and suggestion of appropriate interventions, Source: Own Elaboration

```
Testing alerts with validation data:
⚠ ALERT: High prediction error: 0.11. Predicted glucose: 0.13, actual: 0.14
⚠ Hypoglycemia: Glucose 0.13 mg/dL. Administered insulin: 7.00 U.
⚠ Low activity level: 0.41 g.
⚠ ALERT: High prediction error: 0.22. Predicted glucose: 0.08, actual: 0.11
⚠ Hypoglycemia: Glucose 0.08 mg/dL. Administered insulin: 4.00 U.
⚠ ALERT: High prediction error: 0.19. Predicted glucose: 0.60, actual: 0.75
⚠ Hypoglycemia: Glucose 0.60 mg/dL. Administered insulin: 6.00 U.
⚠ Low activity level: 0.3 g.
```

Evaluation of the CNN Model

The CNN model was designed to integrate food images with textual and nutritional information to classify meal quality and balance, and estimate caloric values. Recent improvements included a complete data pipeline for reorganizing image datasets and implementing transfer learning with fine-tuning using MobileNetV2.

Dataset Reorganization and Preparation

The model was trained using the Food Classification Dataset available on Kaggle, which contains 61 food classes. A Python-based preprocessing script was developed to:

- Read and stratify image-label pairs from the train_img.csv file of the dataset;
- Automatically reorganize images from the train_images directory into class-based folders for training and validation splits using an 80/20 stratified split;
- Compress the reorganized dataset into a reusable ZIP archive, ensuring structured and efficient input for deep learning pipelines.

This preprocessing produced a balanced directory structure across 61 classes, enabling reproducible experiments and streamlined integration with training scripts.

Model Training and Fine-Tuning

A MobileNetV2 model was trained with:

- Initial training using frozen weights for feature extraction;
- Fine-tuning starting at epoch 10 to improve representational learning;
- Strong data augmentation (rotation, zoom, shear, flipping) to prevent overfitting.

The chart in Figure 17 illustrates the accuracy progression, showing a marked improvement after fine-tuning:

- Training accuracy reached above 65%;

- Validation accuracy stabilized between 52–57%, indicating improved generalization compared to the previous version.

The vertical dashed line marks the start of the fine-tuning phase at epoch 10. After an initial drop, the model shows progressive improvements in both training and validation performance, indicating enhanced generalization after fine-tuning.

Figure 17. CNN Model - Training and Validation Accuracy, Source: Own Elaboration

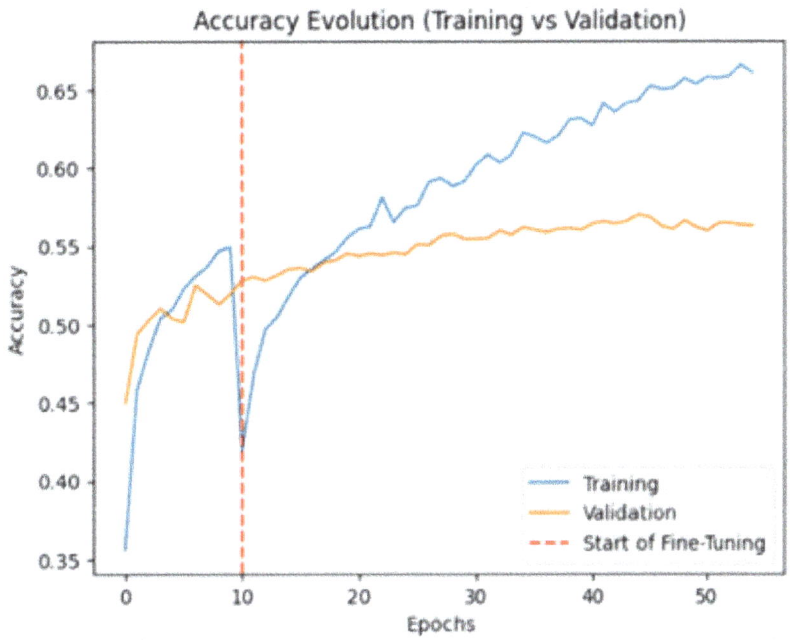

Performance Evaluation

Despite improvements in training and validation accuracy, class imbalance remained a significant challenge. Certain dominant classes, such as bread-white and water-mineral, absorbed predictions from minority or visually similar categories, evidencing persistent data skewness issues. Moreover, visually ambiguous foods (e.g., zucchini, mixed-salad) continued to cause misclassifications.

Although some classes achieved F1-scores above 0.03, the global metrics remained low (accuracy ≈3%), highlighting the need for further balancing strategies and model refinement to improve predictive reliability in real-world scenarios.

Evaluation of the MBP Model

Models developed based on MBP were evaluated on several datasets, covering different application domains such as stress, diabetes, blood pressure, and other physiological indicators. The analyses considered metrics such as accuracy, precision, recall, f1-score, and the overall performance of both classification and regression. Below is a detailed evaluation of the model for the SWELL dataset and the Sleep Health and Lifestyle dataset.

MBP model evaluation for the SWELL dataset

The model developed using the SWELL dataset aims to predict stress conditions in work environments. These conditions were categorized into three main groups:

- No Stress (0) - Work situations without interruptions and without time pressure. Participants could work on their tasks for as long as needed, with a maximum of 45 minutes, but without being aware of this time limit;
- Interruption (1) - Participants received eight emails during the tasks. Some emails were relevant and required specific actions, while others were irrelevant and served merely as distractions;
- Time Pressure (2) - Participants had their task completion time reduced to two-thirds of the time normally required.

Evaluation Process

The model was trained using the MBP technique with data from the SWELL Dataset. During training, the network weights were adjusted to minimize the prediction error for stress conditions.

After training, the model was evaluated using a separate test dataset. The dataset was split using a 70% training and 30% testing ratio, ensuring stratified sampling to maintain the proportion of stress classes in both sets. This approach guaranteed a representative and unbiased evaluation of the model's performance on unseen data.

Obtained Results

The model exhibited high accuracy and robustness in classifying stress levels, as demonstrated by the metrics presented in Table 6, which corresponds to the overall accuracy value of 0,9974.

Table 6. MBP Model for SWELL dataset – Detailed Classification Report, Source: Own Elaboration

Class	Precision	Recall	F1-Score	Support
No Stress (0)	0,9984	0,9999	0,9992	22158
Interruption (1)	0,9991	0,9919	0,9954	11782
Time Pressure (2)	0,9915	0,9987	0,9951	7093
Accuracy	---	---	0,9974	41033
Macro Avg	0,9963	0,9968	0,9966	41033
Weighted Avg	0,9974	0,9974	0,9974	41033

Figure 18 illustrates the confusion matrix for the MBP model trained on the SWELL dataset. The matrix shows the number of correct and incorrect predictions made by the model, indicating excellent performance.

MBP model evaluation for the Sleep Health and Lifestyle dataset

In this case the model was developed to predict systolic and diastolic blood pressure levels based on health metrics related to sleep and lifestyle. This model can be used in applications that:

- Continuously monitor cardiovascular health;

- Assess the impact of factors such as sleep quality and physical activity on cardiovascular health;
- Assist in preventing conditions related to sleep disorders and blood pressure.

Figure 18. MBP Model - Confusion Matrix for the Model Trained on the SWELL Dataset, Source: Own Elaboration

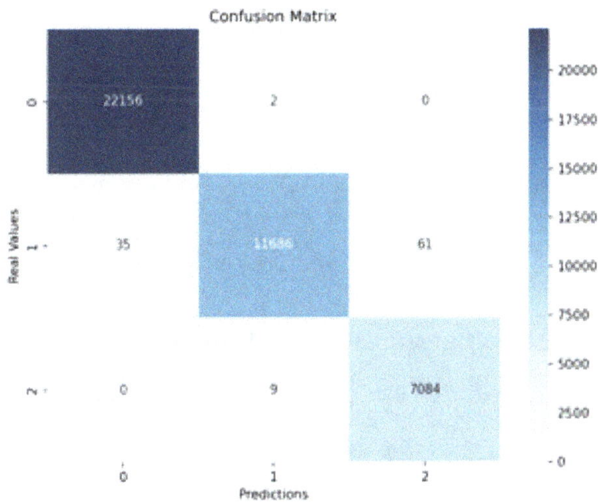

Table 7 presents the evaluation results of the MBP model for the Sleep Health and Lifestyle dataset.

Table 7. MBP Model - Evaluation Results for the Sleep Health and Lifestyle Dataset, Source: Own Elaboration

Pressure Type	**MSE**	**MAE**	**R^2**
Systolic	1,6553	0,5636	0,9698
Diastolic	1,3720	0,3887	0,9615

The model exhibits consistent performance, accurately predicting systolic blood pressure values, as illustrated in Figure 19.

Figure 19. MBP Model: Systolic Pressure - Target vs. Predicted Values, Source: Own Elaboration

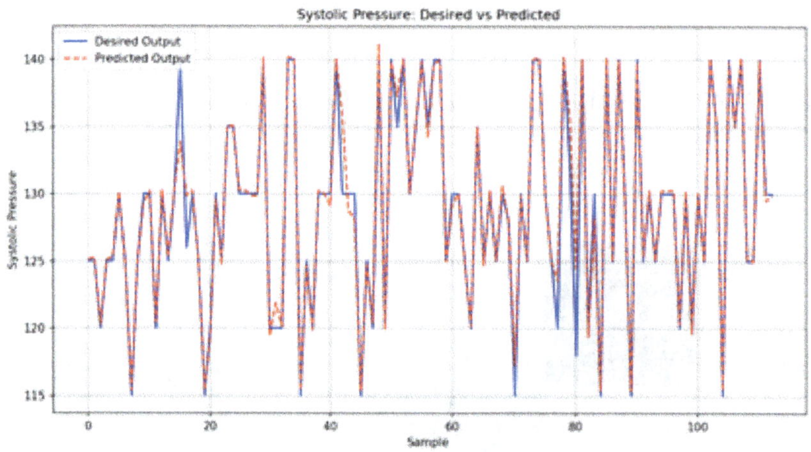

For the prediction of diastolic blood pressure the model also achieves an accurate result, as illustrated in Figure 20.

Figure 20. MBP Model: Diastolic Pressure - Target vs. Predicted Values, Source: Own Elaboration

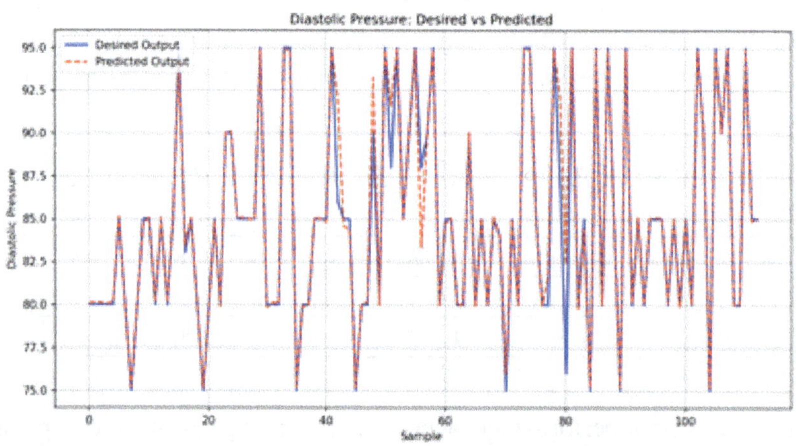

In addition to regression evaluation, the predictions were discretized into clinical categories to assess classification consistency:

- 0: Normal;
- 1: Elevated;
- 2: Hypertension Stage 1;
- 3: Hypertension Stage 2+.

From the perspective of categorical evaluation, the confusion matrix of Figure 21 illustrates the model's classification accuracy across the four systolic blood pressure categories (Normal, Elevated, Hypertension Stage 1, and Hypertension Stage 2+). The model demonstrates high precision in distinguishing between Elevated and Stage 1 classes, with minor misclassifications between Normal and Elevated levels.

Figure 21. MBP Model - Confusion Matrix for Systolic Pressure Prediction, Source: Own Elaboration

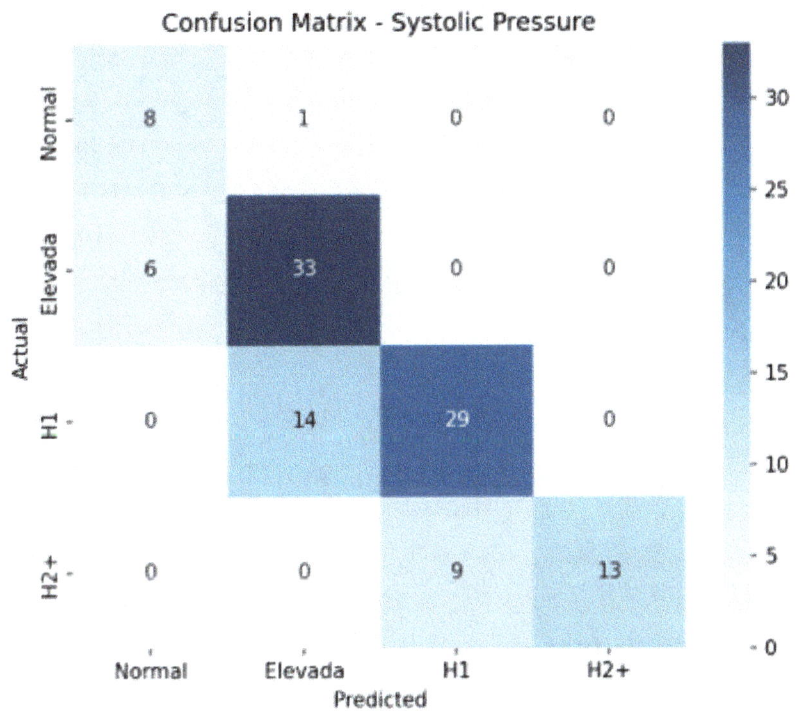

The confusion matrix of Figure 22 highlights the model's performance in classifying diastolic blood pressure categories. The model correctly predicts the majority of Elevated and Stage 1 samples, with only a few misclassifications observed between Normal and Elevated classes.

Figure 22. MBP Model - Confusion Matrix for Diastolic Pressure Prediction, Source: Own Elaboration

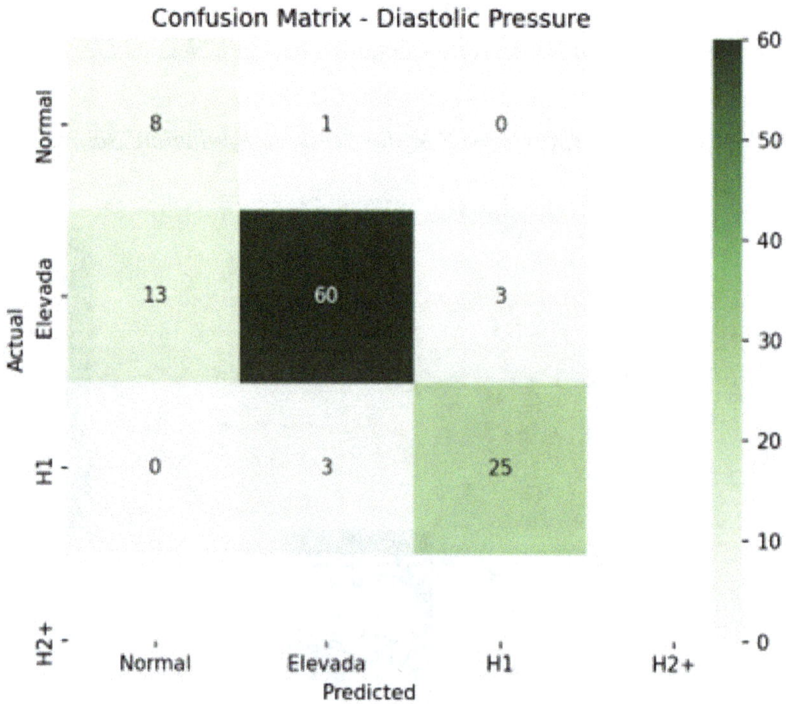

Parallel Processing in the PHA System

The implementation of parallel processing in the proposed system was crucial for improving the efficiency of critical operations, such as data collection, sending alerts, and creating charts. The use of threads and multiprocessing ensured that tasks were carried out simultaneously, significantly reducing overall execution time and increasing the system's scalability. This section presents the specific results of each stage processed in parallel, as well as the benefits achieved.

Evaluation of Results Using Parallel Processing

The use of parallel processing for chart creation and simulations has proven to be an efficient approach for handling large data volumes and significantly reducing the execution time of analyses. This process allows computationally intensive tasks - such as statistical calculations and graphical rendering - to be distributed across multiple cores or machines, maximizing system performance.

This subsection details the methods employed to implement parallelization in chart generation and simulations, highlighting the libraries and frameworks used, as well as the metrics applied to evaluate the effectiveness of the proposed solutions. In addition, practical examples are provided to illustrate the benefits of parallel processing in the context of the analyses performed.

Generating Parallel Charts and Simulations

The implementation of parallel charts and simulations was tested using synthetic physiological data. The system was designed to render and update multiple charts and execute predictive simulations concurrently, using ThreadPoolExecutor and ray.

Test Configuration:

- Four charts: Glucose, Heart Rate (HR), Respiratory Rate (BR), and Physical Activity;
- Five simulations: Glucose evolution under different clinical scenarios.

A series of controlled experiments were conducted using synthetic patient data, simulating real-world physiological parameters like glucose levels, heart rate, respiratory rate, and physical activity. Two execution strategies were compared:

1. Sequential Execution: All tasks (chart rendering) were processed one after the other;
2. Parallel Execution: Tasks were executed concurrently using Python's ThreadPoolExecutor and ray, simulating realistic deployment scenarios where multiple threads monitor patient variables simultaneously.

Real-Time Chart Rendering (Sequential vs. Parallel)

Charts for four vital metrics were created both sequentially and in parallel, with simulated latency using time.sleep() to replicate high-load conditions. Each chart presents a key metric, such as glucose, heart rate, respiratory rate, and physical activity, allowing for a comprehensive analysis. Figure 23 shows the example for the glucose case. The performance test showed:

- Sequential: 8.06 seconds;
- Parallel: 2.07 seconds.

This represents a 74% reduction in execution time, demonstrating how parallelism significantly enhances performance in real-time chart generation.

Figure 23. Parallel Execution - Glucose Levels, Source: Own Elaboration

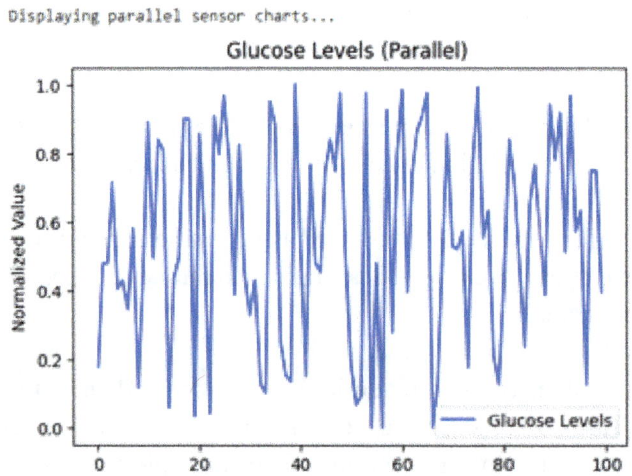

Parallel Glucose Simulations

To test forecasting capabilities under different clinical conditions, five simulations of glucose level evolution were executed in parallel using ray.remote. Each simulation represented a distinct scenario - such as stress, insulin intake, physical activity, or fasting - and modeled how glucose levels would change over 20 time steps. All simulations ran concurrently, reducing computational overhead and enabling the system to deliver real-time predictions. The results are shown in Figure 24.

Figure 24. Parallel simulations of glucose level evolution in five different scenarios, Source: Own Elaboration

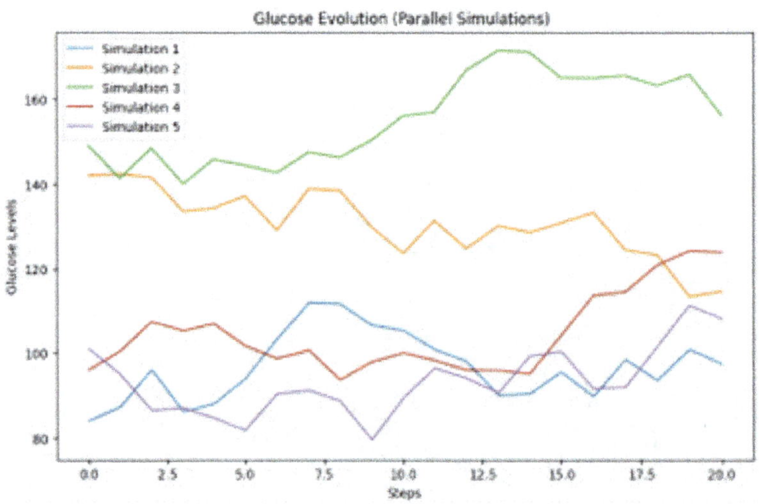

The conducted simulations and chart generation tasks confirm that parallel processing not only accelerates computation but also ensures that the system remains responsive and scalable. This is particularly relevant in mobile or edge-device environments (e.g., Raspberry Pi, smartphones), where computational resources are limited and timing is critical for health alerts.

Triage Execution Time Comparison: Threads vs Sequential

The initial triage process - responsible for collecting, validating, and responding to patient data - was implemented both sequentially and with multithreading. The threaded version distributed data processing across multiple threads responsible for:

- Form data parsing (e.g., glucose, blood pressure, BMI);
- Risk assessment (e.g., K-Means clustering);
- Alert generation (e.g., high glycemia or abnormal vitals).

Performance Results

- Sequential Execution Time: 4.52 seconds;
- Parallel Execution Time: 1.51 seconds.

This 66.6% reduction in execution time allowed the triage module to provide real-time risk classification and faster user feedback, particularly beneficial when dealing with high-frequency inputs from wearables.

Use of Semaphores for Real-Time Alerts

In scenarios involving multiple simultaneous alerts - e.g., high glucose + tachycardia - the system needed to coordinate access to shared alert channels (e.g., Firebase Cloud Messaging, display banners). Semaphores were implemented to ensure:

- Mutual exclusion in alert slots;
- No data races or duplicated alerts;
- Real-time delivery in correct sequence.

This mechanism provided deterministic and conflict-free handling of concurrent alerts, ensuring medical events were processed in the correct order.

Computational Efficiency on Low-Power Devices

To validate system viability in low-resource settings, all modules were tested on:

- Raspberry Pi 4 Model B (4GB RAM);
- Android smartphone with mid-range CPU (Snapdragon 720G).

The results obtained were the following:

- All modules (triage, alert, chart rendering, simulation) remained functional;
- Delays introduced were minimal (e.g., +0.8s in simulations);
- CPU usage remained under 80% in most scenarios.

This confirms the feasibility of deploying the system on portable or edge devices, supporting real-world use in home monitoring and remote healthcare.

DISCUSSION

The results obtained in this study demonstrate substantial progress in the monitoring and proactive management of diabetes, aligning closely with the initial objectives. The implementation of predictive models such as LSTM and MBP enabled highly accurate forecasts of blood glucose levels and other vital health parameters, corroborating findings from prior studies (Rajalakshmi, Sivakumar, Kumari, & Selvi, 2024).

Nevertheless, certain challenges emerged - particularly in the application of the K-Means algorithm for clustering, where the high dimensionality of clinical datasets negatively impacted cluster separation and model interpretability. These limitations reinforce the need to integrate more advanced dimensionality reduction strategies, such as PCA or autoencoders, to improve both computational performance and diagnostic reliability.

A key differentiator of the PHA system was the successful integration of parallel processing techniques. The use of threads during the initial triage process reduced execution time from 4.52 seconds (sequential mode) to 1.51 seconds (parallel mode), accelerating both data collection and real-time report generation. Furthermore, the adoption of semaphores to coordinate personalized alerts allowed for fast, simultaneous system reactions to critical clinical events such as hypoglycemia, hyperglycemia, tachycardia, and bradycardia. This concurrency control ensured high availability and responsiveness in scenarios involving multiple real-time signals.

Despite the system's overall predictive accuracy, some models - particularly when applied to non-linear or noisy datasets like the Physiological Stress Dataset - exhibited reduced performance. This highlights the need for adaptive models that better handle heterogeneous data distributions and context-aware training strategies.

Another notable finding was the system's computational efficiency, even on low-power hardware platforms such as smartphones and Raspberry Pi. The ability to maintain performance under resource constraints demonstrates the solution's feasibility for real-world deployment at scale, particularly in remote or underserved healthcare environments.

Finaly, the integration of PHA data with Electronic Health Records (EHR) and health data standards can be achieved by mapping platform entities to Fast Health Interoperability Resources (FHIR) - e.g., Patient, Observation, Device, Encounter, CarePlan - and exchanging data via secure OAuth2/SMART-on-FHIR API (Benson & Grieve, 2016) (Saripalle, 2019). Streaming signals and summaries can be transformed into standards-based observations using consistent identifiers, provenance, and clinical vocabularies (e.g., LOINC/SNOMED). Where required, HL7 v2 feeds can complement FHIR endpoints, ensuring interoperability while avoiding record duplication (Abdelouahid, Debauche, Mahmoudi, & Marzak, 2023).

Critical Analysis of the Results

The evaluation of the models presented in previous section reveals considerable progress in health monitoring and decision support using IoT and artificial intelligence. However, several limitations must be acknowledged:

- Hardware and Environmental Variability: While performance was promising in controlled tests, real-world deployment will depend heavily on the robustness of IoT devices in diverse environmental and usage conditions;
- Patient Data Variability: Model generalizability may be affected by demographic and physiological variability, which suggests the need for adaptive learning mechanisms or continual retraining based on population-specific data;
- Dimensionality and Algorithm Complexity: As noted in the clustering results, algorithms like K-Means struggled with high-dimensional clinical data, reinforcing the necessity of dimensionality reduction strategies to improve accuracy and explainability;
- Class Imbalance Issues: The confusion matrices, such as that in Section of MBP evaluation, reveal difficulties in classifying underrepresented classes. This underscores the importance of balanced datasets and advanced sampling or loss-weighting techniques;
- Computational Demands: Although CNN and LSTM demonstrated strong predictive capabilities, their complexity and resource consumption may limit scalability, especially on low-power or embedded systems unless optimized or quantized models are employed;
- User Experience and Intrusion: Finally, while the integration of conversational chatbots has shown promise - especially in providing educational support and real-time alerts - the perceived intrusiveness of constant monitoring must be addressed through personalization and adaptive notification systems.

In summary, although the proposed system achieves high performance and offers an innovative approach to personalized health monitoring, future iterations should focus on optimizing model generalization, reducing computational load, and enhancing user engagement strategies.

CONCLUSION

This work presents a comprehensive and scalable solution for continuous diabetes monitoring through the integration of IoT devices, machine learning models, and conversational artificial intelligence. The proposed system, named PHA, successfully combines clinical intelligence with real-time data collection, offering personalized support to both diabetic and non-diabetic patients. By employing advanced models such as LSTM for glucose prediction, MBP for parallel inference, and CNN for dietary analysis, the platform achieves a high level of accuracy and responsiveness.

The implementation of parallel processing techniques significantly improved system performance, reducing execution time and enabling real-time alerts in critical clinical scenarios. The architecture's compatibility with low-resource devices, such as smartphones and Raspberry Pi, further demonstrates its potential for large-scale deployment in both hospital and home environments.

In addition, the system adheres to strict data governance principles, incorporating privacy-by-design strategies aligned with GDPR and ISO/IEC 27001:2022 standards. The integration of a clinically validated LLM-based chatbot reinforces the system's capability to provide personalized, safe, and context-aware health guidance.

This study sets a solid foundation for intelligent, ethical, and scalable health monitoring systems that align with the future of personalized and preventive digital medicine. Future developments will focus on refining model generalization for complex datasets, enhancing fluency in chatbot interactions, and deploying quantized model versions to optimize performance on edge devices and thus considering a possible edge AI configuration (Wang, et al., 2020) of the proposed system. Given the importance and relevance to the system of aspects such as data heterogeneity, access rights and privacy, federated learning may be another path for future development (Nguyen, et al., 2022). On the other hand, digital twins (Vallée, 2025) represents a recent and promising approach that could be considered to the prevention, prediction or proactive and personalized assistance to a chronic disease like diabetes mellitus (Shamanna, et al., 2024).

REFERENCES

Abdelouahid, R., Debauche, O., Mahmoudi, S., & Marzak, A. (2023). Literature review: Clinical data interoperability models. *Information (Basel), 14*(7), 1–21.

Almazrouei, E., Alobeidli, H., Alshamsi, A., Cappelli, A., Cojocaru, R., Debbah, M., . . . Penedo, G. (2023). The Falcon Series of Open Language Models. *arXiv preprint arXiv:2311.16867.*

Alsentzer, E., Murphy, J. R., Boag, W., Weng, W. H., Jin, D., Naumann, T., & McDermott, M. (2019). Publicly Available Clinical BERT Embeddings. *arXiv preprint arXiv:1904.03323.*

American Diabetes Association. (2014). Diagnosis and Classification of Diabetes Mellitus. *Diabetes Care, 37*(Supplement_1), S81–S90. PMID: 24357215

Aymaz, S. (2025). Unlocking the power of optimized data balancing ratios: A new frontier in tackling imbalanced datasets. *The Journal of Supercomputing, 81*(2), 443.

Benson, T., & Grieve, G. (2016). *Principles of health interoperability: SNOMED CT, HL7 and FHIR* (Vol. 3). Springer.

Darabi, P. K. (2023). *Diabetes_Dataset_With_18_Features.* (Kaggle) Retrieved 01 2025, from https://www.kaggle.com/datasets/pkdarabi/diabetes-dataset-with-18-features

Douze, M., Guzhva, A., Deng, C., Johnson, J., Szilvasy, G., Mazaré, P. E., & Jégou, H. (2025). The FAISS Library. *IEEE Transactions on Big Data.*

Dubosson, F., Ranvier, J. E., Bromuri, S., Calbimonte, J. P., Ruiz, J., & Schumacher, M. (2018). The Open D1NAMO Dataset: A Multi-Modal Dataset for Research on Non-Invasive Type 1 Diabetes Management. *Informatics in Medicine Unlocked, 13*, 92–100.

Fagherazzi, G., & Ravaud, P. (2019). Digital diabetes: Perspectives for diabetes prevention, management and research. *Diabetes & Metabolism, 45*(4), 322–329. PMID: 30243616

Fazeli, S. (2018). *ECG Heartbeat Categorization Dataset.* (Kaggle) Retrieved 01 2025, from https://www.kaggle.com/datasets/shayanfazeli/heartbeat

Görer, B., & Aydemir, F. B. (2024). GPT-Powered Elicitation Interview Script Generator for Requirements Engineering Training. *In IEEE 32nd International Requirements Engineering Conference*, 372-379.

Hartigan, J. A., & Wong, M. A. (1979). Algorithm AS 136: A k-means clustering algorithm. *Journal of the royal statistical society. series c (applied statistics), 28(1)*, 100-108.

Hochreiter, S., & Schmidhuber, J. (1997). Long short-term memory. *Neural Computation, 9*(8), 1735–1780. PMID: 9377276

Iniesta, R. (2025). The human role to guarantee an ethical AI in healthcare: A five-facts approach. *AI and Ethics, 5*(1), 385–397.

Ke, G., Meng, Q., Finley, T., Wang, T., Chen, W., Ma, W., & Liu, T. Y. (2017). LightGBM: A Highly Efficient Gradient Boosting Decision Tree. *Advances in Neural Information Processing Systems*, •••, 30.

Koldijk, S., Sappelli, M., Verberne, S., Neerincx, M. A., & Kraaij, W. (2014). The SWELL Knowledge Work Dataset for Stress and User Modeling Research. *In Proceedings of the 16th International Conference on Multimodal Interaction (ICMI '14)*, 291-298.

Kumar, P., Chauhan, S., & Awasthi, L. K. (2023). Artificial intelligence in healthcare: Review, ethics, trust challenges & future research directions. *Engineering Applications of Artificial Intelligence*, *120*, 1–20.

LeCun, Y., Bottou, L., Bengio, Y., & Haffner, P. (2002). Gradient-based learning applied to document recognition. *Proceedings of the IEEE*, *86*(11), 2278–2324.

Lokman, A. S., Zain, J. M., Komputer, F. S., & Perisian, K. (2009). Designing a Chatbot for Diabetic Patients. *In International Conference on Software Engineering & Computer Systems (ICSECS'09)*, 19-21.

Lopes, N., & Ribeiro, B. (2009). GPU Implementation of the Multiple Back-Propagation Algorithm. *In International Conference on Intelligent Data Engineering and Automated Learning. Springer Berlin Heidelberg*, 449-456.

Meigs, J. B. (2019). The genetic epidemiology of type 2 diabetes: Opportunities for health translation. *Current Diabetes Reports*, *19*(8), 1–13. PMID: 31332628

Mottillo, S., Filion, K. B., Genest, J., Joseph, L., Pilote, L., Poirier, P., & Eisenberg, M. J. (2010). The metabolic syndrome and cardiovascular risk: A systematic review and meta-analysis. *Journal of the American College of Cardiology*, *56*(14), 1113–1132. PMID: 20863953

Nassar, C. M., Dunlea, R., Montero, A., Tweedt, A., & Magee, M. F. (2025). Feasibility and preliminary behavioral and clinical efficacy of a diabetes education chatbot pilot among adults with type 2 diabetes. *Journal of Diabetes Science and Technology*, *19*(1), 54–62. PMID: 37278191

Naveed, I., Kaleem, M. F., Keshavjee, K., & Guergachi, A. (2023). Artificial intelligence with temporal features outperforms machine learning in predicting diabetes. *PLOS Digital Health*, *2*(10). PMID: 37878561

Nawabi, A., Tolgyesi, J., Bianchi, E., Toffanin, C., & Dondi, P. (2025). D-Care: A Multi-Tone LLM-Based Chatbot Assistant for Diabetes Patients. *In Proceedings of the 18th International Joint Conference on Biomedical Engineering Systems and Technologies - HEALTHINF, SciTePress, 2*, 766-773.

Nguyen, D. C., Pham, Q. V., Pathirana, P. N., Ding, M., Seneviratne, A., Lin, Z., & Hwang, W. J. (2022). Federated Learning for Smart Healthcare: A Survey. *ACM Computing Surveys*, *55*(3), 1–37.

Rachakonda, L. (2022). *Human Stress Detection in and through Sleep*. (Kaggle) Retrieved 01 2025, from https://www.kaggle.com/datasets/laavanya/human-stress-detection-in-and-through-sleep

Rajalakshmi, R., Sivakumar, P., Kumari, L. K., & Selvi, M. C. (2024). A novel deep learning model for diabetes melliuts prediction in IoT-based healthcare environment with effective feature selection mechanism. *The Journal of Supercomputing*, *80*(1), 271–291.

Rashid, A. (2020). *Diabetes Dataset*. (Mendeley Data) Retrieved 01 2025, from https://data.mendeley.com/datasets/wj9rwkp9c2/1

Ribeiro, D., Gonçalves, C., & Silveira, C. (2025). Personalized Health Assistant: Machine Learning Diabetes Monitoring Integrating IoT and Chatbots. *In: Novais, P., et al. Ambient Intelligence – Software and Applications – 16th International Symposium on Ambient Intelligence (ISAmI 2025).*

Rodríguez-Rodríguez, I., Campo-Valera, M., Rodríguez, J. V., & Frisa-Rubio, A. (2023). Constrained IoT-Based Machine Learning for Accurate Glycemia Forecasting in Type 1 Diabetes Patients. *Sensors (Basel)*, *23*(7), 1–19. PMID: 37050725

Saripalle, R. K. (2019). Fast Health Interoperability Resources (FHIR): Current status in the healthcare system. [IJEHMC]. *International Journal of E-Health and Medical Communications*, *10*(1), 76–93.

Schwaber, K., & Sutherland, J. (2020). The Scrum Guide – The Definitive Guide to Scrum: The Rules of the Game. *Scrum.org*.

Shamanna, P., Joshi, S., Thajudeen, M., Shah, L., Poon, T., Mohamed, M., & Mohammed, J. (2024). Personalized nutrition in type 2 diabetes remission: Application of digital twin technology for predictive glycemic control. *Frontiers in Endocrinology*, *15*, 1–17. PMID: 39634180

Tharmalingam, L. (2023). *Sleep Health and Lifestyle Dataset*. (Kaggle) Retrieved 01 2025, from https://www.kaggle.com/datasets/uom190346a/sleep-health-and-lifestyle-dataset

Toledo-Marín, J. Q., Ali, T., van Rooij, T., Görges, M., & Wasserman, W. W. (2023). Prediction of blood risk score in diabetes using deep neural networks. *Journal of Clinical Medicine*, *12*(4), 1695. PMID: 36836230

UCI Machine Learning. (2016). *Pima Indians Diabetes Database*. (Kaggle) Retrieved 01 2025, from https://www.kaggle.com/datasets/uciml/pima-indians-diabetes-database

Ulianova, S. (2018). *Cardiovascular disease dataset*. (Kaggle) Retrieved 01 2025, from https://www.kaggle.com/datasets/sulianova/cardiovascular-disease-dataset

Vallée, A. (2025). Digital twins for personalized Medicine require epidemiological data and mathematical modeling. *Journal of Medical Internet Research*, *27*(e72411). PMID: 40762974

Wang, X., Han, Y., Leung, V. C., Niyato, D., Yan, X., & Chen, X. (2020). Convergence of edge computing and deep learning: A comprehensive survey. *IEEE Communications Surveys and Tutorials*, *22*(2), 869–904.

Wu, J. H., Li, J., Wang, J., Zhang, L., Wang, H. D., Wang, G. L., & Yuan, J. X. (2020). Risk Prediction of Type 2 Diabetes in Steel Workers Based on Convolutional Neural Network. *Neural Computing & Applications*, *32*, 9683–9698.

Zhao, J., Gao, H., Yang, C., An, T., Kuang, Z., & Shi, L. (2024). Attention-Oriented CNN Method for Type 2 Diabetes Prediction. *Applied Sciences (Basel, Switzerland)*, *14*(10), 1–23.

KEY TERMS AND DEFINITIONS

Chatbot: A software-based conversational agent designed to interact with users through text or voice interfaces. In healthcare, chatbots such as the one integrated in the PHA system provide personalized guidance, collect clinical data, and deliver context-aware alerts using natural language processing and large language models validated for medical use.

Data Analytics: A methodological approach to extract actionable insights from raw data using statistical, computational, and algorithmic techniques. In the case of PHA system, data analytics supports trend detection, anomaly identification, and predictive modeling for patient health monitoring.

Deep Learning: A class of machine learning techniques based on multilayered artificial neural networks capable of modeling complex, non-linear relationships in data. In the PHA system, deep learning models such as LSTM and CNN are employed for tasks like time-series forecasting of glucose levels and dietary image classification.

Diabetes Monitoring: The process of continuously or periodically assessing glycemic levels and associated physiological parameters to ensure proper disease management. PHA system automates this process using IoT devices, predictive models, and personalized alert mechanisms.

Internet of Things: A distributed network of smart, sensor-enabled devices capable of real-time data acquisition, communication, and remote monitoring. In the context of this study, devices such as Fitbit Charge 4 and Dexcom G6 form the backbone of the physiological data stream for continuous health surveillance.

Large Language Model: A type of neural network architecture trained on extensive corpora of textual data to generate coherent, contextually relevant natural language outputs. The Falcon-7B LLM used in the PHA system is integrated with semantic validation pipelines to ensure clinical relevance and safety of generated responses.

Machine Learning: A subfield of artificial intelligence that enables systems to learn patterns from data and improve performance over time without explicit programming. In PHA system, machine learning algorithms are used to segment patients into risk groups, predict vital signs, and support clinical decision-making.

Natural Language Processing: A discipline within artificial intelligence focused on enabling machines to interpret, process, and generate human language. It is central to the operation of the intelligent chatbot in the PHA framework, enabling it to understand user inputs, retrieve relevant context, and generate medical guidance.

Sensor: A physical or virtual device that captures environmental or physiological data such as heart rate, glucose concentration, blood pressure, or activity levels. These sensors form the first layer of the PHA system architecture, enabling the continuous collection of multimodal health indicators.

Chapter 7
Digital Cure or Digital Cage?
Reassessing Wellness in the Age of Algorithmic Mental Health

Unnathi Bhaktharam
O.P. Jindal Global University, India

Kirti Tyagi
https://orcid.org/0000-0001-8454-335X
O.P. Jindal Global University, India

ABSTRACT

This chapter examines the dual effects of digital technology on mental health, looking at how AI-powered tools, telepsychiatry, and mobile applications influence modern experiences of psychological identity, emotional regulation, and self-care. With the utility of tools like natural language processing (NLP), cognitive behavioral therapy (CBT) feedback, and predictive risk assessment algorithms, these digital platforms provide scalable and practical interventions. However, they also carry risks, such as over-reliance, a loss of intrinsic motivation, and an inability to recognize deep human nuances. An elaborate discussion of 'surveillance' in the place of 'support' is portrayed in detail through an analysis of the most common underlying technological mechanisms of different digital intervention tools. The chapter ends with an advocation of optimizing digital care by careful planning, moral supervision, and integration with human-centered assistance to guarantee that technology enhances, rather than harms, mental health outcomes.

INTRODUCTION

Historically, healthcare technology has prioritized physical health, a trend shaped by the biomedical model, which focuses on observable and measurable factors, as well as the traditional clinical separation of the mind and body. This longstanding bias paved the way for mental health neglect, creating a gap in research and innovation for future generations (Engel, 1977). Additionally, most digital health investments, such as the development of diagnostics and therapeutic devices, have been directed towards

DOI: 10.4018/979-8-3373-3531-5.ch007

identifying physical diseases, including cancer, diabetes, and cardiovascular issues, with over 70% of funding allocated to these areas (McKinsey, 2022).

In contrast, mental health has experienced less attention, despite being recognized as a global concern. This gap is particularly stark in low- and middle-income countries, such as India and the Philippines, where the ratio of psychologists to population remains critically low. Several barriers, such as stigma, underreporting, the subjective nature of diagnosis, and the challenges of applying generalized digital algorithms to nuanced mental health conditions, have caused this mental health lag.

This chapter examines how digital mental health technologies, including AI-powered tools, mobile apps, and telepsychiatry, are helping to bridge the gap in mental health care. It critically examines the psychological implications of these technologies for users' identity, behavior, and emotional well-being. The chapter begins with an overview of the evolution of digital mental health technologies and their role in addressing the obstacles of affordability, accessibility, and stigma. It will then analyze the specific technological mechanisms that can influence the human psyche, both positively and negatively. Lastly, using empirical data and key psychological theories, this chapter will examine the advantages and disadvantages of these digital solutions.

Shifting the Digital Focus Towards Mental Health

As a movement and a global crisis, mental health emerged with great attention in the early 20th century globally. Concepts such as mental hygiene, emotional intelligence, and psychological well-being, as well as the simple idea of happiness, have transformed the way people live. The World Health Organization states that one in eight people globally lives with a mental disorder (World Health Organization, 2022). Factors such as pandemics, economic pressures, and social isolation have contributed to a fast-paced lifestyle, with many struggling with depression and generalized anxiety disorder. Global mental health research identifies three significant barriers to care: unawareness about mental health concerns, stigmatization of disorders, and the scarcity of mental health professionals and treatment therapies (Henderson et al., 2013).

Digital mental health solutions stepped in to address all of these problems simultaneously. For example, in India, there is only one psychiatrist for every 100,000 people, as published in the year 2015-2016 by a nationally representative mental health survey (Murthy, 2017). Although this may no longer accurately reflect the current situation, it still highlights the scale of the accessibility gap.

Historical Trajectory of Digital Mental Health Tools

The evolution of digital mental health tools has been shaped by advances in artificial intelligence (AI) and the development of Digital infrastructure. Early, rule-based chatbot therapists, such as "ELIZA", "MoodGym", and "Beating the Blues", transitioned into real-time, responsive, and conversational depth chatbots like "Woebot" and "Wysa".

Digital mental health tool solutions emerged in parallel with the internet revolution in the 1900's and early 2000s. One of the first examples of digital mental health was ELIZA, developed by Joseph Weizenbaum at MIT in the 1960s. The conceptual idea was to replicate/simulate a Rogerian psychotherapist with a machine named a chatbot therapist. Clients or users would engage in written dialogues, emphasizing empathetic reflection. Even though this written method was not a therapeutic tool in the clinical sense, Weizenbaum created a straightforward, rule-based form of communication that paved the way for various subsequent digital discoveries (Weizenbaum, 1966). NLP, or Natural Language Processing, is a field of artificial intelligence that enables computers to understand, interpret, generate, and respond to human language in a practical and meaningful manner. The primary technology of ELIZA utilized NLP in its very initial, not very advanced form.

ELIZA was a revolutionary step towards incorporating digital computers to support discussions about mental health, regardless of its limitations in human depth and engagement, which will be addressed later in this chapter. By the early 2000s, "Beating the Blues", a computerized cognitive behavioral therapy (CBT) program in the UK, demonstrated clinical effectiveness for treating anxiety and depression (Proudfoot et al., 2003). Similarly, the computer-based CBT platform, MoodGYM, launched by the Australian National University in 2001, provided self-guided modules and displayed moderate efficiency in reducing depressive symptoms (Christensen et al., 2002).

These early self-guided computerized platforms, with minimal personalization and no real-time interactions, were soon surpassed by more advanced chatbot therapists. For instance, Woebot, introduced in 2017 and founded by Dr. Alison Darcy, is a mental health chatbot that marked a significant leap in integrating advanced natural language processing (NLP) and generative AI-driven conversation, revolutionizing the responses generated by the system (Sackett et al., 2024). The primary difference between ELIZA's NLP and Woebot's NLP was that the former employed predefined scripts and templates, resulting in machine-like, generic, and invariable responses. For example, when the user typed, *"I feel really down today, what can I do to improve my mood?"*, ELIZA replied, *"Why do you feel really down today?"* (Joseph Weizenbaum's ELIZA, n.d.).

In contrast, the latter was infused with an intellectual segment of context-awareness and emotion detection, which led to adaptive responses. No one answer would be the same as before, just like a conversation. When presented with the same user input, Woebot responded, *"I'm really sorry to hear you're feeling down today. Want to talk about what might be bringing you down? I can also guide you through a quick CBT exercise that might help shift your mood a bit"* (Woebot, personal communication, July 10, 2025). This capacity for emotional detection and adaptive therapeutic suggestions was a game-changer for the new age of AI technology. This was widely adopted and received significant engagement from those who needed support.

AI-powered chatbots like "Wysa" and "Tess" lead the broader ecosystem of next-generation mental health digital technologies. They provided users with 24/7 emotional support and consistent, easy accessibility. With chatbots delivering responses three times faster on average, the 2021 global survey data indicated that 22% of adults and 47% showed a keen interest in using a mental health chatbot (Vyshnevska, 2023). The Woebot users experienced a significant reduction in depression and anxiety symptoms after just two weeks (Fitzpatrick et al., 2017).

This ecosystem has also been expanded to include mobile applications such as Headspace and Calm, which provide guided meditation, mindfulness-based stress reduction, and sleep improvement to enhance emotional regulation and reduce burnout (Huberty et al., 2019). With a growing concern for health in an age of overconsumption and capitalism, wearable integrated devices like Apple Health, FitBit, and Garmin have entered the ecosystem that employs biosensors to track physiological markers (stress levels, sleep patterns, and heart rate variability). Immediate feedback with current health reports and early intervention options is at one's fingertips.

To help bridge the mental health accessibility gap discussed earlier, teletherapy platforms such as BetterHelp and TalkSpace have made licensed mental health experts more accessible through secure audio, video, and chat calls, providing flexible and reasonably priced substitutes for in-person care (Smith et al., 2023).

Chatbot therapists, telepsychiatry, and mobile wellness applications comprise the intricate, self-accessible digital ecosystem integrated into the daily functionality of thousands of people. In 2023, 83% of adult users of wellness apps reported an improvement in well-being, with projections for 2024 indicating a 90% positive impact (Precedence Research, 2024). Digital-based workplace interventions have found consistent reduction in the stress, anxiety, depression, and burnout across employee populations (Cameron et al., 2024). On the Counslr app, where licensed mental health professionals provide 24/7 support, 80.1% of the counseling sessions took place outside conventional hours of 7 am-5 pm, when services were not available, and 88% of the users of this app had never previously sought mental health care before (Morningstar, 2025). More than 4,500 students have benefited from hybrid AI chatbots in schools, such as Sonny (part human and part AI, powered by Sonar Mental Health), which have purportedly reduced negative behavioral occurrences by 26%, indicating real-world emotional and behavioral advantages (Jargon, 2025).

While digital mental health technologies have broadened access and introduced innovative care models, their very strengths of immediacy, personalization, and constant availability can also create ethical and psychological challenges. The following section examines how these tools may blur the line between support and surveillance, potentially undermining the well-being they aim to enhance.

From Empowerment to Surveillance: The Ethical and Psychological Paradoxes of Digital Health Tools

This section critically analyzes the contradictions in digital mental health technologies, particularly the tension between care and control. It examines how instruments designed to empower and assist users may inadvertently foster emotional distress, surveillance, and moral dilemmas related to data privacy and autonomy. By unpacking these contradictions, this section formulates the main argument that digital mental health tools risk undermining the well-being they intend to promote without thoughtful design and regulation.

The line between care and control can be blurry, leading to ambiguity about which entity possesses control - the human or the AI? Prioritizing data collection, adherence, and algorithmic efficiency over emotional support and genuine autonomy. The most fundamental aspects that digital mental health technologies consider a checkmark for completing their algorithm are the *care that needs to be provided*, and the *consistency of upholding that care*. Emerging as powerful tools for psychological support, their intricate and immediate presence in our environment may turn from empowerment into pressure, and support into surveillance. In an attempt to achieve its functions, starkly unhealthy human behaviors often go undetected by algorithms that lack this detection capability in their programming. For accurately assessing mental health, non-verbal cues like physical agitation, paralinguistic features like tone of voice, and psychomotor behavior like fidgeting are vital as they reveal one's emotional states and clinical symptoms that the individuals may be unwilling or unable to articulate verbally (Ambady & Rosenthal, 1992; American Psychiatric Association, 2022). It cannot detect the following vital observable behaviors if it cannot see you.

This underlying limitation explains the paradox of how empowerment can turn into pressure, how support can become surveillance, the constant emotional misalignment, and the battle between developing habits and burnout. The debate over AI's inability to understand emotional nuances raises concerns about false reassurances. Furthermore, the line between behavioral profiling and therapeutic care becomes morally ambiguous when user data, such as journal entries, mood logs, or emotional states, is collected and shared with third parties (outside companies), as found in several studies (Steindl, 2023). Consequently, users start to disengage or self-center, because they think they are being monitored or judged. As these tools are increasingly sophisticated and intelligent, users are lulled into a toxic environment where they assume they possess control. In summary, if not carefully designed and regulated, digital mental health tools can shift *care* and *consistency* into coercion.

Mechanisms of Influence in Digital Mental Health

Behind every algorithmic design of any digital technology lies a foundation rooted in behavioral science and psychological theory. Whether they are chatbot therapists, telepsychiatry services, or mobile wellness applications, they aim to offer innovative care methods, but often overlook significant blind spots regarding risks and unintended consequences. By examining the dual nature of these systems, which encompasses both their potential to promote well-being and unintentionally harm people, this section lays the groundwork for a critical analysis of how digital interventions influence user behavior, emotion, and cognition.

The following subsection discusses popular mechanisms, including self-tracking, gamification, behavioral nudging, and algorithmic feedback, which will be broken down to portray how they work and where they are flawed. This analysis contributes to the broader argument that, without critical evaluation and intentional design, digital mental health tools risk undermining the well-being they intend to promote.

Self-monitoring tools

Self-monitoring tools provide foundational input for more complex therapeutic algorithms. It allows users to systematically track, record, and reflect upon their emotional states and behaviors. Mood diaries, behavior trackers, and journaling features have become essential parts integrated into well-known applications that promote introspection and behavioral insight. They are often paired with charts, streaks, or summaries, encouraging users to draw patterns and identify connections between their life events and emotional responses. The main goal is to promote introspection, emotional regulation, and autonomy in mental health care. Their affordability, confidentiality, and ease of use make them especially alluring, as they allow people to care for their mental health at their own pace and on their own terms. As a supplement to therapy, self-monitoring techniques are also commonly suggested by therapists to assist clients in tracking their progress between sessions or pinpointing triggers.

The appearance of promoting emotional control can backfire by causing anxiety, compulsive self-surveillance, and the idea of perfectionism. (an unattainable and farcical concept, especially in mental health). This dual potential can be explained by the Self-Regulation Theory (Carver & Scheier, 1982), which posits that humans are goal-driven creatures that continually track their progress toward desirable emotional or behavioral states. Simply put, people evaluate the difference between where they are and where they wish to be, and then modify their behavior accordingly.

When functioning well, they are empowered to take control of their mental health and spot trends that would otherwise go unnoticed. Adolescents who used mood tracking applications experienced notable increases in emotional self-awareness by frequently recognizing the links between their emotional shifts and everyday routines (Kauer et al., 2012). This enabled better stress management and earlier help-seeking behavior. However, feedback loops do possess a psychologically detrimental component. Continuous self-monitoring can exacerbate emotional dysregulation rather than lessen it in people who have high levels of anxiety and or self-criticism. Comparing one's current state to an ideal might exacerbate feelings of inadequacy and failure when progress is not rapid or steady. Brülhart and Lalive (2023) highlight in Nature Human Behavior that the overuse of wellness applications can be linked to higher anxiety levels and decreased subjective well-being (Brülhart & Lalive, 2023). This is particularly evident when users feel "trapped" by their data, with some viewing their digital mood charts as objective assessments of their emotional successes or self-worth.

Furthermore, the continual self-tracking and mood monitoring can lead to perfectionism and self-blame, especially when users do not keep up wellness "streaks" or objectives. Digital reminders can start to become stressful, rather than helpful. Features like automatic reminders, behavioral nudging, and AI-driven risk assessments can become progressively invasive pressures, even though they are intended to be assisting tools for mental health care. The impression of support could feel more like monitoring, for instance, when a chatbot labels a user as "high-risk" based on scant textual data without human review, or when a mobile wellness app penalizes missed check-ins. Therefore, the feedback loop turns into a spiral of negative reinforcements rather than empowerment, leaving users feeling worse about not reaching their emotional goals, the more they monitor.

Anecdotal evidence supports this. One user described how her mood app became a source of guilt, as published in the 2025 weekly edition of "The Guardian": "The bot asked me how I was feeling four times a day." I began believing that I had to be in a "good" mood to avoid disappointing the app. This type of false emotional perfectionism aims to achieve the "goal" of constant positivity. It can induce shame by making setbacks seem like personal failures or a lack of self-worth.

Furthermore, persistently recording negative thoughts or depressed moods can promote depressive schemas in rumination-prone individuals. Excessive self-focus, particularly on upsetting material, can accelerate rather than lessen depressive episodes (Nolen-Hoeksema, 2000). In this regard, self-monitoring without contextual emotional support may exacerbate the symptoms it aims to alleviate.

The tracking method is particularly effective when incorporated into evidence-based frameworks, such as cognitive behavioral therapy (CBT). Proceeding to the following sub-section, it becomes evident that self-monitoring is not a stand-alone mechanism but a prerequisite for operating more interactive and interactionist tools, such as digital CBT chatbots and structured cognitive modules.

Cognitive Behavioral Therapy (CBT) Algorithms

Building on the introspection framework established by self-monitoring instruments, CBT algorithms transform user input into personalized therapeutic guidance. They seek to actively intervene in cognitive and emotional patterns by rephrasing skewed thinking and encouraging behavioral change, following the use of mood diaries and trackers, which foster self-awareness and reflection. This section examines the limitations of converting highly human therapeutic processes into standardized code and how CBT algorithms operationalize psychological theories to automate interventions.

Chatbot therapist apps like Wysa and Woebot utilize input from self-monitoring tools to run through a Cognitive Behavioral Therapy (CBT) algorithm, tailoring responses to promote coping strategies, reframing distorted thinking, and implementing specific cognitive-behavioral interventions. Acting as an interactive therapeutic system, the self-monitoring data imputed by the user (sleep patterns, mood changes, physical activity) is processed by underlying algorithms that detect patterns and suggest the CBT strategies. Delivered through push notifications, chatbot dialogues, or structured modules, the chatbot attempts to shift users away from heavy, emotionally loaded thinking patterns to more realistic and productive perspectives.

The underlying therapeutic engine is Beck's Cognitive Theory of emotional disorders, also known as Cognitive Behavioral Therapy (CBT), which highlights how automatic thoughts, intermediate beliefs, and basic schemas shape an individual's emotional and behavioral reactions. Aaron Beck posits that emotional and behavioral problems, like depression, are rooted in how individuals process information and interpret events, rather than being solely caused by external circumstances (Helsen et al., 2000). According to this theory, psychological distress results from people's skewed perceptions of situations, entirely connected to the situations themselves.

In digital apps, this theory is operationalized through algorithmic design, where users are mapped onto recognized cognitive distortions and connected to a decision tree of potential actions. They simulate what might happen in a traditional therapy session, but in a self-directed, modular, and repeated manner.

For instance, users of Woebot might be asked, "What's going through your mind right now?" The bot employs natural language processing (NLP) to identify overgeneralization, a cognitive distortion characterized by similar inputs, such as "I always mess things up at work." A Socratic-style question like "Can you think of a time when that wasn't true?" may be the app's response, or "What evidence is against this or in favor of this idea?" This classic response of cognitive restructuring involves guiding the user to question unreasonable or unhelpful ideas and come up with more sensible alternatives. A revised thought from the cognitive distortion mentioned above would be "I've made mistakes, but I've always completed many projects successfully." Reiterating the purpose of CBT algorithms, this example of a conversation from Woebot has shifted from an emotionally loaded to a more realistic and kinder perspective.

Similarly, MoodGym uses interactive activities and modules to provide CBT-tailored responses. A module may introduce the idea of thought traps, like catastrophizing ("If I fail this assignment, my whole future is ruined"), or mind reading ("They didn't text back as they may be angry with me"). The platform utilizes users' self-reports, responses, and questions to identify these traps, and then offers scenarios and quizzes to help users reframe their ideas. For instance, in the case of catastrophizing, the app may help evaluate the possibility of their feared outcome and envision a more realistic outcome: "Even if I don't do well on this assignment, I can improve in the next one; it is not the end of everything."

While psychoeducational snippets of the basic CBT concept of behavior influencing mood, the effectiveness of the digital apps or tools is an explainable reason for higher mental health levels among users. After just two weeks of its use, Woebot users reported considerably lower depression levels, according to an RCT study that analyzed fully automated conversations with the Woebot (Fitzpatrick et al., 2017). The regularity and immediacy of these digital CBT apps make them very potent. In contrast to human therapists, who may be constrained by availability and scheduling, self-monitoring applications offer on-demand access to coping mechanisms, self-reflection resources, and instructional materials. Frequent engagement may improve users' self-efficacy and emotional resilience over time, which can help them internalize the cognitive and behavioral skills and utilize them outside the app in real-life situations.

There are significant drawbacks to relying solely on standardized CBT methods, especially when used on a digital platform, including the absence of contextual sensitivity, personalization, and emotional nuance. Woebot, Wysa, and other similar applications frequently rely on pre-programmed reactions and responses, in contrast to human therapists who customize the entire therapeutic model based on cultural background, trauma history, or current emotional fluctuations. For users with complex trauma or personality disorders, layered psychological challenges may find the structured, pre-programmed CBT responses invalidating or impersonal. The "one-size-fits-all" strategy can overlook subtleties essential to recovery, such as ingrained emotional needs or relational patterns. Each individual reacts and responds to a therapeutic technique that is suitable for them. According to research, individuals who require more emotional validation than cognitive restructuring or possess high emotional intensity may benefit more from psychodynamic treatments or dialectical behavioral therapy (DBT) (Leichsenring & Leibing, 2005). These subtle interventions are beyond the capabilities of CBT algorithms of digital wellness applications. The wellness market is overly dominated by U.S. and other Western-based companies, leading to linear modules for non-Western cultural frameworks (Market.Us, 2024).

Therefore, while CBT-based apps may be especially effective for users with mild to moderate issues who benefit from structured guidance and behavioral tracking, they are limited by their inability to adapt to the complexity of individual users. There is also a risk of over-reliance on digital tools. Users may feel isolated or dissatisfied without human assistance if their symptoms persist.

Natural Language Processing (NLP): The Core of Conversational AI

While CBT algorithms provide the organized therapeutic foundation for digital interventions, the communicative and user-interactive layer of chatbot functionality is formed by Natural Language Processing (NLP). This subsection expands on the previous discussion by shifting the emphasis from the treatment logic to the therapeutic language. How applications interpret human input, mimic empathy, and foster a sense of connection. It contributes to the overall argument by highlighting how emotional management in chatbot treatment is informed by both technological design and psychological theory. It is a potent tool, but cultural bias, emotional blind spots, and programming limitations also constrain its effectiveness.

NLP is a subfield of artificial intelligence that enables machines to comprehend, analyze, and react to human language. Combining machine learning models with computational linguistics enables the analysis of syntax, semantics, sentiment, and context. The latter is enabled only up to a certain level, as discussed in the previous section regarding CBT's limitation of contextual sensitivity. By identifying keywords and sentiment patterns in user input and selecting from various pre-programmed responses, NLP enables chatbots to engage in encouraging interactions. Open-ended questions, such as "How are you feeling today?" are used to elicit information from users, identify cognitive distortions, and offer recommendations based on the principles of CBT strategies. This automation simulates empathy and promotes behavioral techniques, including journaling, deep breathing, and cognitive reframing.

The social presence theory best explains the psychological impact of NLP, which contends that mediated communication, through different mediums of text, voice, call, video, etc., promotes a sense of interpersonal connection and emotional closeness, even in situations where face-to-face interaction is not viable (Short, 1976). The hypothesis states that a communicator is seen as more socially present if they provide more cues, such as immediacy, warmth, and responsiveness. This theory posits that different media vary in their capacity to convey the perception of a real, physical presence of others. While it suggests that a greater social presence leads to stronger relational communication and deeper trust building, this presence is not restricted to human beings, paving the way for computational entities to mimic these cues commonly found in real-life conversations and human interaction. If the digital apps can provide context-aware, timely, and emotionally responsive messaging that encourages care, comfort, trust, and self-disclosure, viewers and users view the digital platforms as emotionally attuned. Thereby, a social presence is elicited.

This impact is particularly noticeable in chatbots that are driven by NLP that employ emotionally intelligent scripts and warm, validating language. Phrases like "That must be really tough" or "I'm here for you" are programmed to mimic concern and emotional support in their pre-programmed scripts that resemble sympathetic human discourse. Therefore, using affective computing to genuinely understand an emotional nuance, which constitutes the concept of sentiment analysis, is a crucial component in NLP's attempt to mimic a human therapist.

In research by Gale Lucas and her team of researchers, it was found that even when interacting with a system, users were more inclined to divulge private information to virtual entities or humans that employed empathetic language and nonverbal cues. This lends credence to the notion that significant psychological experiences can be produced by successfully stimulated perceived empathy (Lucas et al., 2014). Research also shows that users are more likely to rate virtual health apps and agents as trustworthy and likable when they are accompanied by emotionally expressive and encouraging responses, which leads to higher adherence to the health recommendations of these apps (Bickmore & Picard, 2005).

The illusion of being heard and understood, brought about by emotionally intelligent design, has its own psychological limitations. They lack the emotional nuance and flexibility of human therapists, as they operate on script logic and pattern recognition. According to Boucher et al., these technologies often leave users feeling rejected or misunderstood due to emotionally inappropriate or generic replies, particularly in cases that require nuanced empathy (Boucher et al., 2021). The possibility of a virtual social presence generating an emotional connection, as discussed previously, depends on the advancement and intricacy of the programming, the users' current severe or non-severe mental states, and the users' predispositions to a greater emotional intensity. The digital apps' inability to recognize covert or indirect signs is a significant worry, as many popular AI conversational agents cannot identify more than 40% of the critical mental health indicators. These included subtle allusions to suicidal thoughts ("I wish I could just disappear"), which raises serious questions regarding their dependability in emergencies, as they may be the fastest and accessible resource at that moment (Miner et al., 2016).

Furthermore, by using clichés like "Everything will be okay" without actually addressing the intricacy of the user's concern, chatbots may provide false reassurance, endanger trust, and discourage users from seeking competent assistance. Parasocial relationships can also result from an emotional attachment to these bots, particularly for users who have insecure attachment styles or persistent loneliness. By delaying therapeutic interventions and replacing social connections, this one-sided emotional investment in non-human entities may lead to isolation (Adhikari & Saxena, 2025). The limitation of non-Western cultural sensitivity applies here, as most NLP models are trained on Western-centric and English-language data, leading to culturally biased interpretations. They additionally miss culturally specific idioms or distress cues, which marginalize the non-Western users and lessen the NLP's inclusivity (Meadows & Hine, 2024).

Gamification

While NLP created the illusion of emotional presence and empathy, digital mental health tools significantly rely on behavioral reinforcement to encourage prolonged participation. This sub-section expands on the previous discussion by moving from conversational simulation to motivational design. It examines how gamification, which includes challenges and rewards, motivates users to engage regularly with therapeutic content. This particular digital algorithm will provide insights into how human motivational systems are increasingly used to influence behavior. Like NLP and CBT logic, these motivating techniques have psychological trade-offs that may impact users' autonomy and well-being.

By appealing to the most humanly motivated psychological needs, achievement, progress, and acknowledgement, gamification is a common technique in digital apps. It incorporates game-like features, such as leaderboards, streaks, badges, and points, into non-gaming contexts. Apps like *SuperBetter, Happify, and Fabulous* motivate users to complete wellness activities, such as mindfulness, daily journaling, or cognitive-behavioral training. This digital feature's strongly appealing design and habit-inducing components include visual progress indicators and rewards for consistency, fostering a sense of accomplishment. For example, granting a badge for a week of gratitude practice to reduce mild anxiety symptoms may reinforce the behavior.

The psychological mechanism behind gamification can be viewed through the lens of the Self-Determination Theory (Deci & Ryan, 1985), which posits that human motivation is made up of three fundamental needs, i.e., competence (feeling effective and capable), autonomy (having control over one's actions), and relatedness (feeling connected to others). The theory posits that individuals have innate tendencies towards this growth and psychological needs to experience intrinsic motivation and greater well-being.

These needs are translated into design elements by digital wellness apps. The user's competence is activated when they obtain badges or other visual indicators of their progress, reinforcing their perception of capabilities. The user's autonomy is promoted when they can customize their objectives or select challenges that give them control of how they interact with the app. A sense of relatedness is fostered with community characteristics, common objectives with online friends/members, or uplifting messages that mimic social support.

While gamification can boost adherence and habit formation, the same procedures may have unforeseen adverse consequences. With an increased habit of conditioning oneself to perform any wellness strategy based on external motivation to complete a streak or attain a badge, one's intrinsic motivation, or pursuing an activity for its own sake, becomes less critical. According to a study examining motivational factors over time in gamification, an overemphasis on gamified rewards may exacerbate stress, reduce self-compassion, and lead to internalized pressure if the user fails to achieve their goals (van Roy & Zaman, 2018). Instead of a normal break in one's wellness journey, a missed streak could feel like personal failure.

Offering external rewards for an act that one already finds internally rewarding can reduce their intrinsic motivation to engage in more streaks or challenges, which is the overjustification effect. This is because achievements and trophies can feel overly prescriptive or disconnected from the user's originally internal attached meaning (Sailer et al., 2017). When users associate progress with performance metrics, their initial engagement may decline. A systematic review found that the improper use of leaderboards or badges may lead to fatigue, cheating, and even performance reductions, particularly in settings related to learning and health. These results caution against relying too heavily on gamification without considering user psychology and context (Sailer & Homner, 2019).

Risk Assessment Algorithms: Mental Health Prediction

While gamification builds user habits and sustained participation, this next layer of digital intervention shifts the focus to prediction and prevention. This section examines how risk assessment algorithms based on machine learning function as a real-time diagnostic tool in mental health applications. Examining language, behavior, and sentiment, these algorithms aim to identify severe psychological distress and take appropriate intervention and action. Extending the discussion on NLP's limitations in capturing deeper psychological states, this sub-section demonstrates how risk detection algorithms carry both significant risks and the potential to save lives. This reinforces the chapter's central argument that the impact of these mechanisms depends as much on what is missed as what is detected.

Machine learning technologies are being used more in the rapidly growing field of digital mental health to identify psychological distress and evaluate suicide risk in real time. Building on the inability of NLP to identify subtle allusions or mental health indicators displayed by users, a deeper look into this mechanism is provided by the risk assessment algorithm of digital wellness apps. Through predictive analytics, algorithms trained on massive datasets of anonymized user data, including text inputs, mood ratings, and engagement patterns, are analyzed to recognize language sentiment patterns and behavioral inputs that may indicate emotional crises.

For example, phrases such as "I want to disappear" or "I feel hopeless" may trigger automated escalation procedures, as the NLP matches the user's response to a set of pre-programmed responses designated for immediate intervention by the algorithm. But how does a digital technology that cannot see its user analyze the risk severity through important body language indicators, previous case history, and starkly changing social and personal behavior?

Woebot evaluates risk severity using NLP and decision trees, a core component of its conversational framework that is often visualized as flowcharts mapping out different paths based on user input and predefined rules to assist the chatbot in its interactions (Steele, 2018). This method has a great deal of potential. By providing real-time interventions and early detection that save lives, it alleviates the strain on conventional mental health services and further reaches marginalized communities with little to no access to basic mental health resources. AI-driven technologies can enhance access to care and offer prompt assistance in situations where human aid may not be available (Gutierrez et al., 2024). In a similar vein, machine learning models that analyze language from social media can predict Post-Traumatic Stress Disorder (PTSD) and depression with over 85% accuracy, indicating strong predictive validity in specific situations (Ta et al., 2025).

Flagging individuals who may be at risk is a highly essential function of digital wellness applications; however, it also carries significant drawbacks. False positives, in which non-urgent inputs are marked at high risk, can lead to unwarranted police or emergency interventions. This can have devastating repercussions for the users, developing needless anxiety and suffering. Conversely, missed opportunities for help may arise from false negatives - the inability to identify actual suffering and risk in these critical situations, resulting in neutral or inappropriate responses. The Smart Crisis study, along with other studies on machine-learning assessment of suicide risk prevention through cellphones, discovered that while algorithms had a good overall accuracy (AUC=7.8), they nevertheless missed a significant percentage of cases, highlighting the persistence of false negatives even with passive behavior tracking (María Luisa Barrigón et al., 2023).

Table 1. A synthesis of the dual effect of underlying digital mechanisms in our daily lives

Digital Mechanism	Advantages	Disadvantages
Self-Monitoring Tools	Introspection, autonomy, emotional self-awareness, and affordability	Compulsive self-surveillance, self-criticism, feelings of inadequacy and failure, and unhealthy perfectionism
CBT Algorithms	Regularity and immediacy of care, users' self-efficacy, and emotional self-resilience	Absence of contextual sensitivity, personalization, and emotional nuance
Natural Language Processing (NLP)	Interpersonal connection and emotional closeness	Feeling rejected or misunderstood by emotionally inappropriate or generic replies
Gamification	Sense of accomplishment, increased self-competence, and momentary reduction of mild anxiety symptoms	Internalized pressure and increased stress, fatigue
Risk Assessment Algorithms	Provides care to individuals in areas with no access to support or resources, and an 85% accuracy prediction of symptoms	False positive detection leading to needless anxiety and stress, and false negative detection leading to untreated critical emergencies

These mechanisms, ranging from self-monitoring tools to predictive risk algorithms, display the multi-layered psychological architecture of digital mental health solutions. From behavioral reinforcement and surveillance to therapeutic intervention and emotional management, each builds gradually on the one before. These technologies provide scalable, easily accessible, and life-saving assistance, but they also pose hazards due to oversimplification, dependence, and a lack of human context. As demonstrated in this section, with a comprehensive summary illustrated in Table 1, the exact digital key mechanisms that improve early detection, adherence, or emotional connection can also undermine intrinsic motivation, overlook deep nuances, or even inadvertently exacerbate crises. Therefore, comprehending these psychological foundations is crucial for optimizing the potential for digital care and minimizing its unintended consequences - a dualistic perspective that forms the basis of this paper's argument.

The Algorithmic Turn: From Behavior Change to Identity Shift

The immediate, task-oriented digital mechanisms discussed in the previous section highlight the clinical precision that monitors and intervenes during psychological distress or crises. Digital health technologies, however, are not limited to emergencies; they also subtly yet profoundly influence daily life. The disadvantages of the mechanisms discussed in the previous section reflect only the surface of a much more severe negative transformation on the human mind and body. This section significantly changes the discussion from promoting or destroying mental health to interrogating how the technological algorithms fundamentally alter mental health itself in deeper patterns. Specifically, how they affect users' perception of themselves, reshape behavioral standards, and redefine physical and emotional health. They actively create new identities and value systems through algorithmic design and persuasive architecture, not merely directing behavior.

Figure 1. Pathway illustrating the support-surveillance transition in digital tools

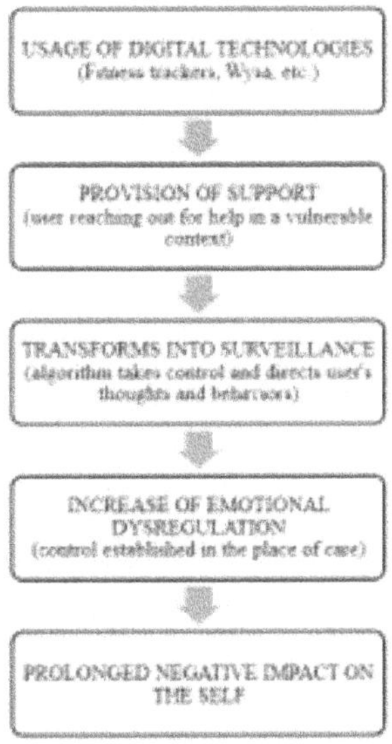

Wearable technology, productivity monitors, fitness trackers, and mental health apps are just a few examples of the digital health technologies that have become normalized in our daily lives. They guarantee discipline, empowerment, and individualized attention. Yet, beneath these promises, however, lies a quieter transformation, as illustrated in Figure 1. We are not just tracking behaviors anymore; we are reshaping identities, motivations, and emotions in relation to digital benchmarks. Digital health, once external, now permeates the psyche, altering how people perceive productivity, rest, self-worth, and health. These algorithmic mechanisms do not merely influence behavior; they modify core psychological frameworks of the human mind.

Internalized Surveillance and Alteration of Core Psychological Processes

Digital goals gradually become anchors, serving as initial reference points that significantly influence user perception and behavior. Users reported a greater likelihood of linking digital goals with self-discipline and health achievement, even when doing so caused physical tiredness or interference with the body's natural activity cycles (Utesch et al., 2022). This reorientation of behavior toward metrics reflects a more profound change, where people submit to the algorithms' authority rather than acting on their intuition.

Digital or algorithmic perfectionism, as defined by digital standards, differs from the traditional concept of perfectionism, which is based on personal estimates and social comparison. Users submissively surrender to the authority of digital mechanisms and unknowingly start to disrupt their authentic well-being. By succumbing to the pressure to optimize every aspect of their day, they begin to neglect their own needs and emotional states. Michael Foucault's work on how institutions shape behavior and identity can be applied to understand how broader digital ecosystems influence lives. It represents a form of biopower - contemporary forms of power that govern populations through subtly internalized norms, such as productivity, health, and sexuality, rather than through overt control or force (Foucault, 1978). In digital health, people optimize and monitor their bodies according to invisible and ingrained digital rules, which are often masked as personal choice by users. Under the illusion that they are in control, they unconsciously surrender to the silent authority of their push notifications and gamified rewards.

The alteration of core psychological processes reveals that digital influence in our daily lives is not just surface-level. From traditional and authentic well-being to potentially disruptive well-being, users are conditioned to equate value with data, rather than experience.

- Self-worth becomes performance-based: Individuals begin to evaluate their value based on metrics like productivity scores, streaks, app feedback, or goal achievement, rather than their emotional well-being and personal growth.
- The rest is perceived as unproductive or ineffective: periods of rest, leisure, and disengagement are viewed as wasted time, as they do not generate measurable progress or data within digital systems. Subsequently, only time spent engaging in activities tracked by digital algorithms is regarded as productive, as it is followed by feedback.
- Discomfort is not seen as feedback, but rather as a failure: Emotional distress or difficulty is viewed as a sign of personal failure, rather than a natural signal for reflection, change, or healing.

Apart from directing users to act or perform differently, there are significant changes and redefinitions in how people think, feel, and perceive themselves. These internal shifts have a profound impact on relationships, identity, and long-term mental health. The moralization of health in the digital culture leads to disordered patterns, such as excessive physical activity to "make up" for calories, sleep anxiety from rigid sleep tracking, and ignoring rest to continue productive streaks. This new form of self-denial, driven by technology's constant demands for improvement, is known as "digital asceticism" (Krzeminska, 2024).

Technoself: Identity Construction

Profound cognitive shifts, including the rewiring of new self-identities, are among the most eminent discoveries in technoself studies, a branch of research dedicated to exploring the technological influence on our core identities. Users start internalizing their data as identity markers, such as "I sleep poorly" or "I am a 10,000-step person". According to studies, the advent of the technoself - a digitally generated selfhood influenced by encounters with technology - is reflected in this transformation (Luppicini, 2013). The gradual entanglement of personal identity with performance metrics explains how users perceive themselves primarily through algorithmic feedback rather than an embodied experience.

This transformation is not accidental but is embedded in the design of the platforms. Many health applications employ "choice architecture". Based on the Nudge Theory, indirect suggestions can influence one's behavior and choices without restricting their freedom (Thaler & Sunstein, 2009). To encourage users to engage in desired behaviors, such as reducing screen time, increasing exercise, and attending sessions regularly, this process may backfire if it is rigorous, directive, and guilt-inducing. This type of persuasive design that compromises mental health raises ethical questions. For example, Noom, an online mobile application strategized for weight loss, uses regular notifications, social pressures, and calorie deficits to promote consistency at the cost of psychological safety (Landsverk, 2022).

IMPLICATIONS AND FUTURE DIRECTIONS: TOWARDS A MORE COMPASSIONATE DIGITAL FUTURE

In response to the need for immediate humanized interventions in the digital sphere, a new way of thinking has emerged as digital technology becomes increasingly integrated into daily life, moving beyond blind adoption or total rejection. Post-digital philosophies have recognized this dilemma by suggesting strategies for "living with and against" technology, integrating its utility while resisting its overreach. In this context, critical digital literacy becomes an essential skill that enables people to access, assess, modify, and co-author their digital experiences, rather than passively consuming them. New design imperatives that prioritize user liberty, ethical persuasion, and emotional well-being are emerging alongside the aforementioned cultural and cognitive changes. Examining these forward-thinking strategies for digital mental health, this section highlights positively influential digital trends, including slow tech, digital minimalism, adaptive therapies, and self-compassion applications.

The human tech movement promotes technology that supports users rather than puts them under strain, while respecting their cognitive boundaries. The idea of continuous optimization is called into question by new cultural movements of digital disobedience (active refusal to conform and internalize algorithms), digital minimalism (intentional and selective use of technology), and slow tech (thoughtful and ethical human-centered tech, Lie, 1996; Newport, 2019; Quadflieg et al., 2022). Pos-digital philosophy, which integrates both human and digital aspects of life, advocates for "living with and against digital systems simultaneously" - acknowledging that digital tools are both essential and inherently faulty, and that agency requires mindful resistance. Studies have shown that blended approaches, combining digital interventions with brief therapist contact, yield higher engagement and effectiveness than purely unguided programs (Baumeister et al., 2014).

The ultimate objective is to use technology on our terms, not to give it up to avoid its negative effects, as humanity has become too intertwined with digital technology to take a step back. Critical digital literacy, adaptable frameworks, and compassionate design will enable users to reclaim their time, focus, and well-being from systems designed for continuous self-evaluation.

A shift from digital tracking to more flexible, human-centered algorithms is an observed digital trend, which modifies workout objectives according to mood, exhaustion, and recuperation, such as those using just-in-time adaptive interventions. These adaptive fitness objectives help strike a balance between feasibility and difficulty, depending on the user's history (Gordon et al., 2019). Meanwhile, with growing digital literacy, users are becoming more active and aware of how to evaluate, filter, and adapt to technology, rather than passively consuming it, according to post-digital theoretical studies (Macgilchrist, 2021).

The extended user independence to incorporate customized goals and the usage of more self-compassion apps, or their incorporation into digital health applications, have become a design imperative. Companion, Mindful Self-Compassion, or Self-Compassion App, are mobile applications that encourage introspection, acceptance, and emotional care, rather than rivalry or productivity. According to Neff and Germer (2013), self-compassion practice is associated with improved emotional regulation, reduced anxiety, and a healthier environment. They provide a vital counterpoint to high-performance trackers.

In synthesizing the various psychological mechanisms found in digital mental health tools - from self-monitoring and CBT algorithms to NLP, gamification, and predictive risk models - it becomes evident that although these tools provide affordable, user-friendly, and clinically and therapeutically practical assistance, they are fundamentally altering motivation, identity, and well-being. Ironically, the exact mechanisms that encourage self-awareness and behavioral control can also strengthen perfectionism, raise anxiety levels, and weaken intrinsic drives. Future directions for digital tools must emphasize individualized flexibility, critical digital literacy, and ethically based design principles that honor users' emotional complexity and sovereignty. Ultimately, technology should empower rather than coerce, providing effectiveness and empathy. It is essential to root its function in mental health within a framework of care rather than control.

LIMITATIONS

While this chapter sheds light on several critical insights into the complex world of digital mental health technologies, several limitations must also be acknowledged. First, the analysis is based purely on a conceptual level and relies on secondary sources, including empirical studies, systematic reviews, and reported user experiences. Subsequently, the use of original empirical data limits the ability to determine causal linkages, correlations, or to evaluate long-term psychological consequences, even while it permits a comprehensive and integrative theoretical framework. Second, the experiences of users are predominantly focused on Western contexts and English-language platforms that reflect structural imbalances in digital mental health research. Consequently, the chapter misrepresents a larger section of non-Western, low-resource, and culturally diverse populations. Third, the findings are limited by the rapidly evolving nature of digital mental health technologies, with continual changes in platform features, algorithms, and regulatory environments, which make it difficult to assess long-term identity-related effects, sustained engagement, and dependency risks. Finally, the chapter primarily focuses on user-level psychological implications and does not entirely address the institutional, commercial, and regulatory factors that influence the implementation and governance of these tools. Future research would benefit from integrative qualitative approaches that capture the subjectivity of the utilization of these technologies, along with a deeper psychological understanding of individual user experiences. Integrating these psychological outcomes with ethical governance frameworks, policy considerations, and lived user experiences spanning across cultures and age through longitudinal and cross-cultural studies would ensure an understanding of creating digital mental health tools that are more responsive to human complexity, rather than algorithmic efficiency.

CONCLUSION

This chapter provides an overview of the era of digital mental health technology, which was invented with the intention of revolutionizing mental health care. It offers critical and systematic examinations of how digital mental health innovations promise important advancements in user mental health, but due to uncritical designs practices and widespread normalization. These very same innovations risk enable surveillance and control rather than support and care. The investigation reveals that digital mental health solutions operate through a layered behavioral mechanism, having dual impacts on users' affect, as they transition from early rule-based systems to AI-powered chatbots, self-monitoring apps, gamified therapies, and predictive algorithms. While the discussed digital solutions have positively improved support by early intervention, they also foster internalized negative patterns of self-surveillance. Beyond these immediate and visually observable behavioral effects, the chapter also examines deeper, less visibile changes in self perception, specifically how algorithmic criteria increasingly shape users' self-worth, productivity, and emotional regulation. Therefore, this chapter draws attention to the deeper psychological and foundational implications of digital mental health technologies that remain largely underexplored in the current literature. Drawing on concepts such as technoself, digital asceticism, and biopower, the chapter suggest that it is the design and administration of these technologies, rather than their mere existence, that pose the most significant challenges.

REFERENCES

Adhikari, V., & Saxena, T. (2025). AI chatbot companions impact on users parasocial relationships and loneliness. *International Journal of Research Publication and Reviews, 6.* https://ijrpr.com/uploads/V6ISSUE5/IJRPR45212.pdf

Ambady, N., & Rosenthal, R. (1992). Thin slices of expressive behavior as predictors of interpersonal consequences: A meta-analysis. *Psychological Bulletin, 111*(2), 256–274. DOI: 10.1037/0033-2909.111.2.256

American Psychiatric Association. (2022). *Diagnostic and statistical manual of mental disorders: DSM-5-TR* (5th ed.). https://psycnet.apa.org/record/2013-14907-000

Barrigon, M. L., Romero-Medrano, L., Moreno-Muñoz, P., Porras-Segovia, A., Lopez-Castroman, J., Courtet, P., & Baca-Garcia, E. (2023). One-week suicide risk prediction using real-time smartphone monitoring: Prospective cohort study. *Journal of Medical Internet Research, 25*, e43719.

Bickmore, T. W., & Picard, R. W. (2005). Establishing and maintaining long-term human-computer relationships. *ACM Transactions on Computer-Human Interaction, 12*(2), 293–327. https://doi.org/DOI: 10.1145/1067860.1067867

Boucher, E. M., Harake, N. R., Ward, H. E., Stoeckl, S. E., Vargas, J., Minkel, J., Parks, A. C., & Zilca, R. (2021). Artificially intelligent chatbots in digital mental health interventions: A review. *Expert Review of Medical Devices, 18*(1), 37–49. DOI: 10.1080/17434440.2021.2013200 PMID: 34872429

Cameron, G., Mulvenna, M., Ennis, E., O'Neill, S., Bond, R., Cameron, D., & Bunting, A. (2024). Effectiveness of digital mental health interventions in the workplace: An umbrella review of systematic reviews (Preprint). *JMIR Mental Health.* Advance online publication. DOI: 10.2196/67785 PMID: 39854722

Carver, C. S., & Scheier, M. F. (1982). Control theory: A useful conceptual framework for personality–social, clinical, and health psychology. *Psychological Bulletin, 92*(1), 111–135. DOI: 10.1037/0033-2909.92.1.111 PMID: 7134324

Christensen, H., Griffiths, K. M., & Korten, A. (2002). Web-based cognitive behavior therapy: Analysis of site usage and changes in depression and anxiety scores. *Journal of Medical Internet Research, 4*(1), e3. DOI: 10.2196/jmir.4.1.e3 PMID: 11956035

Engel, G. L. (1977). The need for a new medical model: A challenge for biomedicine. *Psychodynamic Psychiatry, 40*(3), 377–396. DOI: 10.1521/pdps.2012.40.3.377 PMID: 23002701

Fitzpatrick, K. K., Darcy, A., & Vierhile, M. (2017). Delivering cognitive behavior therapy to young adults with symptoms of depression and anxiety using a fully automated conversational agent (Woebot): A randomized controlled trial. *JMIR Mental Health, 4*(2). Advance online publication. DOI: 10.2196/mental.7785 PMID: 28588005

Foucault, M. (1978). The history of sexuality: Vol. I. *An introduction* (Hurley, R., Trans.). Vintage Books.

Germer, C. K., & Neff, K. D. (2013). Self-compassion in clinical practice. *Journal of Clinical Psychology, 69*(8), 856–867. DOI: 10.1002/jclp.22021 PMID: 23775511

Gordon, M., Althoff, T., & Leskovec, J. (2019). Goal-setting and achievement in activity tracking apps: A case study of MyFitnessPal. *The World Wide Web Conference*, 571–582. https://doi.org/DOI: 10.1145/3308558.3313432

Gutierrez, G., Stephenson, C., Eadie, J., Asadpour, K., & Alavi, N. (2024). Examining the role of AI technology in online mental healthcare: Opportunities, challenges, and implications, a mixed-methods review. *Frontiers in Psychiatry, 15*. Advance online publication. DOI: 10.3389/fpsyt.2024.1356773 PMID: 38774435

Helsen, M., Vollebergh, W., & Meeus, W. (2000). Social support from parents and friends and emotional problems in adolescence. *Journal of Youth and Adolescence*, *29*(3), 319–335. DOI: 10.1023/A:1005147708827

Henderson, C., Evans-Lacko, S., & Thornicroft, G. (2013). Mental illness stigma, help seeking, and public health programs. *American Journal of Public Health*, *103*(5). https://www.ncbi.nlm.nih.gov/pmc/articles/PMC3698814/ PMID: 23488489

Huberty, J., Green, J., Glissmann, C., Larkey, L., Puzia, M., & Lee, C. (2019). Efficacy of the mindfulness meditation mobile app "Calm" to reduce stress among college students: Randomized controlled trial. *JMIR mHealth and uHealth*, *7*(6), e14273. DOI: 10.2196/14273 PMID: 31237569

Jargon, J. (2025, February 22). When school counselors aren't available, a human-AI chatbot answers. *The Wall Street Journal*. https://www.wsj.com/tech/ai/student-mental-health-ai-chat-bots-school-4eb1ba55

Kauer, S. D., Reid, S. C., Crooke, A. H. D., Khor, A., Hearps, S. J. C., Jorm, A. F., Sanci, L., & Patton, G. (2012). Self-monitoring using mobile phones in the early stages of adolescent depression: Randomized controlled trial. *Journal of Medical Internet Research*, *14*(3), e67. DOI: 10.2196/jmir.1858 PMID: 22732135

Khan, S. (2023, April). *What is Telepsychiatry?* Psychiatry.org. https://www.psychiatry.org/Patients-Families/Telepsychiatry

Krzeminska, A. (2024). Balancing self-care and self-control. *Historical Social Research (Köln)*, *49*(3), 77–101. DOI: 10.2307/27331436

Landsverk, G. (2022, December). Noom sells psychology-driven weight loss. Some users expected therapy. *Business Insider*. https://www.businessinsider.com/noom-a-magnet-for-users-with-depression-and-eating-disorders-2022-11

Leichsenring, F., & Leibing, E. (2005). The effectiveness of psychodynamic therapy and cognitive behavior therapy in the treatment of personality disorders: A meta-analysis. *Focus (San Francisco, Calif.)*, *3*(3), 417–428. DOI: 10.1176/foc.3.3.417

Lie, M. (1996). *Making technology our own? Domesticating technology into everyday life*. https://www.researchgate.net/publication/323959352_Making_Technology_Our_Own_Domesticating_Technology_into_Everyday_Life

Lucas, G. M., Gratch, J., King, A., & Morency, L.-P. (2014). It's only a computer: Virtual humans increase willingness to disclose. *Computers in Human Behavior*, *37*, 94–100. DOI: 10.1016/j.chb.2014.04.043

Luppicini, R. (2013). The emerging field of technoself studies (TSS). In *Handbook of research on technoself* (pp. 1–25). IGI Global. https://doi.org/DOI: 10.4018/978-1-4666-2211-1.ch001

Luppicini, R. (2013). *Handbook of research on technoself: Identity in a technological society*. Information Science Reference.

Macgilchrist, F. (2021). Theories of postdigital heterogeneity: Implications for research on education and datafication. *Postdigital Science and Education, 3*(3), 660–667. DOI: 10.1007/s42438-021-00232-w PMID: 40477415

Market.Us. (2024, January 29). Fitness app market surges towards USD 25.9 billion by 2033. *GlobeNewswire*. https://www.globenewswire.com/news-release/2024/01/29/2818703/0/en/Fitness-App-Market-Surges-Towards-USD-25-9-Billion-by-2033-Growth-Driven-By-Increasing-Health-Consciousness.html

Mayo Clinic. (2025, February 26). *Cognitive behavioral therapy*. Mayoclinic.org; Mayo Clinic. https://www.mayoclinic.org/tests-procedures/cognitive-behavioral-therapy/about/pac-20384610

McKinsey & Company. (2022). *McKinsey technology trends outlook 2022*. https://www.mckinsey.com/~/media/mckinsey/business%20functions/mckinsey%20digital/our%20insights/the%20top%20trends%20in%20tech%202022/mckinsey-tech-trends-outlook-2022-full-report.pdf

Meadows, R., & Hine, C. (2024). Entanglements of technologies, agency and selfhood: Exploring the complexity in attitudes toward mental health chatbots. *Culture, Medicine and Psychiatry, 48*(4), 840–857. DOI: 10.1007/s11013-024-09876-2 PMID: 39153178

Miner, A. S., Milstein, A., Schueller, S., Hegde, R., Mangurian, C., & Linos, E. (2016). Smartphone-based conversational agents and responses to questions about mental health, interpersonal violence, and physical health. *JAMA Internal Medicine, 176*(5), 619. DOI: 10.1001/jamainternmed.2016.0400 PMID: 26974260

Morningstar. I. (2025, April 17). New study reveals promise of text-based mental health support app Counslr in decreasing barriers to mental health support. *Morningstar*. https://www.morningstar.com/news/globe-newswire/9423687/new-study-reveals-promise-of-text-based-mental-health-support-app-counslr-in-decreasing-barriers-to-mental-health-support

Murthy, R. S. (2017). National mental health survey of India 2015–2016. *Indian Journal of Psychiatry, 59*(1), 21. DOI: 10.4103/psychiatry.indianjpsychiatry_102_17 PMID: 28529357

Newport, C. (2019). *Digital minimalism: Choosing a focused life in a noisy world*. Portfolio/Penguin.

Nolen-Hoeksema, S. (2000). The role of rumination in depressive disorders and mixed anxiety/depressive symptoms. *Journal of Abnormal Psychology, 109*(3), 504–511. https://pubmed.ncbi.nlm.nih.gov/11016119/ PMID: 11016119

Ordonez, P., & Zhang, X. (2023). *Accelerating Strategic Changes for Digital Transformation in the Healthcare Industry*. Academic Press.

Precedence Research. (2024, November 7). Wellness apps market size to hit USD 45.65 billion by 2034. *Precedence Research*. https://www.precedenceresearch.com/wellness-apps-market

Proudfoot, J., Goldberg, D., Mann, A., Everitt, B., Marks, I., & Gray, J. A. (2003). Computerized, interactive, multimedia cognitive-behavioural program for anxiety and depression in general practice. *Psychological Medicine, 33*(2), 217–227. DOI: 10.1017/s0033291702007225 PMID: 12622301

Quadflieg, S., Neuburg, K., & Nestler, S. (2022). *(Dis)obedience in digital societies: Perspectives on the power of algorithms and data*. Transcript Verlag.

Sackett, C., Harper, D., & Pavez, A. (2024, May 26). Woebot, a mental-health chatbot, tries out generative AI. *IEEE Spectrum*. https://spectrum.ieee.org/woebot

Sailer, M., Hense, J. U., Mayr, S. K., & Mandl, H. (2017). How gamification motivates: An experimental study of the effects of specific game design elements on psychological need satisfaction. *Computers in Human Behavior, 69*, 371–380. DOI: 10.1016/j.chb.2016.12.033

Sailer, M., & Homner, L. (2019). The gamification of learning: A meta-analysis. *Educational Psychology Review, 32*(1), 77–112. DOI: 10.1007/s10648-019-09498-w

Short, J. (1976). *The social psychology of telecommunications*. Wiley.

Smith, K., Blease, C., Faurholt-Jepsen, M., Firth, J., Van Daele, T., Moreno, C., Carlbring, P., Ebner-Priemer, U. W., Koutsouleris, N., Riper, H., Mouchabac, S., Torous, J., & Cipriani, A. (2023). Digital mental health: Challenges and next steps. *BMJ Mental Health, 26*(1), e300670. https://mentalhealth.bmj.com/content/26/1/e300670 PMID: 37197797

Steele, I. (2018, February 22). Journey mapping for chatbots: How to create a chatbot decision tree from scratch. *Comm100*. https://www.comm100.com/blog/journey-mapping-chatbot-decision-tree-from-scratch.html

Stein, O. A., & Prost, A. (2024). Exploring the Societal Implications of Digital Mental Health Technologies: A Critical Review. *SSM. Mental Health, 6*, 100373. DOI: 10.1016/j.ssmmh.2024.100373

Steindl, E. (2023). Safeguarding privacy and efficacy in e-mental health: Policy options in the EU and Australia. *International Data Privacy Law, 13*(3). Advance online publication. DOI: 10.1093/idpl/ipad009

Ta, P., Tran, N., Nguyen, H., & Nguyen, H. D. (2025). Detecting signs of depression on social media: A machine learning analysis and evaluation. *Sustainable Futures : An Applied Journal of Technology, Environment and Society, 10*, 100827. DOI: 10.1016/j.sftr.2025.100827

Thaler, R., & Sunstein, C. (2009). *Nudge: Improving decisions about health, wealth, and happiness*. Penguin.

Utesch, T., Piesch, L., Busch, L., Strauss, B., & Geukes, K. (2022). Self-tracking of daily physical activity using a fitness tracker and the effect of the 10,000 steps goal. *German Journal of Exercise and Sport Research, 52*(2), 300–309. DOI: 10.1007/s12662-022-00821-2

van Roy, R., & Zaman, B. (2018). Need-supporting gamification in education: An assessment of motivational effects over time. *Computers & Education, 127*, 283–297. DOI: 10.1016/j.compedu.2018.08.018

Varnosfaderani, S. M., & Forouzanfar, M. (2024). The Role of AI in Hospitals and Clinics: Transforming healthcare in the 21st century. *Bioengineering (Basel, Switzerland), 11*(4), 1–38. https://www.mdpi.com/2306-5354/11/4/337 PMID: 38671759

Vyshnevska, A. (2023, October 19). Best chatbot statistics for 2024. *Master of Code Global.* https://masterofcode.com/blog/chatbot-statistics

Weizenbaum, J. (1966). ELIZA—A computer program for the study of natural language communication between man and machine. *Communications of the ACM, 9*(1), 36–45. DOI: 10.1145/365153.365168

World Health Organization. (2022, June 8). *Mental disorders.* https://www.who.int/news-room/fact-sheets/detail/mental-disorders

KEY TERMS AND DEFINITIONS

Algorithmic Design: In the context of digital healthcare tools, algorithmic design refers to the methodical process of designing, developing, and implementing complex computer processes (algorithms) that analyze vast amounts of medical data to support and automate various healthcare functions. (Varnosfaderani and Forouzanfar, 2024).

Chatbot Therapy: This involves the use of mental health chatbots to provide psychological support.

Cognitive Behavioral Therapy (CBT): A type of psychotherapy that helps patients manage mental health issues by altering their thought and behavior patterns. It focuses on the relationship between your thoughts, feelings, and actions. It aims to replace negative thoughts with more realistic and optimistic ones, thereby enhancing emotional regulation and building coping mechanisms. (Mayo Clinic, 2025).

Digital Asceticism: It refers to the thoughtful and moderate use of digital technology, serving as a moderate alternative to complete digital escapism. It assists individuals in managing their conscious consumption of information and striking a balance between their online and offline lives.

Digital Mental Health Technologies/Tools: Software-based tools, such as mobile apps and wearable sensors, that rely heavily on artificial intelligence (AI) and big data, and are frequently championed as potential remedies for the scarcity of mental health resources. Services include symptom prediction and detection, personalized treatment, chatbot therapy, and both personal and population-level monitoring. (Stein and Prost, 2024).

Digital/Algorithmic Perfectionism: The ongoing need to project the "best version" of oneself online is the driving force behind digital perfectionism. It is the pressure to attain an idealized, flawless self-image in the digital realm. This is characterized by setting high, and often unrealistic, expectations for digital self-presentation and content creation. (María Pilar Aparicio-Flores et al., 2025).

Mental Health Chatbot: An AI-driven conversational agent that delivers therapeutic techniques and emotional support through simulated dialogue. Using Natural Language Processing (NLP), they guide users through evidence-based strategies with real-time conversations, psychoeducation, and mood tracking.

Mobile Wellness Applications: Digital tools that assist people in tracking health data, including nutritional intake, physical activity, sleep, and stress levels, while offering real-time feedback and recommendations to encourage adherence to a healthy lifestyle. These applications may also integrate interactive technologies and include assessments of mood and familial disease risk. (Ordonez and Zhang, 2023).

Surveillance: In digital mental health tools, surveillance refers to the ongoing and continuous monitoring of users' data and behaviors in ways that may seem and feel invasive and controlling.

Technoself: An academic field that examines how human identity is changing in a technologically advanced society. It analyzes how people interact with technology through various disciplines, including psychology, sociology, and computer science. (Luppicini, 2013).

Telepsychiatry: A subset of telemedicine, which is the process of providing healthcare remotely via technology and often using videoconferencing. Telepsychiatry is the use of digital communication technology to provide services, including psychiatric evaluations, therapy (individual, group, or family), patient education, and medication management. (Khan, 2023).

Chapter 8
Ikigai Play:
Towards an Ikigai Paradigm of Healthy and Active Ageing in Europe

Bruno Giesteira
https://orcid.org/0000-0003-4896-6659
University of Porto, Portugal

Tainá Souza
https://orcid.org/0009-0008-4947-6436
University of Porto, Portugal

Andreia Sousa
https://orcid.org/0000-0001-8070-8970
Lusófona University, Portugal

Liliana Rodrigues
More Than Humans, Portugal

Guilherme Vila Maior
University of Porto, Portugal

ABSTRACT

This chapter is grounded in the results of the ERASMUS+ funded project SmartAgeCare, which investigated active and healthy ageing strategies across eight European countries. The project aims to foster digital inclusion, civic participation, and psychosocial well-being among older adults by exploring innovative models of engagement. This chapter introduces the concept of 'Ikigai Play' as a transdisciplinary framework rooted in a meta-narrative review and inspired by the Japanese philosophy of Ikigai—meaning 'reason for being'. Synthesising evidence from national studies and digital ageing strategies, the chapter identifies regional disparities, psychosocial drivers, and the transformative potential of inclusive technologies. 'Ikigai Play' is proposed as a culturally adaptive model to support autonomy, well-being, and digital health equity.

DOI: 10.4018/979-8-3373-3531-5.ch008

1. INTRODUCTION

This chapter is developed within the framework of the SmartAgeCare project, an international research initiative funded by the Erasmus+ programme of the European Union. The project explores innovative approaches to promote healthy and active ageing across Europe, with a strong focus on digital inclusion, civic engagement, and meaningful participation. Through cross-national collaboration among researchers and institutions from eight European countries, the project addresses how emerging digital technologies and psychosocial paradigms can enhance the autonomy, health, and sense of purpose of older adults.

At the heart of this approach lies the Japanese concept of Ikigai—meaning 'reason for being'—which this chapter proposes as a culturally sensitive and emotionally resonant tool for guiding innovation in age-friendly ecosystems. The main objectives of the SmartAgeCare project are: (1) to investigate the role of digital technologies in improving health outcomes and social participation among older adults; (2) to assess regional disparities in digital and health equity; and (3) to develop a conceptual model that integrates cultural, social, and technological perspectives into a cohesive framework for active ageing.

This chapter proposes the 'Ikigai Play' paradigm — a novel framework that connects health, digital equity, and citizenship with older adults' search for meaning and purpose. Drawing from extensive literature reviews conducted across eight European countries, we argue that Ikigai can serve as a transdisciplinary and humanistic lens for designing inclusive ageing policies and technologies. The global demographic transition toward an ageing population presents both challenges and opportunities for societies across Europe. As populations grow older, the pursuit of healthy and active ageing becomes not only a health imperative but also a social and economic necessity (World Health Organization, 2015). To navigate this shift, new paradigms are required — frameworks that not only support longevity but also emphasize purpose, connection, and wellbeing in later life (Foster & Walker, 2015).

In response to these imperatives, the Ikigai concept—originating from Japanese philosophy—has gained traction in Western health discourse as a model for promoting wellbeing among older adults (García & Miralles, 2017; Imai, 2018). Ikigai, loosely translated as "a reason for being," integrates personal fulfillment, community engagement, and a sense of meaning, making it a powerful lens through which to examine ageing policies and interventions (Sone et al., 2008).

European initiatives focused on active ageing have increasingly turned toward holistic approaches that incorporate psychological, social, and cultural factors (Walker, 2002; WHO, 2020). While biomedical models remain central to healthcare delivery, they are often insufficient to address the multidimensional aspects of ageing. Instead, interdisciplinary and participatory frameworks that center lived experience and purpose are gaining prominence (Buse, Martin, & Nettleton, 2018; Marston & van Hoof, 2019). As a dynamic and context-sensitive concept, *ikigai* also aligns with European ideals of active citizenship, where engagement in community, intergenerational solidarity, and digital participation contribute to a sense of purpose.

Against this backdrop, this chapter addresses the following research question: How can *ikigai* values and approaches be integrated with content on active and healthy ageing, digital transition, and European citizenship to develop a culturally appropriate training program for EU citizens over 65? In answering this question, we seek to bridge psychological well-being, technological innovation, and civic engagement through a unified, human-centered framework.

The chapter is structured as follows: Section 2 outlines the theoretical background, introducing core concepts such as eHealth, digital equity, health literacy, and Ikigai. Section 3 presents the methodology used in conducting a meta-narrative review. Section 4 synthesizes country-specific findings. Section 5 introduces the 'Ikigai Play' conceptual model. Section 6 discusses future research directions. Section 7 concludes with implications for policy, practice, and society. The last section lists the references used throughout the chapter.

2. LITERATURE REVIEW: DIGITAL TRANSFORMATION AND ACTIVE AGEING

This literature review first explores the theoretical foundations of healthy ageing and digital innovation, then focuses on the psychosocial relevance of ikigai, and finally synthesizes recent empirical and policy research across the European digital health landscape.

2.1 Conceptual Foundations: From Deficit to Purpose-Driven Ageing

This section lays the groundwork for the Ikigai Play framework by highlighting the shift from deficit-based to asset-based and purpose-driven approaches to later life. The theoretical framework for this chapter lies at the intersection of four core concepts: healthy and active ageing, digital health innovation, cultural models of wellbeing, and the Japanese concept of Ikigai. Each of these concepts has been studied in various disciplinary contexts, yet their integration remains underexamined in ageing policy and practice (Foster & Walker, 2015; Marston & van Hoof, 2019). As defined by the World Health Organization (WHO, 2015), Healthy and active ageing refers to the process of developing and maintaining the functional ability that enables wellbeing in older age. This approach represents a paradigmatic shift in gerontology and public health, emphasizing autonomy, participation, and functional capacity rather than the mere absence of disease (Steptoe & Fancourt, 2019). For training programs aimed at older adults, this perspective underscores the value of empowerment, engagement, and continuity across physical, social, and emotional domains.

Digital health innovation encompasses a range of technologies—from mobile health (mHealth) applications and telecare services to robotics and smart home ecosystems—that have the potential to support ageing in place, enhance autonomy, and increase access to care (Buse et al., 2018; Marston et al., 2020). However, these technologies often fail to address the sociocultural dimensions of ageing, such as identity, belonging, and a sense of purpose (Neven & Peine, 2017). Bridging this gap is essential for developing human-centered digital tools that are meaningful to diverse older populations. A 2022 scoping review by Kebede et al. further underscores this need by identifying the key barriers and facilitators of digital engagement among older adults. The study conceptualizes digital engagement as a three-stage continuum—from technological nonuse and initial adoption to sustained use. It found that the most cited barriers are a lack of capability (e.g., physical and psychological changes, lack of skill), opportunity (e.g., technological features, environmental context), and motivation (e.g., lack of perceived usefulness or confidence). These findings highlight the importance of designing tailored interventions that account for these intertwined factors, advocating for affordable, usable technologies and lifelong learning opportunities to empower older adults.

Cultural models of wellbeing, including ikigai, provide a more holistic understanding of health by integrating psychological and social factors. Ikigai, a Japanese term loosely translated as "reason for being,", has gained prominence in global ageing discourses. It emphasizes meaning, connectedness, and personal fulfilment (García & Miralles, 2017; Nakanishi, 2019). It blends personal fulfillment, life purpose, and community contribution. Empirical studies have associated Ikigai with increased longevity, mental health, and life satisfaction among older adults (Sone et al., 2008; Imai, 2018).

Recent research by Fukuzawa and Sugawara (2023) highlights that *ikigai*—defined not only as life satisfaction but also as perceived social roles and future orientation—plays a distinct role in wellbeing among older adults. They found that among Japanese individuals aged 75 and older, *ikigai* was significantly more sensitive to loneliness, social support, and participation than life satisfaction. Their findings support the idea that Ikigai uniquely integrates both hedonic and eudaimonic elements of wellbeing and may decline in contexts of low social engagement. Importantly, they found that social support and frequent participation buffered the negative effects of loneliness on ikigai, reinforcing its value as a psychosocial anchor for designing community and health interventions aimed at older adults. This enables a shift from deficit-based to opportunity-driven narratives of ageing, offering a humanistic anchor for innovation.

Furthermore, a 2024 study by Chen et al. demonstrated the efficacy of using a "teachable agent" to enhance Ikigai in seniors. Based on the "learning by teaching" theory, the study introduced a pedagogical agent named Akeso, which seniors could interact with and teach about health-related topics. A user study revealed that this interaction significantly enhanced the participants' sense of fulfilment, fostered a feeling of being needed, stimulated new life goals, and strengthened their self-esteem. The authors argue that by having older adults teach the agent, they experienced a sense of purpose and self-worth, which in turn improved their Ikigai. These findings suggest that human-agent interaction can be a powerful tool for developing interventions that address the psychosocial dimensions of ageing.

Digital Transformation in Health: Europe is experiencing a profound shift toward digital-first healthcare delivery through platforms such as electronic health records (EHRs), mobile health (mHealth), telemedicine, and integrated smart city ecosystems. These tools are designed to increase access, enhance continuity of care, and support data-driven decision-making. However, disparities in adoption remain, particularly among older adults with lower digital literacy or in rural and underserved regions. Addressing these inequities is crucial to ensuring that digital health tools benefit all citizens.

Healthy Life Years (HLY): Healthy Life Years (HLY), a key European Union indicator, measures not only longevity but also the quality of those additional years—free from disability and chronic illness. HLY is central to the EU's active ageing strategies and underlines the necessity of upstream investments in prevention, education, and community health. Integrating *ikigai* into such strategies helps extend their impact beyond physical health, toward purpose and quality of life.

Digital Health Equity and Health Literacy: Digital health equity refers to the fair and inclusive access to health technologies regardless of age, socioeconomic status, or location. Central to this is that health literacy—especially digital health literacy—is critical for ensuring individuals can engage meaningfully with new technologies. Evidence shows strong associations between health literacy and better self-care, chronic disease management, and psychological resilience. Embedding these capacities in training programs for older adults is essential for ensuring their inclusion in digital societies. The challenges identified in the Kebede et al. (2022) study, such as a lack of skills and motivation, are directly tied to the need for improved digital health literacy and equitable access to technology for all citizens.

Together, these interrelated domains provide a robust lens through which to analyze Europe's ageing transition—not only in clinical or technological terms, but as a cultural, ethical, and participatory endeavor. This section establishes the conceptual foundation for the proposed Ikigai Play framework by integrating these interrelated domains. It argues for a shift from deficit-based models of ageing toward asset-based and purpose-driven approaches that reflect the complex realities of older adults' lives across diverse European contexts (Walker, 2002; WHO, 2020).

While Section 2.1 established the theoretical pillars of a purpose-driven approach to ageing, the following section synthesizes how these principles interact with real-world digital health initiatives and governance frameworks across Europe

2.2 A Meta-Narrative of the European Digital Health Landscape

The digital transformation in health has accelerated in recent decades in Europe, driven by technological advances, policy guidelines, and the growing demand for more accessible, efficient, and equitable health systems. In this context, this narrative synthesis examines studies on the implementation of digital technologies such as eHealth, mHealth, telehealth, and smart cities, with an emphasis on promoting active ageing, digital inclusion, and equity for the elderly population. By integrating ethical, legal, financial, technological, and social dimensions, the aim is to understand the structural factors that condition a sustainable and inclusive adoption of these innovations, with a focus on the European context and complementary global references.

Health Outcomes and Digital Equity

Increased longevity is one of the factors driving the ageing of the European population; however, as Liotta et al. (2018) argue, this increase has not been accompanied by proportional gains in Healthy Life Years (HLY), showing ageing marked by fragility. The authors therefore recommend integrated prevention strategies, focusing on promoting healthy habits, combating social isolation, and strengthening digital literacy, emphasizing that the digital transformation in health will only be effective if aligned with education, inclusion, and health promotion actions.

Promoting digital equity is intrinsically linked to people's health literacy. This factor is particularly relevant in active and healthy ageing, as adequate levels of health literacy favor the appropriate use of services, informed decision-making, and autonomous health management.

Based on data from the SHARE project, Terraneo (2015) analyzed educational inequalities in the use of health services by people aged 50 and over in 12 European countries. The results indicate greater use of specialized and preventive services among individuals with more schooling, suggesting that education facilitates access. Tavares (2020), also using SHARE and the DESI index, found that elderly internet users reported better self-perceived health, especially in countries with less developed digital infrastructures.

Barriers and Challenges

Complementing this perspective, Bente et al. (2024) examine the legal, ethical, financial, and technological barriers to the adoption of eHealth in Europe. Legal barriers involve privacy and compliance with regulations such as the GDPR and MDR. Ethical challenges include informed consent and technological validation. Financial sustainability is limited by insufficient reimbursement models, while technical problems of interoperability, usability, and reliability prevail. The study reinforces the need for an integrated and collaborative approach.

Cibin (2023) draws attention to the risks of digital exclusion arising from technological acceleration. European policies, while recognizing this exclusion, tend to be limited to aspects of access and basic technical skills, neglecting socio-cultural barriers faced by vulnerable groups such as the elderly. The analysis of public policies and data from 30 European countries during the pandemic reveals that rapid digitalization has exacerbated inequalities by ignoring contextual needs and offering few analog alternatives.

Inequality also manifests in regional dynamics, as demonstrated by Caravella et al. (2023), who analyzed the distribution of digital skills in 179 European regions. They identified a strong regional polarization, where regions with high digital levels consolidate their advantage, while others face persistent difficulties. This divergence has direct implications for equity in access to digital health. Gullslett et al. (2024), based on WHO data, reveal advances in the adoption of telehealth in Europe, driven by the pandemic. The main obstacles, however, include funding, infrastructure, and professional qualifications. The study highlights the lack of systematic evaluation of initiatives, which jeopardizes evidence-based expansion.

Strategic and Policy Frameworks

In a similar vein, Odone et al. (2019) discuss the strategic role of digital technologies in consolidating the fundamental principles of public health: quality, accessibility, efficiency, and equity. By analyzing the potential and challenges of digitizing European public health, the authors propose a framework that connects innovations such as genomics, artificial intelligence, big data, and mHealth to the fields of promotion, prevention, surveillance, and policy formulation. They highlight five characteristics with high transformative potential: personalization, automation, predictive capacity, data analysis (including interoperability), and interaction.

Bıçakçı (2024) analyze the Digital Europe program (2021-2027), which aims to achieve technological sovereignty for the European Union by investing in AI, high-performance computing, cybersecurity, digital skills, and digital public services. This program is presented as a strategy to consolidate a resilient digital ecosystem.

In the field of urban inclusion, Kolotouchkina et al. (2024) examine smart cities from the perspective of digital equity. The study critiques the technocentric focus of these initiatives, which often prioritize economic efficiency over social well-being, thereby widening existing inequalities. They propose a reflexive framework for inclusive governance to promote more equitable urban policies, guided by digital citizenship, active participation, and social justice.

Bousquet et al. (2015) and Bousquet et al. (2017) highlight the need for a standardized definition of "Active and Healthy Ageing" (AHA) and propose a multidimensional model based on physical, cognitive, and psychosocial capacities. They reinforce the importance of collaborative governance in health innovation. Finally, Falanga et al. (2020) analyzed 37 European initiatives for the civic participation of seniors, finding that most are consultative, while co-decisional forms—though less frequent—have greater potential for empowerment.

Specific Interventions and Tools

Jose et al. (2024) mapped 100 digital technologies for older people with neurocognitive disorders in Europe and Canada. They found that most solutions were not specific to these disorders and that only 28% had scientific evidence of effectiveness, highlighting the need for robust validation. Additionally, Spargo et al. (2021) present the European SHAPES project, which aims to develop an open digital platform to support active and healthy ageing through integrated technological solutions, particularly in supporting medication management among older adults with multimorbidity.

The wide-ranging literature reviewed in this section highlights a complex and fragmented landscape where digital health innovations often fail to align with the psychosocial needs of an ageing population. The presence of legal, ethical, and socio-cultural barriers, coupled with a lack of policy integration, underscores a significant gap between technological potential and real-world implementation. To address this complexity, the present study employs a meta-narrative review methodology, as detailed in the subsequent section. This approach is uniquely suited to synthesizing this diverse and multidisciplinary body of work, allowing us to move beyond siloed findings to identify overarching thematic patterns. By synthesizing the literature through the lens of the Ikigai Play framework and applying a country-specific analysis, our methodology aims to bridge the identified gaps and provide a more holistic, integrated understanding of how to foster purpose-driven and equitable ageing in the digital era.

3. METHODOLOGY

This chapter employs a meta-narrative review methodology, guided by the PRISMA framework for systematic reviews (Moher et al., 2009). This approach is particularly suitable for synthesizing diverse literature across disciplines, allowing the researcher to identify thematic patterns, conceptual shifts, and methodological tensions (Greenhalgh et al., 2005). The procedural steps for literature retrieval and analysis were detailed in a unified methodological guide to ensure a consistent approach among project partners.

Eligibility criteria

The inclusion criteria for the review were: (i) written in English; (ii) full-text available in PDF format; (iii) conducted in a participating SmartAgeing project country; (iv) published within the last 10 years; and (v) addressed at least one of the core thematic axes (ikigai, eHealth, Healthy & Active Ageing, Digital Transition, Inclusion of Older Adults, European Citizenship). To ensure an exploratory and multidisciplinary perspective, no restrictions were placed on the type of document (e.g., scientific articles, reports, policy documents). The exclusion criterion was the failure to meet one or more of the inclusion criteria. All selected documents were read in full, and key information was extracted into a shared digital spreadsheet, General Catalog of Studies, for further thematic organization and analysis.

Information sources and search strategy

A structured search was conducted across academic databases including Scopus, Web of Science, and PubMed, as detailed in the PRISMA flowchart (Figure 1).

Figure 1. PRISMA flowchart outlining identification, screening, eligibility, and inclusion stages of literature selection

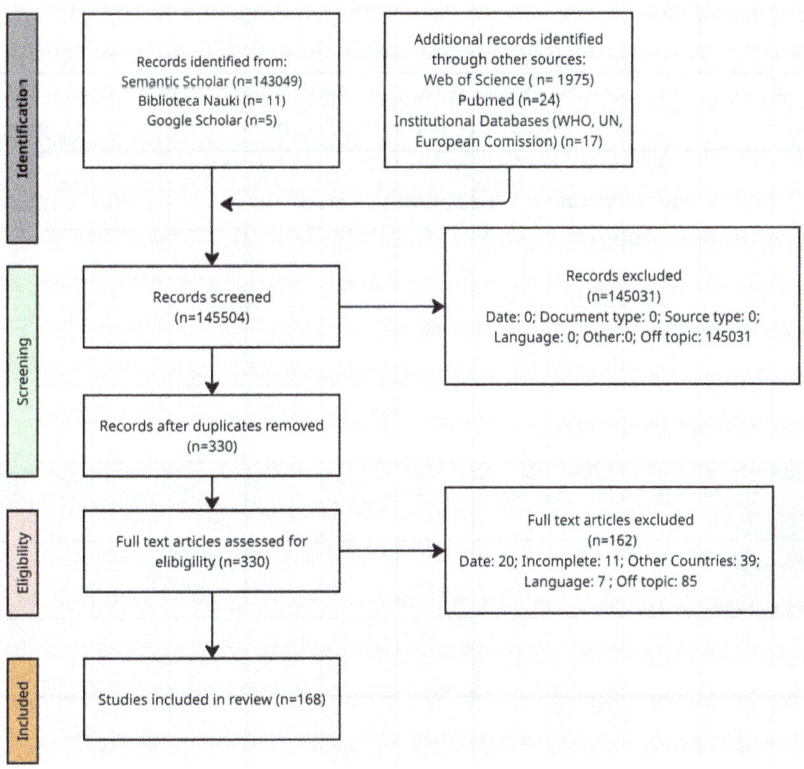

The keywords related to "ikigai," "active ageing," "digital health," and "Europe." Inclusion criteria focused on peer-reviewed studies published within the last 10 years with emphasis on cross-national European initiatives. Exclusion criteria included studies lacking methodological transparency or empirical grounding.

An initial pool of sources was gathered using academic databases (PubMed, Scopus, Google Scholar), project deliverables from the SmartAgeCare initiative, grey literature, and policy documents from EU and national bodies. Keywords included: healthy ageing, digital health, active ageing, eHealth, mHealth, citizenship, ikigai, and digital literacy.

Each partner was instructed to carry out an initial search using Semantic Scholar, which was selected for its open-access nature and broad disciplinary coverage. However, it was later realized that Semantic Scholar does not support Boolean operators, which necessitated a refined approach. Concurrently, each partner conducted complementary searches in national databases specific to their respective countries. Poland accessed the national scientific repository Biblioteka Nauki, while Latvia expanded its research using Google Scholar. As the coordinating partner, Portugal further expanded the scope by incorporating Web of Science and PubMed, along with institutional and policy-related databases such as WHO Europe, the United Nations, and the European Commission. This broadened the geographic and thematic coverage to include both national and European perspectives.

Notably, the original review protocol did not include the term ikigai among predefined keywords or thematic categories. As the review progressed, a need emerged to explore this concept in greater depth due to its conceptual alignment with the project's goals. Consequently, an additional exploratory search was conducted. Initial searches for ikigai in Semantic Scholar and Web of Science yielded limited results, indicating the need for a more comprehensive strategy. A refined and extended advanced search was then carried out on Web of Science and PubMed. The Web of Science was selected for its multidisciplinary nature, and the PubMed database was used to deepen the investigation of links between digital health and older adult well-being. All selected documents were read in full, and key information was extracted into a shared digital spreadsheet and the Notion platform for further thematic organization and synthesis. The final set of 60+ sources was included across the eight European countries (Figure 2). These were synthesized narratively within country-specific profiles, and the ikigai literature, largely from Japan, was reviewed separately and integrated conceptually. Thematic axes—health, digital transition, and citizenship—structured the synthesis.

Figure 2. Papers by Country

Number of Papers by Partner

	Belgium	Cyprus	Germany	Italy	Latvia	Poland	Portugal	Slovenia	TOTAL
Papers **Before** Filtering	338	110	138 866	414	1 314	666	2 661	248	144 876
Papers **After** Filtering	22	11	66	17	33	26	199	12	386
Papers **After** Duplicates	20	11	56	14	32	14	161	9	317

- **Step 1: Identification**

An initial pool of sources was gathered using academic databases (PubMed, Scopus, Google Scholar), project deliverables from the SmartAgeCare initiative, grey literature, and policy documents from EU and national bodies. Keywords included: *healthy ageing*, *digital health*, *active ageing*, *eHealth*, *mHealth*, *citizenship*, *ikigai*, and *digital literacy*.

- **Step 2: Screening**

Duplicate entries were removed, followed by a title and abstract screening to assess relevance. Inclusion criteria: (1) published between 2015–2025; (2) focused on older adults or ageing; (3) related to digital health, well-being, citizenship, or purpose. Exclusion criteria included language barriers (non-English/Portuguese), lack of full-text access, or limited empirical detail.

- **Step 3: Eligibility**

Full-text articles were then assessed for eligibility. Studies were categorized by country, methodology (quantitative, qualitative, mixed), and thematic relevance (digital access, health outcomes, social participation, psychosocial models).

- **Step 4: Inclusion and Synthesis**

A final set of over 60 sources was included across the eight European countries. These were synthesized narratively within country-specific profiles. The Ikigai literature, largely from Japan, was reviewed separately and integrated conceptually. Thematic axes—health, digital transition, and citizenship—structured the synthesis.

Data extraction followed PRISMA guidelines and incorporated thematic synthesis techniques as outlined by Thomas and Harden (2008). Each study was coded according to population, intervention, context, and outcomes, enabling comparative analysis across different health systems and cultural settings. Documents were grouped thematically for analysis, based on their alignment with the core domains.

Figure 3. Types of Study

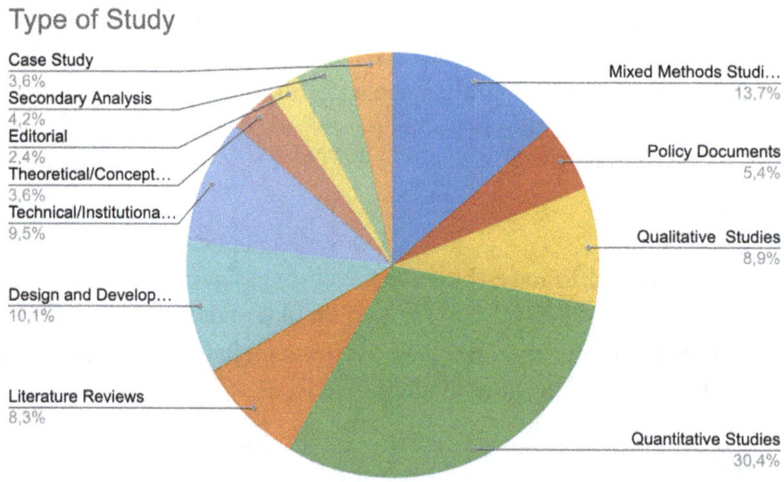

The study types were classified based on the methodologies explicitly stated in the publications. In cases where the methodology was not clearly specified, an informed classification was conducted by the researchers (Figure 3).

Based on the provided data, the global distribution of study types is dominated by quantitative research, which accounts for the largest share at 30.4%. Following this, mixed methods studies represent a significant portion at 13.7%, indicating a strong preference for research that combines both quantitative and qualitative approaches. Other notable study types include design and development (10.1%), technical/institutional (9.5%), and qualitative studies (8.9%). The remaining categories, which each make up less than 10% of the total, include literature reviews (8.3%), policy documents (5.4%), secondary analysis (4.2%), as well as a small number of theoretical/conceptual studies (3.6%), case studies (3.6%), and editorials (2.4%).

The results confirm that this approach yielded a robust and multidisciplinary literature review grounded in empirical evidence. The distribution of study types—quantitative, mixed methods, design/development, and qualitative—demonstrates that the review captures a comprehensive spectrum of research. It reflects not only statistical rigor but also practical applicability and contextual understanding.

Ethical considerations were addressed by following the principles of informed consent, data anonymization, and responsible reporting, in line with the Helsinki Declaration (World Medical Association, 2013).

This PRISMA-informed approach supports clarity in the review process and facilitates cross-country comparison while respecting contextual specificity. It also accommodates diverse types of evidence, aligning with the transdisciplinary goals of the SmartAgeCare project.

4. RESULTS AND SYNTHESIS

This section presents a meta-narrative synthesis of the literature, exploring key findings across different European countries and their connection to the ikigai paradigm. The analysis highlights regional disparities, digital inclusion, health promotion, and the potential for ikigai as a unifying framework for health, digital transition, and citizenship goals.

4.1 Ikigai Literature Review

The meta-narrative synthesis revealed four primary clusters of empirical research related to the ikigai paradigm and healthy ageing: (1) longitudinal cohort studies from Japan, (2) cross-national studies comparing European and Japanese populations, (3) psychometric evaluations of ikigai-related instruments, and (4) technology-supported ageing interventions.

Studies from Japan, such as the Ohsaki Cohort Study, have consistently demonstrated a positive correlation between ikigai and longevity, with findings suggesting that older adults who report a strong sense of purpose have significantly lower mortality rates (Sone et al., 2008). Similarly, longitudinal analyses by the Japan Gerontological Evaluation Study (JAGES) reinforce the importance of psychological and social determinants in health outcomes among older populations (Kondo et al., 2009).

Cross-national studies conducted in Portugal, Germany, and the United States have attempted to validate the ikigai-9 instrument in Western contexts, showing moderate to strong reliability and construct validity (Fido et al., 2019; Schnell, 2020). These studies highlight the cultural adaptability of the ikigai construct, while also revealing nuances in how purpose and fulfilment are culturally expressed.

In these countries, ikigai is adapted to reflect purpose through work, recognition, or personal fulfillment. Digital tools supporting ikigai include conversational AI, learning platforms, and therapeutic games; however, ethical concerns—such as dependency and data privacy—remain. The integration of ikigai with technology must respect cultural expectations, focusing on user-centered, values-driven design.

Standardized psychometric tools such as the Geriatric Depression Scale (GDS-15), Mini-Mental State Examination (MMSE), and Purpose in Life Test (PIL) have been used in tandem with ikigai measures to explore mental health correlations (Yesavage et al., 1982; Ryff & Keyes, 1995; Lawton et al., 2002). For instance, findings from SmartAgeCare pilot studies in Ireland and Portugal indicate that digital interventions can improve cognitive scores and ikigai-related outcomes among older adults.

The synthesis also indicates a growing trend toward integrating social technologies into healthy ageing strategies. Social participation, emotional bonds, and health behaviors reinforce ikigai. Community-based programs like the Chofu-Digital-Choju Movement integrate digital and in-person socialization to boost subjective well-being. Cultural differences are evident: Japanese participants embrace assistive technologies like social robots more openly than Western counterparts, where autonomy and privacy concerns dominate. Initiatives in Sweden, the Netherlands, and Denmark have incorporated serious games, digital storytelling, and social robots into elder care programs with measurable psychosocial benefits (Neven & Peine, 2017; Marston et al., 2020). These approaches align with the ikigai Play framework by emphasizing engagement, creativity, and meaning-making in later life.

Overall, the findings suggest that the ikigai paradigm is not only measurable and transferable across cultures, but also offers a promising framework for aligning digital innovation with well-being–enhancing strategies that foster purpose, motivation, and healthy ageing across cultures supporting ageing populations in a more human-centered and purposeful manner.

4.2 Portugal

The methodological analysis of studies related to Portugal includes a total of 82 initially identified documents, of which 36 were excluded based on pre-established criteria. The main reasons for exclusion were: different country of origin (n=17), lack of adherence to the topics (off-topic; n=12), publication prior to the 10-year time limit (n=4), incomplete document (n=1), and incompatible language (n=1). Thus, 46 studies were deemed eligible and included in the final analysis (Figure 4).

Figure 4. PRISMA, Portugal

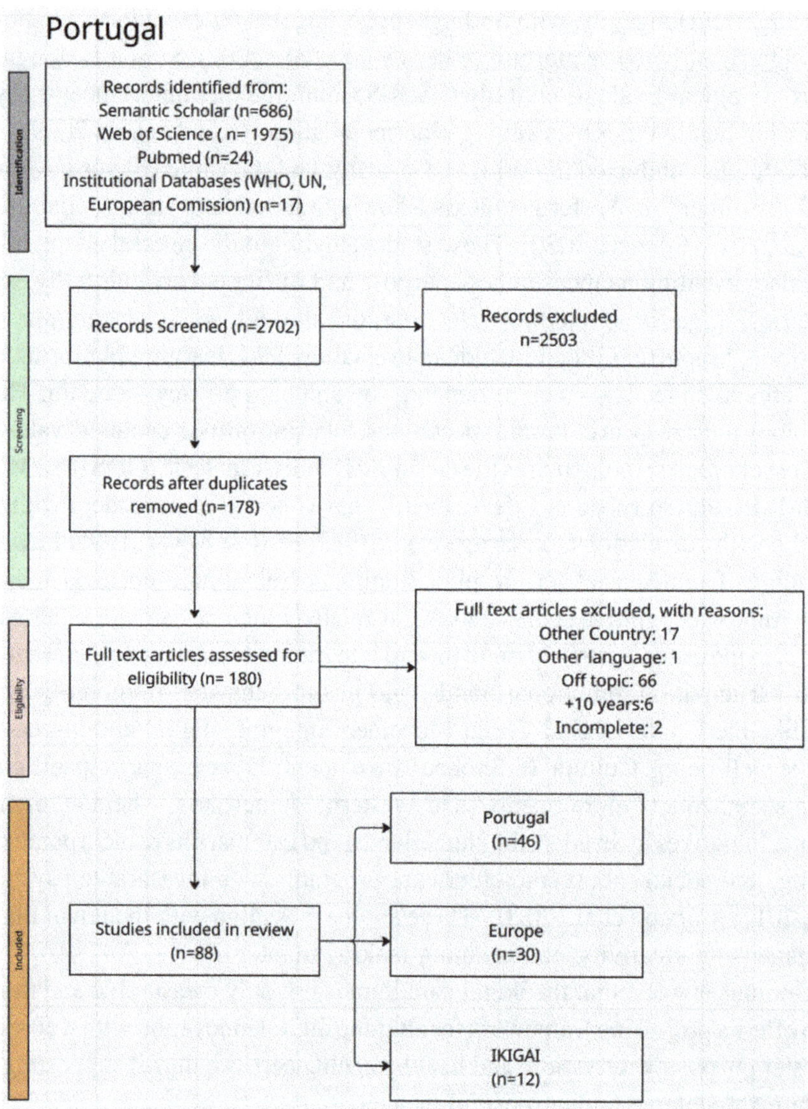

Among the included studies, there is a predominance of quantitative approaches (28.3%), followed by mixed-methods studies (17.4%) and design and development research (17.4%). Literature reviews accounted for 15.2% of the sample, while qualitative methods represented 10,9%. Case studies (6.5%), one public policy document (2.2%), and one secondary data analysis (2.2%) were also identified, demonstrating the diversity of Portuguese scientific output in the field of active ageing and digital inclusion (Figure 5).

Figure 5. Types of Data Resources in Portugal

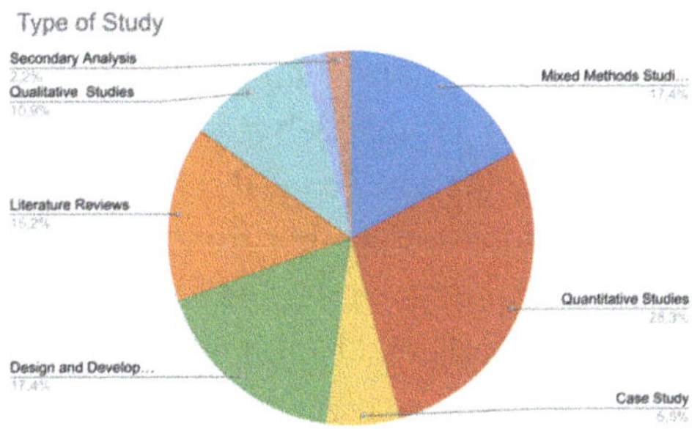

Portugal presents a complex case for active ageing due to persistent inequalities in income, health, and digital literacy (Eurostat, 2022). Older adults, especially in rural areas, face limited access to digital infrastructure and public health services (Loureiro et al., 2021). Nonetheless, regional projects like Ageing@Coimbra and +TV4E have made significant strides in promoting digital inclusion among elderly populations (Barros et al., 2020). The AGAPE initiative in Lisbon illustrates how digital storytelling and social technologies can enhance wellbeing and a sense of purpose among older adults (Ferreira et al., 2018).

Portugal is facing one of the most significant ageing transitions in Europe, marked by increased longevity and declining birth rates. Between 2010 and 2019, life expectancy at age 60 rose— from 23.1 to 24.3 years— but, this was accompanied by a decline in health-related quality of life (HRQoL), particularly among older individuals with multimorbidity and excess weight. Education and physical activity have been shown as protective factors, while self-perception of health reveals gender differences, with women reporting worse health but greater engagement in active ageing activities.

Beyond clinical metrics, ageing in Portugal is shaped by psychosocial determinants. Mental health and subjective well-being, especially after age 75, emerge as stronger predictors of active ageing than physical conditions. Longitudinal evidence links anxiety and depression to lower quality of life, while retirement stress impacts life purpose. These findings affirm the 'ageing paradox'—a tendency for subjective well-being to remain stable or even improve with age.

Portugal's social networks among older adults are categorized into family, friendship, neighborhood, and institutional ties, with varying degrees of emotional and practical support. Yet, over 1.2 million Portuguese seniors live alone or only with other elderly people, increasing risks of isolation and institutionalization, particularly in rural areas. Community initiatives show promise but struggle against demographic decline. Programs like Ageing@Coimbra embody intersectoral strategies through mobile units, brain health education, and citizen engagement. Participants have acknowledged improvements in health and support services but also point out gaps in housing and social participation.

Despite progress, national policy remains fragmented. Only 4.3% of Portuguese municipalities have local ageing plans. The national system is marked by weak coordination, low effectiveness, and heavy reliance on informal networks. The COVID-19 pandemic exposed these vulnerabilities but also spotlighted new directions in digital health, like telemedicine, user portals, and mobile applications. However, there is still no structured national strategy for using big data, and the regulation of wellness apps remains underdeveloped.

Digital literacy is a crucial enabler for active ageing. Programs like AUDID and OITO have increased older adults' confidence with digital tools, though gains in health literacy were limited. Television-based platforms (e.g., +TV4E) show promise by aligning with familiar user habits. Yet barriers persist, including sensory limitations, design mismatches, and trust in digital services. Effective strategies include tailored pedagogies, simplified interfaces, and long-term user support.

The role of mHealth is also expanding. Apps that deliver short videos or reminders have been shown to improve adherence and knowledge. Training caregivers through platforms like Help2CARE indirectly benefits elderly users. Game-based solutions are another frontier—digital games have shown potential for supporting mental health, emotional expressiveness, and social connectedness. Platforms developed by Costa et al. and Regalado et al. improved mental health indicators and digital skills aligned with EU standards (e.g., DigComp).

Portugal is also leading the way in smart health ecosystems. Projects like AGAPE and My-AHA integrate IoT and predictive analytics to personalize monitoring and care. Other platforms, such as CoaFEld and HELASCOL, blend AI, gamification, and environmental data. These systems share a commitment to co-design and usability evaluation with and for the elderly.

Ultimately, ageing in Portugal is a multidimensional experience shaped by intersecting physical, digital, and psychosocial factors. Despite a strong research ecosystem and innovative practices, national fragmentation hinders widespread impact. Bridging digital and social inclusion with culturally sensitive design—especially through concepts like ikigai—can offer pathways to more purposeful, connected, and equitable ageing futures.

4.3 Poland

Of the 14 articles initially selected for full-text reading, 11 met the eligibility criteria: publication within the last 10 years, written in English, authorship linked to Poland, and relevance to at least one of the central themes of the review *(e-health/digital health, healthy & active ageing, digital transition, digital inclusion, citizenship, and ikigai).* The three excluded studies were removed for the following reasons: one was conducted in other countries, and two were written in a language other than English (Figure 6).

Figure 6. PRISMA, Poland

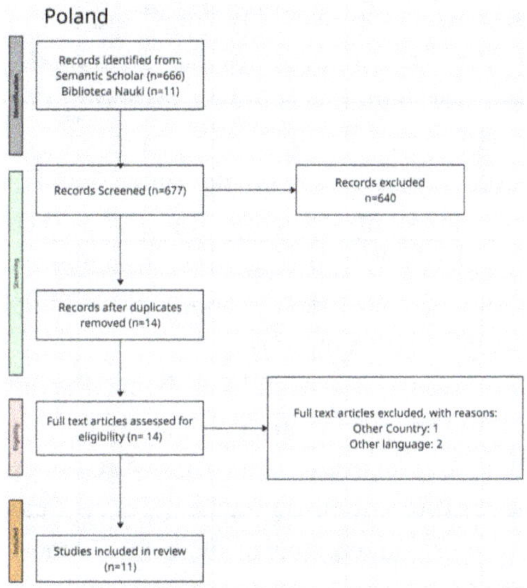

The analysis of these studies revealed a clear predominance for quantitative methods, which represented 54.5% of the total sample. The remaining studies were evenly distributed, at 9.1% each, among qualitative research, literature reviews, policy analyses, mixed methods, and secondary data studies. This distribution is shown in Figure 7, highlighting the central role that statistical and numerical approaches still play in the Polish academic production related to digital inclusion and ageing.

Figure 7. Types of Data Resources in Poland

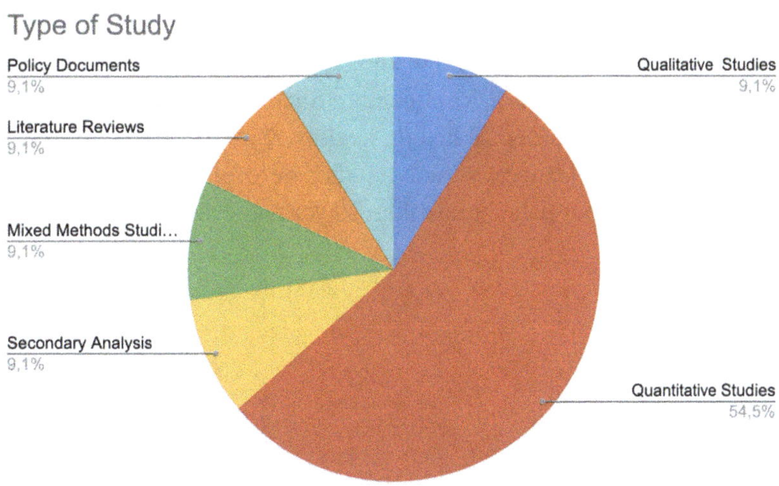

Poland's ageing population faces systemic health inequalities and fragmented care services, particularly in post-industrial regions (OECD, 2021). While digital health strategies have been introduced, implementation is uneven. Local projects such as "Aktywni+" and Senior+ initiatives emphasize digital education and intergenerational activities that align with the ikigai model by fostering social connection and purpose (Kubiak, 2020). However, high levels of ageism and limited digital trust remain key challenges (Domagała & Wilk, 2020).

Poland is undergoing rapid demographic ageing, marked by regional imbalances and structural limitations in health, social services, and digital infrastructure. Rural areas such as the Opole Voivodeship face population shrinkage, prompting calls for "silver economy" strategies to view ageing as an opportunity. Despite progress in eHealth policies, digital literacy among older adults remains low, and inequalities in access are widespread, especially between regions.

Studies reveal that digital inclusion supports mental well-being. For example, internet use among older adults correlates with reduced depression symptoms, particularly for those living alone. Participation in lifelong learning programs, such as Universities of the Third Age, plays a critical role in boosting ICT skills and digital confidence. Factors influencing digital health acceptance include perceived usefulness, ease of use, and social influence—core dimensions of the UTAUT model.

Local governments play a mixed role in promoting active ageing, with some initiatives in small towns fostering healthy lifestyles despite limited budgets. However, smart ageing strategies are underutilized, and there is often a disconnect between digital and social policies. Policy analysis reveals fragmented governance, weak integration of health and digital strategies, and a lack of funding for age-friendly infrastructure.

Cultural values and priorities are central. Older adults value independence, privacy, strong social connections, and access to healthcare—values that shape their willingness to engage with digital tools. Poland's digital health transformation, while promising, requires deeper alignment with these individual motivations and regional needs, ensuring equity and long-term effectiveness.

4.4 Slovenia

Of the 11 articles initially selected for full-text reading, 8 met the eligibility criteria: publication within the last 10 years, written in English, authorship linked to Slovenia, and relevance to at least one of the central themes of the review (e-health/digital health, healthy & active ageing, digital transition, digital inclusion, citizenship, and ikigai). The three excluded studies were removed for the following reasons: one was considered off topic, one was published more than 10 years ago, and one was incomplete (Figure 8).

Figure 8. PRISMA, Slovenia

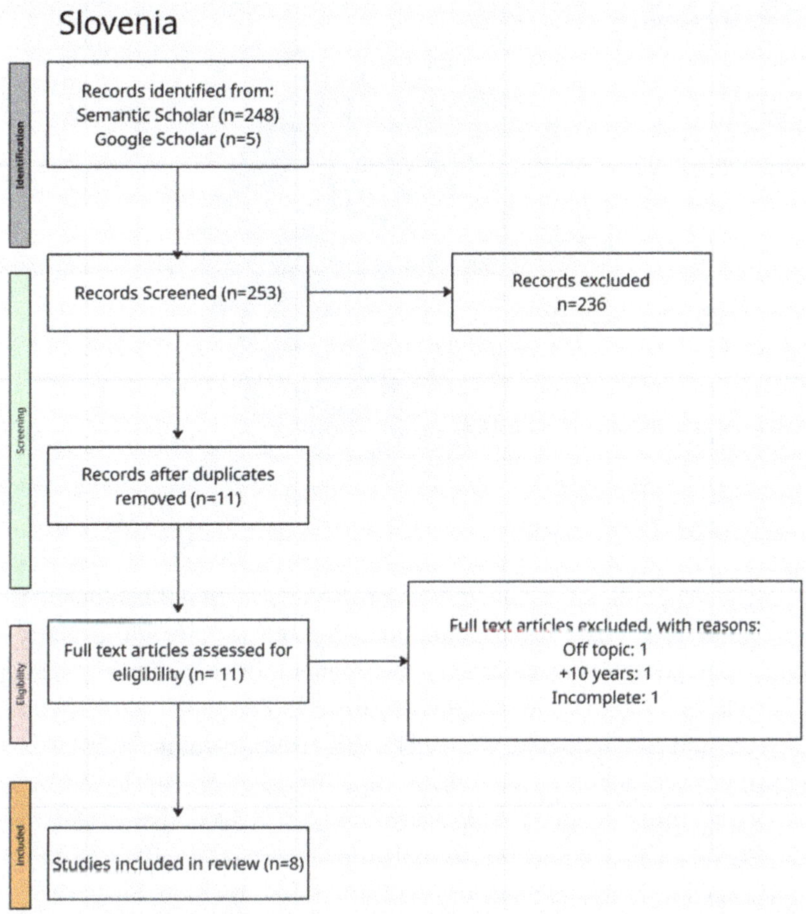

A methodological analysis of these 8 selected studies revealed that mixed methods designs were predominant, accounting for 50% of the sample (Figure 9). These studies combined qualitative and quantitative techniques with the aim of capturing both measurable results and the depth of individual and contextual experiences. In addition to the mixed-methods studies, 25% of the sample was made up of quantitative investigations, and the other types of studies were case study (12.5%) and also policy document (12,5%).

Figure 9. Types of Data Resources in Slovenia

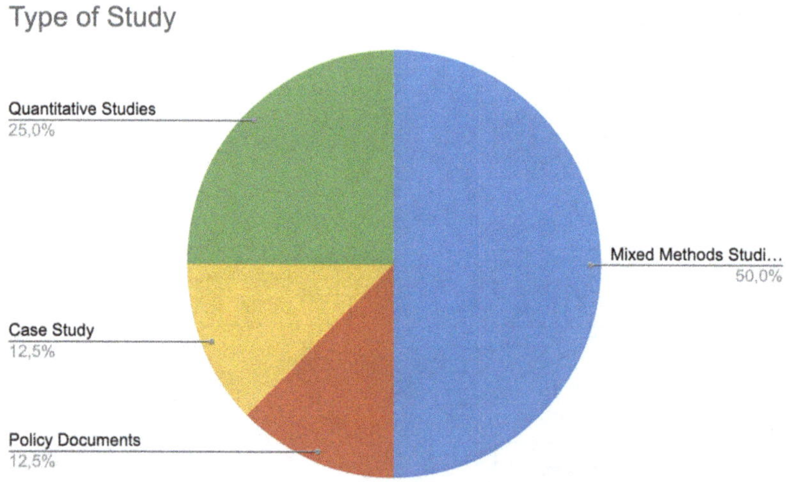

In Slovenia, active ageing policies are integrated into broader national health and innovation frameworks (European Commission, 2020). Programmes like "Simbioza" have successfully increased digital competence among older people by encouraging intergenerational mentoring (Novak et al., 2017). Studies indicate that Slovenian older adults value ikigai-related domains such as autonomy and social participation, although rural-urban disparities persist (Hribernik & Dolničar, 2019).

Slovenia demonstrates considerable progress in digital health, characterized by robust electronic health records (EHR), integrated patient data platforms like zVEM, and national registries such as CRPD. During the COVID-19 pandemic, these tools proved essential, although limitations remain in infrastructure, professional training, and user digital skills.

Mixed-methods research reveals strong civic engagement in digital design, such as gardening apps co-created with older users and intergenerational mentorships where senior entrepreneurs support young NEETs. These programs foster well-being and social inclusion across age groups.

Social isolation and unhealthy behaviors remain challenges, especially in home care environments. Preferences lean toward informal caregiving, with low coverage of formal services. Despite campaigns like the European Year for Active Ageing (2012), long-term care reform remains stalled. Less than 3% of older people receive home care.

Slovenia's strategic direction is promising, but implementation requires better coordination and evaluation. Bridging digital literacy gaps, supporting caregivers, and expanding inclusive participation are key to sustaining progress in active ageing and digital equity.

4.5 Latvia

Of the 32 articles initially selected for full-text reading, 19 met the eligibility criteria: publication within the last 10 years, written in English, authorship linked to Latvia, and relevance to at least one of the central themes of the review *(e-health/digital health, healthy & active ageing, digital transition, digital inclusion, citizenship, and ikigai).*The thirteen excluded studies were removed for the following reasons: five were conducted in other countries, five were considered off topic, three were published more than 10 years ago, and four were written in a language other than English (Figure 10).

Figure 10. PRISMA, Latvia

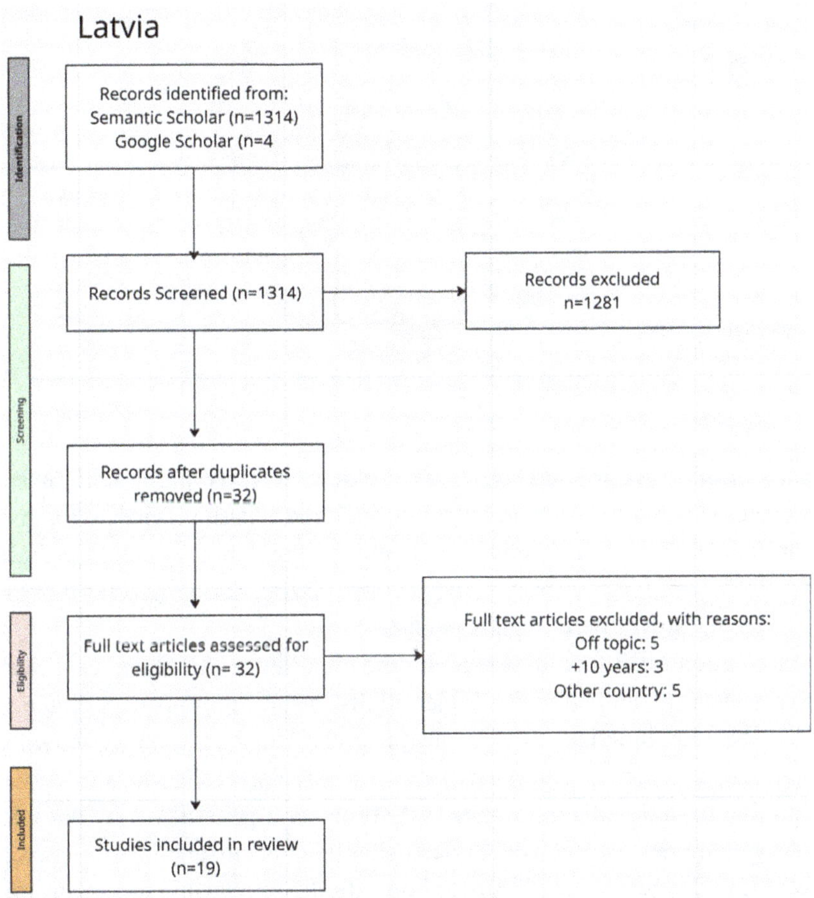

The methodological review of the 19 selected studies from Latvia highlights a clear predominance of quantitative research (47.4%), qualitative designs accounted for 21.1%. Additional contributions included a mixed methods study, a case study, a design and development, a secondary analysis, a theoretical/conceptual studies and a technical/institutional each representing 5.3% of the total (Figure 11).

Figure 11. Types of Data Resources in Latvia

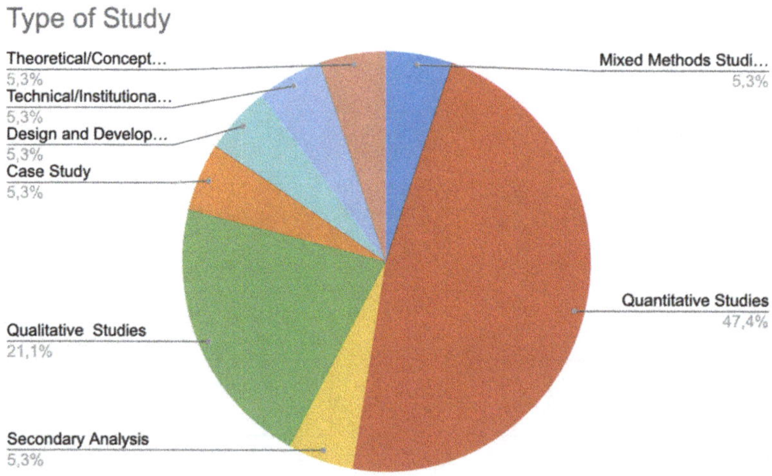

Latvia faces demographic decline and high rates of elderly poverty, particularly in rural regions (European Commission, 2021). Access to digital technologies and health services remains uneven, despite national eHealth initiatives. Local programs like "Senioru Skola" aim to enhance digital skills among older adults, promoting a sense of community and purpose (Ozola & Lapiņa, 2020). However, structural barriers such as broadband infrastructure gaps persist.

Latvia faces stark structural inequalities shaping the experience of ageing, especially along dimensions of geography, education, and ethnicity. Older adults in rural regions experience social exclusion, economic precarity, and poor digital access. Despite these challenges, Latvia has made strides in eHealth infrastructure, telemedicine, and patient portal expansion, particularly following the COVID-19 pandemic.

Research shows that digital skills among older Latvians are generally low, but peer-led and intergenerational learning methods are effective. Civic engagement is closely linked to perceived health and autonomy. Projects like "Connect, Latvia!" aim to boost digital citizenship in regions impacted by youth migration and ageing.

The economic need drives many seniors to remain in or return to the workforce. However, this does not necessarily reflect active ageing but rather financial insecurity. Retirement migration to other EU countries is also common.

Care initiatives—such as intergenerational programs in care homes—show emotional and cognitive benefits but are often underfunded. Overall, Latvia shows potential for transformative ageing strategies, but current efforts remain fragmented and unevenly distributed across the country.

4.6 Italy

Of the 14 articles initially selected for full-text reading, 12 met the eligibility criteria: publication within the last 10 years, written in English, authorship linked to Italy, and relevance to at least one of the central themes of the review *(e-health/digital health, healthy & active ageing, digital transition, digital inclusion, citizenship, and IKIGAI).*The two excluded studies were removed for the following reasons: one were considered off topic, one were published more than 10 years ago (Figure 12).

Figure 12. PRISMA, Italy

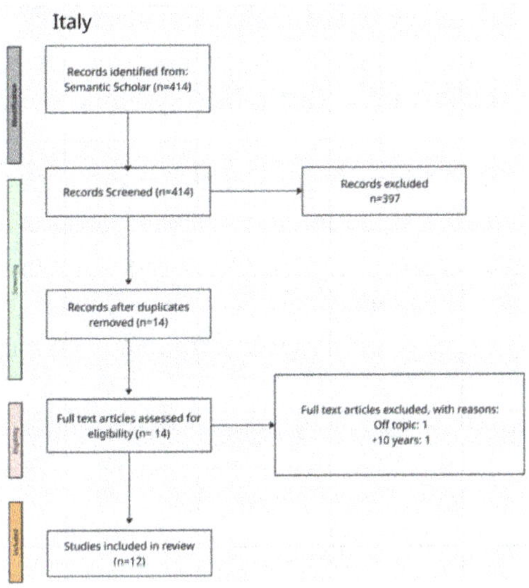

The methodological analysis of the 12 selected records indicates a predominance of quantitative studies, representing 41.7% of the total. Mixed methods, qualitative, and design and development studies each accounted for 16.7% of the records. One literature review (8.3%) (Figure 13).

Figure 13. Types of Data Resources in Italy

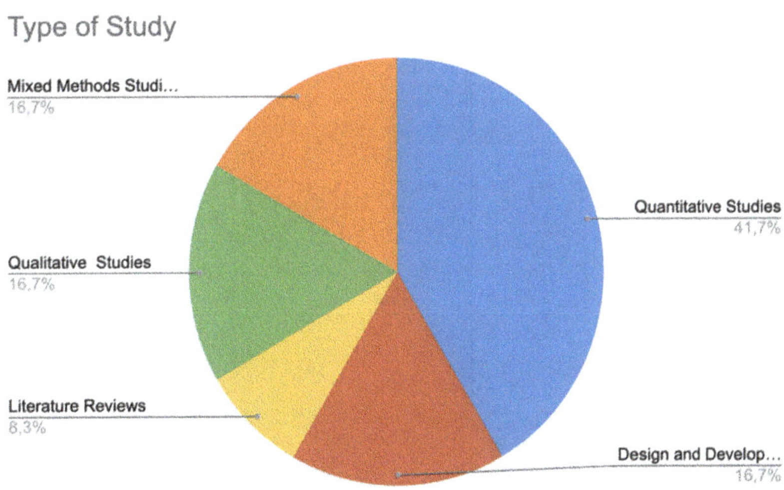

Italy's ageing population reflects strong intergenerational caregiving practices but also significant regional disparities in access to care and technology (ISTAT, 2021). Northern regions demonstrate higher uptake of telemedicine and social innovation platforms, whereas southern areas lag behind (Santoni et al., 2015). Community-based digital storytelling projects, such as "Nonni Digitali," have fostered a sense of ikigai among participants by highlighting meaningful life narratives and intergenerational.

Italy's ageing population is one of the oldest globally, with over 23% aged 65 or older. Challenges include limited digital literacy among older adults and pronounced regional disparities in healthcare and connectivity. Rural regions, especially in the South, face systemic exclusion from eHealth and digital services.

Policy responses include national telemedicine initiatives and regional eHealth portals, but implementation is inconsistent. Civic participation in digital design remains limited. Cultural norms around familial caregiving dominate, placing stress on informal carers without adequate state support.

Educational attainment and socioeconomic status greatly influence digital engagement. Projects addressing digital inclusion through intergenerational learning and community hubs have shown promise but lack national scale.

Italy's success in ageing well will depend on bridging North-South divides, investing in digital health infrastructure, and fostering inclusive models that respect local culture while empowering older adults through purpose and agency.

4.7 Germany

From the initial selection of 54 full-text articles, 15 met the eligibility criteria: published within the last 10 years, written in English, authored or co-authored by researchers affiliated with institutions in Germany, and aligned with at least one of the central themes of this review (e-health/digital health, healthy & active ageing, digital transition, digital inclusion, citizenship, and ikigai). The thirty-nine excluded studies were removed for the following reasons: thirteen were conducted in other countries, eight were considered off topic, eight were published more than 10 years ago, eight were incomplete, and four were written in a language other than English.

Figure 14. PRISMA, Germany

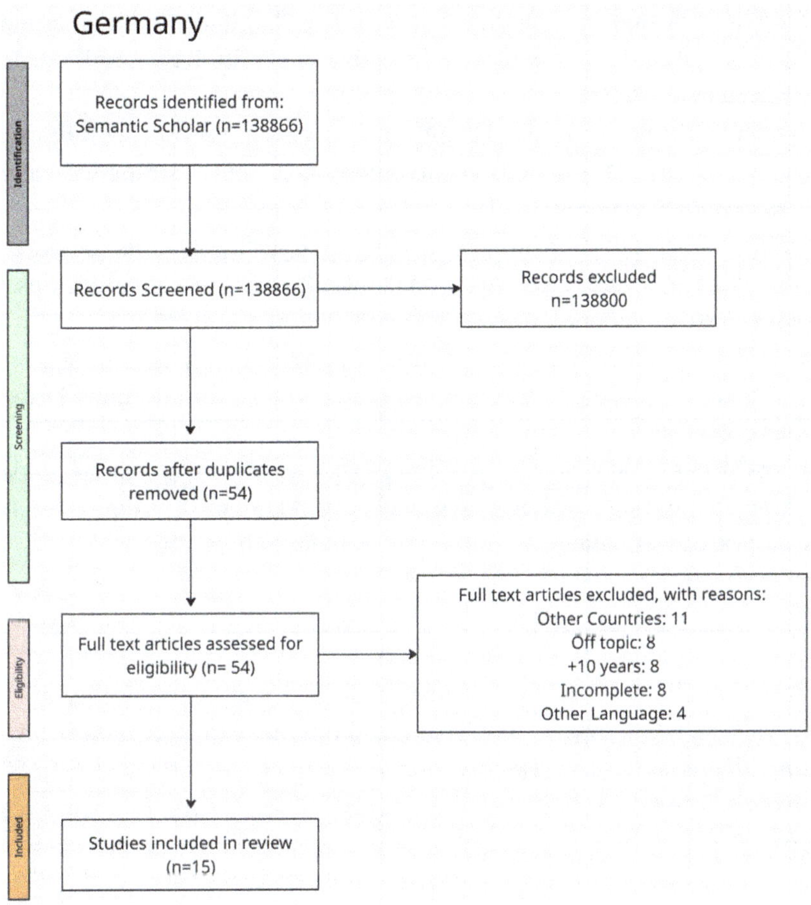

The methodological overview of the 15 studies from Germany reveals notable diversity, with a predominance of quantitative approaches (26.7%), followed by editorials and secondary analyses (20% each). Design and development studies accounted for 13.3%, while mixed methods, conceptual, institutional, and case studies each represented 6.7% of the total (Figure 15).

Figure 15. Types of Data Resources in Germany

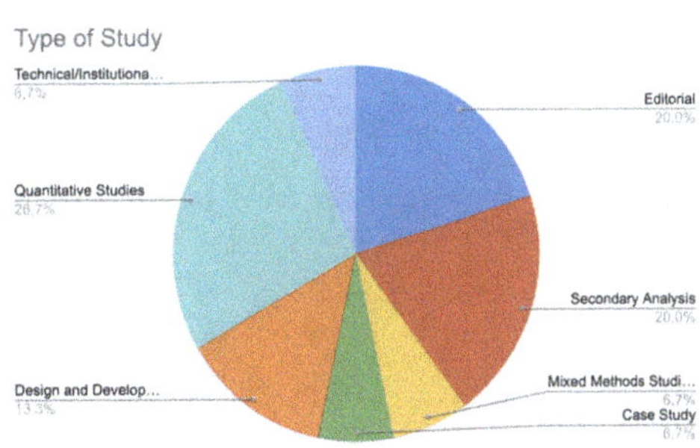

Germany has a robust ageing policy landscape supported by strong institutional frameworks and funding mechanisms (BMFSFJ, 2020). Nevertheless, disparities persist between urban and rural regions in terms of digital inclusion and healthcare access. The "DigitalPakt Alter" program is one of the flagship initiatives aimed at bridging these gaps through community-based digital learning centers for older adults (von Eitzen et al., 2021).

Germany offers one of the most advanced healthcare systems in Europe, with substantial investment in eHealth, yet ageing populations still face gaps in digital inclusion. A strong federal system results in regional differences in implementation.

SHARE data indicates that education, income, and region significantly affect seniors' access to digital tools and healthcare. Ikigai-relevant research shows that health and close relationships are predictors of life satisfaction, with German seniors scoring high on valuation of life (VOL).

Digital health initiatives include smart health cards, patient portals, and regional telemedicine networks. Public awareness campaigns and senior-focused education programs have made strides in improving digital engagement.

However, barriers persist: older adults with lower socioeconomic status are underrepresented in digital transformation. Integrating psychosocial models like ikigai into Germany's healthcare narrative can help address subjective well-being and participation more holistically.

4.8 Cyprus

Of the 11 articles initially selected for full-text reading, 9 met the eligibility criteria: publication within the last 10 years, authorship linked to Cyprus, and relevance to at least one of the central themes of the review *(e-health/digital health, healthy & active ageing, digital transition, digital inclusion, citizenship, and ikigai).* The two excluded studies were removed for the following reasons: two were considered off topic.

Figure 16. PRISMA, Cyprus

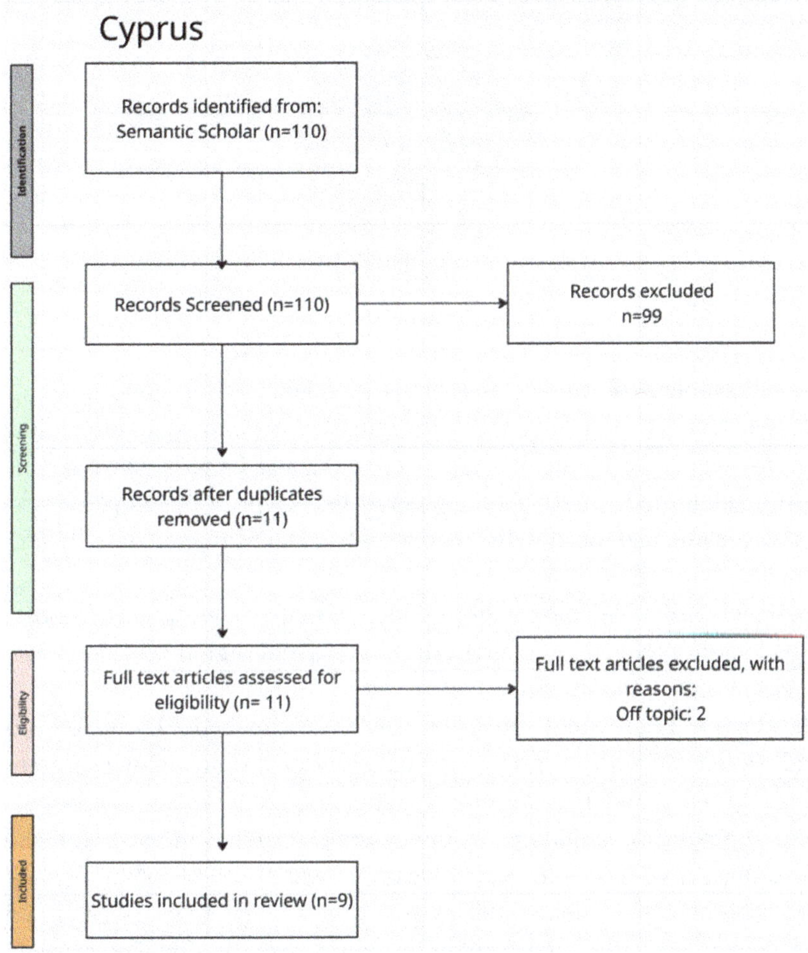

The analysis of the 9 selected records reveals a predominance of design and development studies, representing 44.4% of the total. Technical and institutional reports account for 22.2% of the records. The remaining studies are distributed between qualitative studies (11.1%), teoreticat/concepts (11,1%) and literature review (11.1%) (Figure 17).

Figure 17. Types of Data Resources in Cyprus

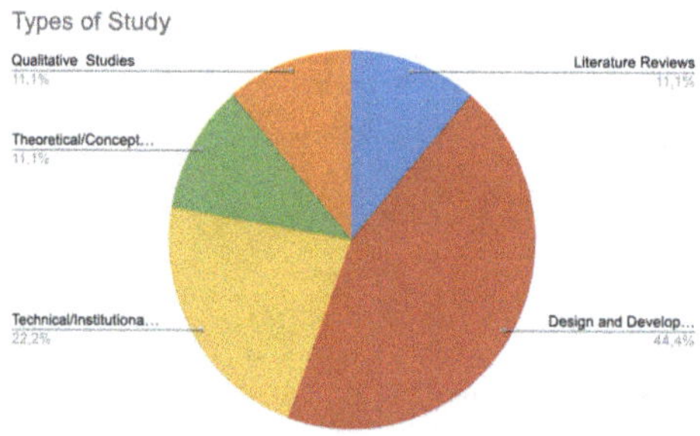

Cyprus faces a unique blend of rural ageing, high dependency ratios, and fragmented service delivery systems (European Commission, 2022). While digital literacy among older adults remains limited, EU-funded programs such as "e-Inclusion" and "Active Ageing Cyprus" have begun addressing this gap (Theodoulou-Loizidou et al., 2020). Studies report that Cypriot elders place strong emphasis on family, spiritual engagement, and meaningful routines—key tenets aligned with ikigai values (Kouta & Kaite, 2011).

Cyprus is experiencing steady demographic ageing, particularly in rural and semi-urban areas. The health system is undergoing reform, including efforts to expand digital services, yet older adults face persistent challenges in access and usability.

Digital health adoption is growing, driven by new platforms and EU-funded projects. However, health literacy and confidence with digital tools remain low, especially among those over 70. Regional inequality, language diversity, and underdeveloped public transport hinder inclusion.

Community-based programs, including senior centers and digital literacy workshops, have shown effectiveness in bridging gaps. Cross-generational learning and gamified apps are emerging as key tools.

To align with European active ageing goals, Cyprus must invest in user-centered digital solutions, enhance caregiver support, and tailor interventions that emphasize meaning, interdependence, and social connectivity—aligning with ikigai principles.

4.9 Belgium

Of the 20 articles initially selected for full-text reading, 12 met the eligibility criteria: publication within the last 10 years, written in English, authorship linked to Belgium, and relevance to at least one of the central themes of the review *(e-health/digital health, healthy & active ageing, digital transition, digital inclusion, citizenship, and IKIGAI).* The seven excluded studies were removed for the following reasons: five were conducted in other countries, two were considered off topic, and one was published more than 10 years ago (Figure 18).

Figure 18. PRISMA, Belgium

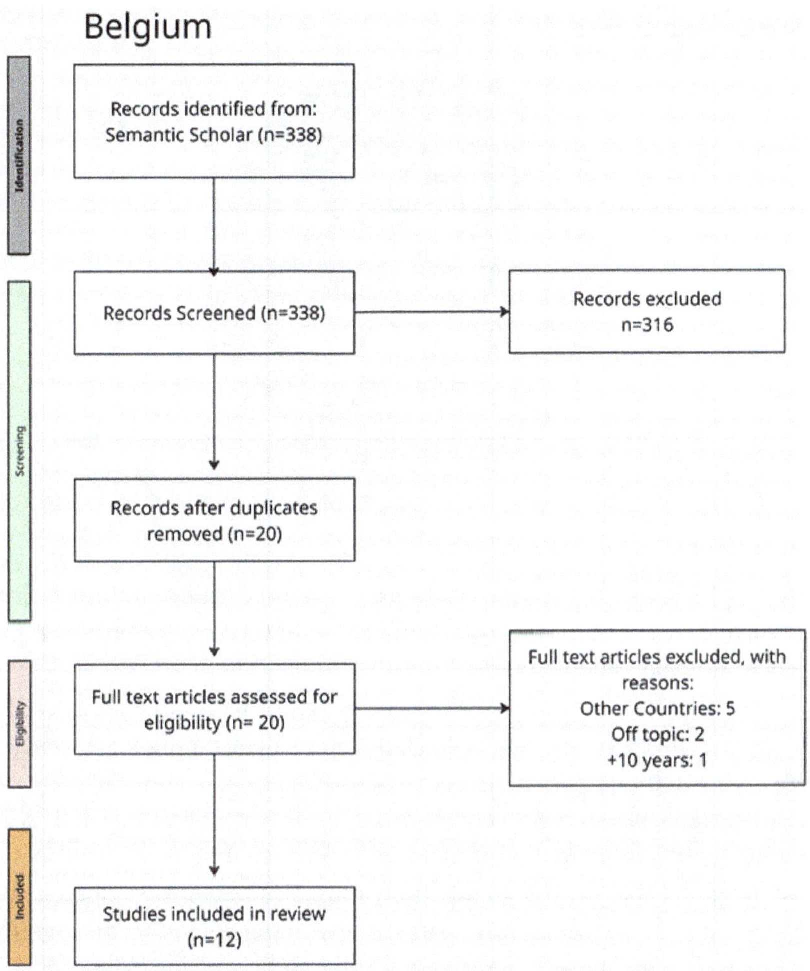

The methodological analysis of the 12 studies from Belgium indicates a predominance of quantitative approaches (33.3%), followed by mixed methods and qualitative designs (25% each), and public policy analyses (16.7%) (Figure 19).

Figure 19. Types of Data Resources in Belgium

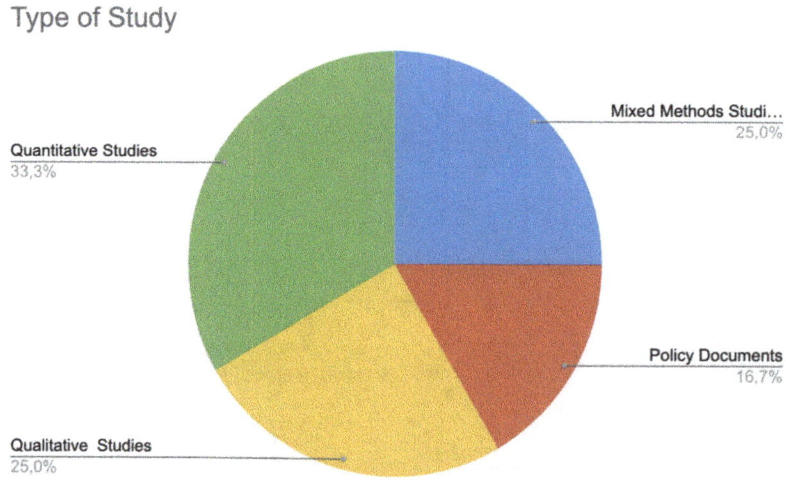

Belgium's digital health landscape is well-developed, with coordinated public policies and technology initiatives. The national digital health strategy, combined with robust regulations, supports large-scale services such as telehealth and patient portals.

A key focus is on solutions co-created with users, aligning with citizen-centered design. Studies demonstrate how regional projects and data utilization can influence policy and practices, thereby improving care integration and participation.

Digital applications emphasize subjective well-being, promoting autonomy and creating new opportunities for older adults. The integration of digital tools with social networks is also a key theme, with one study demonstrating that internet use significantly mitigates feelings of loneliness.

However, barriers to access and use remain, particularly for older adults with cognitive impairments. Challenges related to ageism and health literacy can compound exclusion. The need for ongoing adaptation to users' evolving needs is also a recognized challenge.

In summary, Belgium stands out for its technological infrastructure and its integration with public policies and user-focused research. The country's ecosystem offers insights into creating inclusive, adaptive, and supportive digital systems for lifelong well-being, with strong ties to the pillars of ikigai.

This section synthesizes literature across eight European countries and ikigai-specific studies. The analysis highlights regional disparities, digital inclusion, health promotion, and the potential for ikigai as a framework to unify health, digital transition, and citizenship goals.

A summary of findings, reflection on the 'Ikigai Play' paradigm as a response to ageing inequalities, and implications for European policy and innovation.

5. DISCUSSION

The analysis of ikigai-related initiatives across diverse European contexts highlights both shared challenges and context-specific innovations. The findings of this chapter suggest that national health systems, digital infrastructures, and sociocultural norms have a profound impact on the ageing experience in Europe. Across the eight countries reviewed, distinct patterns emerge that influence how purpose, participation, and digital health coverage are approached.

Figure 20. Ikigai Conceptual Framework

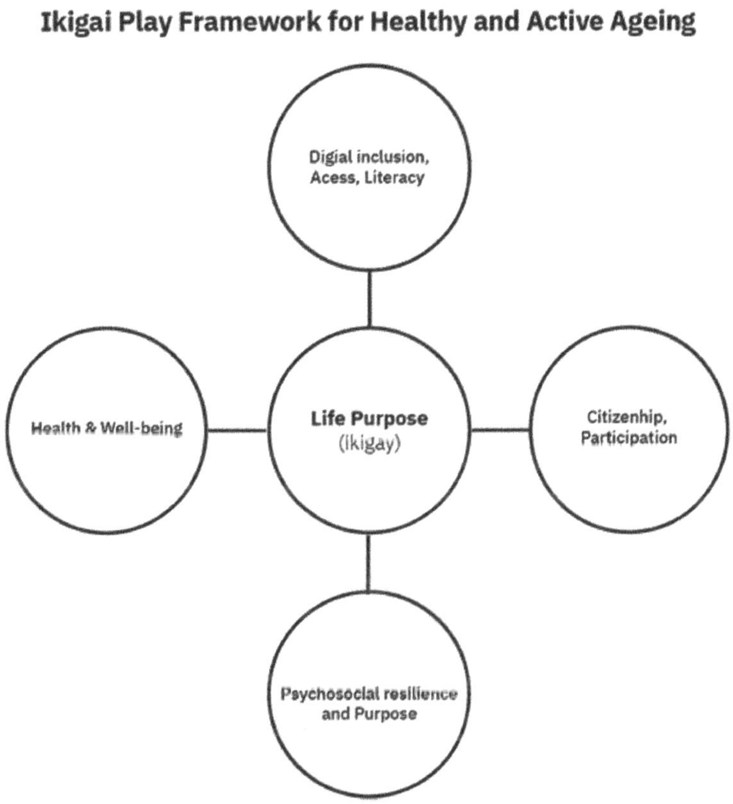

A key theme that emerged is the importance of cultural sensitivity in applying the ikigai paradigm. While the core elements of ikigai—purpose, community, and meaningful engagement—are widely applicable, their interpretation varies considerably across national and regional contexts (Mathews, 1996; Kumano, 2018).

The country-specific findings illustrate this:

- **Portugal:** Ageing is challenged by institutional fragmentation and low digital literacy, yet enriched by local innovations like Ageing@Coimbra and emotionally resonant digital games.
- **Poland:** Active ageing is closely tied to the role of local governments and peer networks, but is often hindered by structural disparities and weak integration of ageing and digital policy.
- **Slovenia:** The country offers a model of civic co-design and strong eHealth infrastructure, but lags in formal care provision and long-term system reform.

- **Latvia:** Digital exclusion, rural ageing, and economic stress dominate the narrative, yet peer learning and intergenerational programs show promise.
- **Italy:** Regional inequalities and overburdened informal carers are significant challenges, but community hubs and digital upskilling efforts are growing.
- **Germany:** The country has a robust policy landscape and flagship initiatives like the "DigitalPakt Alter," but disparities persist between urban and rural regions and among different socioeconomic groups.
- **Cyprus:** This context highlights the need for culturally tailored interventions and regional sensitivity to infrastructure gaps, with a strong emphasis on family and spiritual engagement.
- **Belgium:** Belgium stands out for its well-developed digital health infrastructure and coordinated public policies that support user-centered co-design and the integration of digital tools with social networks.

The findings support prior research emphasizing that psychological well-being and perceived purpose are crucial determinants of active ageing (Ryff, 1989; Steptoe et al., 2015). Countries with robust community-based programs, such as Portugal's Ageing@Coimbra and Germany's DigitalPakt Alter, demonstrate stronger alignment with ikigai principles. These cases suggest that purpose-driven ageing can be promoted through inclusive, localized digital health interventions (Marston et al., 2020).

Moreover, the role of technology as an enabler, rather than a replacement, for human connection was evident in several national case studies. This reflects critiques of techno-solutionism and highlights the importance of co-creation, storytelling, and intergenerational dialogue (Neven & Peine, 2017). For example, projects such as Nonni Digitali in Italy and Simbioza in Slovenia demonstrate how digital tools can reinforce rather than undermine human-centered values in ageing.

The discussion also raises broader implications for European health policy. While frameworks such as the WHO Decade of Healthy Ageing promote integrated approaches, practical implementation still faces fragmentation at the local level (WHO, 2020). The ikigai paradigm offers a heuristic that may help unify biomedical, psychological, and sociocultural aspects of ageing strategies.

Ultimately, the findings suggest that ikigai is not merely a cultural curiosity but a potentially transformative concept for rethinking healthy ageing. The Ikigai Play framework (Figure 20), grounded in local realities, offers a framework that can help unify biomedical, psychological, and sociocultural aspects of ageing strategies. When tailored to context and embedded in community innovation, it offers a foundation for more meaningful and humanized digital health ecosystems, inviting each country to cultivate purpose through digital inclusion, civic design, and psychosocial resilience. When tailored to context and embedded in community innovation, it offers a foundation for more meaningful and humanized digital health ecosystems.

The Ikigai Play Framework

The insights from the country reviews confirm that a humanistic, integrative model is needed to address these local realities. In response, this chapter introduces the concept of Ikigai Play as an integrative and transdisciplinary framework for promoting healthy, active, and meaningful ageing in the digital era. Drawing from country-specific literature across eight European nations and grounded in psychosocial theory, 'Ikigai Play' advances a model where ageing well is tied to life purpose, digital empowerment, civic engagement, and equitable access to health technologies.

The framework is composed of four core pillars:

- **Digital Inclusion**: Older adults require not only access to devices and connectivity, but also tools tailored to their preferences, limitations, and learning styles. Digital literacy efforts must move beyond traditional training to include co-design and human-centered development.
- **Health and Well-being**: Digital health (eHealth/mHealth) must integrate mental and emotional dimensions, emphasizing prevention, autonomy, and usability across socioeconomic strata.
- **Citizenship and Participation**: Ageing populations must be included as rights-bearing contributors in policymaking, digital innovation, and knowledge production. Their involvement ensures more ethical, relevant, and sustainable outcomes.
- **Psychosocial Resilience and Purpose**: The ikigai concept enables a humanistic view of ageing—focusing on meaning, connection, and self-worth as primary health outcomes.

Together, these dimensions shape Ikigai Play, a vision of ageing where purpose, participation, and technology converge. The model challenges current silos in health, digital strategy, and social inclusion by proposing an integrated approach rooted in equity, dignity, and motivation.

Ultimately, the findings suggest that ikigai is not merely a cultural curiosity but a potentially transformative concept for rethinking healthy ageing. The Ikigai Play framework, grounded in local realities, offers a framework that can help unify biomedical, psychological, and sociocultural aspects of ageing strategies. When tailored to context and embedded in community innovation, it offers a foundation for more meaningful and humanized digital health ecosystems, inviting each country to cultivate purpose through digital inclusion, civic design, and psychosocial resilience.

6. LIMITATIONS AND FUTURE RESEARCH DIRECTIONS

6.1 Limitations of the Study

This chapter, grounded in a meta-narrative review for the SmartAgeCare project, provides a comprehensive conceptual framework but is subject to methodological and conceptual limitations:

The inclusion criterion of a 10-year publication window (2015–2025) is broad for the field of Digital Health. Given the rapid pace of technological change and the profound acceleration of digital adoption post-2020, data from the earlier part of the decade may reflect outdated digital contexts, policies, and literacy rates, potentially limiting the immediate currency of findings related to eHealth and digital equity.

To meet the transdisciplinary goals, the review placed no restrictions on document type (including reports and policy documents), thereby introducing heterogeneity in the evidence. While necessary for contextual breadth (European Citizenship axis), the synthesis relies on data with varying levels of methodological rigour, compared to evidence sourced exclusively from highly indexed, peer-reviewed databases. Furthermore, the search strategy was affected by inconsistencies across partner countries (e.g., limitations of Semantic Scholar; uneven use of national databases), potentially resulting in asymmetrical depth in the national literature profiles.

The core empirical evidence for the psychosocial benefits of Ikigai, as acknowledged in the review, is sourced mainly from the Japanese cultural context. Although the chapter proposes a culturally sensitive adaptation, the transferability and precise interpretation of Ikigai across the highly diverse social and political landscapes of Europe (Mediterranean, Central/Eastern, Northern) remain conceptual challenges requiring future empirical validation.

The primary contribution of this chapter is the conceptual model, 'Ikigai Play,' which is grounded in synthesis rather than primary data collection or empirical validation. Consequently, the synthesised relationships among the three core axes (meaning/Ikigai, digital equity, and citizenship) constitute theoretical integrations that require comprehensive testing through mixed-methods and longitudinal studies to confirm their efficacy in developing training programs.

6.2 Future Research Directions

To consolidate the conceptual and empirical advances proposed in this chapter, several future research directions should be prioritized. The exploration of ikigai as a framework for digital health and active ageing opens promising avenues for interdisciplinary inquiry. Future research should focus on empirically validating the impact of ikigai-oriented interventions on physical health, psychological well-being, and social inclusion across diverse ageing populations (Kumano, 2018; Schnell, 2020). Cross-cultural studies are particularly necessary to understand how ikigai is interpreted and enacted in various European contexts. While Japanese origins provide a strong conceptual foundation, adaptations must be sensitive to local values, identities, and socio-political conditions (Mathews, 1996; Gordon, 2022). Such comparative research could inform culturally competent policy and program development. Further investigation is needed into the role of digital storytelling, intergenerational platforms, and participatory design in enhancing purpose among older adults. These methods may offer innovative ways to translate ikigai principles into practice (Marston et al., 2020; Neven & Peine, 2017). Lastly, future studies should evaluate long-term outcomes of ikigai-based interventions, including metrics related to quality of life, healthcare usage, and civic engagement. Mixed-method and longitudinal designs would provide deeper insights into how ikigai contributes to sustainable and inclusive ageing models within Europe.

The following research directions should be prioritized:

- **Comparative longitudinal studies** across EU member states that measure changes in digital health access, purpose-driven well-being, and civic participation among older adults.
- **Development and validation of ikigai-based interventions**, including mobile apps, social prescribing models, and culturally adapted digital content aimed at enhancing meaning and mental health.
- **Evaluations of co-design methodologies** that engage older adults in the development of smart health systems, ensuring that age-friendly technologies reflect their life experience and capabilities.
- **Policy research on digital equity**, analyzing how public infrastructure, subsidies, and education policy support or hinder inclusive digital ageing.
- **Cross-cultural adaptation of the ikigai model,** exploring its resonance in Mediterranean, Central/Eastern European, and Northern contexts to define common ground and divergent values.

Research in this space must go beyond measuring deficits and instead center older people as agents of change, wisdom, and innovation. The Ikigai Play model offers not only a research lens but also an agenda for policy and practice that dignifies ageing as an active, connected, and purposeful life stage.

7. CONCLUSION

This chapter has explored the potential of the ikigai paradigm as a holistic and culturally resonant framework for advancing healthy and active ageing in Europe. By synthesizing evidence across diverse national contexts, the findings suggest that ikigai can enrich existing models of digital health, community engagement, and purpose-driven policy (Kumano, 2018; Marston et al., 2020).

Key themes that emerged include the importance of intergenerational connectivity, the value of local digital storytelling projects, and the need for inclusive co-design in technology development. These approaches align with contemporary calls for more person-centered and participatory paradigms in ageing research (Neven & Peine, 2017; WHO, 2020).

Importantly, the ikigai model invites a shift away from deficit-based narratives of ageing toward an emphasis on meaning, dignity, and lifelong potential. Future digital innovation in ageing must build upon this foundation, incorporating both technological and humanistic dimensions to support resilient and inclusive ageing societies.

As Europe continues to grapple with demographic transitions, the ikigai paradigm offers a timely and adaptable lens to promote well-being, equity, and flourishing in later life.

Our study proposed a new way to frame ageing in Europe: not simply as a challenge to be managed, but as an opportunity to empower older citizens to lead lives filled with purpose, connection, and health. Based on a meta-narrative review conducted through the SmartAgeCare project, we identified disparities and innovations across eight countries in areas of digital access, health outcomes, civic engagement, and psychological well-being.

Ikigai Play offers a conceptual framework to unify diverse efforts across sectors, highlighting that successful ageing is not only about preventing disease, but also about cultivating meaning, agency, and community belonging in later life. Digital health tools, participatory governance, and purpose-centered interventions must be designed inclusively, embracing the diversity of ageing experiences in Europe.

To move forward, researchers and policymakers must reframe technology not as a solution imposed on older people, but as a set of co-created tools that empower them. Embedding Ikigai as a guiding paradigm offers the potential to build more inclusive, joyful, and equitable futures for ageing societies.

ACKNOWLEDGMENTS

Research has been conducted within the ambit of the project "SmartAgeCare" Cofunded by the ERASMUS+ KA220-ADU – Cooperation for innovation and the exchange of good practices – Capacity Building in the field of Higher Education (2023-1-PT01-KA220-ADU-000166402 - S05597-202307)

This work was funded by Fundação para a Ciência e Tecnologia (FCT), under HEI-Lab R&D Unit (UIDB/05380/2020, https://doi.org/10.54499/UIDB/05380/2020).

The authors acknowledge the use of OpenAI's ChatGPT-4 (March 14 version) and Google's Gemini for assistance with refining the language and grammar of this manuscript. The authors reviewed and edited the content as needed and took full responsibility for the final publication.

REFERENCES

Barros, P. P., Machado, S. R., & Simões, J. A. (2020). Portugal: Health system review. *Health Systems in Transition*, *22*(2), 1–122. PMID: 22222781

Bente, B. E., Van Dongen, A., Verdaasdonk, R., & van Gemert-Pijnen, L. (2024). eHealth implementation in Europe: A scoping review on legal, ethical, financial, and technological aspects. *Frontiers in Digital Health*, *6*, 1332707. DOI: 10.3389/fdgth.2024.1332707 PMID: 38524249

Bıçakçı, A. S. (2024). Digital Europe Program: Nurturing Technological Sovereignty for a Resilient European Digital Ecosphere. *Ankara Avrupa Çalışmaları Dergisi, 23*(Özel Sayı-Future of Europe: Reflections from Türkiye), 135–174. https://doi.org/DOI: 10.32450/aacd.1439811

BMFSFJ. (2020). *DigitalPakt Alter*. Federal Ministry for Family Affairs, Senior Citizens, Women and Youth.

Bousquet, J., Bewick, M., Cano, A., Eklund, P., Fico, G., Goswami, N., Guldemond, N. A., Henderson, D., Hinkema, M. J., Liotta, G., Mair, A., Molloy, W., Monaco, A., Monsonis-Paya, I., Nizinska, A., Papadopoulos, H., Pavlickova, A., Pecorelli, S., Prados-Torres, A., & de Oliveira-Alves, B. (2017). Building bridges for innovation in ageing: Synergies between action groups of the EIP on AHA. *The Journal of Nutrition, Health & Aging*, *21*(1), 92–104. DOI: 10.1007/S12603-016-0803-1 PMID: 27999855

Bousquet, J., Kuh, D., Bewick, M., Standberg, T., Farrell, J., Pengelly, R., Joel, M. E., Rodriguez Mañas, L., Mercier, J., Bringer, J., Camuzat, T., Bourret, R., Bedbrook, A., Kowalski, M. L., Samolinski, B., Bonini, S., Brayne, C., Michel, J. P., Venne, J., & Zins, M. (2015). Operational Definition of Active and Healthy Ageing (AHA): A Conceptual Framework. *The Journal of Nutrition, Health & Aging*, *19*(9), 955–960. DOI: 10.1007/s12603-015-0589-6 PMID: 26482699

Caravella, S., Cirillo, V., Crespi, F., Guarascio, D., & Menghini, M. (2023). The diffusion of digital skills across EU regions: Structural drivers and polarisation dynamics. *Regional Studies, Regional Science*, *10*(1), 820–844. DOI: 10.1080/21681376.2023.2265498

Cibin, R. (2023). When Sociotechnical Imaginaries Become True: Digital Transition of Public Services and Inequalities during the Pandemic. *Societies (Basel, Switzerland)*, *13*(10), 220. DOI: 10.3390/soc13100220

European Commission. (2020). The 2020 Ageing Report: Economic and Budgetary Projections for the EU Member States (2019–2070).

Falanga, R., Cebulla, A., Principi, A., & Socci, M. (2020). The Participation of Senior Citizens in Policy-Making: Patterning Initiatives in Europe. *International Journal of Environmental Research and Public Health, 18*(1), 34. DOI: 10.3390/ijerph18010034 PMID: 33374566

Foster, L., & Walker, A. (2015). Active and successful aging: A European policy perspective. *The Gerontologist, 55*(1), 83–90.

Fukuzawa, A., & Sugawara, I. (2023). Social Support and Participation as Factors Relating to Ikigai and Life Satisfaction in Lonely Older Japanese. *Ageing International, 48*(2), 465–481. DOI: 10.1007/s12126-022-09486-6

Gordon, C. (2022). The anthropology of purpose: Ikigai and cultural translation. *Journal of Cross-Cultural Studies, 33*(1), 55–72.

Gullslett, M. K., Ronchi, E., Lundberg, L., Larbi, D., Lind, K. F., Tayefi, M., Ngo, P. D., Sy, T. R., Adib, K., & Hamilton, C. (2024). Telehealth development in the WHO European region: Results from a quantitative survey and insights from Norway. *International Journal of Medical Informatics, 191*, 105558. DOI: 10.1016/j.ijmedinf.2024.105558 PMID: 39084085

ISTAT. (2021). *Italy's demographic trends and projections.* Italian National Institute of Statistics.

Jose, A., Sasseville, M., Gorus, E., Giguère, A., Bourbonnais, A., Abbasgholizadeh Rahimi, S., Balley, C., Buyl, R., & Gagnon, M.-P. (2024). Existing Digital Health Technology Index Summary Report for Older Adults Living with Neurocognitive Disorders (Mild and Major) and Their Informal Caregivers: An Environmental Scan. *Geriatrics (Basel, Switzerland), 9*(4), 85. DOI: 10.3390/geriatrics9040085 PMID: 39051249

Kebede, A. S., Ozolins, L. L., Holst, H., & Galvin, K. (2022). Digital Engagement of Older Adults: Scoping Review. In Journal of Medical Internet Research (Vol. 24, Issue 12). JMIR Publications Inc. https://doi.org/DOI: 10.2196/40192

Kolotouchkina, O., Ripoll González, L., & Belabas, W. (2024). Smart Cities, Digital Inequalities, and the Challenge of Inclusion. *Smart Cities, 7*(6), 3355–3370. DOI: 10.3390/smartcities7060130

Kondo, N., Sembajwe, G., Kawachi, I., Van Dam, R. M., Subramanian, S. V., & Yamagata, Z. (2009). Income inequality, mortality, and self rated health: Meta-analysis of multilevel studies. *BMJ (Clinical Research Ed.)*, •••, 339.

Kouta, C., & Kaite, C. (2011). Spirituality and ageing in Cyprus: A qualitative study. *Journal of Religion and Health, 50*(4), 869–878.

Kumano, M. (2018). On the concept of ikigai: A psychosocial perspective. *The Japanese Psychological Research, 60*(4), 205–217.

Liotta, G., Canhao, H., Cenko, F., Cutini, R., Vellone, E., Illario, M., Kardas, P., Poscia, A., Sousa, R. D., Palombi, L., & Marazzi, M. C. (2018). Active Ageing in Europe: Adding Healthy Life to Years. *Frontiers in medicine, 5*, 123. DOI: 10.3389/fmed.2018.00123 PMID: 29780804

Loureiro, A., Brites, R., & Domingues, M. (2021). Ageing and digital participation: A case study of Portuguese older adults. *Gerontechnology (Valkenswaard)*, *20*(2), 100–108.

Marston, H. R., & Van Hoof, J. (2019). "Who doesn't think about technology when designing urban environments for older people?" A case study approach to a proposed extension of the WHO's age-friendly cities model. *International Journal of Environmental Research and Public Health*, *16*(19), 3525.

Marston, H. R., Musselwhite, C., & Hadley, R. (2020). Active ageing and the role of technology: A critical review. *The Gerontologist*, *60*(7), e294–e305.

Mathews, G. (1996). *What makes life worth living? How Japanese and Americans make sense of their worlds*. University of California Press.

Nakanishi, M. (2019). Purpose in life and health outcomes among older Japanese adults. *Aging & Mental Health*, *23*(8), 1010–1016. DOI: 10.1080/13607863.2018.1471587

Neven, L., & Peine, A. (2017). From triple win to triple sin: How a problematization approach can help re-imagine care technology innovation. *Technological Forecasting and Social Change*, *118*, 153–160.

Odone, A., Buttigieg, S., Ricciardi, W., Azzopardi-Muscat, N., & Staines, A. (2019). Public health digitalization in Europe. *European Journal of Public Health*, *29*(Supplement_3), 28–35. DOI: 10.1093/eurpub/ckz161 PMID: 31738441

OECD. (2021). [OECD Publishing.]. *Health at a Glance. Europe*, •••, 2021.

Ryff, C. D. (1989). Happiness is everything, or is it? Explorations on the meaning of psychological well-being. *Journal of Personality and Social Psychology*, *57*(6), 1069–1081.

Ryff, C. D., & Keyes, C. L. M. (1995). The structure of psychological well-being revisited. *Journal of Personality and Social Psychology*, *69*(4), 719.

Santoni, G., Marengoni, A., & Calderón-Larrañaga, A.. (2015). Defining health trajectories in older adults with multimorbidity. *BMC Geriatrics*, *15*, 1–10.

Schnell, T. (2020). *The psychology of meaning in life*. Routledge.

Spargo, M., Goodfellow, N., Scullin, C., Grigoleit, S., Andreou, A., Mavromoustakis, C. X., Guerra, B., Manso, M., Larburu, N., Villacañas, Ó., Fleming, G., & Scott, M. (2021). Shaping the Future of Digitally Enabled Health and Care. *Pharmacy (Basel, Switzerland)*, *9*(1), 17. DOI: 10.3390/pharmacy9010017 PMID: 33445509

Steptoe, A., Deaton, A., & Stone, A. A. (2015). Subjective wellbeing, health, and ageing. *Lancet*, *385*(9968), 640–648. PMID: 25468152

Steptoe, A., & Fancourt, D. (2019). Older adults' electronic media use and loneliness: Time trends and associations, 2012–18. *EClinicalMedicine*, *9*, 42–49. DOI: 10.1016/j.eclinm.2019.08.015

Terraneo, M. (2015, February). Inequities in health care utilization by people aged 50+: Evidence from 12 European countries. *Social Science & Medicine*, *126*, 154–163. DOI: 10.1016/j.socscimed.2014.12.028 PMID: 25562311

Theodoulou-Loizidou, M., Polycarpou, A., & Stylianou, A. (2020). Digital inclusion and older adults in Cyprus. *European Journal of Ageing Studies*, *9*(1), 22–34.

Thomas, J., & Harden, A. (2008). Methods for the thematic synthesis of qualitative research in systematic reviews. *BMC Medical Research Methodology*, *8*(1), 45.

von Eitzen, S., Schroeder, K., & Braun, A. (2021). Community-based ageing and digital inclusion in Germany. *Social Policy and Administration*, *55*(3), 394–409.

WHO. (2020). *Decade of Healthy Ageing: 2020–2030.* World Health Organization.

World Medical Association. (2013). World Medical Association Declaration of Helsinki: Ethical principles for medical research involving human subjects. *Journal of the American Medical Association*, *310*(20), 2191–2194. DOI: 10.1001/jama.2013.281053 PMID: 24141714

Yesavage, J. A., Brink, T. L., Rose, T. L., Lum, O., Huang, V., Adey, M., & Leirer, V. O. (1982). Development and validation of a geriatric depression screening scale: A preliminary report. *Journal of Psychiatric Research*, *17*(1), 37–49.

KEY TERMS AND DEFINITIONS

Ikigai: A Japanese term loosely translated as "a reason for being." It represents the intersection of personal fulfillment, life purpose, community engagement, and a sense of meaning that drives daily activities and contributes to long-term well-being.

Ikigai Play: A novel, transdisciplinary conceptual framework proposed in this chapter that integrates the psychosocial pursuit of meaning (Ikigai) with the challenges of digital equity, active health, and European citizenship among older adults.

Digital Health Equity: The fair and inclusive access to, and meaningful use of, health technologies (e.g., eHealth, mHealth) regardless of an individual's age, socioeconomic status, location, or digital literacy level.

Active European Citizenship: In the context of ageing, this refers to the meaningful engagement of older adults in social, cultural, and political life—including intergenerational solidarity and active participation in digital decision-making and services—contributing to both personal purpose and democratic vitality.

Health & Active Ageing (HAA): As defined by the WHO, it is the process of developing and maintaining the functional ability that enables well-being in older age, emphasizing autonomy, participation, and functional capacity rather than just the absence of disease.

Healthy Life Years (HLY): A key European Union indicator that measures the expected number of years a person will live free from disability or chronic illness. It serves as a metric for the success of active aging and public health strategies.

Chapter 9
Transforming Healthcare Delivery:
The Role of Digital Technologies in Disease Prevention and Health Monitoring

Vishal Kumar
https://orcid.org/0009-0001-7600-0600
GD Goenka University, India

Prateek Jain
https://orcid.org/0000-0002-6410-9713
GD Goenka University, India

ABSTRACT

Digital health technologies are reshaping healthcare by improving disease prevention, early diagnosis, and continuous health monitoring. This chapter delves into the expanding role of digital tools—from e-health and telemedicine to AI and ML—in advancing preventive healthcare. It emphasizes the use of wearable devices and biosensors for real-time monitoring, empowering both patients and providers to detect early health risks. The shift to AI-powered systems enables personalized care, automated diagnostics, and proactive engagement, but also raises concerns around data privacy, ethical use, adoption challenges, and equity in access—especially in underserved regions. Through global case studies, the chapter highlights successful digital health interventions and explores future directions, including digital integration in national health policies, regulation, and literacy. It also examines trends like virtual care, remote monitoring, and AI-linked EHRs, offering insights into how digital health can foster a more inclusive, responsive, and future-ready healthcare system.

1. INTRODUCTION

1.1 AI with Healthcare

In the healthcare industry, artificial intelligence (AI) has revolutionized patient monitoring, diagnosis, and treatment. With more precise diagnoses and more individualized treatments made possible, it

DOI: 10.4018/979-8-3373-3531-5.ch009

is significantly enhancing healthcare research and results. Because AI can swiftly scan large volumes of clinical data, it assists healthcare workers in spotting trends and illness signs that could otherwise go unnoticed. AI and healthcare have a wide range of possible uses, from predictive results from electronic health records to early detection using radiological image scanning. Millions of people all over the world might get care more intelligently, quickly, and efficiently if medical facilities use artificial intelligence in hospitals and clinics. The future of healthcare is clearly looking to artificial intelligence that will enhance patient outcomes, slash costs for providers, and change the manner in which patients obtain high-quality treatment (Mahmud & Riley, 2021).

In several fields, particularly healthcare, artificial intelligence (AI) has become a more reliable and valuable tool. Physicians' practices could be improved by it by enabling better organization and efficiency that would improve patient care and outcomes. AI may help patients gain better access to care, which should lead to improved follow-up and patient satisfaction.

Artificial intelligence (AI), supported by timely and accurate data and evidence, has the potential to transform health care delivery by improving health outcomes, patient safety, and the affordability and accessibility of high-quality care. AI integration is critical to building an infrastructure capable of caring for an increasingly aging population, utilizing an ever-increasing knowledge of disease and options for precision treatments, and combatting workforce shortages and burnout of medical professionals (Abernethy et al., 2022) (Akpakwu, 2018).

The integration of Artificial Intelligence (AI) in healthcare has emerged as a transformative force, reshaping the way medical professionals diagnose diseases, develop treatment plans, and manage healthcare systems. AI-driven technologies, including machine learning (ML), deep learning (DL), natural language processing (NLP), and robotics, are paving the way for enhanced accuracy, efficiency, and personalized care. As global healthcare systems strive to improve patient outcomes, reduce costs, and optimize workflows, AI is playing a crucial role in addressing the challenges of modern medicine. With the rapid advancement of AI algorithms and the availability of vast medical datasets, AI-powered solutions are revolutionizing fields such as medical imaging, drug discovery, robotic surgery, predictive analytics, virtual health assistants, and patient management. From early disease detection and risk assessment to automated administrative processes, AI offers immense potential to improve the overall quality of healthcare services (Ma & Vervoort, 2020).

The opportunities of AI in healthcare extend beyond diagnosis and treatment; they also include public health monitoring, personalized medicine, and healthcare accessibility in remote areas. AI-driven predictive models are being used to foresee potential health crises, enabling proactive interventions.

Similarly, AI chatbots and virtual assistants are assisting patients with routine medical inquiries, reducing the burden on healthcare professionals. However, while AI offers numerous advantages, its implementation in healthcare presents challenges, including ethical considerations, data privacy concerns, regulatory compliance, and the need for human-AI collaboration. Ensuring bias-free AI models, maintaining patient confidentiality, and integrating AI seamlessly into existing healthcare infrastructures are critical factors that must be addressed to maximize its benefits. This article explores the opportunities, roles, and implementation strategies of AI in healthcare, shedding light on its transformative potential while also discussing the hurdles that need to be overcome. As AI continues to evolve, its responsible and strategic deployment will be crucial in shaping the future of medicine and healthcare delivery worldwide (Mannucci E, Silverii GA, et al., 2020).

AI applications in healthcare can be classified to the following domains: surgery, nursing assistant, medical consultation, administration and workflow, treatment design, cyber security, machine vision, automatic and preliminary diagnosis, health monitoring, medication management, and clinical trials. All these domains have applications utilizing AI in their operations. The authors focused on quantitative studies wherein they collected some services using AI with a high impact on care outcomes and proposed a collection of services that could provide the best outcomes in preventive healthcare and in clinical work.

1.2 Digital Healthcare

Digital health has the potential to revolutionize the way healthcare is delivered, particularly in resource-limited settings. The WHO has outlined the potential benefits of digital health, including increased access to healthcare, improved quality and safety of healthcare, and increased efficiency in healthcare delivery. However, it is important to address the challenges and ethical considerations associated with the implementation of digital health solutions. These challenges include issues related to data security and privacy, the digital divide, and the need for adequate regulation (Falzon D, et al. 2016).

Figure 1. Digital Healthcare

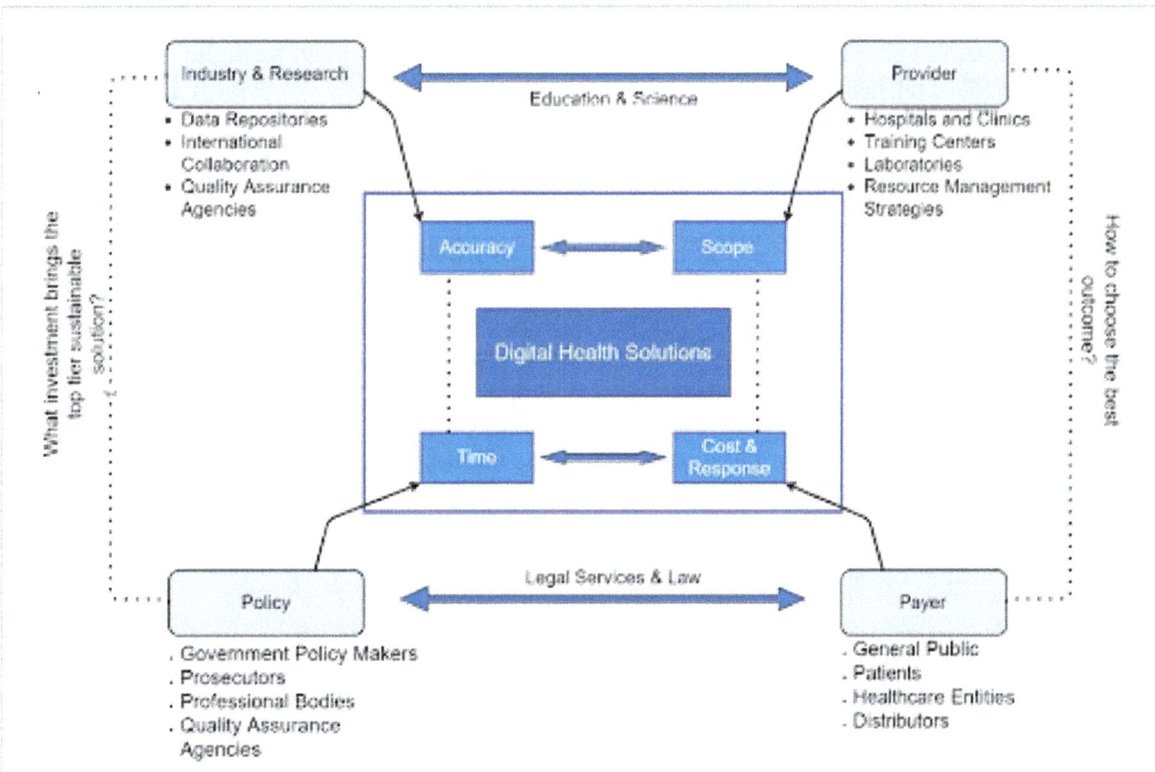

Figure 1 shows a conceptual demonstration of a remote monitoring system that uses wearable sensors to collect data on the wearer's physiological indicators and monitor the patient's condition in real time. The patient's data is passed on to the mobile device through wireless communication, and then the data is passed to the remote center via the Internet. When the system detects a patient's sudden condition, such as a fall, it sends an alert message to the emergency service center to provide timely assistance to

the patient. In an emergency, the data-linked family members and caregivers are also alerted to each other, notifying the relevant personnel of the patient's status.

2. LITERATURE REVIEW

Digital health technologies are reshaping healthcare delivery globally, particularly in disease prevention, early diagnosis, and real-time health monitoring. Recent studies indicate that e-health platforms, telemedicine systems, wearable devices, biosensors, artificial intelligence (AI), and machine learning (ML) have shifted healthcare from reactive treatment toward proactive and preventive approaches (Vishal et al., 2022). In this digital transformation, patients are becoming more empowered, actively engaging in their own health management through mobile health apps and AI-driven personalized recommendations (Sharma et al., 2023).

Multiple research works have highlighted that the adoption and acceptance of such technologies depend not only on technical capability, but also on human, behavioural, psychological, and organisational factors. For this reason, the Technology Acceptance Model (TAM) has been widely used to understand end-user behaviour regarding digital health solutions (Davis, 1989). TAM argues that Perceived Usefulness (PU) and Perceived Ease of Use (PEOU) significantly influence acceptance behavior for digital health systems, including wearables, telehealth platforms, and electronic medical records (Venkatesh & Davis, 2000). In the healthcare domain, studies confirm that PU and PEOU remain dominant predictors of technology adoption both for patients and healthcare professionals (Gagnon et al., 2010; Strudwick, 2015).

Although TAM is widely used, recent studies argue that digital health adoption requires consideration of external factors, such as privacy concerns, data protection, digital literacy, and social influence, especially in low-resource settings where the digital divide persists (Ahlan & Isma'eel, 2014; Garavand et al., 2016). In disease prevention and monitoring, wearable biosensors and AI-enabled dashboards have demonstrated significant potential. Still, ethical and access issues remain challenges that must be addressed through robust data governance and policy support (Vishal et al., 2024).

Therefore, literature clearly suggests that digital technology-enabled prevention systems can improve healthcare outcomes and reduce cost burden. Still, successful implementation depends equally on technological innovation and user-centred adoption frameworks. This literature also highlights the need for continued research that integrates TAM theory with digital health policy, cybersecurity, equity, and data ethics to build sustainable and inclusive healthcare ecosystems.

3. ROLE OF WEARABLE DEVICES & BIOSENSORS FOR HEALTH MONITORING

Artificial Intelligence (AI) has revolutionized healthcare by bringing about advancements in patient monitoring, personalized treatment plans, diagnostics, and healthcare administration. AI-driven technologies, including machine learning (ML), deep learning (DL), natural language processing (NLP), and predictive analytics, are being integrated into healthcare systems, which are changing to become more accurate, efficient, and data-driven. Medical decision-making, resource optimization, and early disease detection are all aided by AI's ability to process enormous volumes of data rapidly.(Hill C, Martin J, Thomson S, et al. 2017)

3.1 Biosensors: Revolutionizing Health Monitoring

Biosensors are devices designed to detect and measure biological signals, often integrated into wearables or standalone devices. These sensors continuously monitor specific biomarkers in the body, such as glucose levels, blood pressure, saliva content, or cortisol levels. AI plays an essential role in improving the accuracy and efficiency of biosensors, thus enhancing health management and disease prediction. One of the key contributions of AI in biosensors is real-time data processing. AI algorithms analyze data from biosensors as it is generated, identifying any abnormalities in biomarker levels. For example, AI is integral in continuous glucose monitoring systems, which are vital for individuals with diabetes, providing actionable insights to help regulate blood sugar levels. AI also enables predictive analytics by examining historical data from biosensors to forecast potential health risks.

Table 1. Types of Biosensors

Sensor Name	Description	Uses	Impact with AI on Healthcare
Disease Detection Biosensors	Sensors designed to detect the presence of specific disease biomarkers.	Early detection of diseases like cancer, infections, and metabolic disorders.	AI helps identify patterns in biomarker data, improving early diagnosis accuracy and enabling predictive healthcare.
Retinal Prostheses	Biosensors interfacing with retinal cells to restore partial vision.	Treatment of vision loss due to retinal diseases like retinitis pigmentosa.	AI optimizes image processing for better visual experiences, enhances adaptive response to different lighting conditions.
Enzyme Biosensors	Sensors that detect biological reactions involving enzymes.	Monitoring glucose in diabetes, detecting pathogens or toxins.	AI enhances real-time monitoring and predictive alerts for conditions like diabetes and infections.
Phenotypic Diagnostics for Cancer	Biosensors analyzing cellular phenotypes to detect cancer.	Early cancer detection and classification.	AI analyzes complex phenotype patterns to distinguish cancer types faster and more accurately than manual methods.
Rapid DNA and RNA Diagnostics	Sensors that detect DNA and RNA sequences for disease identification.	Quick genetic testing for infections, hereditary diseases, and cancer.	AI accelerates genomic analysis, improving the speed and precision of diagnoses and personalized treatment planning.
Medical Mycology Biosensors	Sensors designed to detect fungal pathogens.	Diagnosis of fungal infections(e.g.,candidiasis, aspergillosis).	AI aids in differentiating fungal infections from bacterial/viral ones, leading to faster, targeted treatments.
Optical DNA Diagnostic Biosensors	Optical sensors detecting DNA changes.	Detection of genetic mutations and hereditary diseases.	AI interprets optical signals faster, improving genetic disorder diagnosis and enabling tailored therapies.
Heart Disease Diagnosis Biosensors	Sensors that monitor cardiovascular health indicators.	Detection of heart diseases like arrhythmias,heart attacks.	AI predicts cardiovascular events by analyzing heart patterns, allowing preventive actions and reducing hospitalizations.

continued on following page

Table 1. Continued

Sensor Name	Description	Uses	Impact with AI on Healthcare
Overall Health Monitoring Biosensors	General biosensors tracking vital health metrics(e.g.,temperature, heart rate).	Continuous health status monitoring for wellness and disease prevention.	AI aggregates multi-sensor data to provide real-time alerts, health trend predictions, and personalized healthcare insights.
MRI Contrast Imaging Biosensors	Biosensors used to enhance MRI imaging quality.	Better imaging for tumor detection, brain scans, and internal injuries.	AI improves image reconstruction and interpretation, leading to more accurate diagnostics and early disease discovery.

3.2 Clinical applications are just one aspect of AI's role in healthcare

other areas include drug development, public health monitoring, healthcare administration, and operational efficiency. AI improves the capacity to anticipate disease outbreaks, optimize hospital operations, and enhance patient interaction through chatbots and virtual assistants. Though AI has many advantages, there are also significant obstacles to its use in healthcare, including concerns about data privacy, ethical dilemmas, legal restrictions, and a lack of trust between AI and medical practitioners.

3.3 Enhancing Medical Decision-Making

Because AI can analyze large datasets and give healthcare practitioners evidence-based recommendations, it is greatly enhancing medical decision-making. AI models support the optimization of treatment regimens, the prediction of patient outcomes, and the identification of illness trends. Doctors can diagnose patients more quickly and accurately because AI can process complex medical data and generate actionable insights. The possibility of medical errors is also decreased and patient outcomes are improved with AI-driven Clinical Decision Support Systems (CDSS), which allow physicians to evaluate treatment alternatives based on genetic information, historical patient data, and predictive analytics.

Figure 2. Clinical Decision Support System

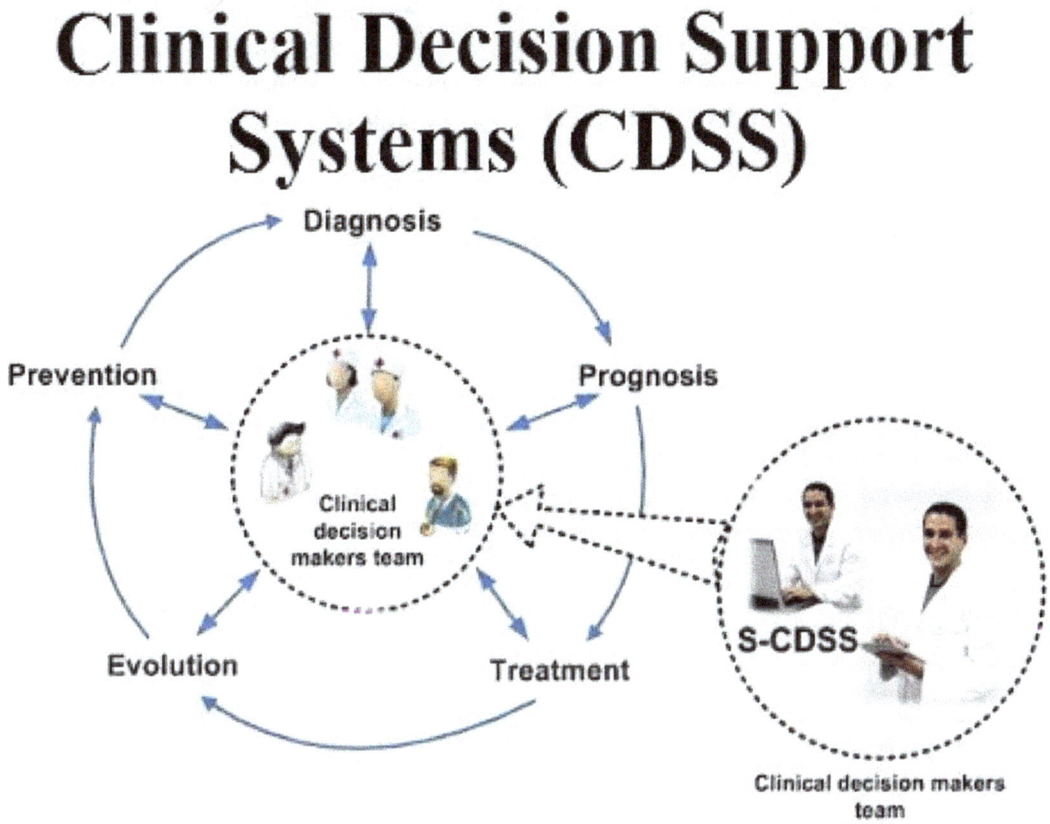

3.4 Advancing Precision Medicine and Personalized Healthcare

Through the customization of medicines according to each patient's genetic profile, lifestyle, and medical history, artificial intelligence is transforming precision medicine. While traditional treatment methods frequently take a generic approach, artificial intelligence (AI) enables individualized healthcare by forecasting a patient's reaction to particular drugs and treatments. By reducing adverse drug responses and increasing treatment efficacy, this results in safer and more efficient care. AI-enabled genomic analysis enables researchers to identify genetic markers linked to illnesses, opening the door to targeted treatments and early disease diagnosis for conditions including cancer, heart disease, and neurological disorders.

3.5 Improving Healthcare Efficiency and Administration

Beyond therapeutic uses, artificial intelligence is essential to healthcare management and operational effectiveness. AI-driven automation frees up healthcare personnel to concentrate more on patient care by easing the workload associated with manual recordkeeping, appointment scheduling, and resource allocation. By automating data entry, summarising clinical notes, and detecting potential medical errors, artificial intelligence (AI) improves the management of Electronic Health Records (EHRs). Virtual assistants and chatbots driven by AI also assist in managing patient relations, responding to medical questions, and offering round-the-clock assistance with appointment scheduling and prescription reminders. Hospitals and clinics may decrease administrative workloads and increase patient engagement with these AI-driven solutions.

3.6 AI in Public Health and Epidemiology

In order to monitor disease outbreaks, forecast epidemiological trends, and enhance pandemic response plans, artificial intelligence (AI) is processing enormous volumes of data. The COVID-19 pandemic saw widespread use of AI-powered models to forecast virus transmission, evaluate risk variables, and maximize vaccination, delivery. AI is also useful for tracking trends in population health, evaluating environmental influences on public health, and spotting new illness trends. AI-driven epidemiological models enable governments and healthcare institutions to better prevent and manage infectious diseases through proactive approaches.

Figure 3. role of AI in healthcare

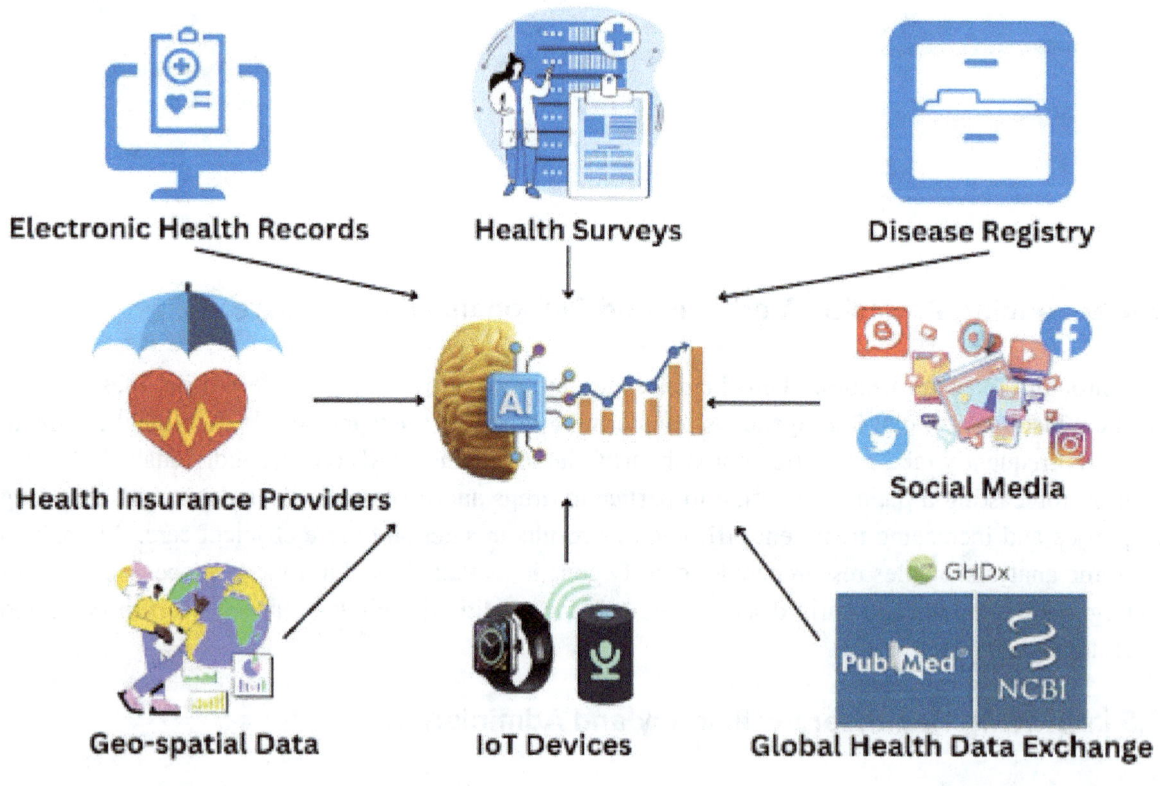

3.7 Wearable Devices in Healthcare:

Wearable technology has revolutionized the landscape of patient monitoring, offering a dynamic and real-time approach to healthcare.

1. Wearables enable real-time monitoring of vital signs, providing a continuous stream of data on parameters such as heart rate, blood pressure, and respiratory rate (Dias et al., 2018).
2. It facilitates remote patient monitoring, enabling healthcare providers to access real-time health data without being physically present. This capability is particularly valuable for individuals with chronic conditions, post-surgery recovery, or those requiring ongoing medical attention.
3. They also help reduce hospital readmissions by providing a seamless means of continuous monitoring post-discharge. Patients equipped with wearables can be remotely monitored for signs of deterioration or complications, enabling timely interventions and preventing unnecessary hospital visits (Rumschlag et al., 2018). (Rossi R, Socci V, Talevi D, et al. 2020).

Figure 4. Wearable Devices in Healthcare

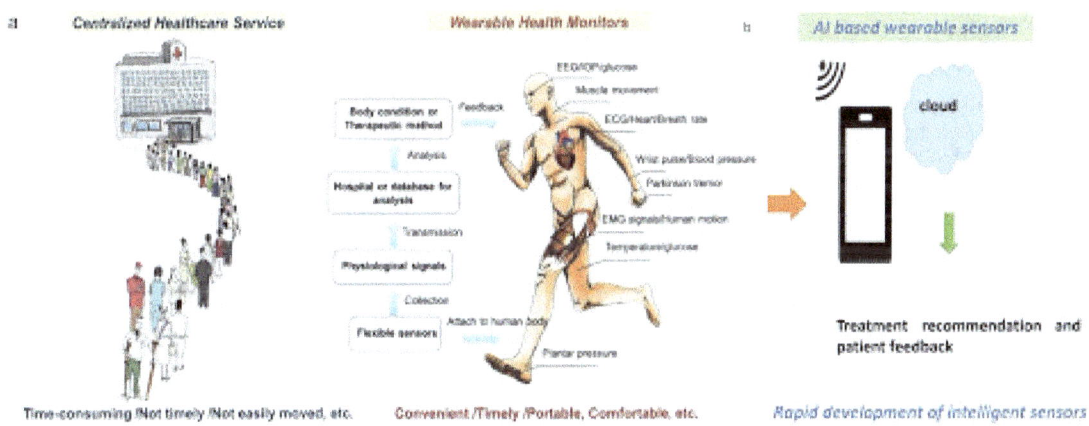

4. TRANSFORMATION FROM TRADITIONAL TO DIGITAL TECHNOLOGIES

4.1 How Digital Technologies Transform Workforce Structures, Financing Models, and Patient–Provider Dynamics

Digital technologies are fundamentally reshaping healthcare systems by transforming workforce structures, financing models, and patient–provider dynamics. The increasing adoption of artificial intelligence (AI), telemedicine, and data analytics has led to a reconfiguration of workforce roles, emphasizing interdisciplinary collaboration and digital literacy among healthcare professionals. Routine administrative tasks are increasingly automated, enabling clinicians to focus on patient-centered care and decision-making (Socha-Dietrich et al., 2021).

In terms of financing models, digital transformation promotes value-based care frameworks that reward outcomes rather than service volume. The integration of electronic health records and predictive analytics allows for better resource allocation, performance monitoring, and cost optimization (Ghosh et al., 2023). These innovations foster sustainable financial ecosystems, supporting efficiency and transparency in healthcare operations.

Furthermore, patient–provider dynamics are evolving due to the proliferation of digital platforms and remote monitoring technologies. Patients are no longer passive recipients of care but active participants who manage their health through mobile applications, wearable devices, and teleconsultations. This shift enhances patient autonomy, shared decision-making, and personalized healthcare delivery (Sætra, Fosch-Villaronga,et al. 2021).

Collectively, these transformations demonstrate that the digital revolution in healthcare is not merely technological but deeply strategic, redefining the relationships, roles, and resources that underpin modern health systems.

4.2 How Digital Technologies Promote Health Equity, Digital Inclusion, and Accessibility for Underserved Communities

Digital technologies play a transformative role in promoting health equity, digital inclusion, and accessibility for underserved communities. Through innovations such as telemedicine, mobile health (mHealth) platforms, and artificial intelligence-driven diagnostics, healthcare access has become more geographically and economically inclusive. These technologies bridge the gap for rural and low-income populations who traditionally face barriers to physical healthcare facilities (Alami et al., 2020).

Digital inclusion initiatives ensure that vulnerable groups—such as older adults, people with disabilities, and individuals in remote areas—can effectively use and benefit from digital health tools. Programs focusing on digital literacy, low-cost connectivity, and multilingual platforms are key enablers of inclusive healthcare systems (OECD, 2021). Furthermore, assistive technologies and accessible design frameworks empower patients with disabilities, enhancing independent living and active participation in their own care (Sharma et al., 2023).

In terms of health equity, data-driven public health systems and remote monitoring technologies facilitate early disease detection, continuous care, and equitable distribution of resources. Digital transformation thus reduces disparities by decentralizing healthcare services and fostering patient engagement across diverse populations (Mehta et al., 2022).

Overall, digital technologies act as catalysts for equitable healthcare, advancing accessibility, affordability, and inclusion for underserved communities worldwide.

5. ECONOMICAL BENEFITS OF DIGITAL TECHNOLOGIES

Detailed Economic Evaluation of Digital Technologies:

The integration of digital technologies into healthcare has been widely recognized not only for improving clinical outcomes but also for reshaping the economics of health systems. A detailed economic evaluation highlights three critical dimensions: cost-effectiveness, return on investment (ROI), and long-term financial impacts.

Cost-Effectiveness:

Digital technologies often prove cost-effective by reducing the burden of preventable diseases, hospital readmissions, and unnecessary diagnostic tests. For example, telemedicine reduces the need for travel and in-person consultations, lowering direct costs for both patients and providers. Similarly, wearable devices and remote monitoring tools help detect early symptoms of chronic diseases, allowing timely intervention and reducing expensive emergency care. Cost-effectiveness is especially pronounced in resource-constrained settings, where digital tools bridge gaps in accessibility and improve efficiency by maximizing limited healthcare resources.

Return on Investment (ROI):

Although the initial investment in digital infrastructure—such as cloud systems, data management platforms, and AI-driven analytics—can be high, the ROI is typically favorable over time. Digital technologies improve workflow efficiency, optimize resource allocation, and enhance patient engagement, all of which translate into financial savings. For instance, automated diagnostic tools powered by AI can reduce the workload on radiologists, leading to cost savings in staffing and operational expenses. ROI is also reflected in the ability of health organizations to reach larger populations with fewer resources through mobile health (mHealth) platforms and teleconsultations.

Long Term Financial Impacts:

Over the long term, digital transformation contributes to financial sustainability by shifting healthcare toward preventive care rather than costly curative interventions. Predictive analytics, powered by big data and AI, enable risk stratification and targeted interventions that can substantially reduce the incidence of high-cost chronic diseases. Moreover, digital systems improve record-keeping and data accuracy, thereby reducing financial losses from medical errors, fraud, and inefficiencies. On a macroeconomic scale, healthier populations supported by digital health innovations also contribute to higher workforce productivity and lower public health expenditures. However, the economic benefits are contingent upon effective implementation, equitable access, and the ability of systems to adapt to technological change without excessive dependence on private platforms.

Health Equity & Digital Divide

While digital technologies promise efficiency and accessibility, their uneven distribution risks widening existing healthcare inequalities. Health equity refers to the principle that all individuals should have fair access to healthcare services, regardless of socioeconomic status, geography, or digital literacy. The digital divide—the gap between those with access to digital resources and those without—poses one of the most significant barriers to achieving this equity.

Access to Infrastructure:

In high-income countries, robust digital infrastructure ensures widespread adoption of telemedicine, electronic health records, and AI-driven applications. Conversely, in low- and middle-income countries, inadequate internet penetration, unreliable electricity supply, and high device costs hinder access to digital health services. Rural and marginalized populations are disproportionately affected, reinforcing disparities in health outcomes.

Digital Literacy:

Even when digital tools are available, varying levels of digital literacy can affect their practical use. Elderly patients, for instance, often struggle with navigating mobile health applications or wearable devices. Lack of training and support creates exclusion, limiting the benefits of digital transformation to younger, more technologically adept populations.

Affordability:

The cost of digital health services and devices can act as another barrier. Subscription fees, data costs, or the price of wearable sensors may be prohibitive for low-income groups. Without targeted subsidies or public programs, digital healthcare risks becoming a privilege for the affluent rather than a universal solution.

Cultural and Language Barriers:

Health technologies often fail to address cultural diversity or language differences. Applications designed in dominant languages may not be accessible to minority groups, creating further inequities in usage.

Policy Implications:

To close the digital divide, policymakers must invest in digital infrastructure, provide subsidies for devices and services, and implement inclusive training programs. Public–private partnerships can help scale affordable digital solutions, while regulatory frameworks should ensure equitable distribution of technological resources. Addressing the digital divide is not only an ethical imperative but also essential for realizing the full potential of digital transformation in healthcare.

5.1 Emerging system risks of digital transformation such as e waste, data ownership or dependence on private platforms

Emerging System Risks of Digital Transformation

The rapid shift toward digital transformation in healthcare and other sectors has introduced new systemic risks that require careful consideration. While digital tools enhance efficiency, accessibility, and innovation, they also create vulnerabilities that may compromise sustainability, equity, and trust in modern systems. Some of the key risks include:

- **E-Waste:**

The accelerated deployment of digital devices—ranging from smartphones and tablets to medical sensors, diagnostic equipment, and data servers—has significantly increased the volume of electronic waste. Many of these devices have short lifespans due to rapid technological advancements and planned obsolescence. Improper disposal of e-waste can release toxic substances, threatening ecosystems and human health. Without strong recycling infrastructures, digital healthcare risks contributing to long-term environmental degradation.

- **Data Ownership and Privacy:**

The widespread use of digital health platforms generates vast amounts of sensitive personal data. However, ownership and control over this data often rest with corporations or service providers rather than individuals. This raises ethical concerns about transparency, informed consent, and the commercialization of patient information. Cases of unauthorized data sharing, breaches, or misuse highlight the urgent need for stronger governance frameworks to safeguard privacy and empower individuals to retain ownership of their digital identities.

- **Dependence on Private Platforms:**

Many healthcare systems and governments rely heavily on private companies for digital infrastructure, cloud services, and AI-driven analytics. This dependency creates vulnerabilities in cases where providers alter service terms, restrict interoperability, or prioritize profit motives over public interest. Moreover, monopolization by a few dominant tech companies can limit innovation, lock institutions into costly vendor contracts, and make healthcare systems dependent on external entities for continuity of essential services.

6. IMPACT OF FACTORS ON TECHNOLOGY ADOPTION

The adoption of digital health technologies is not uniform across populations and is heavily shaped by contextual factors. In low- and middle-income countries (LMICs), three interrelated determinants—**internet access, device** affordability, and digital literacy play a particularly critical role in shaping the extent and effectiveness of technology adoption.

Internet Access

Reliable and affordable internet access is the backbone of digital health adoption. In many LMICs, poor connectivity and high data costs remain key barriers. Rural and remote areas often lack adequate broadband infrastructure, limiting access to telemedicine platforms, electronic health records, or AI-driven applications. This creates uneven adoption patterns where urban populations benefit more from digital health, while rural communities remain underserved. Initiatives such as low-bandwidth applications, offline functionality, and satellite internet services can help mitigate these barriers, but widespread adoption still depends on national infrastructure investment (World Health Organization, 2022; Zhang et al., 2024).

Device Affordability

Smart phones, tablets, and wearable devices are essential tools for accessing modern digital health systems. However, in LMICs, the high cost of devices relative to average household income significantly restricts adoption. Even when mobile phones are available, they are often basic feature phones with limited internet or application capability. Affordability challenges also extend to maintenance, charging (especially in areas with unreliable electricity), and replacement costs. Public-private partnerships and subsidy programs are essential to ensure that low-income populations are not excluded from digital health innovations (GSMA, 2020)

Digital Literacy

Digital literacy—knowledge and confidence in using digital tools—directly influences technology adoption. In LMICs, low levels of digital literacy, particularly among older adults, rural populations, and women, pose significant challenges. Lack of training prevents individuals from effectively using health apps, online consultation platforms, or wearable monitoring devices. Moreover, limited awareness of data privacy and security issues may increase vulnerability to misuse or mistrust of digital systems. Programs that integrate community-based digital literacy training, multilingual support, and culturally relevant content are critical to bridging this gap (van Dijk, 2020; Ahmed et al., 2022).

Interconnected Challenges

These three factors are deeply interconnected. Without affordable devices, internet access cannot translate into meaningful use; without digital literacy, neither devices nor connectivity will result in effective adoption. Addressing them requires a holistic strategy that combines infrastructure investment, financial support, and community education (International Telecommunication Union, 2021; Chen, Y. & Huang, W., 2023).

Implications for Policy and Practice

For policymakers, prioritizing universal internet coverage, subsidized device access, and scalable digital literacy programs is key to inclusive digital health adoption. For practitioners and technology developers, creating low-cost, user-friendly, and locally adaptable digital health solutions can help ensure that innovations reach the populations who need them most (World Health Organization, 2022).

Table 2. Comparative Impact of Factors on Technology Adoption

Factor	High-Income Countries (HICs)	Low- and Middle-Income Countries (LMICs)
Internet Access	Nearly universal broadband/mobile internet; high-speed connections widely available. Main challenges include rural coverage gaps and high data consumption needs.	Limited infrastructure in rural areas, high data costs, and inconsistent service quality. Adoption often restricted to urban centers.
Device Affordability	Smartphones, wearables, and tablets widely affordable; frequent upgrades common. Subsidy programs exist for disadvantaged groups.	High cost relative to income restricts adoption. Populations rely on low-end phones or shared devices. Limited access to advanced health wearables.
Digital Literacy	High baseline digital literacy, especially among younger populations. Elderly and marginalized groups may still face challenges.	Low digital literacy rates, especially in rural communities, older adults, and women. Lack of training limits effective use of digital health tools.
Overall Impact on Technology Adoption	Widespread adoption with minor equity gaps. Policies and subsidies help address residual challenges.	Uneven adoption with significant rural-urban divide. Barriers in affordability, access, and literacy slow down large-scale integration of digital health.

7. TRENDS OF DIGITAL FIRST HEALTHCARE SYSTEM

It is important to ensure that telehealth becomes a permanent part of national healthcare systems, rather than just being used in emergency situations (Montague E, Perchonok J, et al. 2012) . This would allow for more widespread use of telehealth during epidemics. Investment in 5G technology and the development of modern communication infrastructure in developing countries can also facilitate the implementation of telehealth in these regions (Fagherazzi G, Goetzinger C, Rashid MA, et al. 2020). Digital health has evolved from simply digitizing medical records to implementing comprehensive information and communication solutions for delivering high-quality healthcare across the care continuum. Companies are using connected sensors, smartphones, diagnostic algorithms, and wearables to capture health data, provide feedback, and facilitate proactive care models (Bouabida K, Lebouché B, Pomey MP, et al 2022). Patient-centric systems that promote patient engagement are becoming more important as consumers become more empowered. Health companies and leaders should embrace new approaches presented by the emerging health ecosystem (Kaihlanen AM, Virtanen L, Buchert U, et al. 2022)

Machine Learning in Biopharma and Medtech

Starting in 2025, the pharmaceutical industry is poised to harness the full potential of artificial intelligence (AI) to accelerate drug discovery and align with emerging medical technology trends. A groundbreaking example occurred in January 2020, when scientists from the UK and Japan developed and patented the first drug molecule created entirely by AI, which was approved for human trials to treat obsessive-compulsive disorder. Today, many pioneering projects are integrating AI and machine learning to optimise chemical research and drug development processes, such as molecular modelling and simulating complex chemical reactions under variable conditions. This digital approach significantly reduces the need for costly reagents and sophisticated lab equipment by enabling virtual experimentation, thereby cutting research expenses and accelerating scientific innovation.

Automate Hospital Workflows

Robotics is transforming the healthcare sector by streamlining hospital workflows, improving efficiency, accuracy, and patient care. Technologies like robotic process automation (RPA) manage routine administrative functions such as appointment scheduling, billing, and patient intake, while physical robots support tasks like delivering medications, maintaining cleanliness, and assisting in surgeries. These innovations help reduce the likelihood of human error and allow healthcare professionals to dedicate more time to patient-centred services. Additionally, robotic systems enhance inventory control by ensuring essential supplies are replenished promptly. By automating repetitive duties, robotics boosts overall hospital performance, speeds up services, and strengthens the healthcare system's adaptability and effectiveness.

Symptom Checker Chatbots & Virtual Health Assistants

Chatbots are AI-backed computer applications (sometimes not full-blooded AI but sophisticated algorithms) that conduct human-like, meaningful conversations via voice, text, or option-based input. One trend in digital health innovation is that the concept of AI-supported chatbots or AI chat boxes extends far beyond simple symptom checking or consultation. A more advanced evolution of these online services is known as Virtual Health Assistants, sophisticated AI-powered tools designed to provide personalized healthcare support, automate patient interactions, manage medical documentation, facilitate scheduling, and enhance overall patient engagement and care coordination.

Facial Recognition with Masks

Facial recognition has emerged as a widely adopted technology in healthcare, enabling secure access for authorized medical personnel to mobile devices and computer systems. During the COVID-19 pandemic, the need for advanced facial recognition systems became even more crucial, as deep learning algorithms were required to identify staff members wearing face masks accurately. Reports indicate that certain companies have successfully developed systems capable of recognising masked individuals with up to 99.9% accuracy.

Wearables and Mobile Apps in Medical Practice

Remote health monitoring and wellness applications are experiencing significant growth, a trend expected to accelerate through 2025 and beyond. A glance at platforms like Google Play or the Apple App Store reveals a wide selection of both professional and semi-professional mobile apps focused on health and well-being. Many of these apps integrate seamlessly with wearable devices—such as fitness trackers and heart rate monitors—to collect real-time biometric data. This data, including pulse rate, body temperature, blood pressure, and other key health indicators, is used to monitor and analyze a user's overall health status. A notable example is TATEEDA GLOBAL, which has developed a cross-platform tablet application for iOS and Android. This app provides healthcare professionals with instant access to ECG data and diagnostic reports from advanced devices known for their high-accuracy arrhythmia detection capabilities.

Figure 5. Major AI APIS for Healthcare

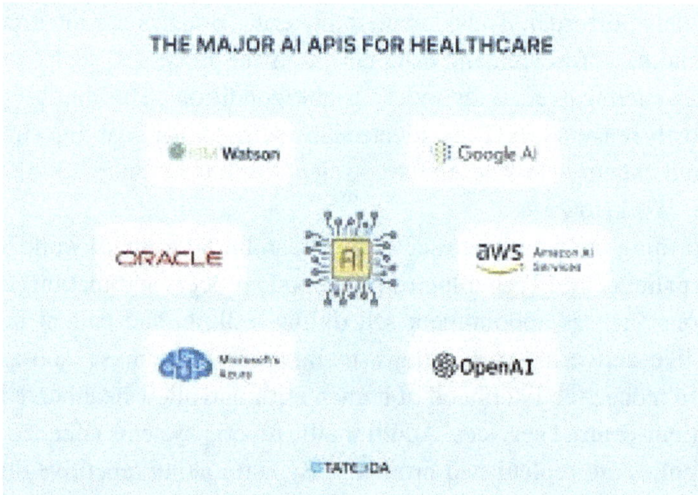

7.1 Health prevention through behavioural health tools

Digital health technologies (DHTs) have become vital tools in strengthening preventive health systems. They enhance early detection, enable continuous health monitoring, and support behavioural change through scalable, cost-effective interventions. According to the World Health Organization (WHO), integrating DHTs into national strategies is crucial for achieving equitable and sustainable health outcomes (WHO, 2020).

Surveillance and Early Detection

Technologies such as mobile apps, wearables, and cloud-based analytics provide valuable data for population-level surveillance. These tools help detect early symptoms or behavioural changes, prompting timely public health interventions. For instance, digital screening tools have successfully identified individuals at risk of chronic diseases such as diabetes and guided them into prevention programs (CDC, 2023).

Behavior Change Interventions

Mobile health (mHealth) applications and SMS-based interventions deliver reminders, goal-setting tools, and personalized recommendations that promote healthier lifestyles. Systematic reviews show that well-designed apps incorporating behavior-change techniques effectively increase physical activity and improve dietary habits (Milne-Ives et al., 2020). Wearable devices further strengthen this process by providing real-time feedback on activity, sleep, and heart rate (Sun et al., 2021).

Behavioral Health Tools

Digital Cognitive Behavioral Therapy (dCBT) and internet-based interventions are effective in managing depression, anxiety, and insomnia. Meta-analyses reveal that guided iCBT produces significant improvements in mental health outcomes, making it a valuable tool for both prevention and early intervention (Karyotaki et al., 2017). Additionally, AI-powered chatbots and telehealth platforms expand access to psychological support while optimizing healthcare resources.

Integration with Public Health Actions

Digital technologies can be integrated into public health workflows through mechanisms like digital screening, automated follow-ups, and adaptive interventions. For example, wearable-based monitoring can trigger customized coaching messages when activity levels drop, while dCBT programs can be scaled across universities and workplaces (WHO, 2020).

Implementation and Policy Considerations

To ensure effective adoption, public health systems must address several critical factors: 1) promoting digital equity and accessibility, 2) maintaining robust data privacy and governance, 3) integrating digital tools into traditional care systems, and 4) providing digital literacy training for healthcare professionals. Moreover, rigorous evaluation and monitoring are essential to assess cost-effectiveness and health impact (WHO, 2020)

7.2 Social and policy trends in digital healthcare transformation

The transformation of healthcare through digital technologies is not only a technical shift but also a social and policy evolution. Governments, insurance systems, and health education institutions play pivotal roles in either accelerating or constraining this transformation. Their actions determine how effectively digital health solutions can be implemented, scaled, and sustained across populations.

Role of Governments

Governments are central to setting the regulatory and infrastructural foundation for digital healthcare. They shape national digital health strategies, data governance frameworks, and reimbursement policies that guide innovation. According to the World Health Organization (WHO, 2020), government leadership is crucial for ensuring interoperability, privacy protection, and equitable access to digital tools. Countries such as the United Kingdom and Singapore have successfully implemented nationwide electronic health record systems and telemedicine frameworks through government-driven initiatives.

Role of Insurance Systems

Insurance systems, both public and private, influence the adoption of digital healthcare through reimbursement models and coverage policies. When insurance providers reimburse for telemedicine visits, remote monitoring, or digital therapeutics, patients and providers are more likely to use these services (OECD, 2021). However, inconsistent reimbursement standards and a lack of recognition for digital interventions in traditional billing codes often hinder widespread adoption.

Role of Health Education

Health education institutions are vital in preparing the workforce for digital transformation. Integrating digital literacy, data analytics, and telehealth competencies into medical and nursing curricula ensures that future professionals can effectively use technology in clinical and public health practice (Frenk et al., 2020). Public education campaigns also play a role by improving health literacy and empowering citizens to use digital tools responsibly and effectively.

Social Trends and Public Acceptance

Societal attitudes toward technology, privacy concerns, and digital inclusion strongly influence healthcare digitization. Increased reliance on mobile health apps and wearable devices reflects a cultural shift toward self-monitoring and preventive care. However, disparities in digital access—often shaped by socioeconomic status, geography, and age—can widen health inequalities if not addressed through inclusive policies (Van Dijk, 2020).

Policy Challenges and Recommendations

Key policy challenges include data protection, cybersecurity, interoperability, and ethical use of AI in healthcare. Governments and health agencies must develop regulatory frameworks that encourage innovation while safeguarding patient rights. Collaborative public–private partnerships can accelerate digital health adoption by combining government oversight with industry innovation. Furthermore, insurance incentives and educational reforms should align to support a cohesive and sustainable digital healthcare ecosystem.

7.3 Comparison of Global Health Systems in different countries according to income levels

Digital transformation in healthcare manifests differently across regions, reflecting variations in economic capacity, infrastructure, governance, and health priorities. Comparing global health systems shows that while high-income countries often lead in technology adoption, low- and middle-income countries (LMICs) are innovating in unique ways to address local challenges.

Digital Healthcare in High-Income Countries

High-income nations such as the United States, the United Kingdom, Germany, and Japan have made substantial progress in integrating digital health. They benefit from advanced digital infrastructure, strong research ecosystems, and robust regulatory frameworks. For example, the UK's National Health Service (NHS) has implemented nationwide electronic health records (EHRs) and telehealth services that enhance coordination and patient engagement (NHS Digital, 2022). Similarly, countries like Japan are leveraging artificial intelligence for predictive analytics and elderly care management (OECD, 2021). These countries also emphasize data privacy, cybersecurity, and interoperability across digital platforms.

Digital Healthcare in Low- and Middle-Income Countries

In contrast, LMICs face challenges such as limited infrastructure, unequal internet access, and insufficient funding. However, innovation is thriving through mobile health (mHealth) solutions that are often low-cost and community-driven. For instance, India's Ayushman Bharat Digital Mission (ABDM) aims to create a unified digital health ecosystem connecting citizens, providers, and insurers (Government of India, 2021). Kenya's M-TIBA platform enables patients to manage healthcare payments and insurance via mobile phones, expanding financial inclusion in health (GSMA, 2020). These models demonstrate how resource-constrained settings can leapfrog traditional systems using mobile and cloud technologies.

Comparative Analysis of Trends

The primary distinction between high- and low-income settings lies in focus and implementation. High-income countries prioritise system integration, precision medicine, and data analytics, while LMICs emphasize accessibility, affordability, and scalability. Furthermore, policy environments differ: high-income nations invest heavily in research, regulation, and cybersecurity, whereas LMICs rely on public–private partnerships and donor-funded programs to sustain digital health initiatives (World Bank, 2022).

Lessons and Opportunities for Global Health

Cross-country learning offers valuable insights. High-income nations can adopt frugal innovations from LMICs to reduce costs and improve efficiency, while LMICs can benefit from the governance and data protection models developed by wealthier countries. International collaboration, knowledge sharing, and global funding mechanisms—such as those led by WHO, World Bank, and USAID—can help bridge gaps and accelerate equitable digital health transformation worldwide (WHO, 2020).

8. THE PILLARS OF SUSTAINABILITY

Green Tech:

The increasing reliance on digital health technologies requires sustainable approaches to minimise environmental impact. Green technology emphasises the use of energy-efficient data centres, eco-friendly manufacturing processes, and software optimisation to reduce power consumption. For instance, AI algorithms can be designed to require fewer computational resources, making healthcare systems more sustainable. By integrating renewable energy sources such as solar or wind power into health infrastructures, digital healthcare can align with global climate goals while still delivering reliable services.

Low Energy Solutions:

Continuous health monitoring via wearables, biosensors, and telemedicine platforms often relies on portable devices that consume substantial energy. Developing low-power hardware and lightweight software applications extends device life and reduces energy consumption. For example, edge-computing devices can process data locally rather than transmitting large volumes to servers, lowering both energy use and operational costs. Low-energy solutions also make digital health more accessible in low-resource settings where the electricity supply is limited.

E-Waste:

With the rapid advancement of medical devices, diagnostic equipment, and wearable sensors, electronic waste has become a pressing concern. Outdated or discarded technologies contribute to pollution, as they contain hazardous materials such as lead, mercury, and cadmium. Improper disposal poses serious risks to ecosystems and human health. The challenge is particularly severe in developing countries where recycling facilities and e-waste management systems are underdeveloped. Addressing e-waste is critical to ensuring that technological progress in healthcare does not create long-term ecological harm. Figure 6 shows **the** Major pollutants and hazardous materials that can be generated from e-waste when improperly dumped or managed.

Figure 6. Negative impact of Electronic waste

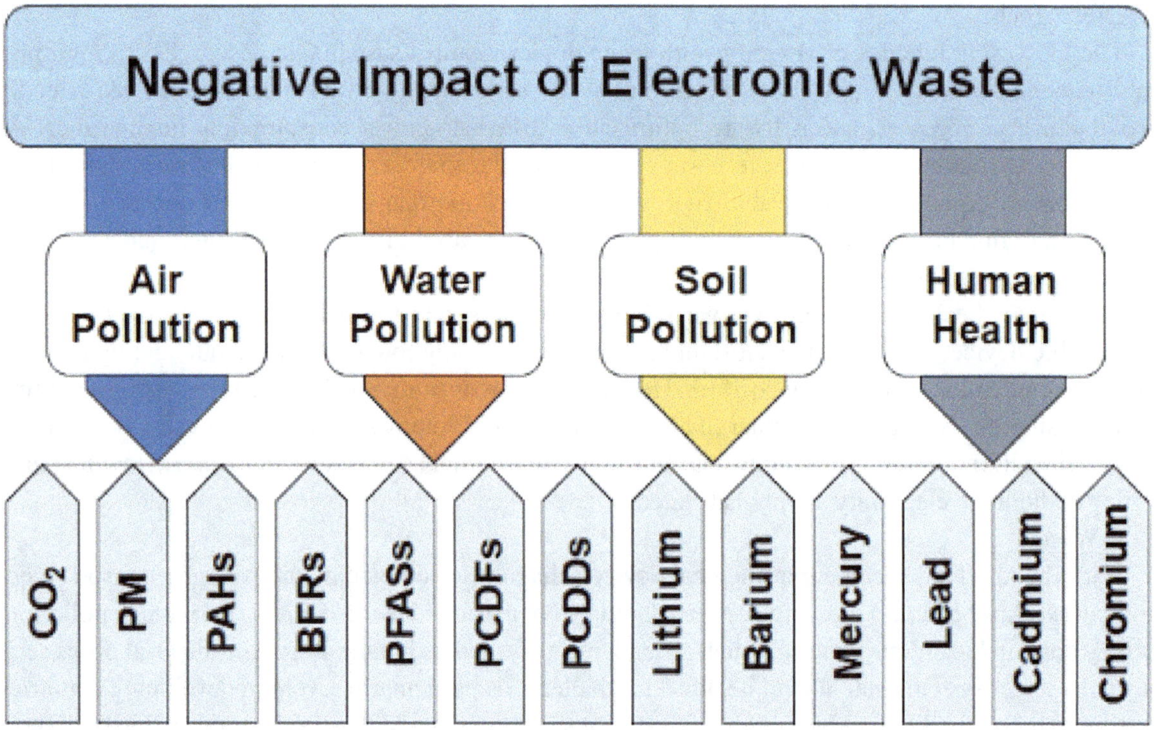

Soil Pollution: E-waste also has a significant impact on soil and its biological component. The accumulation of e-waste in mountains and dumping sites, particularly **in** countries such as India, China, Pakistan, and African nations, has affected the microbial communities present at contaminated sites. Alterations in microbial communities can significantly impact soil ecological function. For example, e-waste contains heavy metals such as mercury, lead, cadmium, nickel, arsenic, and chromium, as well as persistent organic pollutants, which can reduce the normal soil microbial biota (Salam & Varma, 2019).

Device Recycling:

Recycling and reusing medical devices can significantly reduce the burden of e-waste. Components such as circuit boards, batteries, and rare earth metals can be recovered and repurposed for new devices. Establishing take-back programs and encouraging manufacturers to adopt circular economy principles are vital steps toward sustainability. In addition, healthcare institutions can partner with certified e-waste recyclers to ensure safe disposal. Effective recycling not only helps protect the environment but also lowers production costs by reducing the need for raw materials.

9. CHALLENGES OF DIGITAL HEALTH AND PREVENTION

Digital health offers many benefits, but it also poses important challenges that require attention. These challenges can be divided into two main types:

Technical Challenges: These involve problems with technology, such as a Lack of awareness of AI technologies, Data security and privacy issues, unreliable data, Infrastructure gaps, and Suboptimal design and implementation of digital technologies.

Non-Technical Challenges: These include Societal factors, Ethical challenges; Increased connected health solutions, Resource and economic interest barriers, Policy and governance challenges

9.1 Technical Challenges

9.1.1 Lack of awareness on AI technologies

Building trust with patients is crucial in healthcare, and this is especially true when it comes to AI-based technologies. Doctors and policy makers acknowledge that the public may be reluctant to rely on AI-generated recommendations, given the long-standing importance of face-to-face interaction with physicians (Sun TQ, Medaglia R. 2019). To complicate matters, there is often a lack of understanding among the general population about the potential benefits and limitations of AI in healthcare, leading to unrealistic expectations that can make it difficult for physicians to adopt these technologies (Vollmer S, Mateen BA, Bohner G, et al., 2020).

9.1.2 Data security and privacy issues

The application of artificial intelligence in healthcare generates and stores vast amounts of sensitive personal and medical information, making data security and privacy a paramount concern (Price & Cohen, 2019). Various data security risks exist, such as data breaches where hackers or malicious actors gain unauthorized access to patient data (like medical records or insurance information), potentially causing significant financial and reputational damage to healthcare providers. Inadequate data encryption, whether at rest or in transit, can leave patient data vulnerable to unauthorized access or misuse. Lack of access control, failing to manage user access to patient data properly, can also lead to unauthorized access or misuse. Without proper data retention strategies, the storage period of patient data may extend beyond what is necessary, increasing the risk of unauthorized access or misuse. Furthermore, the absence of data breach prevention and response plans can leave healthcare providers unprepared in the event of a data breach.

Thus, healthcare providers need to ensure their systems and processes are secure and that patient data is protected from unauthorized access or misuse. A combination of technical and organizational measures can be employed to tackle these issues, including data encryption, access control, and data breach prevention and response planning (Figueroa-Lorenzo S, Anorga J, Arrizabalaga S, 2019). Beyond technical measures, healthcare providers must comply with legal requirements such as the Health Insurance Portability and Accountability Act (HIPAA) in the United States, which regulates the use and disclosure of patient data. Adherence to such regulations is crucial to protecting patient data. Data security and privacy concerns are critical issues in the healthcare sector, and healthcare providers must take steps to ensure that data used for training and deploying deep learning models is secure and that patient privacy is safeguarded (Boyce B. 2014).

9.1.3 Unreliability of available data

The heterogeneous nature of data sources and large volumes of data including epidemiologic, surveillance, and health services data required for public health services gathered across various health systems without broad standards for reporting and consistency was emphasized as a problem of data reliability. (O'Mahony C, Jichi F, Pavlou M, et al. (2014). Further, data quality issues, including incomplete data, were said to be a challenge (Deo RC. 2015). especially for big data in public health surveillance and research, where noisy data (i.e. poor quality data) reduces efficiency (Aapro et al., 2020) Further, the unreliability of unvalidated or anonymous user-generated and/or observational data (Kruse, et al.,. 2019) were said to bias reports. For example, reports on social media could misrepresent the general public health situation, as significant portions of the population, including people suffering disparities in access to digital technologies, are excluded from the data.(HealthITAnalytics. 2020; Pattichis & Panayides, 2019; Owoyemi et al., 2022).

9.1.4 Infrastructure gaps

Public health increasingly relies on complex, high-volume data from heterogeneous sources. Ensuring the promise of better public health precision in a digital era imposes new infrastructure requirements to enable operations (Brown, 2021; Vollmer et al., 2020). More robust computing infrastructure (Connor CW. et al. 2019). including high-bandwidth, low-latency computer networks and clusters of machines for computation are required to take advantage of high-volume data Zucker & Regehr, 2002; Connor et al., 2019; Obermeyer et al. 2016). This was mostly emphasized in the use of big data and artificial intelligence for public health surveillance, epidemiology, and research. Capacity for ongoing maintenance of infrastructure and access to repair parts also constitute a barrier(Murthy S, Leligdowicz A, et al,. 2015). Many public health agencies lack access to such computing or IT power (LeCun, Y., Bengio, Y., & Hinton, G. et al. 2015) Further, in resource-limited settings, unreliable power supply is a complicating factor. In addition to providers, public health service users also require access to computers, smartphones, and Internet services, which are often disparately distributed along socioeconomic gradients. These infrastructure requirements are closely related to funding and human resource needs, as the development of infrastructure needed to implement effective information systems has been slow, especially in financially limited local health departments(MIT Sloan. et al . 2021).

9.1.5 Suboptimal design and implementation of digital technologies

Many digital technologies in public health are characterized by overenthusiastic and sometimes complex designs that neglect basic foundations of digital health, including attention to users' needs rather than needs perceived by the implementers, and implementation of interventions that are based on proven behavioral theories (agrabi F, Ammenwerth E, Craven CK, et al. 2021). Further, the focus on using digital interventions for data collection, without due consideration to the value they might offer to frontline health providers and other user potentially limits engagement (Manogaran & Lopez, 2017). User contexts have also been oversimplified and not well accounted for in the development of digital tools, with limited evaluation of the usability and acceptability of the tools among targeted users (Cai, Y., Clinto, M., & Xiao, Z.et al. 2021) (Daskalopoulou, A., & Palmer, M. et al . 2021)

9.2 Non-technical challenges

9.2.1 Societal factors

While technology is at the heart of any digital health system, the related transformations cannot be viewed purely through a technological lens (Asahi K, Undurraga EA, Valdés R, Wagner R. 2021). Digital technologies need to deliver affordable, easy-to-use healthcare solutions to a growing and aging population in which new technologies are often slow to be adopted and accepted by the general populace (Nicola M, Alsafi Z, Sohrabi C, et al. 2020). Factors that influence this lack of acceptance include regulatory factors, such as uncertainties surrounding digital health policies and legislation, as well as a perceived lack of accountability within the commercial sector. The commercial industry itself has challenges related to the complexity of the multinational nature of the digital health market and the need to operate within the constraints of a multitude of different health systems (Carter et al., 2020).

Figure 7. Social Factors in Healthcare

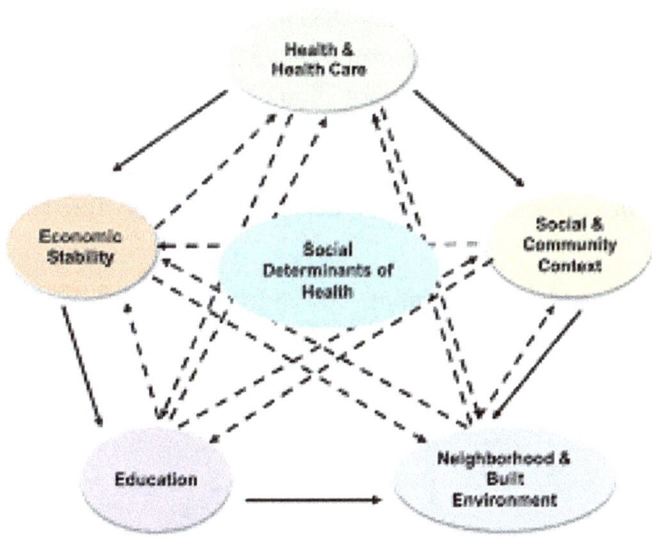

9.2.2 Ethical challenges

The increasing digitisation of healthcare and the growth of mobile and IoT devices as data collection tools raise many ethical issues. One recurring theme concerns the exact nature of the roles of consumer tech companies, such as Amazon, Apple, Google, Facebook, and Samsung, which have all entered the digital health domain (HealthITAnalytics, 2020).

Figure 8. Ethical challenge

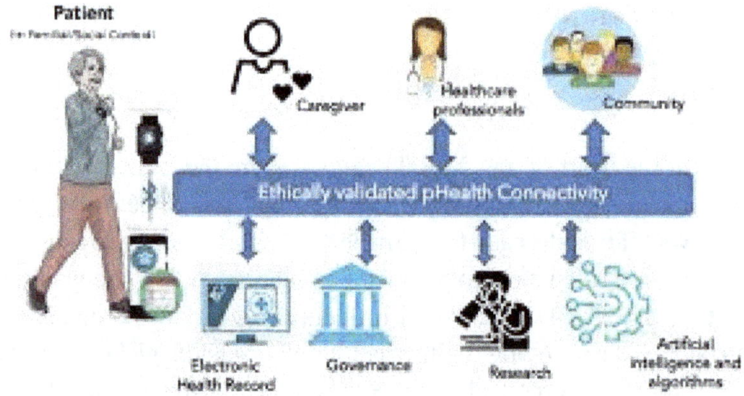

9.2.3. Increased Connected Health Solutions

A core aim of digital health is to help facilitate the circulation of data between patients, devices, and clinicians Peiffer-Smadja N, Rawson TM, Ahmad R, et al. 2020). Increasing this connectivity enables more innovative and more timely sharing of information between clinicians and patients and has strong links to the predictive, preemptive, and personalized principles of digital health (Currie G, Hawk KE, Rohren E, Vial A, Klein R. et al. 2019). Connected health solutions are also a key element in response to the COVID-19 pandemic Ahmad MA, Patel A, Eckert C, Kumar V, Teredesai A. et al. 2020).

Figure 9. Increased Connected Health Solutions

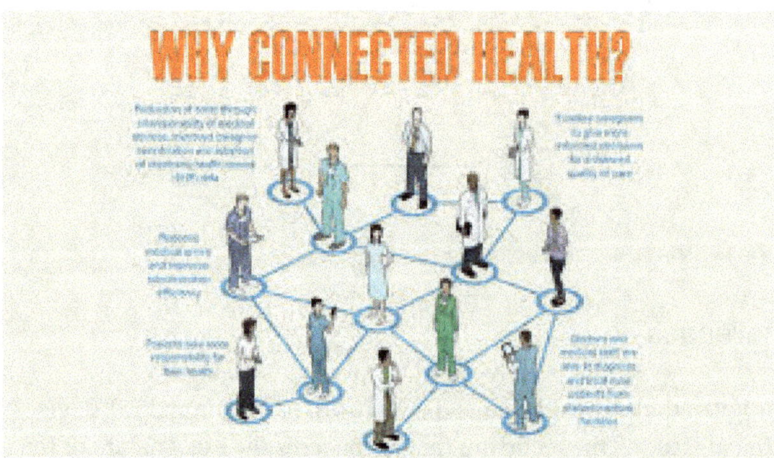

9.2.4 Resource and economic interest barriers:

The lack of long-term economic investments required to maintain essential infrastructure and human resources were said to complicate the sustainability of digital innovations in public health (HealthI-TAnalytics. 2020) especially with limited public health funding. (Zucker & Regehr, 2002). (Awan SE, Sohel F, Sanfilippo FM, Bennamoun M, Dwivedi G. 2018). Difficulties establishing clear cost–benefit outcomes and accountability strategies were also identified.(Fatehi, F., Samadbeik, M., & Kazemi, A. 2020) (World Health Organisation, 2024). These difficulties were reported to be worse among public health practitioners working in resource-limited settings (Vollmer S, Mateen BA, Bohner G, et al. (2020)) Current innovations in public health were described as driven by commercial interests of for-profit organizations, often targeting populations serving these interests, worsening existing health disparities, and limiting opportunities for widespread impact in line with public health principles (Morris, B. B., Rossi, B., & Fuemmeler, B. 2022)(Anderson-Lewis et al., 2018)

9.2.5 Environmental & Sustainability Considerations / Challenges

Environmental and sustainability challenges arise when integrating advanced digital and AI-based technologies in healthcare and public health monitoring. Firstly, the high computational power required to train and deploy Artificial Intelligence models significantly increases energy consumption, contributing to carbon emissions and environmental degradation (Vishal et al., 2023). Secondly, rapid software and hardware upgrade cycles generate more electronic waste (e-waste) because old sensors, wearables, and IoT devices are frequently discarded. This improper disposal of electronic components can pollute soil and water resources.

Additionally, sustainability challenges include the heavy reliance on cloud storage and data centres, which require continuous electricity and cooling systems, further increasing the ecological footprint. Another challenge is developing environmentally friendly supply chains for digital devices, as sustainable sourcing of materials (e.g., rare minerals used in chips) is still limited. Therefore, it is essential to promote the use of green AI approaches, energy-efficient algorithms, and recyclable device design standards to ensure long-term, sustainable technology deployment (Vishal et al., 2023). In Fig. 10 below, we have shown the Environmental & Sustainability Considerations. It highlights differences in accuracy among methods and clearly shows that the proposed model delivers better predictive performance, improved efficiency, and superior classification performance in disease detection.

Figure 10. Environmental & Sustainability Considerations/ Challenges

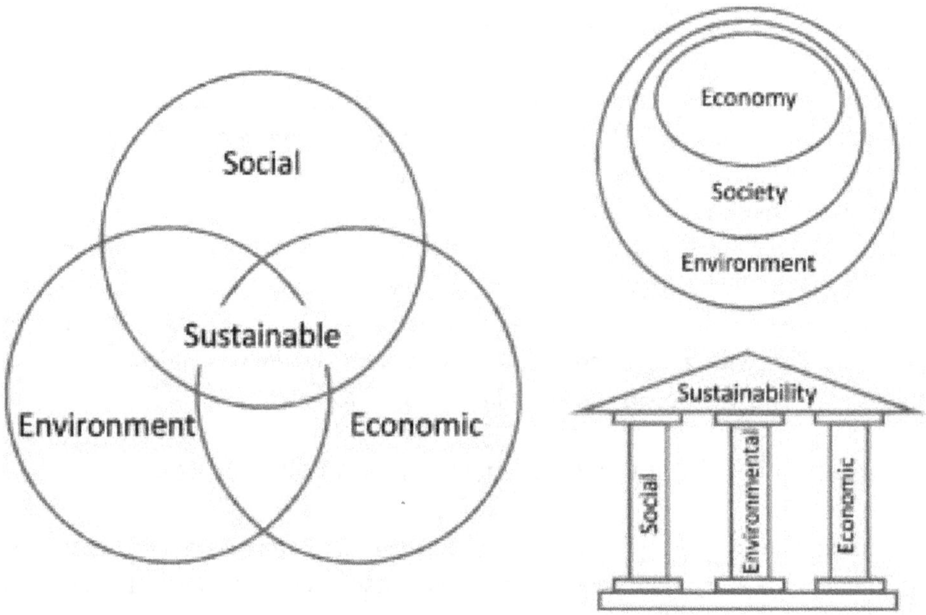

9.3: Regional Perspectives on Health System Strength

Regional perspectives on health system strength highlight the diverse capacities, challenges, and priorities that shape healthcare delivery worldwide. Each region's health system strength is influenced by its governance structure, financing mechanisms, workforce distribution, and digital readiness (World Health Organization, 2022).

In high-income regions, strong infrastructure, robust financing, and advanced digital integration enable efficient service delivery and health data management. These regions increasingly focus on preventive care, precision medicine, and sustainable financing models supported by digital health ecosystems (Kruk et al., 2018).

Conversely, low- and middle-income regions face challenges such as inadequate funding, workforce shortages, and inequitable access to healthcare services. However, digital technologies and community-based health programs are emerging as powerful tools to strengthen resilience and accessibility (Tausch et al., 2022). The regional adoption of telehealth, mobile health (mHealth), and interoperable data systems has improved disease surveillance, remote consultations, and primary care in resource-limited settings.

Ultimately, analyzing regional health system strength provides strategic insight into how countries can leverage local innovations and global partnerships to build more equitable, efficient, and digitally empowered healthcare systems.

9.4: Ethical, Policy Integration & Data Governance issues:

Ethical, policy integration, and data governance issues are central to the responsible adoption of digital technologies in healthcare. As data-driven systems, artificial intelligence (AI), and digital health platforms become more prevalent, they introduce complex ethical challenges related to privacy, consent, bias, and accountability. Ensuring patient autonomy and maintaining trust are vital, especially when personal health data are collected and analyzed by algorithmic systems (Floridi et al., 2018).

Policy integration is another crucial concern, as healthcare digitalization often outpaces regulatory frameworks. Fragmented or outdated policies can hinder interoperability, cross-border data exchange, and equitable access to innovations (Leslie et al., 2021). Effective policy integration requires alignment between technological innovation, public health objectives, and ethical principles, ensuring that digital solutions benefit all sections of society without discrimination.

Data governance issues emerge from the massive volumes of sensitive health data generated through electronic health records, wearable devices, and AI systems. Robust data governance frameworks must ensure transparency, data quality, cybersecurity, and equitable data sharing while protecting individual rights (Gostin et al., 2019). The adoption of international standards, such as the GDPR and WHO digital governance guidelines, provides a foundation for ethical and secure digital transformation.

In summary, addressing these issues requires a multidisciplinary approach that balances innovation with integrity, promoting fairness, inclusivity, and trust in digital health ecosystems.

9.5 Privacy as a Fundamental Right in India

The concerns around the protection of personal data and the right to privacy in India are further complicated by the judicial discourse on the issue. Privacy has been intensely contested and litigated in India since the 1950s. In 2017, the Supreme Court ruled in a landmark nine-judge bench decision that the right to privacy is a fundamental right in India. The Puttaswamy decision was the outcome of a constitutional challenge to the Aadhaar biometric identity scheme. Before this, the Supreme Court had held in MP Sharma v. Satish Chandra and Kharak Singh v. State of UP that privacy was not a fundamental right.

9.6 Health Data Protection and Privacy Concerns

In India, one of the most critical challenges in the digital health ecosystem is the protection and maintenance of data privacy, primarily due to the ambiguities and loopholes present in the existing legal frameworks (Reddy, 2023). The Information Technology Act, 2000, and the corresponding Data Protection Rules offer only a fundamental level of data protection and are not healthcare-specific, as they mandate only that individuals be informed about the intended use of their data (Section 43A, IT Act, 2000; Reddy, 2023). Although the National Digital Health Blueprint (NDHB) recommends the adoption of ISO 22600:2014 for Health Informatics—Privilege Management and Access Control (ISO, et al. 2014), the actual operationalization of ISO standards is highly challenging for most healthcare providers in India, and ensuring compliance at the provider level remains uncertain (Pinto, 2022).

Table 3. Indian policies affecting the digitisation of healthcare:

Type of Regulation	Title of Regulation	Date Effective	Relevant Clauses
Law	The Drugs and Cosmetics Act ("D&C Act")	10 April 1940	—
Law	Information Technology Act and Rules (IT Act)	9 June 2000	Section 2(w), Section 43A, Section 79
Regulations	The Clinical Establishments (Registration and Regulation) Act	9 August 2010	Section 38(1) and 38(2)
Law	The Information Technology Reasonable security practices and procedures and sensitive personal data or information Rules ("Data Protection Rules")	1 April 2011	Rule 3, Rule 4(1), Rule 5(1), Rule 5(3), Rule 5(7), Rule 7
National Standards	The Information Technology (Intermediaries Guidelines) Rules ("Intermediary Guidelines")	1 April 2011	Rule 3
Law	The Medical Devices Rules ("MDR")	5 May 2017	—
Regulations	DNA Technology (Use and Application) Regulation Bill	8 July 2019	—
Regulations	Digital Personal Data Protection Bill (DPDP Bill)	18 November 2022	Clause 8

10. CASE STUDIES OF AI IN HEALTHCARE

10.1 Helmets for the treatment of depression

Danish researchers have designed a helmet that helps reactivate parts involved in depression and enables rapid recovery in patients by transmitting weak electrical pulses to the brain. Scientific Services of Iranian Students' News Agency (ISNA) reported that the performance of this helmet differed from the controversial method of electroconvulsive therapy (ECT), in which very weak electrical pulses are transmitted to parts of the brain associated with depression. Electrical pulses activate capillaries by mimicking the body's natural mechanism for forming new blood vessels. In this method, patients do not feel electrical pulses, whereas in ECT, the electrical pulses are so severe that they may cause patients to lose their memory in some cases. Professor Steen Dissing from Copenhagen University states that electrical pulses affect capillaries in the brain. Depression symptoms disappear in most patients after 7 days, and they achieve better scores on the depression test. A clinical test of this helmet was performed on 65 patients with depression in Denmark and New Zealand; for 34 patients, half an hour per day and for others, one hour per day of treatment was prescribed using this helmet. In 65% of patients, depression symptoms disappeared after 1 week; depression improvement in patients who had received a half-hour treatment was reported 73% and in the second group 67%. The only side effect of this helmet is mild nausea, which resolves after treatment. The results of this study help in the development of new treatment methods for disorders such as posttraumatic stress disorder (PTSD) (Ajami, S., & Teimouri, F. 2015) (Singh, R. P., Hom, G. L., Abramoff, M. D., Campbell, J. P., & Chiang, M. F. 2020)

Figure11. Major AI for Healthcare

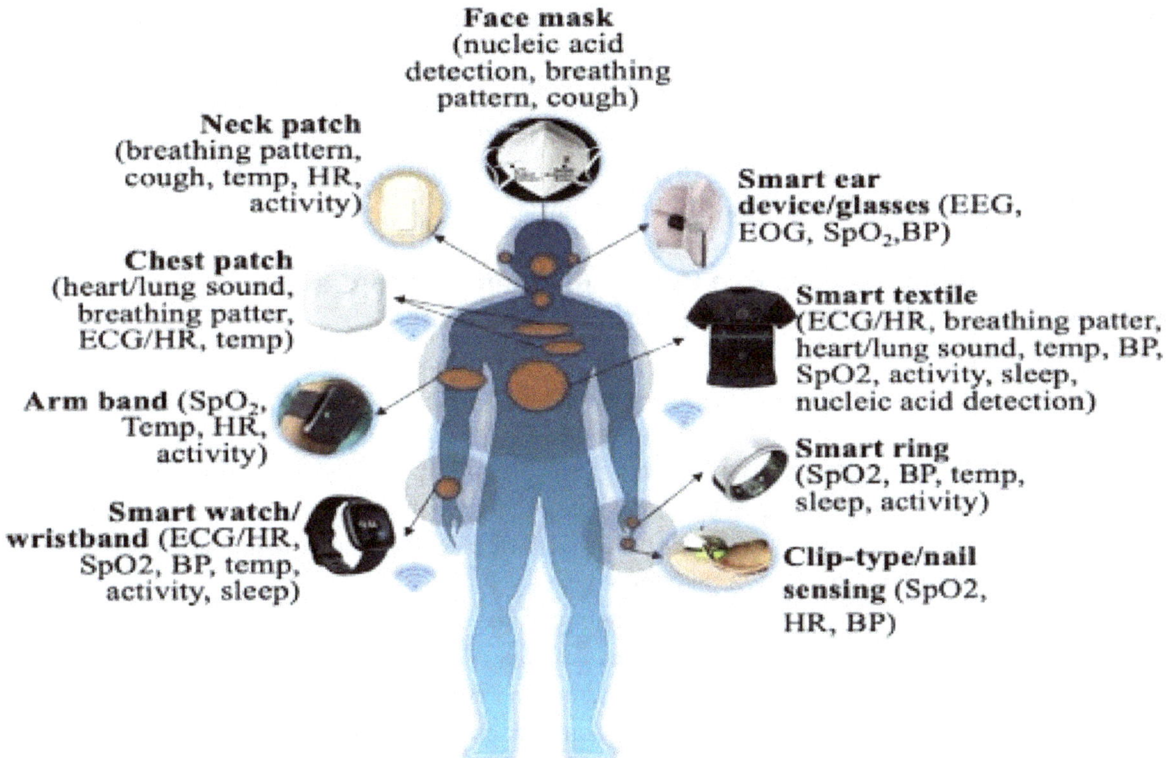

10.2 Case Study on AI-Powered Wearable ECG for Early Cardiac Risk Detection and Remote Monitoring in the U.S.

Problem: Cardiovascular diseases, especially arrhythmias like atrial fibrillation (AFib), require timely detection and continuous monitoring. However, many patients, particularly the elderly or those in remote areas, lack access to regular hospital-based ECG testing. Traditional monitoring devices, such as Holter monitors, are bulky, require clinic visits, and typically monitor for only 24–48 hours. This results in missed early warning signs, delayed diagnosis, and increased risk of stroke, heart failure, or even sudden cardiac arrest. The absence of accessible, real-time data further limits physicians' ability to make informed treatment decisions.

Solution: Wearable devices like Kardia Mobile, a pocket-sized ECG device, revolutionised how patients monitor heart health. It allows users to take on-demand ECG readings at home in under 30 seconds. These readings are synced with a mobile app and analyzed using AI algorithms, which detect abnormalities like AFib, bradycardia, or tachycardia. Patients can share these ECG reports instantly with their cardiologists, enabling timely interventions. The tool supports remote cardiac monitoring, reduces the need for in-person checkups, and promotes preventive care by identifying risks before they become emergencies (Turakhia, et al.2019)

Tools/ Techniques Used:

- KardiaMobile (1-lead and 6-lead) wearable ECG device, Mobile application for recording and syncing ECGs
- Cloud-based dashboard for physician access, Real-time alert system for abnormal readings
- Remote Patient Monitoring (RPM) platforms
- Logistic Regression: For basic arrhythmia classification (e.g., AFib detection)
- Convolutional Neural Networks (CNNs): For analyzing ECG waveform patterns
- Signal Processing Algorithms: To extract heart rate variability features
- Time-Series Analysis: For continuous monitoring and trend analysis

10.3 Transforming Diabetic Eye Care: AI-Driven Retinopathy Screening in Thailand's Primary Healthcare System

Problem: Thailand has a growing population of people with type 2 diabetes, and diabetic retinopathy (DR) is one of the most common and severe complications leading to preventable blindness. However, there is a critical shortage of trained ophthalmologists, particularly in rural and semi-urban regions. As a result, diabetic patients often miss annual screenings or receive delayed diagnoses, causing progressive and irreversible vision loss. Primary care centres lacked the tools and expertise to handle early screening, creating a large care gap in preventive ophthalmology.

Solution: To address this, the Thai government partnered with Google Health to deploy a deep learning-based AI system in primary health centers. Trained nurses or general practitioners capture retinal images using fundus cameras, and the AI system analyses the images in real-time to detect signs of diabetic retinopathy. The AI model provides instant risk classification (e.g., no DR, mild, moderate, severe), allowing clinicians to refer high-risk patients to specialists immediately. This automated screening process improves early detection, ensures timely treatment, and significantly reduces the burden on eye care specialists (Gulshan et al., 2016). In Figure 12 below, we have illustrated the ROC curves for different models. It clearly shows that the proposed model achieves the highest AUC, demonstrating better sensitivity, specificity, and overall predictive performance in disease classification.

Tools/ Techniques Used:

- **Digital Fundus Cameras**: For capturing high-quality retinal images
- **Google Health AI Platform**: For analyzing fundus images
- **Local mobile or desktop applications** for image upload and viewing
- **Cloud infrastructure**: For secure data storage and access
- **Clinical Decision Support System (CDSS)**: For triaging and referral suggestions
- **Convolutional Neural Networks (CNNs)**: For feature extraction and image classification
- **Transfer Learning**: Using pre-trained image models for better accuracy with limited local data
- **Supervised Learning**: Trained on large annotated datasets of retinal images
- **Binary and Multiclass Classification Algorithms**: To categorise DR severity levels

Figure 12. Technology Acceptance Model (TAM)

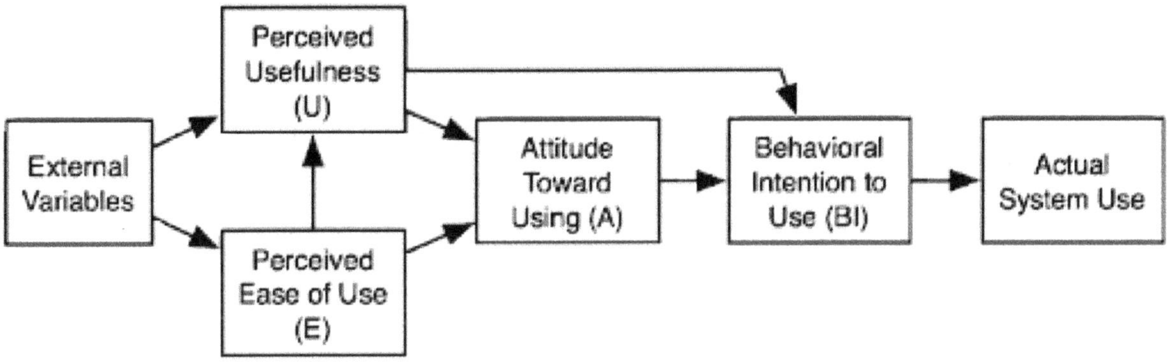

TAM has been divided into five categories: (i) information technology in health, (ii) acceptance of e-health, (iii) telemedicine, (iv) security of e-health, and (v) education impact of e-health.

11. CONCLUSION

In recent years, digital health technologies—powered by Artificial Intelligence—have emerged as transformative forces in shifting healthcare from reactive treatment to proactive prevention. This chapter has underscored how tools like wearable devices, biosensors, and AI-driven platforms are enabling earlier detection, personalized health insights, and continuous monitoring. These innovations are reshaping modern healthcare into a more dynamic, data-driven, and preventive ecosystem. However, the full potential of this transformation hinges on addressing key challenges: protecting patient privacy, ensuring algorithmic fairness, improving digital access, and strengthening regulatory frameworks. As case studies from around the world demonstrate, when implemented thoughtfully, digital health solutions can improve health outcomes, support clinicians, and empower individuals. Looking ahead, the integration of AI with national health strategies, increased investment in digital infrastructure, and advances in health tech innovation will be critical. Ultimately, by embracing a digital-first mindset, we can foster a more inclusive, efficient, and forward-looking healthcare system—one where prevention is prioritised, care is personalized, and public health is proactively protected.

A proactive, well-rounded strategy is required for practitioners and policymakers in light of the digital transformation of healthcare. To reduce environmental harm, e-waste management regulations and sustainable technology design must be given top priority. Establishing unambiguous data governance rules is the second step to ensuring individuals maintain control and ownership of their medical records. Third, to reduce reliance on private platforms, governments should encourage interoperability, open standards, and public-private partnerships that protect the public interest. Fourth, regular audits, encryption standards, and employee training are necessary to increase cybersecurity protocols and lower risks. Last but not least, inclusive healthcare requires tackling the digital divide by funding infrastructure and digital literacy initiatives. The integration of sustainability, security, equity, and accountability can optimise the advantages of digital health while reducing systemic dangers.

REFERENCES

Aapro, M., Bossi, P., & Dasari, A.. (2020). Digital health for optimal supportive care in oncology. *Supportive Care in Cancer*, *28*(10), 4589–4612. DOI: 10.1007/s00520-020-05539-1 PMID: 32533435

Abernethy, A.. (2022). The promise of digital health: Then, now, and the future. *NAM Perspectives*, •••, 6. PMID: 36177208

Advancing Remote Monitoring for Patients With Alzheimer Disease and Related Dementias: Systematic Review. (2025). *JMIR Aging*, *8*, e69175. https://doi.org/JMIR AgingDOI: 10.2196/69175 PMID: 40367504

Ahlan, A. R., & Isma'eel, M. (2014). Patient acceptance of information and communication technology in healthcare: A systematic review. *Procedia Technology*, *16*, 1314–1323.

Ahmad, M. A., Patel, A., Eckert, C., Kumar, V., & Teredesai, A. (2020). Fairness in machine learning for healthcare. In: *Proceedings of the 26th ACM SIGKDD International Conference on Knowledge Discovery & Data Mining*, 3529–3530.

Ahmadi, A. (2024). Digital health transformation: Leveraging ai for monitoring and disease management. [IJBLS]. *International Journal of BioLife Sciences*, *3*(1), 10–24.

Ahmed, S., Irfan, S., Kiran, N., Masood, N., Anjum, N., & Ramzan, N. (2023). Remote health monitoring systems for elderly people: A survey. *Sensors (Basel)*, *23*(16), 7095. DOI: 10.3390/s23167095 PMID: 37631632

Ajami, S., & Teimouri, F. (2015). Features and application of wearable biosensors in medical care. *Journal of Research in Medical Sciences : the Official Journal of Isfahan University of Medical Sciences*, *20*(12), 1208–1215. PMID: 26958058

Akpakwu, E. (2018). Four ways AI can make healthcare more efficient. World Economic Forum. https://www.weforum.org/agenda/2018/05/four-ways-ai-is-bringing-down-the-cost-of-healthcare/

Alami, H., Rivard, L., Lehoux, P., Hoffman, S. J., & Fortin, J. P. (2020). Telemedicine in low-income countries: Challenges and opportunities in the COVID-19 era. *Frontiers in Public Health*, *8*, 556. DOI: 10.3389/fpubh.2020.00556

Alim, A., & Imtiaz, M. H. (2023). Wearable Sensors for the Monitoring of Maternal Health—A Systematic Review. [MDPI]. *Sensors (Basel)*, *23*(5), 2411. DOI: 10.3390/s23052411 PMID: 36904615

Anderson-Lewis, C., Darville, G., Mercado, R. E., Howell, S., & Di Maggio, S. (2018). mHealth technology use and implications in historically underserved and minority populations in the United States: Systematic literature review. *JMIR mHealth and uHealth*, *6*(6), e8383. PMID: 29914860

Anjum, N., Kumar, R., & Singh, P. (2024). An architectural framework of elderly healthcare monitoring and tracking through wearable sensor technologies. *Multimedia Tools and Applications*, *83*(15), 67825–67870. DOI: 10.1007/s11042-024-18177-0

Asahi, K., Undurraga, E. A., Valdés, R., & Wagner, R. (2021). The effect of COVID-19 on the economy: Evidence from an early adopter of localized lockdowns. *Journal of Global Health*, *11*, 05002. DOI: 10.7189/jogh.11.05002 PMID: 33643635

Awan, S. E., Sohel, F., Sanfilippo, F. M., Bennamoun, M., & Dwivedi, G. (2018). Machine learning in heart failure: Ready for prime time. *Current Opinion in Cardiology*, *33*(2), 190–195. DOI: 10.1097/HCO.0000000000000491 PMID: 29194052

Bhardwaj, R., Nambiar, A. R., & Dutta, D. (2017). A study of machine learning in healthcare. In: *2017 IEEE 41st Annual Computer Software and Applications Conference (COMPSAC)*, Vol. 2, pp. 236–241.

Bhatia, R. (2023). The DPDP Bill and the future of privacy in India. *Journal of Law and Policy Studies*, *12*(3), 45–62.

Biosensors and AI for Mental Health Monitoring: A Systematic Review. (2025). *Biosensors*, *15*(4), 202. https://doi.org/ MDPIDOI: 10.3390/bios15040202 PMID: 40277515

Bouabida, K., Lebouché, B., & Pomey, M. P. (2022). Telehealth and COVID-19 pandemic: Overview. *Healthcare (Basel)*, *10*(11), 2293. DOI: 10.3390/healthcare10112293 PMID: 36421617

Boyce, B. (2014). HIPAA compliance from a private practice purview. *Journal of the Academy of Nutrition and Dietetics*, *114*(9), 1341. PMID: 25053183

Brown, S. (2021, April 21). Machine learning, explained. MIT Sloan School of Management. https://mitsloan.mit.edu/ideas-made-to-matter/machine-learning-explained

Cai, Y., Clinto, M., & Xiao, Z. (2021). Artificial intelligence assistive technology in hospital professional nursing technology. *Journal of Healthcare Engineering*, *2021*(1), 1721529. PMID: 34873437

Carter, S. M., Rogers, W., Win, K. T., Frazer, H., Richards, B., & Houssami, N. (2020). The ethical, legal and social implications of using artificial intelligence systems in breast cancer care. *The Breast : Official Journal of the European Society of Mastology*, *49*, 25–32. PMID: 31677530

Centers for Disease Control and Prevention. (2023). *Mobile technologies for public health*. CDC. https://www.cdc.gov

Chen, X., Wang, F., & Zhang, H.. (2025). Effectiveness of wearable activity trackers on physical activity among adolescents in school-based settings: A systematic review and meta-analysis. [BioMed Central]. *BMC Public Health*, *25*, 1050. DOI: 10.1186/s12889-025-22170-z PMID: 40102761

Chiang, D.-L., Huang, Y.-T., Chen, T.-S., & Lai, F.-P. (2020). Applying time-constraint access control of personal health record in cloud computing. *Enterprise Information Systems*, *14*, 266–281. DOI: 10.1080/17517575.2018.1522452

Cohen, I. G., Evgeniou, T., Gerke, S., & Minssen, T. (2020). European AI strategy: Implications for digital health. *The Lancet. Digital Health*, *2*(7), e376–e379. PMID: 33328096

Collage of Community Physicians of Sri Lanka. (2021). Elementor #4517. Available at: https://ccpsl.org/elementor-4517/ (Accessed May 31, 2021).

Connor, C. W. (2019). Artificial intelligence and machine learning in anesthesiology. *Anesthesiology*, *131*(6), 1346–1359. DOI: 10.1097/ALN.0000000000002694 PMID: 30973516

Currie, G., Hawk, K. E., Rohren, E., Vial, A., & Klein, R. (2019). Machine learning and deep learning in medical imaging: Intelligent imaging. *Journal of Medical Imaging and Radiation Sciences*, *50*(4), 477–487. DOI: 10.1016/j.jmir.2019.09.005 PMID: 31601480

Daskalopoulou, A., & Palmer, M. (2021). Persistent institutional breaches: Technology use in healthcare work. *Social Science & Medicine*, *289*, 114399. PMID: 34583147

Davis, F. D. (1989). Perceived usefulness, perceived ease of use, and user acceptance of information technology. *Management Information Systems Quarterly*, *13*(3), 319–340.

Davis, F. D. (1989). Perceived usefulness, perceived ease of use, and user acceptance of information technology. *Management Information Systems Quarterly*, *13*(3), 319–340.

Deo, R. C. (2015). Machine learning in medicine. *Circulation*, *132*(20), 1920–1930. DOI: 10.1161/CIRCULATIONAHA.115.001593 PMID: 26572668

Fagherazzi, G., Goetzinger, C., & Rashid, M. A.. (2020). Digital health strategies to fight COVID-19 worldwide. *Journal of Medical Internet Research*, *22*(6), e19284. DOI: 10.2196/19284 PMID: 32501804

Falzon, D., Timimi, H., & Kurosinski, P.. (2016). Digital health for the End TB strategy. *The European Respiratory Journal*, *48*(1), 29–45. DOI: 10.1183/13993003.00424-2016 PMID: 27230443

Fang, Y. (2015). Visualizing the structure and the evolving of digital medicine: A scientometrics review. *Scientometrics*, *105*, 5–21. DOI: 10.1007/s11192-015-1696-1

Fatehi, F., Samadbeik, M., & Kazemi, A. (2020). What is digital health? Review of definitions. In *Integrated citizen centered digital health and social care* (pp. 67–71). IOS Press.

FDA. (2022). Digital Health Center of Excellence. https://www.fda.gov/medical-devices/digital-health-center-excellence

Figueroa-Lorenzo, S., Anorga, J., & Arrizabalaga, S. (2019). Role-based access control in SCADA systems. *Sensors (Basel)*, *19*(20), 4455. PMID: 31615147

Floridi, L., Cowls, J., Beltrametti, M., Chatila, R., Chazerand, P., Dignum, V., Luetge, C., Madelin, R., Pagallo, U., Rossi, F., Schafer, B., Valcke, P., & Vayena, E. (2018). AI4People—An ethical framework for a good AI society: Opportunities, risks, principles, and recommendations. *Minds and Machines*, *28*(4), 689–707. DOI: 10.1007/s11023-018-9482-5 PMID: 30930541

Frenk, J.. (2020). Health professionals for a new century: Transforming education to strengthen health systems. *Lancet*, *376*(9756), 1923–1958. DOI: 10.1016/S0140-6736(10)61854-5 PMID: 21112623

Frenk, J., Chen, L., & Bhutta, Z. A.. (2020). Health professionals for a new century: Transforming education to strengthen health systems. *Lancet*, *376*(9756), 1923–1958. DOI: 10.1016/S0140-6736(10)61854-5 PMID: 21112623

Gagnon, M.-P., Desmartis, M., Labrecque, M., Car, J., Pagliari, C., Pluye, P., Frémont, P., Gagnon, J., Tremblay, N., & Légaré, F. (2010). Systematic review of factors influencing the adoption of information and communication technologies by healthcare professionals. *Journal of Medical Systems*, *36*(1), 241–277. PMID: 20703721

Gagnon, M. P., Orruño, E., Asua, J., Abdeljelil, A. B., & Emparanza, J. (2010). Patient and professional factors influencing teleconsultation acceptance. *International Journal of Medical Informatics*, *79*(8), 539–548. PMID: 20538514

Garavand, A., Mohseni, M., Asadi, H., Etemadi, M., & Moradi-Joo, M. (2016). Factors influencing the adoption of health information technologies: A systematic review. *Electronic Physician*, *8*(8), 2713–2721. PMID: 27757179

Garcia-Moreno, F. M., Bermudez-Edo, M., & Pérez-Mármol, J. M.. (2023). Systematic design of health monitoring systems centered on older adults and ADLs. [BioMed Central]. *BMC Medical Informatics and Decision Making*, *23*(Suppl 3), 300. DOI: 10.1186/s12911-024-02432-3 PMID: 38350979

Gerke, S., Minssen, T., & Cohen, I. G. (2020). Ethical and legal challenges of AI-driven healthcare. In Artif Intell Healthc, 295–336.

Ghosh, S., Dutta, A., & Chatterjee, S. (2023). Digital transformation of healthcare enterprises in the era of disruptions—A structured literature review. *Sustainability*, *17*(13), 5690.

Gochhait, S., Singh, T., Bende, A., Thapliyal, M., Vemulapalli, H., Shukla, G., Ghosh, D., & Chinta, D. Implementation of EHR using Digital Transformation: A study on Telemedicine; *Proceedings of the 2020 International Conference for Emerging Technology (INCET)*; Belgaum, India. 5–7 June 2020; pp. 1–4.

Gostin, L. O., Halabi, S. F., & Wilson, K. (2019). Health data and privacy in the digital era. *Journal of the American Medical Association*, *322*(3), 207–208. DOI: 10.1001/jama.2019.4311 PMID: 31199429

Government of India. (2021). *Ayushman Bharat Digital Mission (ABDM)*. National Health Authority. https://abdm.gov.in

Government of India. (2021). *Ayushman Bharat Digital Mission (ABDM)*. National Health Authority. https://abdm.gov.in

GSMA. (2020). *Mobile for Development: M-TIBA case study*. GSM Association. https://www.gsma.com/mobilefordevelopment

Gulshan, V., Peng, L., Coram, M., Stumpe, M. C., Wu, D., Narayanaswamy, A., & Webster, D. R. (2016). Development and validation of a deep learning algorithm for detection of diabetic retinopathy in retinal fundus photographs. *Journal of the American Medical Association*, *316*(22), 2402–2410. DOI: 10.1001/jama.2016.17216 PMID: 27898976

Gunasekeran, D. V., Tseng, R. M. W. W., Tham, Y. C., & Wong, T. Y. (2021). Applications of digital health for public health responses to COVID-19: A systematic scoping review. npj. *Digital Medicine*, *4*, 36–41. DOI: 10.1038/s41746-021-00412-9 PMID: 33637833

Hamadani, J. D., Hasan, M. I., & Baldi, A. J.. (2020). Immediate impact of stay-at-home orders to control COVID-19 transmission on socioeconomic conditions, food insecurity, mental health, and intimate partner violence in Bangladeshi women and their families. *The Lancet. Global Health*, *8*, e1380–e1389. DOI: 10.1016/S2214-109X(20)30366-1 PMID: 32857955

Healthcare, I. T. News. (2017). 86% of healthcare companies use some form of AI. https://www.healthcareitnews.com/news/86-healthcare-companies-use-some-form-ai

HealthITAnalytics. (2020). Over 80% of health execs have artificial intelligence plans in place. https://healthitanalytics.com/news/over-80-of-health-execs-have-artificial-intelligence-plans-in-place

Hill, C., Martin, J., & Thomson, S.. (2017). Navigating the challenges of digital health innovation. *The British Journal of Psychiatry*, *211*(2), 65–69. DOI: 10.1192/bjp.bp.115.180372 PMID: 28522435

Hinton, G. (2018). Deep Learning - A Technology with the Potential to Transform Health Care. *Journal of the American Medical Association*, *320*(11), 1101–1102. PMID: 30178065

Homayounfar, S. Z., & Andrew, T. L. (2020). Wearable Sensors for Monitoring Human Motion. *SLAS Technology*, *25*, 9–24. PMID: 31829083

Hopfield, J. J. (1982). Neural networks and physical systems with emergent collective computational abilities. *Proceedings of the National Academy of Sciences of the United States of America*, *79*(8), 2554–2558. PMID: 6953413

Hourani, D., Darling, S., & Cameron, E.. (2021). What makes for a successful digital health integrated program of work? *Frontiers in Digital Health*, *3*, 661708. DOI: 10.3389/fdgth.2021.661708 PMID: 34713136

Ibeneme, S., Karamagi, H., & Muneene, D.. (2022). Strengthening health systems using innovative digital health technologies in Africa. *Frontiers in Digital Health*, *4*, 854339. DOI: 10.3389/fdgth.2022.854339 PMID: 35434700

IMA. (2012). *Indian Medical Association Protest Against Clinical Establishment Rules*. Indian Medical Association.

Information Technology Act, No. 21 of 2000, Acts of Parliament, India. (2000). https://www.indiacode.nic.in/handle/123456789/1999

ISO. (2014). *ISO 22600-1:2014 Health informatics — Privilege management and access control*. International Organization for Standardization.

Joseph, T. (2021). Digital health and discriminatory data practices in India. *Economic and Political Weekly*, *56*(40), 22–27.

Joseph, T. (2021). Digital health and discriminatory data practices in India. *Economic and Political Weekly*, *56*(40), 22–27.

Kahar, A. (2020). Adoption barriers in telemedicine in India: A systematic assessment. *Journal of Health Informatics in Developing Countries*, *14*(2), 1–13.

Kaihlanen, A. M., Virtanen, L., & Buchert, U.. (2022). Towards digital health equity. *BMC Health Services Research*, *22*, 188. DOI: 10.1186/s12913-022-07584-4 PMID: 35151302

Kapoor, A., Guha, S., & Kanti Das, M.. (2020). Digital healthcare: The only solution for better healthcare during COVID-19 pandemic? *Indian Heart Journal*, *72*, 61–64. DOI: 10.1016/j.ihj.2020.04.001 PMID: 32534691

Karyotaki, E., Efthimiou, O., & Miguel, C.. (2017). Internet-based cognitive behavioral therapy for depression: A network meta-analysis. *JAMA Psychiatry*, *74*(4), 351–359. DOI: 10.1001/jamapsychiatry.2017.0044 PMID: 28241179

Khosla, S., Tepie, M. F., & Nagy, M. J.. (2021). The alignment of real-world evidence and digital health: Realising the opportunity. *Therapeutic Innovation & Regulatory Science*, *55*, 889–898. DOI: 10.1007/s43441-021-00288-7 PMID: 33914297

Kim, J., Park, Y., & Choi, S. (2025). Wearable sensors and artificial intelligence for sleep apnea detection: A systematic review. *Journal of Medical Systems*, *49*(3), 66. DOI: 10.1007/s10916-025-02199-8 PMID: 40387964

King, W. R., & Jun, H. (2001). A meta-analysis of the technology acceptance model. *Information & Management*, *38*(1), 27–36.

Kruk, M. E., Gage, A. D., Arsenault, C., Jordan, K., Leslie, H. H., Roder-DeWan, S., Adeyi, O., Barker, P., Daelmans, B., & Doubova, S. V. (2018). High-quality health systems in the Sustainable Development Goals era: Time for a revolution. *The Lancet. Global Health*, *6*(11), e1196–e1252. DOI: 10.1016/S2214-109X(18)30386-3 PMID: 30196093

Kruse, C., Betancourt, J., Ortiz, S., Luna, S. M. V., Bamrah, I. K., & Segovia, N. (2019). Barriers to the use of mobile health in improving health outcomes in developing countries: Systematic review. *Journal of Medical Internet Research*, *21*(10), e13263. PMID: 31593543

Kushwaha, S., Bahl, S., Bagha, A. K., Parmar, K. S., Javaid, M., Haleem, A., & Singh, R. P. (2020). Significant applications of machine learning for COVID-19 pandemic. *J Ind Integr Manag*, *5*(4), 453–479.

LeCun, Y., Bengio, Y., & Hinton, G. (2015). Deep learning. nature, 521(7553), 436-444.

Lee, Y., Kozar, K. A., & Larsen, K. R. T. (2003). The technology acceptance model: Past, present, and future. *Communications of the AIS*, *12*(1), 752–780.

Legris, P., Ingham, J., & Collerette, P. (2003). Why do people use information technology? A critical review of the technology acceptance model. *Information & Management*, *40*(3), 191–204.

Leslie, D., Mazumder, A., Peppin, A., Wolters, M. K., & Hagerty, A. (2021). Does AI ethics need ethical AI? *Philosophy & Technology*, *34*(4), 1115–1140. DOI: 10.1007/s13347-021-00470-2

Ma, X., & Vervoort, D. (2020). Critical care capacity during the COVID-19 pandemic: Global availability of intensive care beds. *Journal of Critical Care*, *58*, 96–97. DOI: 10.1016/j.jcrc.2020.04.012 PMID: 32408107

Magrabi, F., Ammenwerth, E., & Craven, C. K.. (2021). Managing pandemic responses with health informatics. *Yearbook of Medical Informatics*, *30*(1), 56–60. DOI: 10.1055/s-0041-1726490 PMID: 33882604

Mahmud, M., & Riley, E. (2021). Household response to an extreme shock: Evidence on the immediate impact of the Covid-19 lockdown on economic outcomes and well-being in rural Uganda. *World Development*, *140*, 105318. DOI: 10.1016/j.worlddev.2020.105318 PMID: 34548741

Mannucci, E., Silverii, G. A., & Monami, M. (2020). Saturation of critical care capacity and mortality in patients with the novel coronavirus (COVID-19) in Italy. *Trends in Anaesthesia & Critical Care, 33*, 33–34. DOI: 10.1016/j.tacc.2020.05.002 PMID: 38620165

Manogaran, G., & Lopez, D. (2017). A survey of big data architectures and machine learning algorithms in healthcare. *International Journal of Biomedical Engineering and Technology*, *25*(2–4), 182–211.

Marazziti, D., & Stahl, S. M. (2020). The relevance of COVID−19 pandemic to psychiatry. *World Psychiatry; Official Journal of the World Psychiatric Association (WPA)*, *19*, 261. DOI: 10.1002/wps.20764 PMID: 32394565

Mehta, S. J., Dacso, C., & Jain, S. H. (2022). Digital health equity: Addressing the digital determinants of health in practice. *NPJ Digital Medicine*, *5*(1), 119. DOI: 10.1038/s41746-022-00660-6 PMID: 35982146

Milne-Ives, M., Lam, C., de Cock, C., Van Velthoven, M., Osei, E., Meinert, E., & Meinert, E. (2020). Mobile apps for health behavior change: Systematic review. *JMIR mHealth and uHealth*, *8*(3), e16915. DOI: 10.2196/16915 PMID: 32186518

Montague, E., & Perchonok, J.. (2012). Health and wellness technology use by underserved health consumers: Systematic review. *Journal of Medical Internet Research*, *14*(3), e2095. PMID: 22652979

Morris, B. B., Rossi, B., & Fuemmeler, B. (2022). The role of digital health technology in rural cancer care delivery: A systematic review. *The Journal of Rural Health*, *38*(3), 493–511. PMID: 34480506

Mukherjee, S., & Shah, I. (2021). The social consequences of labelling Tablighi Jamaat as "super spreader". *Asian Journal of Social Science*, *49*(4), 356–372.

Mukherjee, S., & Shah, I. (2021). The social consequences of labelling Tablighi Jamaat as "super spreader". *Asian Journal of Social Science*, *49*(4), 356–372.

Murthy, S., Leligdowicz, A., & Adhikari, N. K. J. (2015). Intensive care unit capacity in low-income countries: A systematic review. *PLoS One*, *10*, e0116949. DOI: 10.1371/journal.pone.0116949 PMID: 25617837

Nagase, F. I., Stafinski, T., & Avdagovska, M.. (2022). **Effectiveness of remote home monitoring for patients with Chronic Obstructive Pulmonary Disease (COPD):** Systematic review. *BMC Health Services Research*, *22*, 646. BioMedCentralDOI: 10.1186/s12913-022-07938-y PMID: 35568904

Nagase, K., Tanaka, Y., & Saito, M. (2022). AI-enabled wearable devices for chronic disease management: Opportunities and challenges. *Journal of Healthcare Engineering*, *2022*, 1–12. DOI: 10.1155/2022/9876543

NDHM. (2020). *Health Data Management Policy*. National Health Authority, Government of India.

Nguyen, A., Paustian, M., & Ibarra, J. (2021). Digital transformation in healthcare systems: Assessing adoption and readiness in post-COVID era. *Journal of Medical Internet Research*, *23*(6), e28865.

NHS Digital. (2022). *Digital transformation strategy*. NHS England. https://digital.nhs.uk

Nicola M, Alsafi Z, Sohrabi C, et al. (2020). The socio-economic implications of the coronavirus pandemic

O'Mahony, C., Jichi, F., & Pavlou, M.. (2014). A novel clinical risk prediction model for sudden cardiac death in hypertrophic cardiomyopathy (HCM risk-SCD). *European Heart Journal*, *35*(30), 2010–2020. DOI: 10.1093/eurheartj/eht439 PMID: 24126876

Obermeyer, Z., & Emanuel, E. J. (2016). Big Data, Machine Learning, and Clinical Medicine. *The New England Journal of Medicine*, *375*(13), 1216–1219. PMID: 27682033

OECD. (2021). *Empowering the health workforce to make the most of the digital revolution.* OECD Health Working Paper No. 129. https://doi.org/DOI: 10.1787/4a9f0ad5-en

OECD. (2021). *Health at a Glance: Digital Health Insights.* OECD Publishing., DOI: 10.1787/ae3016b9-

OECD. (2021). *Health at a Glance: Digital Health Insights.* OECD Publishing., DOI: 10.1787/ae3016b9-

Owoyemi, A., Osuchukwu, J., & Azibuike, C.. (2022). Digital solutions for community and primary health workers: Lessons from implementations in Africa. *Frontiers in Digital Health*, *4*, 876957. DOI: 10.3389/fdgth.2022.876957 PMID: 35754461

Pattichis, C. S., & Panayides, A. S. (2019). Connected health. *Frontiers in Digital Health*, *1*, 1–3. DOI: 10.3389/fdgth.2019.00001 PMID: 34713013

Peiffer-Smadja, N., Rawson, T. M., & Ahmad, R.. (2020). Machine learning for clinical decision support in infectious diseases: A narrative review of current applications. *Clinical Microbiology and Infection*, *26*(5), 584–595. DOI: 10.1016/j.cmi.2019.09.009 PMID: 31539636

Pinto, R. (2022). Implementation challenges of ISO standards in Indian healthcare. *Health Informatics Journal*, *28*(2), 211–225.

Price, W. N., & Cohen, I. G. (2019). Privacy in the age of medical big data. *Nature Medicine*, *25*(1), 37–43. PMID: 30617331

Qudah, B., Albrecht, U. V., & Schoech, E. (2022). Factors influencing adoption of mobile health applications: An extended TAM approach. *International Journal of Medical Informatics*, *159*, 104691.

Reddy, A. (2023). Legal gaps in India's digital health transformation. *Indian Journal of Medical Ethics*, *8*(1), 13–19. PMID: 35695849

Reddy, A. (2023). Legal gaps in India's digital health transformation. *Indian Journal of Medical Ethics*, *8*(1), 13–19. PMID: 35695849

Remote Monitoring and Holistic Care of Home-Isolated COVID-19 Positive Healthcare Workers During the Omicron Wave: Prospective Cohort Study From India. Jain, Agarwal, Bhardwaj, Lakshmi, Singh, Chauhan, Singh. (2022). Frontiers in Public Health etc. *Frontiers*.

Remote Patient Monitoring Applications in Healthcare: Lessons from COVID-19 and Beyond. Khan, A., & Duncan, D. (2025). *Electronics*, *14*(15), 3084. https://doi.org/MDPIDOI: 10.3390/electronics14153084

Rossi, R., Socci, V., & Talevi, D.. (2020). COVID-19 pandemic and lockdown measures impact on mental health among the general population in Italy. *Frontiers in Psychiatry*, *11*, 790. DOI: 10.3389/fpsyt.2020.00790 PMID: 32848952

Roth, J. A., Battegay, M., Juchler, F., Vogt, J. E., & Widmer, A. F. (2018). Introduction to machine learning in digital healthcare epidemiology. *Infection Control and Hospital Epidemiology*, *39*(12), 1457–1462. PMID: 30394238

Rudin, C., & Ustun, B. (2018). Optimized scoring systems: Toward trust in machine learning for healthcare and criminal justice. *Interfaces*, *48*(5), 449–466.

Sætra, H. S., & Fosch-Villaronga, E. (2021). Healthcare digitalisation and the changing nature of work and society. *Humanities & Social Sciences Communications*, *8*, 219. DOI: 10.1057/s41599-021-00859-9 PMID: 34442144

Salam, M., & Varma, A. (2019). A review on impact of e-waste on soil microbial community and ecosystem function. *Pollution*, *5*(4), 761–774. DOI: 10.22059/poll.2019.277556.592

Shajari, S., Kuruvinashetti, K., Komeili, A., & Sundararaj, U. (2023). The emergence of AI-based wearable sensors for digital health technology: A review. *Sensors (Basel)*, *23*(23), 9498. DOI: 10.3390/s23239498 PMID: 38067871

Sharma, N., Kaur, S., & Singh, P. (2023). Digital inclusion and accessibility: Bridging the gap for persons with disabilities in healthcare systems. *Journal of Health Informatics in Developing Countries*, *17*(2), 45–59.

Sharma, S. (2019). Time constraints and patient load in primary healthcare settings in India. *Indian Journal of Community Medicine : Official Publication of Indian Association of Preventive & Social Medicine*, *44*(3), 240–244. PMID: 31602100

Singh, R. P., Hom, G. L., Abramoff, M. D., Campbell, J. P., & Chiang, M. F. (2020). Current challenges and barriers to real-world artificial intelligence adoption for the healthcare system, provider, and the patient. *Translational Vision Science & Technology*, *9*(2), 45–45. PMID: 32879755

Socha-Dietrich, K., Vujicic, M., & Weideman, M. (2021). *Empowering the health workforce to make the most of the digital revolution.* OECD Health Working Paper No. 129. OECD Publishing. https://doi .org/DOI: 10.1787/4a9f0ad5-en

Strudwick, G. (2015). *Predicting nurses' use of healthcare technology using the Technology Acceptance Model: An integrative review.* CIN: Computers, Informatics. *Nursing*, *33*(5), 189–198. PMID: 25974361

Strudwick, G. (2015). Predicting nurses' use of healthcare technology using the Technology Acceptance Model (TAM). *Computers, Informatics, Nursing*, *33*(5), 189–198. PMID: 25974361

Sun, T. Q., & Medaglia, R. (2019). AI in the public sector: Evidence from healthcare. Gov Inf Q, 36(2), 368–383.Turakhia, M. P., Desai, M., Perez, M. V., Apple, Watch Study Investigators. (2019). Diagnostic utility of a smartwatch for atrial fibrillation detection. *Journal of the American Medical Association*, *321*(3), 247–257. DOI: 10.1001/jama.2018.20045 PMID: 30570663

Sun, Y., Wang, Y., Wang, L., & Zhang, Z. (2021). Wearable technologies for health promotion and disease prevention. *Journal of Medical Internet Research*, *23*(5), e25642. DOI: 10.2196/25642 PMID: 34028359

Sun, Y., Wang, Y., Wang, L., & Zhang, Z. (2021). Wearable technologies for health promotion and disease prevention. *Journal of Medical Internet Research*, *23*(5), e25642. DOI: 10.2196/25642 PMID: 34028359

Tausch, A., Heshmati, A., & Brand, U. (2022). Regional health system performance and digital transformation in developing economies. *International Journal of Health Policy and Management*, *11*(7), 1382–1393. DOI: 10.34172/ijhpm.2021.25

Van Dijk, J. (2020). *The digital divide: Understanding inequality in the information society*. Sage Publications.

Van Dijk, J. (2020). *The digital divide: Understanding inequality in the information society*. Sage Publications.

Venkatesh, V., & Bala, H. (2008). Technology acceptance model 3 and a research agenda on interventions. *Decision Sciences*, *39*(2), 273–315.

Venkatesh, V., & Davis, F. D. (2000). A theoretical extension of the technology acceptance model: Four longitudinal field studies. *Management Science*, *46*(2), 186–204.

Venkatesh, V., & Davis, F. D. (2000). A theoretical extension of the technology acceptance model: Four longitudinal field studies. *Management Science*, *46*(2), 186–204.

Venkatesh, V., Morris, M. G., Davis, G. B., & Davis, F. D. (2003). User acceptance of information technology: Toward a unified view. *Management Information Systems Quarterly*, *27*(3), 425–478.

Vishal, K.. (2022). Transforming healthcare delivery: The role of digital technologies in disease preven tion and health monitoring. *Journal of Digital Health Innovation*, *4*(2), 45–56.

Vishal, K.. (2024). AI-driven preventive healthcare frameworks in low-resource environments. *International Journal of AI in Health Systems*, *6*(1), 22–38.

vishal, K., Sharma, R., & Kaur, P. (2023). Environmental impacts and sustainability challenges of advanced digital health technologies. *International Journal of Green Technology and Sustainable Computing*, 11(4), 55–68.

Voigt, P., & Von dem Bussche, A. (2017). *The EU General Data Protection Regulation (GDPR)*. Springer Publications.

Vollmer, S., Mateen, B. A., & Bohner, G.. (2020). ML for patient benefit: 20 questions. *BMJ (Clinical Research Ed.)*, *368*. Advance online publication. DOI: 10.1136/bmj.l6927 PMID: 32198138

Wang, T., Lee, S., & Kim, H. (2023). Barriers and facilitators of AI adoption in clinical decision support systems: A systematic review. *BMC Medical Informatics and Decision Making*, *23*(1), 17–29. PMID: 36691014

Wang, X., Liu, Z., & Zhang, T. (2017). Flexible Sensing Electronics for Health Monitoring. *Small*, *13*, 1602790. PMID: 28306196

Watts, D. J., & Strogatz, S. H. (1998). Collective dynamics of 'small-world' networks. *Nature*, *393*(6684), 440–442. PMID: 9623998

Wearable technologies used in the monitoring of cardiovascular diseases in the community: A systematic review of randomizedcontrolledtrials. (2025). [journal details]. PubMed

Wei, S., & Wu, Z. (2023). The application of wearable sensors and machine learning algorithms in rehabilitation training: A systematic review. *Sensors (Basel), 23*(18), 7667. DOI: 10.3390/s23187667 PMID: 37765724

World Bank. (2022). *Individuals using the Internet (% of population)*. World Bank Open Data.

World Bank. (2022). *Digital-in-health: Unlocking the value for everyone*. World Bank Group. https://documents.worldbank.org

World Bank. (2022). *Digital-in-health: Unlocking the value for everyone*. World Bank Group.

World Health Organization. (2020). *Operational Planning Guidelines To Support Country Preparedness and Response*. WHO.

World Health Organization. (2020). *Global strategy on digital health 2020–2025*. World Health Organization. https://www.who.int/docs/default-source/documents/global-strategy-on-digital-health-2020-2025

World Health Organization. (2020). *Global strategy on digital health 2020–2025*. World Health Organization. https://www.who.int/docs/default-source/documents/global-strategy-on-digital-health-2020-2025

World Health Organization. (2024). *Health equity for persons with disabilities: guide for action*. World Health Organization.

World Health Organization (WHO). (2022). *Tracking universal health coverage: 2021 global monitoring report.* Geneva: World Health Organization. https://www.who.int/publications/i/item/9789240061269

Wu, J.-Y., Wang, Y., Ching, C. T. S., Wang, H.-M. D., & Liao, L.-D. (2023). IoT-based wearable health monitoring device and its validation for potential critical and emergency applications. *Frontiers in Public Health, 11*, 1188304. DOI: 10.3389/fpubh.2023.1188304 PMID: 37397724

Yang, X., & Yu, Y.. (2020). Clinical course and outcomes of critically ill patients with SARS-CoV-2 pneumonia in Wuhan, China: A single centered, retrospective, observational study. *The Lancet. Respiratory Medicine, 8*, 475–481. DOI: 10.1016/S2213-2600(20)30079-5 PMID: 32105632

Zdravković, S. (2008). Telemedicine: Perspectives and expectations. *Archive of Oncology, 16*, 69–73. DOI: 10.2298/AOO0804069Z

Zhang, L., Chen, H., & Zhao, M. (2024). Internet access and digital health adoption: Global comparative insights. *Telemedicine Journal and e-Health, 30*(1), 12–25.

Zhang, L., He, J., & Wang, Y. (2024). Wearable sensor-enabled systems for early detection of depression: A systematic review. *IEEE Access : Practical Innovations, Open Solutions, 12*, 54321–54335. DOI: 10.1109/ACCESS.2024.3456789

Zucker, R. S., & Regehr, W. G. (2002). Short-term synaptic plasticity. *Annual Review of Physiology, 64*(1), 355–405. PMID: 11826273

KEY TERMS AND DEFINITIONS

API: An interface that allows different software applications to communicate, share data, and perform functions smoothly, enabling integration, automation, and efficient interaction between systems and digital services.

Binary Classification: Binary Classification is a supervised learning method that categorises data into two classes (e.g., diabetic/non-diabetic), enabling transparent decision-making, prediction, and medical diagnosis using labelled input features.

Chatbots: AI-driven virtual assistants that understand user queries, provide instant responses, automate tasks, offer healthcare guidance, and improve communication by interacting via text or voice in real time.

Convolutional Neural Networks: A Convolutional Neural Network (CNN) is a deep learning model that automatically extracts features from images using convolutional layers, enabling accurate classification, disease detection, and pattern recognition in medical imaging.

Cloud Computing: Cloud Computing provides on-demand storage, processing power, and services over the internet, enabling scalable data management, remote access, real-time analytics, and efficient deployment of healthcare or AI applications.

Digital Health: Digital Health uses technologies such as mobile apps, wearables, telemedicine, and AI to monitor health, enhance diagnosis, improve patient care, and support data-driven healthcare delivery.

Digital Transformation: The process of integrating digital technologies into systems or services to improve efficiency, enhance decision-making, automate workflows, and deliver faster, smarter, and more innovative operations.

Environmental & Sustainability: Environmental and Sustainability focuses on protecting natural resources, reducing pollution, promoting renewable energy, and ensuring long-term ecological balance for a healthier planet and future generations.

Epidemiology: The scientific study of the spread and control of diseases

Interoperability: The ability of different systems, devices, or applications to exchange, interpret, and use data seamlessly, enabling coordinated healthcare, efficient workflows, and integrated digital solutions.

KardiaMobile: A pocket-sized medical device that records medical-grade ECG in seconds, detects heart rhythm abnormalities, and syncs results to a smartphone for quick cardiac monitoring anywhere.

Logistic Regression: A supervised ML algorithm that predicts the probability of a binary outcome, helping classify diseases, assess risks, and support medical decision-making using input features.

Multiclass Classification: A supervised learning method that assigns input data to more than two categories, enabling prediction, diagnosis, and analysis across multiple disease types or outcomes.

Patient Centric: Patient-centric is a healthcare model focused on individual patient needs, preferences, and experiences, promoting personalised care, active engagement, improved outcomes, and better communication between patients and providers.

Sensors: Electronic components that detect and measure physical or biological signals, such as temperature, heart rate, movement, or glucose levels, converting them into data for monitoring, analysis, and innovative healthcare applications.

Supervised Machine Learning: Supervised Machine Learning uses labelled data to train models that learn input–output relationships, enabling accurate prediction, classification, and early disease detection by mapping patient features to known health outcomes.

Technology Acceptance Model: The: Technology Acceptance Model (TAM) explains how users adopt and use technology, emphasising perceived usefulness and ease of use to predict acceptance and effective integration in healthcare or other systems.

Transformation: The process of converting data, signals, or systems from one form to another, enabling better analysis, improved understanding, enhanced performance, and effective decision-making across various applications.

Unsupervised Machine Learning: Unsupervised Machine Learning automatically discovers hidden patterns, clusters, and relationships in unlabeled data, helping identify anomalies, group similar patients, support diagnosis patterns, and reveal insights without predefined output labels.

Wearable Devices: Wearable devices use advanced sensors to monitor real-time health parameters such as glucose, heart rate, activity, and sleep, enabling early disease detection, continuous tracking, timely alerts, and personalised healthcare support.

Chapter 10

From Self Reports to Sensors in Machine Learning and Multimodal Advances in Chronic Stress Detection

Mamta Nag
IIIT Naya Raipur, India

J. Vijaya
https://orcid.org/0000-0002-9948-8573
IIIT Naya Raipur, India

K. Mallikharjuna Rao
https://orcid.org/0000-0002-6096-3963
IIIT Naya Raipur, India

ABSTRACT

Traditional stress assessment methods rely on self-reports, which are subjective and lack real-time responsiveness. Recent advances in multimodal stress detection address these limits by integrating physiological, behavioral, and environmental data, improving accuracy and robustness. This review synthesizes findings from 50+ recent peer-reviewed studies, highlighting the role of wearable sensors and AI models in high-stress environments. Physiological markers such as Electrodermal Activity (EDA), Heart Rate Variability (HRV), and respiration emerge as reliable indicators, with EDA distinguishing stress from cognitive load in mobile contexts. Machine learning and deep learning methods—including Random Forests, CNNs, LSTMs, and federated learning—report accuracies above 90%. Key challenges remain in data collection, feature extraction, fusion, and interpretability, alongside ethical concerns over privacy and fairness. Finally, a roadmap is proposed toward explainable, privacy-preserving stress monitoring systems tailored for chronic stress management.

DOI: 10.4018/979-8-3373-3531-5.ch010

INTRODUCTION

Because of the speed of modern life, a significant portion of the global population now experiences chronic stress, which is an undesirable but inevitable part of their lives. It is a silent epidemic, a constant unease of both physiological and psychological pressure: an insidious layer of stress at an experiential level that is far more than just feeling overwhelmed. The clinical evidence is clear: chronic and uncontrolled stress is one of the main causes of serious physical and mental health problems, and is potentially the largest comorbid factor in nearly every serious health condition. Stress is also an established precursor to the development and maintenance of main depressive and anxiety disorders, which often trap the individual in a detrimental cycle that is virtually impossible to break (Aqajari et al., 2024). Stress does not impact just the mind. The physiological wear and tear on the body (physiological damage) caused by recurrent activation of the "fight-or-flight" situations produces a cost to health, contributing to accelerated cellular aging, higher risk of cardiovascular disease, immune dysregulation, and metabolic syndrome. The social and economic cost is staggering: decreased productivity and increased rate of employee 'burnout' for employers and stakeholders globally, and the increased costs in health and social services makes it urgent for governments and public policy to make better progress on strategies to manage stress globally.

At the core of any effective strategy is the capacity to see the problem clearly, to accurately and continuously measure it. The reality is however, we have been poorly equipped to assess stress for decades. Until recently, psychological assessment of stress has primarily relied on retrospective clinical interviews of varying quantifiable importance at formal assessment as well as self-report questionnaires that are wildly inaccurate (Archana & Devaraju, 2020). Our reliance on outdated measures either legitimately or under social pressure (social acceptance bias) understate stressors when presenting data. Regardless, none of the stress measures when reviewing the data dynamically address the timeline or time resolution and suffer from inherent inaccuracies in regards to time. While clinical interviews, administration of self-report questionnaires or some combination of both provides a snapshot of a single period of time, (i.e., weeks, or months) at best that is somewhat wrong since the problem is actually dynamic not static and is therefore best represented as a fluid experience. As such, it does not take into consideration how individuals, clinicians and employers navigate experiences if they do not have a current and accurate map especially if the map is outdated and wholly inaccurate. A deep technological revolution is filling the long-lasting diagnostic gap, revolution stemming from the combination of two technological innovations: the proliferation of biosensors worn on the body and the intelligence of applied machine learning. The first pillar is hardware. Wearable devices have effectively placed a research-quality physiological laboratory on the wrist of millions (AristiZabal et al., 2021). The sophisticated sensors that previously only existed within constrained or controlled research parameters are now applied in consumer-grade smartwatches, fitness trackers, and smart rings. These devices now turn the body's small, analog language (the elegant dance of heart rate variability (HRV), skin conductance (eds), ethnic patterns (like counts of breaths or sleep stages)), into a continuous fidelity digital story. All of the objective real-world data from these continuous streams will be the basis for a new digital data-driven science for mental health monitoring.

This influx of raw physiological data, however is noise without T whisker was or guides someone capacious learning) is signal could mean work is due, a heated argument, walk up a flight of stairs, or pure joy. This dimension to the revolution: a second pillar - the interpretation engine that is as necessary to find the signal in the noise. This added complexity: the amount of data can (require computational brain) many machine learning (ML) algorithms can learn the nuance, multidimensional patterns that consistently distinguish the physiology signature form negative psychological distress from these confusing states. The initial work in the field demonstrated proof of concept using traditional, interpretable models like Support Vector Machines (SVM) and Random Forest (RF) the field established a minimum of performance on publicly available datasets, WESAD [3] at acceptable levels.

Building on this, momentum quickly transitioned into deep learning. Model architectures like one-dimensional Convolutional Neural Networks (1D-CNNs) and Long Short-Term Memory (LSTMs) shifted paradigms towards end-to-end learning, enabling models to learn how to find the most important predictive features directly from raw sensor data, eliminated manual feature engineering, and furthermore offer potential fund and accuracy previously not realized (Bobade & Vani, 2020), (Bodaghi et al., 2024). A perhaps equally important evolutionary track, running in parallel with this algorithmic development, has been a real paradigmatic shift toward a more holistic approach to stress. Researchers quickly came to understand that stress is a very broad, whole-body experience that one single data stream can never fully encapsulate, no matter how clean it may be. This understanding has forced the field decisively into multimodal systems that are capable of tying together data from many sources to create a stronger, more contextually relevant model. Such multimodal systems can combine both internal physiological signals with external behaviours (e.g. rich information such as the slight flinch of a facial expression as encoded by a camera (Bolpagni et al., 2024) and even examine the linguistic content or the sentiment included in the text of social media postings in order to understand the context surrounding a spike in physiological measurements. As these systems become stronger and more accurate, the field is also maturing, shifting focus to the "last-mile" challenges of deploying them in the real world. The nature of complex deep learning models is non-transparent, black-box in nature, creating a pressing need to explore Explainable AI (XAI) to ensure systems are transparent, trustworthy and auditable especially within clinical applications. Simultaneously, there are the well-known and evident privacy risks associated with collecting and storing such intimate and personal data; these privacy risks underscore why privacy-preserving architectures such as Federated Learning, which enables model development while the raw data remains on the user's device, are necessary and unobjectionable areas of research (Booth et al., 2022).

This survey provides an organized and comprehensive introduction to this exciting and rapidly changing field. We synthesize the results from a selection of key seminal and recent research studies, to give a coherent account of this field, and its evolution from first principles to cutting edge. We will systematically organize the various methodological approaches, describe the emergent evolution of the core technologies, and critically analyse real-world applications of these tools, which are beginning to fundamentally change how we approach the understanding and management of well-being. We will position and address the hardest problems we face and then lay out the most promising future directions for intelligent systems and how they can help us manage stress not solely in reactive ways, but also in responsible and proactive ways, and as effectively as possible.

BACKGROUND

The shift toward automated systems powered by machine learning (ML) and deep learning (DL) offers a more objective and scalable solution to stress and affect detection. One of the foundational studies by Can et al. (2019) utilized physiological signals including blood volume pulse, skin conductivity, skin temperature, electromyography, and respiration to recognize emotions in human–machine interaction. Classifiers such as Support Vector Machines (SVM) and Fisher Discriminant Analysis achieved high accuracy, demonstrating the effectiveness of physiological markers in affect recognition. Building on this, studies by Chen et al. (2020) and Cuevas et al (2019) underscored the critical role of feature selection techniques in enhancing classification accuracy while reducing computational complexity, a key requirement when working with high-dimensional multimodal datasets. Expanding beyond human affect detection, Gedam & Paul (2021) explored the application of ML tools in plant stress phenotyping, a novel and rapidly developing area in plant sciences. Their work highlights the importance of integrating ML into data collection, processing, and curation workflows to increase efficiency and accuracy in agricultural practices. In another domain, Geeta et al. (2024) investigated the potential of Virtual Reality (VR) and Brain–Computer Interaction (BCI) technologies to improve immersive experiences by directly linking to users' brains. Leveraging affective computing and psychophysiological methods, their study measured and influenced emotional engagement, thereby paving the way for ML-based approaches capable of detecting stress more reliably and dynamically. Hasib et al. (2023) presented the Tesserae project, which employs large-scale, longitudinal, multimodal wearable sensing to monitor well-being in information workers. Their findings illustrate how wearable data can uncover real-world patterns in stress, anxiety, and affect. Complementing this, Hosseini et al. (2022) conducted a comparative analysis showing that ensemble learning techniques significantly enhance stress detection accuracy using physiological signals, emphasizing the benefits of combining multiple models to improve robustness and generalization. Beyond stress detection, Jaber et al. (2022) proposed a hybrid optimization algorithm that integrates quantum-behaved simulated annealing with moth-flame optimization. This method demonstrated faster convergence and higher solution accuracy in complex mathematical modeling, showcasing the adaptability of ML-driven optimization methods. Finally, Je et al. (2021) provided a comprehensive review of ML applications for identifying risk factors associated with obesity and overweight. Their work demonstrates the potential of ML techniques in analyzing complex health datasets for early risk prediction and preventive healthcare. Applying machine learning to human stress is the result of a long-standing scientific quest for ongoing, individualized, and impartial mental health monitoring; it is not just a computational challenge. It is necessary to first comprehend the biological phenomenon being measured and then follow the intellectual development of the research intended to decode it in order to completely appreciate the contemporary approaches, their inherent challenges, and their potential for the future. After exploring the physiological underpinnings of the stress response—the "digital footprint" it leaves on the body this section offers a systematic summary of the relevant literature, tracing the development of the field from basic ideas to the state-of-the-art.

A Digital Footprint of Stress: The Body's Alarm System

The autonomic nervous system (ANS) and the Hypothalamic-Pituitary-Adrenal (HPA) axis are the primary regulators of stress, which is defined biologically as the body's complex and highly coordinated response to any demand or perceived threat. The "fight-or-flight" branch of the ANS, the Sympathetic Nervous System (SNS), sets off a quick series of physiological reactions in response to stressors, preparing the body for quick action. This activation generates a variety of concrete, measurable signals that contemporary sensors can pick up, so it's not just an abstract idea. Almost all machine learning models in this field use these signals as their raw input (Hosseini et al., 2023) .

- **Rhythm of the Heart (HRV):** The heart system is extremely reactive to stress, so the most researched modality. SNS activation naturally elevates HR and blood pressure and at the same time inhibits the activity of the Parasympathetic Nervous System (PNS), the "rest-and-digest" division that is tasked with relaxation and restoration. This dynamic interplay is best described by Heart Rate Variability (HRV), which quantifies the small, millisecond-order fluctuation in interval between heartbeats. A high HRV, reflecting an ideal equilibrium between SNS and PNS, reflects a flexible, resilient, and responsive physiological state. Low HRV is an old and reliable marker for a stressed body, associated with impaired physiological resilience. Due to this, HRV from either clinical-grade electrocardiography (ECG) or the photoplethysmography (PPG) sensors used in most smartwatches provides a foundation for recent research on stress detection.

- **Skin Reaction (EDA):** Electrodermal Activity (EDA), or Galvanic Skin Response (GSR), gives a "pure" and unbiased measure of sympathetic activation. Sweat glands are rare in being innervated almost solely by the SNS. Tiny, imperceptible variations in perspiration that occur during episodes of emotional or physical activation change the electrical conductivity of the skin. Since it is very resistant to the parasympathetic nervous system, EDA is an instant and unambiguous body measure of "fight-or-flight" state activation. Its sensitivity and resilience make it a primary feature in the majority of multimodal stress datasets, e.g., the WESAD benchmark, which is widely used, and a focal point for on-body sensing (KS S, 2022).
- **Electrical Activity of the Brain (EEG):** In attempting to get nearer to the central nervous system's function in stress, researchers resort to electroencephalography. By inserting electrodes upon the scalp to record electrical activity of the brain, EEG is able to identify characteristic alterations in brainwave patterns during stress. This may involve alterations in the amplitude of particular frequency bands, i.e., a reduction in alpha wave amplitude (which is related to relaxed, quiet states) and an increase in beta wave amplitude (which is related to active, anxious thinking). The high temporal resolution and informativeness of EEG make it a strong modality, albeit rather less convenient for general use than wearables. It has but brought about the advent of advanced deep learning models tasked with attributing its very intricate spatiotemporal patterns
- **Peripheral and Behavioral Manifestations:** The response to stress is not solely internal; it occurs in our behavior and other peripheral cues. Algorithms of computer vision are today learned to detect the telltale signs of stress on our face the furrowing of an eyebrow, the stiffening of a jaw, or the alteration of eye-blink rate giving a strong behavioral cue. In a very recent and pioneering set of studies, postural change and motion kinematics, recorded using full-body sensor suits, have proven to be trustworthy indicators of acute psychosocial stress. A variety of other peripheral measures, including skin temperature, respiratory rhythm, and even sleep-pattern disruption, are standardly incorporated into large-scale models to create an enhanced physiological picture (Korkmaz et al., 2025)

A Digital Footprint of Stress: Psychological Dimensions of Stress

- **Cognitive processes (Thinking Pattern):** Cognitive processes refer to the way individuals perceive, interpret, and mentally evaluate stressors. These include thought patterns such as anticipation, rumination, attention allocation, and perceived controllability of a situation. Cognitive appraisal determines whether a stimulus is interpreted as threatening, manageable, or neutral, thereby directly influencing the stress response. Differences in cognitive processing explain why identical situations may elicit varying stress levels across individuals (Vallone, 2024)

Methods for Integration with Machine Learning:

- o **Self-report and Cognitive Assessment Modeling:** Structured questionnaires and cognitive scales (e.g., perceived stress or cognitive load measures) can be encoded as features and combined with physiological signals in supervised learning models.
- o **Text and Speech-Based Cognitive Analysis:** Natural Language Processing (NLP) techniques applied to speech transcripts, written responses, or diary entries can capture cognitive markers such as negative thought patterns, uncertainty, or rumination.
- o **EEG-Based Cognitive Load Estimation:** EEG features related to attention and mental workload can be modeled using deep learning architectures to infer cognitive stress levels.
    - **Emotional state:** Emotional state refers to the affective responses associated with stress, such as anxiety, fear, frustration, or sadness. Emotional reactions mediate the relationship between cognitive appraisal and physiological activation. Prolonged negative emotional states can intensify stress responses and contribute to chronic stress conditions. Emotional variability and regulation capacity are therefore critical components of stress dynamics (Vallone, 2024)

Methods for Integration with Machine Learning:

- o **Emotion Recognition from Facial Expressions:** Computer vision–based models, including convolutional neural networks (CNNs), can detect emotional states from facial cues and micro-expressions.
- o **Speech and Voice Emotion Analysis:** Acoustic features such as pitch, tone, and speech rate can be analyzed using machine learning classifiers to infer emotional stress indicators.
- o **Multimodal Affective Fusion Models:** Emotional features from facial, vocal, and physiological data can be fused using multimodal deep learning frameworks to improve stress detection accuracy.
    - **Situational appraisal(Contextual Understanding):** Situational appraisal involves the individual's interpretation of environmental context, including task demands, social setting, time pressure, and perceived support. Contextual factors strongly influence how stress is experienced and expressed. Ignoring situational context may lead to misinterpretation of physiological stress signals, as elevated responses can also occur during non-stressful but demanding activities (Vallone, 2024).

Methods for Integration with Machine Learning:

- o **Context-Aware Modeling:** Sensor data such as location, activity level, and time-based information can be incorporated into machine learning models to contextualize physiological stress signals.
- o **Behavioral Pattern Analysis:** Wearable and mobile data capturing movement, interaction patterns, and daily routines can be used to infer situational stressors through unsupervised or semi-supervised learning.

- o **Hybrid Physiological–Contextual Models:** Combining physiological signals with contextual metadata enables machine learning models to distinguish stress-related responses from context-driven arousal.

By integrating cognitive processes, emotional states, and situational appraisal with physiological data, machine learning–based stress models can move beyond a purely biological perspective. Such integrative approaches address the psychological complexity of stress and reduce the risk of reductionist interpretations, thereby aligning computational models more closely with contemporary stress theory.

A Field in Motion:

A clear and logical evolutionary trajectory is revealed by the corpus of research aimed at deciphering this rich digital footprint. From early proof-of-concept tests employing traditional algorithms to extremely complex, multimodal deep learning frameworks made to manage the subtleties and complexity of practical application, research has methodically advanced.

This development can be viewed as a sequence of intellectual movements that build on one another to produce increasingly strong, reliable, and powerful systems.

- **Phase 1: Using classical ML to demonstrate that it is feasible:** A basic question that motivated the first wave of research was whether stress could be accurately predicted from sensor data at all. Researchers used reliable, computationally efficient, and reasonably interpretable algorithms from the classical machine learning toolkit to address this. Sensor data, frequently from controlled laboratory experiments or survey-based datasets, was subjected to models such as Random Forest (RF), Support Vector Machines (SVM), and K-Nearest Neighbors (KNN).

In addition to demonstrating the concept's feasibility through their consistent success in stress classification, they also set critical performance benchmarks on publicly available datasets such as WESAD, which are still used to assess new models today (Kyamakya et al., 2021).

- **Phase 2: The DL Breakthrough for Automated Feature Learning:** Although early models demonstrated the feasibility, their performance began to level off and required researchers to choose and pick the best predictive features from the data—ideally a hard, time-consuming, and expert-demanding task. The deep learning breakthrough presented an attractive alternative: end-to-end learning. Architectures such as Convolutional Neural Networks (CNNs) might be able to learn the most significant hierarchical features from raw time-series or 2D representations such as spectrograms. Meanwhile, Recurrent Neural Networks (RNNs) and their enhanced variant, Long Short-Term Memory (LSTM) networks, were set to capture temporal evolution and interdependence in physiological signals in an explicit way [8]. This resulted in much higher predictive accuracy and spawned powerful hybrid models such as the CNN-LSTM, which leverage the strengths of both spatial feature extraction in the CNNs and sequential modeling in LSTMs, and are today a standard approach to solving difficult sensor data (Mathur & Sethia, 2024).
- **Phase 3: The Multimodal Imperative for Robustness:** After the algorithms became stronger, the essential philosophical transformation happened. The researchers began to understand increasingly that dependence on one signal was inherently weak. A heart rate monitor will not know

the distinction between the physiological excitement of fear and excitement from a great run. This ambiguity in it leads to a high false positive rate and undermines the trust of the users. This awareness resulted in the unapologetic experimentation with multimodal fusion. What one stands to gain is an enhanced and context-rich image through the enlightened integration of different data streams—integrating more than one physiological signal, integrating internal biology with external behavior signals such as facial expressions, or even inspecting the social media post's language to learn more about the reason for a physiological spike (Medina Fernández et al., 2021).

- **Phase 4: Maturing to Meet Real-World Challenges:** The intersection of very powerful but black-box models compelled the community to grow up and confront the practical and ethical issues of real-world use. This imposed novel architectural mandates. The "black box" model of deep learning established an urgent need for Explainable AI (XAI) to provide enough transparency for models to be used in healthcare settings and instill user confidence. Likewise, the enormous privacy hazards of homogenizing massive amounts of personal health information have made it that privacy-friendly paradigms such as Federated Learning (FL), where models are collaboratively trained on users' devices without their raw data ever exiting them, are an indispensable and non-negotiable field of study for any ethically-mandated rollout.

MAIN FOCUS OF THE CHAPTER

Building a machine learning model for stress detection is an algorithmic, step-by-step process that can be thought of as a data-driven pipeline. The pipeline starts with the first and often daunting task of obtaining relevant data, moves on to data cleaning and feature representation, and ends with the careful training and testing of a predictive model which shown in Figure 1. Every step in this pipeline entails a unique set of methodological choices and trade-offs that significantly impact the strength, accuracy, and finally the usability of the final system in real-world scenarios

Figure 1. Framework for Stress predition model

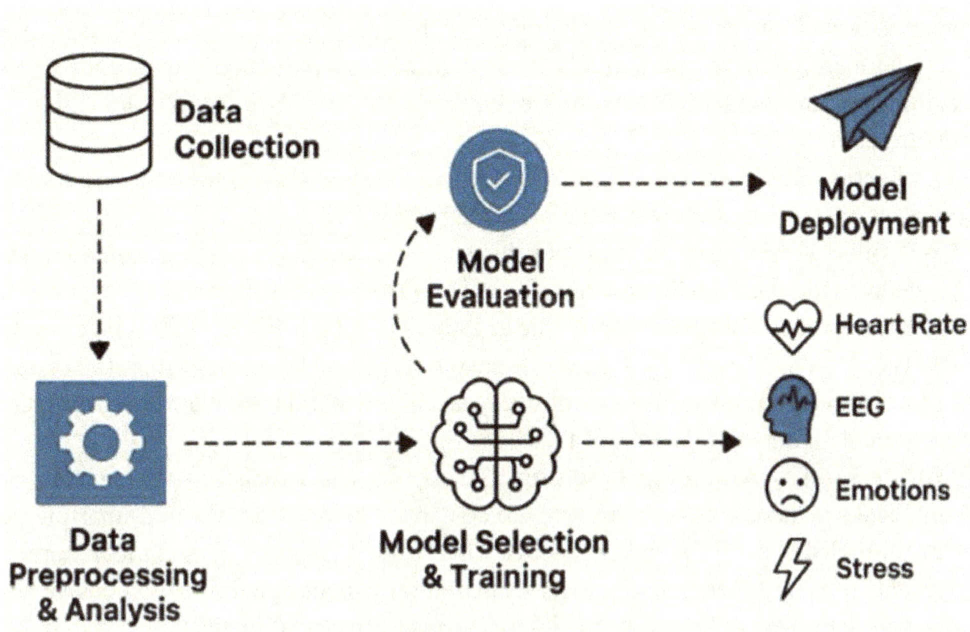

1. Data Acquisition:

The entire stress detection system is built upon the data used to train and test it. The selection of data modalities and the environment in which they are collected represent the first and most critical decisions in the research process, defining the boundaries of what the model can ultimately achieve.

a. **Data Sources and Modalities:** Researchers leverage a diverse array of data streams to capture the complex physiological, behavioral, and contextual correlates of stress. These can be broadly categorized as follows:
   i. **Physiological Signals:** This category, which measures the body's autonomic response directly, is the most common. Cardiovascular information (heart rate, heart rate variability) from ECG or PPG sensors, electroencephalography (EEG) for brain activity, and electrodermal activity (EDA) as a direct indicator of sympathetic arousal are important signals. A complete physiological profile often includes other signals such as skin temperature, respiration, and electromyography (EMG) ((Minaee et al., 2021).
   ii. **Behavioral Signals:** Observable behaviors and expressions that are influenced by our internal stress state fall under this category. Inertial Measurement Units (IMUs) are used to detect changes in body posture and motion kinematics, computer vision is used to analyze facial expressions and muscle movements from images or videos, and Natural Language Processing (NLP) is used to analyze the sentiment and linguistic content of text from sources such as social media (Mishra & Vijaya, 2024).

iii. **Contextual and Self-Reported Data:** The crucial "ground truth" labels and contextual knowledge are provided by this data. In order to provide timely (albeit subjective) labels for supervised learning, the most popular approach is Ecological Momentary Assessment (EMA), which asks users to provide quick, real-time self-reports of their perceived stress levels through a smartphone app. Numerous studies, particularly those that focus on particular populations like students or employees, are also based on extensive demographic surveys and psychological questionnaires (Mitro et al., 2023).

b. **Data Collection Environments:** The setting where data is collected presents a fundamental trade-off between experimental control and real-world realism.

i. **Controlled Laboratory Settings:** In this setting, researchers employ validated, standardized procedures like the Trier Social Stress Test (TSST) to consistently cause a particular kind of acute stress in subjects. This makes it possible to gather clear, high-fidelity data with clear, time-locked labels ('stress' vs. 'baseline'). A model trained on an acute lab stressor might not generalize well to the chronic, complex stressors of everyday life, which is the main disadvantage of limited ecological validity (Mynoddin et al., 2025).

ii. **"In-the-Wild" / Ambulatory Settings:** A popular and expanding strategy to overcome the drawbacks of laboratory research is to use consumer-grade wearables and smartphones to gather data in realistic, everyday environments. This method captures stress in its natural state, but it presents significant labeling challenges and motion artifact signal noise. Extensive "in-the-wild" datasets are essential tools for creating real-world-functional models (Nag & Vijaya, 2025).

iii. **Publicly Available Benchmark Datasets:** In order to enable reproducible research and enable direct comparison between various machine learning models, several publicly accessible benchmark datasets have become the standard within the community.

Datasets, increasingly gathered in lab or semi-controlled settings but publicly released, provide a shared ground for validation. The most impactful and commonly used is WESAD (Wearable Stress and Affect Detection). WESAD records multimodal physiological signals (ECG, EDA, EMG, temperature, respiration, accelerometer) with chest-mounted and wrist-mounted sensors for 15 participants. Baseline, amusement, and stress (induced by the TSST) conditions are included in the experiment and thus comprise explicit labels for three different affective states. Its multimodal and widespread use has rendered it the de facto standard for measuring new algorithms, with almost all research employing it to test their models and report relative performance (Nath et al., 2020).

iv. **Survey-Based and Public Health Datasets:** A unique but extremely valuable class of datasets is derived from self-reported data from questionnaires and extensive public health surveys rather than sensor readings. These datasets offer a distinct but complementary viewpoint to physiological monitoring and are essential for developing models that can forecast stress risk based on demographic, lifestyle, and psychological factors. Many studies use standardized tools like the Perceived Stress Scale (PSS) or create and distribute custom surveys to target particular populations. This method is widely used to study stress in specific groups, like working employees or college students (Oesten et al., 2023).

v. **The Emergence of Synthetic Datasets:** The use of synthetic data generation is a new and extremely promising strategy to address the widespread issues of data scarcity, class imbalance, and privacy concerns. This approach uses generative models (such as Generative Adversarial Networks, or GANs) to generate new, artificial data points that replicate the statistical characteristics of a real dataset, rather than gathering more real data, which is costly and morally challenging. Using data from actual wearable devices, one groundbreaking study showed that an ensemble machine learning model trained on a freshly synthesized dataset could effectively generalize for stress prediction. Without sacrificing user privacy, this method offers a potent path forward for balancing unbalanced classes, enhancing the limited amount of real-world data, and creating more resilient models (Onim et al., 2025).

2. **Data Preprocessing and Feature Engineering**

Raw sensor data is inherently noisy and rarely suitable for direct use in machine learning models, especially classical ones. It must first be cleaned, transformed, and engineered into a meaningful and robust representation.

a. **Signal Cleaning and Artifact Removal:** This is an important first step. In order to prevent any one feature from unfairly controlling the learning process, it entails applying digital filters (such as band-pass filters for EEG signals), employing complex algorithms to identify, eliminate, or reduce motion artifacts from PPG or ECG signals, and normalizing or standardizing the data to a common scale (Oryngoaha et al., 2024).
b. **Feature Engineering vs. End-to-End Learning:** This represents a key methodological divergence in the field.
   i. **Manual Feature Engineering:** Researchers with substantial domain expertise are required to manually extract a set of predictive features from the raw signals for classical models such as Random Forest and SVM. These can include frequency-domain features (like power in various HRV or EEG spectrum frequency bands), time-domain features (like HR mean and standard deviation), and non-linear features that convey the signal's complexity. Although this process is time-consuming and may overlook new patterns, it produces interpretable features (Ouyang, 2025)
   ii. **Automated Feature Learning:** CNNs and other deep learning models perform exceptionally well in end-to-end learning. The most pertinent hierarchical features are automatically learned by the model in this paradigm from the raw or minimally processed data (e.g., a 2D spectrogram image or a 1D signal sequence) [8]. Although it often results in better performance and avoids the need for manual feature engineering, model interpretability is sacrificed in the process (OuZar, 2020).

3. **Model Selection and Training Paradigms:**

Once the data is prepared, an appropriate machine learning model must be selected and trained. The literature showcases a clear progression of algorithmic choices.

a. **Classification by Data Modality:** The most fundamental choice a researcher makes is what data to feed the model. This decision dictates everything from the system's accuracy to its intrusiveness in a user's life.
   i. **Unimodal Approaches:** These systems use a single, particular kind of data to create their predictive models. They are essential for foundational research because they enable scientists to identify and comprehend the predictive potential of individual biomarkers and behaviors, even

though they may not be as reliable as multimodal systems. Systems that rely solely on physiological signals, such as HRV or EDA, those that rely on behavioral cues, such as body posture or facial expressions, systems that use natural language processing (NLP) to analyze social media text, or models that were trained solely on data from psychological surveys are a few examples (Priya, 2020).

ii. **Multimodal Approaches:** The prevalent trend in contemporary research is the use of multimodal approaches, which acknowledge that stress is a complex psycho-physiological construct that cannot be adequately captured by a single signal. These systems combine information from various sources to produce a predictive model that is more reliable, contextually aware, and accurate. Context-Integrated Fusion, which attempts to comprehend not only that a user is stressed, but also why, by incorporating contextual information, Behavioral-Physiological Fusion, which connects internal states with external expressions (e.g., fusing facial landmark data with biometric signals), or Physiological Sensor Fusion, which combines multiple sensor streams (e.g., HR, EDA, and temperature from a smartwatch)(Rastgoo, 2018).

b. **Classification by Modeling Paradigm:** This axis sorts approaches by the type of algorithm doing the predictive work.

i. **Classical Supervised Learning:** These studies make use of well-known machine learning algorithms, such as Random Forest (RF) and Support Vector Machines (SVM), which are praised for their interpretability and computational effectiveness. They continue to be very competitive in many situations and are frequently used for benchmarking (RaZavi, 2024).

ii. **Ensemble and Hybrid Learning:** Ensemble methods combine several models to improve robustness and predictive power. This includes training ensembles on artificially enhanced datasets to enhance their capacity to generalize to new data and scenarios or systematic hybrid approaches that combine various algorithms for a more potent predictor (Reddy, 2018).

iii. **Deep Learning:** For managing the complexity and volume of stress data, this paradigm—which employs multi-layered neural networks for end-to-end learning—has taken center stage. The most popular architectures are Long Short-Term Memory (LSTM) networks for modeling temporal dynamics and Convolutional Neural Networks (CNNs) for feature extraction; these are frequently combined to create potent hybrid models (Saylan, 2023).

c. **Classification by System-Level Architecture:** This final category looks beyond prediction to the system's real-world function and addresses critical implementation challenges.

i. **Real-Time and IoT-Based Systems:** Here, operational deployment for ongoing observation and feedback is the main focus. In order to provide prompt alerts, these systems usually make use of an Internet of Things (IoT) architecture, which streams data from wearables for immediate processing. This is essential for applications that require safety or for prompt interventions(Schniidt, 2018) .

ii. **Explainable AI (XAI) Frameworks:** The "black box" nature of increasingly complicated and opaque models can be a major deterrent to trust, particularly in clinical settings. The goal of XAI-focused research is to make these models transparent by offering concise, intelligible justifications for their predictions, as this is thought to be a necessary condition for clinical adoption (Song, 2024).

iii. **Privacy-Preserving Systems (Federated Learning):** To address the profound privacy risks of centralizing vast amounts of sensitive health data, Federated Learning (FL) has emerged as a critical architectural solution. FL is a fundamental idea for any ethical healthcare application since it enables the cooperative training of models on decentralized user devices without ever letting the user control the raw data (Thapliyal, 2017).

4. **Model Evaluation and Validation**

Thoroughly assessing the trained model's performance and, most crucially, its capacity to generalize to new, unseen data is the pipeline's last and most crucial step.

a. **Performance Metrics:** The particular task (i.e., regression or classification) determines which evaluation metric is used. Although classification accuracy is frequently reported, it can be very deceptive for datasets that are unbalanced (where "stress" events are significantly less common than "non-stress" events). As a result, the majority of thorough studies also include Precision, Recall, and the F1-Score, which offers a more impartial assessment of a model's performance .
b. **Validation Strategies:** Robust validation techniques are necessary to make sure a model isn't only "memorizing" the training data, which is a problem known as overfitting. K-Fold Cross-Validation is the standard method. Leave-One-Subject-Out (LOSO) Cross-Validation is a more rigorous and practical validation technique for studies with several participants (Vijaya, 2026).

Applications and domains of stress detection

Automated stress detection has applications that go well beyond scholarly studies and have the potential to revolutionize a wide range of real-world industries. These technologies have the potential to change entire fields from a reactive, post-hoc intervention model to a proactive, data-driven management and prevention model by offering objective, ongoing, and personalized insights into an individual's mental state. The application domains are incredibly varied, spanning from the routines of personal life and education to high-stakes clinical and occupational settings. The fundamental value proposition is the same across all domains: using data to address particular issues, lessen the detrimental effects of ongoing stress, and eventually enhance human outcomes by bringing the invisible into the open.

1) **Clinical, m-Health, and Biomedical Applications:** This domain represents one of the most significant and immediately impactful areas for stress detection technology. Chronic stress is a major risk factor for numerous mental and physical disorders, and the ability to objectively monitor it can serve as a powerful tool for clinicians, researchers, and patients alike.
   a) **Augmented Diagnostics and Personalized Treatment Monitoring:** The sparse and subjective information obtained from self-reports during appointments can be greatly enhanced by machine learning systems, which can give clinicians a continuous, longitudinal view of a patient's physiological stress levels. In between visits, this enables a far more nuanced understanding of a patient's condition. In this regard, the emergence of medically focused Explainable AI (XAI) is a key facilitator since it offers the clarity and justification required for physicians to have faith in and confidently incorporate these systems into their diagnostic process (Wahab, 2024).
   b) **Proactive Mental Health and Population Screening (m-Health):** The development of mobile health (m-Health) platforms that leverage consumer wearable data for early-stage screening and general population wellness is a major and expanding area of focus. By identifying people who display recurring physiological or behavioral patterns of stress and may be at risk of developing

more severe stress-related disorders like anxiety or depression, these systems can act as effective early warning tools (Xu, 2023).

2) **Occupational Health and High-Stakes Workplaces:** A large percentage of the world's workforce experiences chronic stress primarily from their modern workplace, which has been linked to well-documented increases in employee burnout, absenteeism, decreased productivity, and safety hazards. Automated stress detection gives businesses data-driven tools to create safer, healthier, and more productive workplaces.
    a) **General Workplace Well-being and Burnout Prevention:** Predicting and tracking stress in general working employees is the focus of a substantial amount of research . Platforms at the enterprise level are being created especially to give businesses the means to track and handle workplace stress on a systemic, anonymous basis.
    b) **Enhancing Safety in Critical Operations:** Unmanaged stress can be a serious safety risk in some situations where human error can have disastrous results, in addition to being a wellness concern. In order to reduce the risks of stress-induced cognitive impairment, real-time stress monitoring is being actively developed as an essential safety tool for pilots, air traffic controllers, and long-haul truck drivers. In high-stress emergency evacuation situations, it is also being investigated to guarantee safe and orderly reactions (Zhai, 2006).
3) **Academic and Educational Settings:** Students, especially those in higher education, deal with a special combination of social, academic, and financial demands, which puts them at risk for mental health issues that could affect their long-term wellbeing and academic performance. Creating models to forecast stress levels in college students in particular has been the subject of a sizable number of studies. The creation of proactive support systems is the main use case. To promote a campus culture where student well-being is actively managed, university wellness centers can use these systems to identify individuals displaying data-driven signs of high stress and reach out with targeted resources, rather than waiting for students to seek help (Zhang, 2023).
4) **Personal Wellness, Ubiquitous Computing, and Smart Environments:** Personal health and lifestyle management is the largest and fastest-growing application domain, driven by the consumer wearables market's explosive growth. People are empowered by this "Quantified Self" movement to actively and intelligently monitor and manage their own well-being. Users receive real-time feedback on their stress levels throughout the day thanks to stress detection systems built into smartwatches and other personal electronics. In order to provide real-time stress assessment and feedback, the technology aims to establish seamless, Internet of Things (IoT)-based ecosystems where wearable data is continuously and intelligently processed. The development of context-aware, closed-loop systems that can actively control the user's surroundings to be more restorative in addition to detecting stress is the key to the future of personal wellness (Alfredo et al., 2023).

Challenges and open issues

The unresolved issues cover basic concerns about data integrity, human subjectivity, model generalizability, and significant ethical obligations; they are not just technical obstacles that can be solved with more data or improved algorithms. Whether or not this technology evolves from a promising academic field into a reliable and significant real-world tool will depend on how the research community handles these challenges.

1) **The Elusive Ground Truth: The Unresolved Challenge of Labeling Stress:** Establishing the "ground truth" is the most basic and enduring challenge in stress research, and it forms the basis of almost all other problems. The quality and accuracy of the labels that a model is trained on determines its performance in supervised machine learning. It is very challenging to come up with a clear, impartial, and widely accepted label for stress.
   a) **The Confounding Variable Problem:** The physiological reactions of the body to psychological stress, such as an elevated heart rate and increased skin conductance, are frequently indistinguishable from those to a variety of other non-stressful stimuli. A moment of pure joy, the metabolic effects of caffeine, or physical exertion can all produce physiological signatures that are almost exactly the same as those of negative stress. This undermines user trust because a model trained only on physiological data can easily misclassify a brisk walk as a moment of high anxiety.
   b) **The Subjectivity and Burden of Self-Reports:** Ecological Momentary Assessment (EMA), in which participants self-report their perceived stress levels on a regular basis, is the most widely used method for resolving the labeling issue. Although this offers useful, timely labels, the approach is fundamentally flawed. The self-reports are subjective by nature and impacted by mood, personality, and self-awareness, and it places a heavy participatory burden on the user, resulting in survey fatigue.
   c) **The Lab-to-Life Validity Gap:** Although rigorously regulated laboratory procedures such as the TSST [6] can yield clear, unambiguous labels for acute stress that has been induced, these settings are not ecologically valid. Because they have not been trained to withstand the noise and complexity of real-world stress, models that attain near-perfect accuracy in the lab frequently suffer a sharp decline in performance when used "in the wild." .((Xu, 2023), (Schniidt, 2018), (Bolpagni et al., 2024))
2) **The Generalizability Crisis: Building Models That Work for Everyone:** The idea that a model is only as good as the data it was trained on is fundamental to machine learning. The widespread dearth of extensive, varied, and openly accessible datasets is a major unresolved problem in stress detection. A generalizability crisis results from this.
   a) **Pervasive Population Bias:** It is extremely unlikely that a model developed solely using data from college students will translate well to working IT sector employees, whose stressors and daily schedules differ greatly.
   b) **The Data Scarcity and Privacy Paradox:** Because personal health data is extremely sensitive, building sizable, publicly accessible benchmark datasets is a costly, time-consuming, and morally challenging undertaking.
   c) **The Intractable Problem of Inter-Subject Variability:** The physiological reaction to stress varies greatly from person to person, and stress is a very personal experience. A single, generalized model may not work well for any particular person due to this high inter-subject variability. Research into highly customized models that are tailored to each person's particular physiology and lifestyle has increased as a result of this.
3) **The "Black Box" Dilemma and the Imperative for Trust:** Researchers encounter the "black box" problem as they use more intricate models, such as deep neural networks, to attain cutting-edge accuracy. Although the internal decision-making processes of these models are frequently totally opaque, they are capable of producing remarkably accurate predictions. Real-world adoption is directly and significantly hampered by this lack of transparency.

a) **The Barrier to Clinical and Professional Adoption:** If a system is unable to support its recommendations, a clinician will not trust it, much less follow through on it. Because of this, Explainable AI (XAI) is now one of the most important open research topics in the whole field. Developing interpretable and accurate systems that offer medically relevant and comprehensible explanations for a model's predictions is a challenge .

4) **Practical Hurdles: The Final Mile to Real-World Deployment:** There are numerous practical and logistical issues that need to be addressed in addition to the fundamental data and modeling challenges.
   a) **Computational Efficiency and Battery Life:** Complex models that are computationally demanding and have the potential to rapidly deplete a wearable device's limited battery are necessary for continuous real-time monitoring. Research on creating accurate and power-efficient lightweight machine learning models is ongoing and crucial.
   b) **Data Security and Profound Ethical Considerations:** There are serious ethical and privacy issues and m any important questions are still unresolved: Who is the owner of this data? How is it protected from intrusions? One technological component of the solution is the creation of privacy-preserving architectures such as Federated Learning, but it must be combined with the implementation of strong legal frameworks and clear user-consent models ((Nath et al., 2020), (Nag & Vijaya, 2025), (Misra, 2024), (Vijaya, 2026)..

SOLUTIONS AND RECOMMENDATIONS

Proposed stress prediction System (Case Study of Nurse stress analysis)

Stress is a physiological response to internal and external demands, categorized into eustress (positive) and distress (negative). While eustress enhances creativity and productivity, distress occurs when coping capacity falls short, causing harmful effects. Stressors may be acute, episodic, or chronic, with chronic stress posing severe health risks. Nursing, among the most stressful professions, exposes individuals to heavy workloads, emotional strain, and long shifts, leading to psychological and physical problems such as anxiety, exhaustion, cardiovascular issues, and reduced patient care quality is shown in Figure 2. Recent research highlights physiological indicators like heart rate variability, electrodermal activity, and skin temperature to better understand stress and develop workplace interventions that support nurses' well-being and healthcare safety.

Figure 2. Framework for Stress predition model

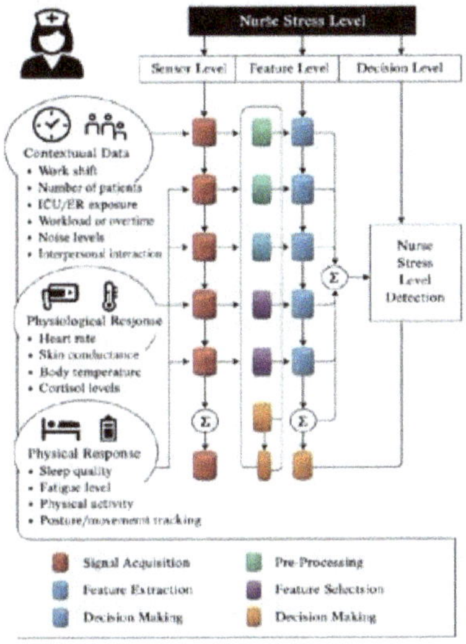

- **Impact of Stress on Nurses' Performance:** Stress significantly affects nursing performance in high-pressure healthcare environments. Nurses must make rapid decisions, regulate emotions, and maintain physical stamina under demanding conditions. Prolonged stress often leads to cognitive overload, impairing attention, memory, and clinical judgment—factors associated with increased medical errors and reduced efficiency. Emotional strain manifests as anxiety, exhaustion, and reduced empathy, diminishing both care quality and nurse-patient relationships. Ultimately, sustained stress contributes to burnout, compromised care delivery, and poor job satisfaction.
- **Consequences of Chronic Stress in Professional Nursing:** Chronic stress poses serious risks to the physical and mental health of nurses. Long-term exposure to occupational stressors such as emotional labor, time pressure, and high patient acuity elevates the risk of cardiovascular conditions, including hypertension and arrhythmias. Gastrointestinal issues and musculoskeletal pain are also common, exacerbated by stress responses and extended physical demands. Mental health consequences include burnout, anxiety, depression, and, in severe cases, post-traumatic stress disorder (PTSD), particularly in emergency and critical care settings. These outcomes reduce quality of life, contribute to workforce attrition, and impair patient care outcomes.
- **Stress Response and Measurement in Nursing:** Nurses frequently work in high-stress conditions marked by long shifts, emergencies, and emotional demands. Stress activates sensory nerves that transmit signals to the central nervous system (CNS), triggering responses via the autonomic and somatic nervous systems. Stress assessment modalities in nursing include psychological self-reporting, physiological biomarkers, and behavioral observation, each offering insights into how nurses respond to workload, patient outcomes, and interpersonal challenges.
  - o Psychological Evaluation: Self-report tools such as the Perceived Stress Scale (PSS) and Nursing Stress Scale (NSS) remain widely used. However, recall bias may reduce accuracy when surveys are completed after intense shifts. lternatives include Likert scales (e.g., 1 =

no stress, 6 = extreme stress) or categorical ratings (low, medium, high). These methods are simple but less practical during real-time clinical tasks. Annotation-based approaches enhance accuracy, using offline event labeling (e.g., EMR logs) or online tagging supported by wearables. Hybrid systems combining retrospective and real-time data offer greater flexibility

- Measuring Physiological Responses:
  - **Cortisol Levels:** Cortisol is a reliable stress biomarker, measurable via non-invasive salivary tests. However, its natural diurnal rhythm—peaking after waking and declining through the day—requires careful timing to avoid confounding results.
  - **Electrodermal Activity (EDA):**EDA measures skin conductance, which rises with sweat gland activity driven by the autonomic nervous system. It is particularly useful in high-pressure nursing scenarios, such as trauma care, where stress-induced arousal is acute. Wearable EDA sensors enable real-time monitoring and inform stress-reduction strategies.
  - **Heart Activity:** Stress activates the sympathetic nervous system, raising heart rate (HR) and reducing heart rate variability (HRV)—key indicators of strain [43–45]. HR and HRV can be derived from electrocardiogram (ECG) or photoplethysmogram (PPG) signals, the latter commonly used in wearables. Continuous monitoring of HR and HRV helps detect stress early, enabling timely interventions and supporting nurses' well-being.
- External Physical Responses: Stress in nurses also manifests through observable behaviors such as changes in posture, facial expressions, gait, tremors, and repetitive movements. Technologies like computer vision, inertial sensors, and accelerometers detect these subtle cues, which often indicate fatigue or psychological strain. Wearable and ambient systems allow continuous tracking of such markers, facilitating early detection of burnout and improving occupational health.

Stress detection in nurses through machine learning and deep learning follows a structured framework that begins with **preprocessing**, where raw physiological signals are cleaned, normalized, and denoised, while missing values are imputed to ensure data quality and reliability. Next, **feature extraction and selection** are applied using filter, wrapper, embedded, or hybrid methods to identify the most relevant physiological and contextual features for accurate modeling. A range of **machine learning algorithms**—including Support Vector Machines (SVM), Random Forests (RF), Naïve Bayes Classifiers (NBC), K-Nearest Neighbors (KNN), and Artificial Neural Networks (ANNs)—are employed to classify stress, with deep learning architectures like **Convolutional Neural Networks (CNNs)** and **Long Short-Term Memory (LSTM) networks** further enhancing performance by capturing spatial and temporal dependencies in biosignals. More advanced strategies, such as **federated learning** for privacy-preserving model training, **semi-supervised learning** to leverage scarce labeled data, and **multimodal deep learning** to integrate heterogeneous inputs (ECG, EDA, HR, respiration, skin temperature), improve adaptability and personalization. Finally, **fusion techniques**—whether early, late, hybrid, or adaptive—combine information across modalities to strengthen robustness, mitigate sensor noise, and boost classification accuracy.

Proposed Evolutionary-based Deep learning models

There is no single cause for a nurse to experience stress, which is the main challenge in predicting stress levels among healthcare professionals. Nurse stress is typically influenced by multiple contributing factors, such as workload, shift patterns, patient interactions, work environment, and personal lifestyle, all of which can affect the nurse's overall well-being. Identifying these factors is difficult because it depends on both the nurse's personal history and the unique aspects of their work environment. The combination of these variables makes accurate stress classification challenging and requires in-depth analysis of the nurse stress prediction system. To address these challenges, we propose an alternative optimized deep learning solution for nurse stress management in India. In the proposed approach, stress prediction is treated as an optimization problem, identifying the optimal solution using evolutionary-based deep learning, as represented in Figure 3.

Evolutionary Algorithms: Evolutionary algorithms are optimization techniques inspired by natural selection and biological evolution. In the context of nurse stress prediction, these algorithms help identify the most influential factors contributing to stress by iteratively selecting, combining, and refining candidate solutions. By simulating processes such as mutation, crossover, and selection, evolutionary algorithms can efficiently explore complex datasets and optimize predictive models, ensuring that the final system highlights the most critical stressors for individual nurses.

Deep Learning: Deep learning is a subset of machine learning that uses multi-layered neural networks to automatically extract features and learn complex patterns from large datasets which shown in Figure 4. For nurse stress prediction, deep learning models can analyze multimodal data, including physiological signals, behavioral patterns, and environmental information, to predict stress levels with high accuracy. When combined with evolutionary optimization, deep learning can be fine-tuned to focus on the most relevant features, resulting in a robust and adaptive stress prediction system.

Figure 3. Proposed Nurse stress prediction system

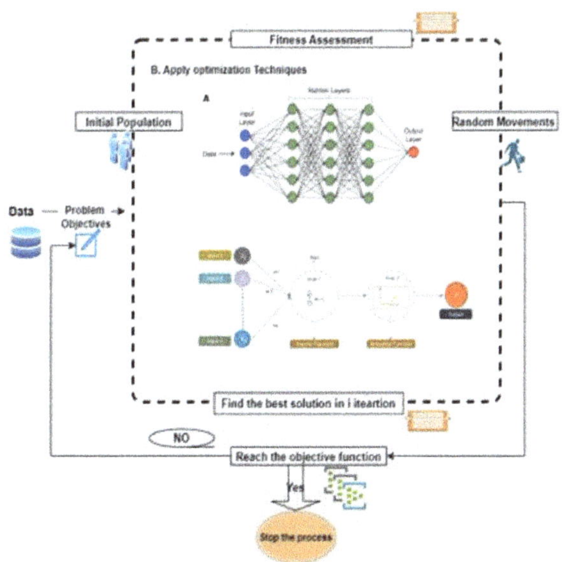

Figure 4. The working principles of two nodes in every layer of the architecture Source: Springer (2020)

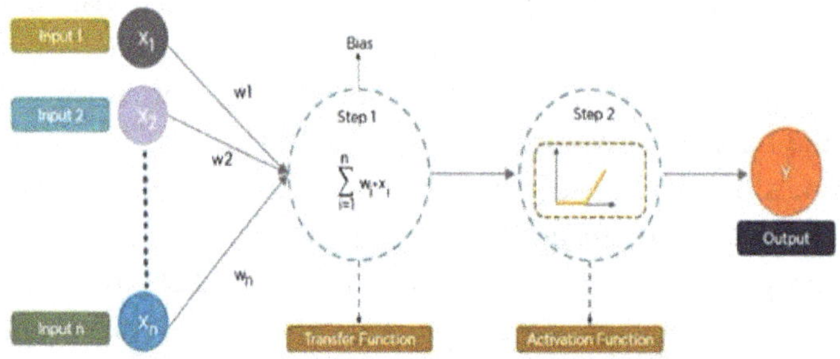

In this proposed model, optimization principles are applied to various deep learning models (GANs, RBFNs, MLPs, SOMs, DBNs, RBMs, and Autoencoders) to enhance the performance of the nurse stress prediction system and overcome the limitations of conventional deep learning models. Using this approach, each optimization technique can be analyzed along with its advantages and disadvantages to determine its suitability for predicting nurse stress. Finally, multiple experimental setups are employed to validate the performance of the evolutionary-based deep learning models (E-DL) and to identify the most effective model for a robust and accurate nurse stress prediction system.

FUTURE RESEARCH DIRECTIONS

The fundamental ideas of applying machine learning to stress detection have been clearly established by the corpus of research reviewed in this paper. From early proofs of concept to the creation of incredibly precise, multimodal systems that can decode the intricate language of human physiology, the field has advanced. But the path from fruitful research prototypes to genuinely revolutionary, commonplace technology is only getting started. In order to develop systems that are more intelligent, individualized, reliable, and smoothly woven into everyday life, this domain must go beyond simple classification. The most promising avenues for the future are those that directly tackle the fundamental issues of context, privacy, personalization, and actionability with the goal of creating intelligent wellness partners rather than merely stress detectors.

- **Hyper-Contextualization: The Fusion of Signals and Semantics:** One of the worst flaws in systems today in general is that they are not capable of distinguishing stress-induced physiological arousal from arousal due to other stimuli such as exercise or excitement. The future is to develop hyper-contextualized models not only knowing what the body is doing but why it is doing it. This means a more profound and smarter kind of multimodal fusion far beyond simple and basic sensor stream merging. The recent merging of Large Language Models (LLMs) with multimodal frameworks gives a very distinct vision of this future. Upcoming systems will probably be end-to-end data aggregators, silently combining an extensive set of contextual clues—everything from calendar entries ("Board Meeting") and e-mail, to GPS information (at the gym versus at the office), to ambient audio levels and even phone call vocal prosody—to create an abundant, dynamic portrait of a user's existence. This brings in the important semantic richness otherwise missing and enables models to make much more precise and subtle judgments.

- **Privacy-Preserving Personalization at Scale:** The combined scarcity of data and the deep aspirational requirement for personalization demand a paradigm shift in model training and deployment. The future is not one monolithic "stress model" that can be applied to everyone. Rather, it will move towards hybrid solutions that marry the strengths of large population dataset power with deep individualized adaptation, all while carefully maintaining user anonymity. Federated Learning (FL) will be the preferred architecture to train base models over decentralized health data, resolving the privacy paradox in a beautiful manner. A new device user might download such a base model and subsequently employ Transfer Learning or any other fine-tuning methods to quickly adapt it within a few days through his/her own personalized physiological data. This "generalize-then-personalize" process derives the strength of big data and makes the ensuing model strategically adapted to the individual's own stress response, addressing the core issue of inter-subject variance. Synthetic data generation may make this even more rapid by giving robust and varied training material without ever infringing on the privacy of actual individuals.
- **From Explainable AI (XAI) to Actionable and Adaptive AI (A^2I):** Building user trust on the foundation of openness is non-negotiable, and Explainable AI (XAI) has the key to opening the "black box" of complex models. Future direction, however, is to move beyond explanation per se to create Actionable and Adaptive AI. It is not sufficient for a system to inform a user, "You are stressed because your HRV has decreased." A truly useful system must respond to the all-important follow-up question, "So what do I do about it?" That means building closed-loop, adaptive systems that can monitor a user's state, predict a stress event is about to occur, respond by providing a timely and targeted intervention (such as a guided breathing exercise or a walk suggestion), and then adapt based on the body's feedback about whether or not it succeeded. This "sense-infer-act-learn" cycle generates a system that learns and evolves with the user over time, changing the technology from a static detector to an active and discerning wellness coach.

CONCLUSION

Machine learning's journey in stress detection has been rapid and remarkable, evolving from simple proofs-of-concept to sophisticated, multimodal systems capable of capturing the subtle signals of human physiology. Literature indicates a clear progression toward more advanced deep learning models, integrative data fusion, and a growing focus on critical real-world challenges such as privacy, trustworthiness, and personalization. Despite these advances, establishing reliable ground truth data and creating universally applicable models remain essential. The future points toward hyper-contextualized, privacy-preserving, and actionable AI that goes beyond detection to develop intelligent wellness companions, capable of understanding, interpreting, and supporting stress management in a deeply personalized and adaptive way. Such technology holds immense potential not only to measure well-being but also to actively enhance it meaningfully. Stress is a significant factor affecting nurses' health and performance due to demanding work environments and critical responsibilities. Long-term exposure to work-related stress can lead to serious health issues, lower job satisfaction, and a decline in patient care quality. Multimodal stress detection systems using wearable physiological sensors—capturing signals like HR, HRV, EDA, RSP, PPG, and skin temperature—have shown strong performance in real-time monitoring and prediction of high-stress episodes. Advanced machine learning techniques, including CNNs, LSTMs, GANs, ensemble models, and federated learning, have achieved high accuracy and robustness, often exceeding 90%, and address challenges such as limited labeled data and privacy concerns. Overall, combining wearable sensor data with machine learning offers a viable approach for proactive nurse stress management, improving employee well-being and contributing to enhanced patient care outcomes.

REFERENCES

Alfredo, R. D., Nie, L., Kennedy, P., Power, T., Hayes, C., Chen, H., . . . Martinez-Maldonado, R. (2023, March). " That Student Should be a Lion Tamer!" StressViz: Designing a Stress Analytics Dashboard for Teachers. In *LAK23: 13th International Learning Analytics and Knowledge Conference* (pp. 57-67). https://dl.acm.org/doi/abs/10.1145/3576050.3576058

Aqajari, S. A. H., Wang, Z., Tazarv, A., Labbaf, S., Jafarlou, S., Nguyen, B., & Rahmani, A. M. (2024). Enhancing performance and user engagement in everyday stress monitoring: A context-aware active reinforcement learning approach. *arXiv preprint arXiv:2407.08215*. https://doi.org//arXiv.2407.08215DOI: 10.48550

Archana, V. R., & Devaraju, B. M. (2020). Stress detection using machine learning algorithms. *International Journal of Research in Engineering, Science and Management, 3*(8), 251-256. https://journal .ijresm.com/index.php/ijresm/article/view/171

Aristizabal, S., Byun, K., Wood, N., Mullan, A. F., Porter, P. M., Campanella, C., & Bauer, B. A. (2021). The feasibility of wearable and self-report stress detection measures in a semi-controlled lab environment. *IEEE Access : Practical Innovations, Open Solutions*, *9*, 102053–102068. https://ieeexplore.ieee .org/document/9483899/

Bobade, P., & Vani, M. (2020, July). Stress detection with machine learning and deep learning using multimodal physiological data. In *2020 Second International Conference on Inventive Research in Computing Applications (ICIRCA)* (pp. 51-57). IEEE. https://ieeexplore.ieee.org/document/9183244

Bodaghi, M., Hosseini, M., & Gottumukkala, R. (2024, April). A multimodal intermediate fusion network with manifold learning for stress detection. In *2024 IEEE 3rd International Conference on Computing and Machine Intelligence (ICMI)* (pp. 1-8). IEEE. https://ieeexplore.ieee.org/abstract/document/10586177/

Bolpagni, M., Pardini, S., Dianti, M., & Gabrielli, S. (2024). Personalized stress detection using biosignals from wearables: A scoping review. *Sensors (Basel)*, *24*(10), 3221. https://www.mdpi.com/1424 -8220/24/10/3221 PMID: 38794074

Booth, B. M., Vrzakova, H., Mattingly, S. M., Martinez, G. J., Faust, L., & D'Mello, S. K. (2022). Toward robust stress prediction in the age of wearables: Modeling perceived stress in a longitudinal study with information workers. *IEEE Transactions on Affective Computing*, *13*(4), 2201–2217. https://par .nsf.gov/servlets/purl/10356010

Can, Y. S., Arnrich, B., & Ersoy, C. (2019). Stress detection in daily life scenarios using smart phones and wearable sensors: A survey. *Journal of Biomedical Informatics*, *92*, 103139. https://www.sciencedirect .com/science/article/pii/S1532046419300577 PMID: 30825538

Chen, Y., Qin, X., Wang, J., Yu, C., & Gao, W. (2020). Fedhealth: A federated transfer learning framework for wearable healthcare. *IEEE Intelligent Systems*, *35*(4), 83–93. https://arxiv.org/abs/1907.09173

Cuevas, A. G., Chen, R., Thurber, K. A., Slopen, N., & Williams, D. R. (2019). Psychosocial stress and overweight and obesity: findings from the Chicago community adult health study. *Annals of Behavioral Medicine, 53*(11), NP-NP. https://pubmed.ncbi.nlm.nih.gov/30917198/

Gedam, S., & Paul, S. (2021). A review on mental stress detection using wearable sensors and machine learning techniques. *IEEE Access : Practical Innovations, Open Solutions*, *9*, 84045–84066. https://ieeexplore.ieee.org/document/9445082

Hasib, K. M., Islam, M. R., Sakib, S., Akbar, M. A., Razzak, I., & Alam, M. S. (2023). Depression detection from social networks data based on machine learning and deep learning techniques: An interrogative survey. *IEEE Transactions on Computational Social Systems*, *10*(4), 1568–1586. https://ieeexplore.ieee.org/document/10108975/

Hosseini, M., Bodaghi, M., Bhupatiraju, R. T., Maida, A., & Gottumukkala, R. (2023). Multimodal stress detection using facial landmarks and biometric signals. *arXiv preprint arXiv:2311.03606*. https://arxiv.org/abs/2311.03606

Hosseini, S., Gottumukkala, R., Katragadda, S., Bhupatiraju, R. T., Ashkar, Z., Borst, C. W., & Cochran, K. (2022). A multimodal sensor dataset for continuous stress detection of nurses in a hospital. *Scientific Data*, *9*(1), 255. https://pubmed.ncbi.nlm.nih.gov/35650267/ PMID: 35650267

Jaber, D., Hajj, H., Maalouf, F., & El-Hajj, W. (2022). Medically-oriented design for explainable AI for stress prediction from physiological measurements. *BMC Medical Informatics and Decision Making*, *22*(1), 38. https://bmcmedinformdecismak.biomedcentral.com/articles/10.1186/s12911-022-01772-2 PMID: 35148762

Korkmaz, A. Ç., Korkmaz, A., & Koşunalp, S. (2025). Predicting Nurse Stress Levels Using Time-Series Sensor Data and Comparative Evaluation of Classification Algorithms. *Engineering Proceedings*, *104*(1), 30. https://www.mdpi.com/2673-4591/104/1/30

KS. S., & HD, P. (2022). Stress Prediction in Working Employees using Artificial Intelligence of Things. *Journal of Pharmaceutical Negative Results, 13*. https://www.pnrjournal.com/index.php/home/article/view/1570

Kyamakya, K., Al-Machot, F., Haj Mosa, A., Bouchachia, H., Chedjou, J. C., & Bagula, A. (2021). Emotion and stress recognition related sensors and machine learning technologies. *Sensors (Basel)*, *21*(7), 2273. https://www.mdpi.com/1424-8220/21/7/2273 PMID: 33804987

Mathur, A., & Sethia, D. (2024). Body sensor-based multimodal nurse stress detection using machine learning. In *2024 16th International Conference on COMmunication Systems & NETworkS (COMSNETS)* (pp. 67-73). IEEE. https://ieeexplore.ieee.org/document/10427006/

Medina Fernández, I. A., Carreño Moreno, S., Chaparro Díaz, L., Gallegos-Torres, R. M., Medina Fernández, J. A., & Hernández Martínez, E. K. (2021). Fear, stress, and knowledge regarding COVID-19 in nursing students and recent graduates in Mexico. *Investigacion y Educacion en Enfermeria*, *39*(1). https://pubmed.ncbi.nlm.nih.gov/33687809/ PMID: 33687809

Minaee, S., Minaei, M., & Abdolrashidi, A. (2021). Deep-emotion: Facial expression recognition using attentional convolutional network. *Sensors (Basel)*, *21*(9), 3046. https://www.mdpi.com/1424-8220/21/9/3046 PMID: 33925371

Mishra, A. S., & Vijaya, J. (2024). Data Mining and Knowledge Discovery: Transforming Healthcare Through Biomedical Intelligence. In *Machine Learning and Generative AI in Smart Healthcare* (pp. 23-40). IGI Global. https://www.igi-global.com/chapter/data-mining-and-knowledge-discovery/355614

Mitro, N., Argyri, K., Pavlopoulos, L., Kosyvas, D., Karagiannidis, L., Kostovasili, M., & Amditis, A. (2023). AI-enabled smart wristband providing real-time vital signs and stress monitoring. *Sensors (Basel)*, *23*(5), 2821. https://pubmed.ncbi.nlm.nih.gov/36905025/ PMID: 36905025

Mynoddin, M., Dev, T., & Chakma, R. (2025). Brain2Vec: A Deep Learning Framework for EEG-Based Stress Detection Using CNN-LSTM-Attention. *arXiv preprint arXiv:2506.11179*. https://doi.org//arXiv.2506.11179DOI: 10.48550

Nag, M., & Vijaya, J. (2025, June). Enhanced Stress Prediction among nurses in their work environment using Clustered Chameleon Swarm Algorithm. In *2025 3rd Cognitive Models and Artificial Intelligence Conference (AICCONF)* (pp. 1-6). IEEE. https://ieeexplore.ieee.org/document/11064058/

Nath, R. K., Thapliyal, H., Caban-Holt, A., & Mohanty, S. P. (2020). Machine learning based solutions for real-time stress monitoring. *IEEE Consumer Electronics Magazine*, *9*(5), 34–41. https://scholars.uky.edu/es/publications/machine-learning-based-solutions-for-real-time-stress-monitoring

Oesten, M., Richer, R., Abel, L., Rohleder, N., & Eskofier, B. M. (2023, October). VoStress–voice-based detection of acute psychosocial stress. In *2023 IEEE EMBS International Conference on Biomedical and Health Informatics (BHI)* (pp. 1-4). IEEE. https://ieeexplore.ieee.org/abstract/document/10313458

Onim, M. S. H., Humble, T. S., & Thapliyal, H. (2025, January). Quantum Hybrid Support Vector Machines for Stress Detection in Older Adults. In *2025 IEEE International Conference on Consumer Electronics (ICCE)* (pp. 1-4). IEEE. https://ieeexplore.ieee.org/abstract/document/10929873

Oryngozha, N., Shamoi, P., & Igali, A. (2024). Detection and analysis of stress-related posts in reddit's acamedic communities. *IEEE Access : Practical Innovations, Open Solutions*, *12*, 14932–14948. https://ieeexplore.ieee.org/abstract/document/10412045

Ouyang, Q. (2025). Speech emotion detection based on MFCC and CNN-LSTM architecture. *arXiv preprint arXiv:2501.10666*. https://doi.org/DOI: 10.54254/2755-2721/5/20230570

Ouzar, Y., Lagha, L., Bousefsaf, F., & Maaoui, C. (2022, August). Multimodal stress state detection from facial videos using physiological signals and facial features. In *International Conference on Pattern Recognition* (pp. 139–150). Springer Nature Switzerland., https://link.springer.com/chapter/10.1007/978-3-031-37745-7_10

Priya, A., Garg, S., & Tigga, N. P. (2020). Predicting anxiety, depression and stress in modern life using machine learning algorithms. *Procedia Computer Science*, *167*, 1258–1267. https://www.sciencedirect.com/science/article/pii/S1877050920309091

Rastgoo, M. N., Nakisa, B., Rakotonirainy, A., Chandran, V., & Tjondronegoro, D. (2018). A critical review of proactive detection of driver stress levels based on multimodal measurements. *ACM Computing Surveys*, *51*(5), 1–35. https://dl.acm.org/doi/abs/10.1145/3186585

Razavi, M., Ziyadidegan, S., Mahmoudzadeh, A., Kazeminasab, S., Baharlouei, E., Janfaza, V., & Sasangohar, F. (2024). Machine learning, deep learning, and data preprocessing techniques for detecting, predicting, and monitoring stress and stress-related mental disorders: Scoping review. *JMIR Mental Health, 11*(1), e53714. https://pubmed.ncbi.nlm.nih.gov/39167782/ PMID: 39167782

Reddy, U. S., Thota, A. V., & Dharun, A. (2018, December). Machine learning techniques for stress prediction in working employees. In *2018 IEEE International Conference on Computational Intelligence and Computing Research (ICCIC)* (pp. 1-4). IEEE. https://ieeexplore.ieee.org/document/8782395/

Saylam, B., & İncel, Ö. D. (2023). Quantifying digital biomarkers for well-being: Stress, anxiety, Positive and negative affect via wearable devices and their time-based predictions. *Sensors (Basel), 23*(21), 8987. https://www.mdpi.com/1424-8220/23/21/8987 PMID: 37960685

Schmidt, P., Reiss, A., Duerichen, R., Marberger, C., & Van Laerhoven, K. (2018, October). Introducing wesad, a multimodal dataset for wearable stress and affect detection. In *Proceedings of the 20th ACM international conference on multimodal interaction* (pp. 400-408). https://dl.acm.org/doi/10.1145/3242969.3242985

Song, Y., Zhang, X., Luo, D., Shi, J., Zang, Q., Wang, Y., & Bai, Y. (2024). Predicting nursing workload in digestive wards based on machine learning: A prospective study. *BMC Nursing, 23*(1), 908. https://bmcnurs.biomedcentral.com/articles/10.1186/s12912-024-02570-z PMID: 39696189

Thapliyal, H., Khalus, V., & Labrado, C. (2017). Stress detection and management: A survey of wearable smart health devices. *IEEE Consumer Electronics Magazine, 6*(4), 64–69. https://ieeexplore.ieee.org/document/8048734/

Vallone, F., Cattaneo Della Volta, M. F., & Zurlo, M. C. (2024). Stress dimensions, patterns of coping, and psychopathological risk among nurses: A person-centred approach. *BMC Nursing, 23*(1), 569. https://link.springer.com/article/10.1186/s12912-024-02250-y PMID: 39148064

Vijaya, J., Verma, P. K., Thakur, R., Soni, S., Sharma, T., & Chauhan, B. (2026). Overview of ML and Optimization Algorithms in Disease Prediction and a Comprehensive Review. *Integrative Machine Learning and Optimization Algorithms for Disease Prediction*, 63-98. https://www.igi-global.com/chapter/overview-of-ml-and-optimization-algorithms-in-disease-prediction-and-a-comprehensive-review/384902

Wahab, O., Adda, M., & Zrira, N. (2024). Serenisens: A multimodal ai framework with llms for stress prediction through sleep biometrics. *Procedia Computer Science, 251*, 342–349. https://linkinghub.elsevier.com/retrieve/pii/S1877050924033532

Xiang, J. Z., Wang, Q. Y., Fang, Z. B., Esquivel, J. A., & Su, Z. X. (2025). A multi-modal deep learning approach for stress detection using physiological signals: Integrating time and frequency domain features. *Frontiers in Physiology, 16*, 1584299. https://www.frontiersin.org/journals/physiology/articles/10.3389/fphys.2025.1584299/full PMID: 40236827

Xu, J., Zhang, L., Ji, Q., Ji, P., Chen, Y., Song, M., & Guo, L. (2023). Nursing students' emotional empathy, emotional intelligence and higher education-related stress: A cross-sectional study. *BMC Nursing, 22*(1), 437. https://bmcnurs.biomedcentral.com/articles/10.1186/s12912-023-01607-z PMID: 37981672

Zhai, J., & Barreto, A. (2006, August). *Stress detection in computer users based on digital signal processing of noninvasive physiological variables. In 2006 international conference of the IEEE engineering in medicine and biology society*. IEEE., https://pubmed.ncbi.nlm.nih.gov/17946041/

Zhang, X., & Zhang, L. (2023). Risk prediction of sleep disturbance in clinical nurses: A nomogram and artificial neural network model. *BMC Nursing*, *22*(1), 289. https://bmcnurs.biomedcentral.com/articles/10.1186/s12912-023-01462-y PMID: 37641040

ADDITIONAL READING

Badr, Y., Tariq, U., Al-Shargie, F., Babiloni, F., Al Mughairbi, F., & Al-Nashash, H. (2024). A review on evaluating mental stress by deep learning using EEG signals. *Neural Computing & Applications*, *36*(21), 12629–12654. https://link.springer.com/article/10.1007/s00521-024-09809-5

Oliver, E., & Dakshit, S. (2025). Cross-Modality Investigation on WESAD Stress Classification. *arXiv preprint arXiv:2502.18733*. https://doi.org//arXiv.2502.18733DOI: 10.48550

Rashid, N., Mortlock, T., & Al Faruque, M. A. (2023). Stress detection using context-aware sensor fusion from wearable devices. *IEEE Internet of Things Journal*, *10*(16), 14114–14127. https://ieeexplore.ieee.org/abstract/document/10097874/

Vos, G., Ebrahimpour, M., van Eijk, L., Sarnyai, Z., & Azghadi, M. R. (2025). Stress monitoring using low-cost electroencephalogram devices: A systematic literature review. *International Journal of Medical Informatics*, *105859*, •••. https://www.sciencedirect.com/science/article/pii/S1386505625000760 PMID: 40056845

KEY TERMS AND DEFINITIONS

CNN (Convolutional Neural Network): A deep learning model often used to analyze images and facial expressions.

Edge Computing: Running AI on devices like phones or wearables instead of cloud servers—fast and private.

Ethical AI: AI systems designed with fairness, privacy, and user trust in mind.

Explainable AI (XAI): AI that can explain its decisions in a human-understandable way.

Federated Learning: Training AI across many devices without sharing personal data.

Fusion Strategy: The method of combining data from different sources to make better predictions.

LSTM (Long Short-Term Memory): A neural network that learns from time-based data like heartbeat or voice.

Multimodal System: AI system using multiple data types (e.g., voice, face, physiology) to improve accuracy.

Physiological Signals: Body signals like ECG, EDA, and EEG used to detect internal stress responses.

Stress Detection: Identifying physical or emotional stress through data like heart rate, speech, or facial expressions.

Sustainability in AI: Building AI that is energy-efficient, reusable, and low-cost.

Transfer Learning: Reusing a model trained on one task for a new but related task.

Transformer Model: A deep learning architecture good at understanding sequences in text and signals.

Chapter 11
From Virtual Care to Real Satisfaction:
A Narrative Review on the Impact of Service Quality in Telemedicine

N. Kavipriya
https://orcid.org/0000-0003-4246-7568
Sri Ramachandra Institute of Higher Education and Research, India

Selvam Jesiah
Sri Ramachandra Institute of Higher Education and Research, India

ABSTRACT

The COVID-19 pandemic significantly accelerated the adoption of telemedicine, making it vital for safe and accessible healthcare delivery. This narrative review explores the relationship between service quality and patient satisfaction in telemedicine, synthesizing findings from 49 studies. Using the SERVQUAL model—tangibility, reliability, responsiveness, assurance, and empathy—the study identifies key dimensions affecting patient experience. Results highlight improved communication, convenience, reduced wait times, and cost savings as critical satisfaction drivers. Functional and technical quality aspects are both crucial in evaluating service quality. While demographic factors had minimal impact, increased telemedicine use correlated with higher satisfaction. The review underscores the need for more nuanced, qualitative research to refine measurement tools and better understand patient perspectives. Findings offer insights for healthcare providers and policymakers aiming to enhance telemedicine services in a patient-centered care landscape.

INTRODUCTION

Rationale

With the advent of the COVID-19 pandemic and the quick development of digital technology, telemedicine has become an essential part of contemporary healthcare. The integration of telemedicine into healthcare systems requires careful alignment with national and international regulatory guidelines to

DOI: 10.4018/979-8-3373-3531-5.ch011

ensure safe and effective delivery of care. The necessity for social distancing and the lack of definitive treatments during the early stages of the pandemic made telemedicine a vital mode of communication between healthcare professionals and both infected and non-infected individuals (Monaghesh et al., 2020). Due in large part to the growing dependence on and advancement of digital platforms, telemedicine—which serves as a diagnostic and screening tool—has become increasingly relevant in recent years.

These technologies enable healthcare providers to monitor patients remotely, particularly those with chronic conditions who require ongoing medical supervision but face barriers in accessing in-person care (Bitar et al., 2021).

In India, the Telemedicine Society of India (TSI) has played a pivotal role in promoting telemedicine through regular updates, training programs for healthcare and allied professionals, and publications highlighting advancements in telehealth (Telemedicine Society of India, Tamil Nadu, 2020). In India, telemedicine usage was sparse and irregular before to 2020. However, under the 'Digital India' initiative, the Government of India launched the eSanjeevani telemedicine platform on August 9, 2020. During the COVID-19 crisis, healthcare providers leveraged video conferencing to offer remote consultations, enhancing accessibility and continuity of care (Porecha, 2021).

The eSanjeevani platform supports both patient-to-doctor (eSanjeevani OPD) and doctor-to-doctor consultations (eSanjeevani 95), aiming to connect tertiary care institutions with primary health centers, particularly in rural and underserved areas. As of March 2021, the platform had facilitated over three million consultations, underscoring its role in delivering essential non-COVID healthcare services during the pandemic (Ministry of Health & Family Welfare, Govt. of India, 2022). Both public and private sector efforts to expand telemedicine access are seen as potential solutions to address India's longstanding healthcare delivery challenges.

In the fiercely competitive and quickly changing global healthcare industry of today, patient satisfaction is becoming a key metric for evaluating the quality of services. Research has consistently emphasized the importance of incorporating patient perspectives in assessing healthcare performance (Fatima et al., 2018; Mosadeghrad, 2014). Patient satisfaction influences healthcare utilization decisions and reflects the extent to which services meet or exceed user expectations. The SERVQUAL model, introduced by Parasuraman et al. (1985), is widely employed for evaluating service quality across various industries. While originally developed for the service sector, its relevance has been established in healthcare settings as well, including hospitals (Aghamolaei et al., 2014). However, its applicability should be contextually validated to ensure accurate assessment across different environments.

Table 1. Applications of SERVQUAL dimensions and descriptions to the quality of telemedicine services.

Dimensions	Descriptions	Example of Telemedicine Services
Tangibility	The visible and physical characteristics of buildings, equipment, staff, and communication materials that represent service excellence.	The physical facilities of a health-care facility would be visually appealing. e.g., background, appearance of physician,
Responsiveness	Willingness to support patients and provide required services	Doctors express genuine interest in resolving issues and are eager to assist patients who live in remote areas.
Assurance	Employees' skills to communicate trust and confidence, as well as their knowledge and respect.	Physicians have the ability to respond to queries of the patients in a polite manner.

continued on following page

Table 1. Continued

Dimensions	Descriptions	Example of Telemedicine Services
Empathy	Customer service that is caring and personalized.	Doctors and support personnel care about the patients' well-being and form long- term connections with them.
Reliability	Doctors and support staff are concerned about the well-being of their patients and develop long-term relationships with them.	Medical investigations, treatment, connection, follow-up, and other services are provided when they promise to be provided.

How SERVQUAL is Applied to Telemedicine?

Though SERVQUAL is used conventionally in face-to-face healthcare, its application to telemedicine means reinterpreting every dimension in the cyber care setup:

1.**Tangibility** → Physical infrastructure in telemedicine is substituted by digital tangibility. This incorporates clearness of video/audio, ease-of-use teleconsultation platforms, physician's professional appearance on the screen, and access to digital health records.
2.**Reliability** → Expands beyond punctuality and proper diagnoses to encompass system reliability (reliable internet, secure websites) and the provider's consistency in completing digital prescriptions, test orders, and follow-ups.
3.**Responsiveness** → In telehealth, responsiveness encompasses technical support, on-time digital correspondence, and prompt answering of online inquiries, as opposed to medical responsiveness.
4.**Assurance** → Patients are greatly dependent on trust in clinical competence and digital safety. Assurance thus addresses data privacy, patient data encryption, and trust in the provider's capacity to provide safe care virtually.
5.**Empathy** → The telemedicine challenge is to recreate a feeling of personalized, caring interaction in spite of physical distance. Adaptation entails employing verbal cueing, active listening, and visual engagement tactics to transmit empathy digitally.

Thus, telemedicine adaptation of SERVQUAL entails redefining service quality dimensions for a blended "clinical + digital" environment. This involves incorporating technology-centric subdimensions like system usability, platform accessibility, and information security.

The SERVQUAL framework is widely regarded as a practical, multidimensional, and comprehensive tool for evaluating users' subjective perceptions of service quality. It has demonstrated acceptable validity and has been applied extensively across various service sectors such as banking, healthcare, telecommunications, higher education, and information technology (Sohail, 2007; Butt & De Run, 2008; Niranjan & Metri, 2008; Sritharan, 2013). Its conception and evaluation of service quality are its strongest points. A review of literature examining SERVQUAL from 1998 to 2013 affirms its continued relevance and identifies it as a significant area of interest in academic research, contributing meaningfully to the broader understanding of service quality (Wang Binliang, 2021).

Patients have a unique chance to assess the quality of healthcare services received since their experiences provide direct information about the efficacy of care.Service quality is a key concern not only for patients but also for healthcare providers and institutions. However, perceptions of care quality can often obscure the actual value of services rendered. One effective approach to bridging this gap is incorporating patient perspectives to refine and enhance healthcare delivery processes. Recognizing the critical role of service quality is essential for ensuring operational efficiency and reliability in hospitals. This in turn forms the basis for providing value-added patient care and attaining a long-term competitive advantage. Given the growing use of telemedicine during the COVID-19 pandemic, it is more important than ever to assess patient satisfaction and service quality in this evolving healthcare model. Understanding patients' telemedicine experiences can provide valuable information about the efficacy, acceptability, and potential of digital health services.

Consequently, the present study aims to: (a) review the literature on the relationship between service quality and patient satisfaction in telemedicine-based healthcare settings; (b) evaluate the key findings of studies on patient satisfaction with telemedicine applications; and (c) look into the connection between telemedicine usage and patient satisfaction levels. In addition, the project seeks to address the following research topics in order to fulfill these objectives: (1) In the healthcare industry, which elements of service quality are most important? (2) Is there a measurable relationship between patient happiness and telehealth services? (3) Are telemedicine consultations preferred by patients over traditional methods?

THEORETICAL FRAMEWORK

Quality of Service

Service quality is the core concern of every service industry and is essentially the dynamic interaction between the service firm and the consumer (Johns, 1999). There are many studies in various industries like hospitality and food services that have delved into how service quality can effect customer satisfaction and consumer behavior (Cao & Kim, 2015; Cronin & Taylor, 1994; Zaibaf et al., 2013; Cynthia et al., 2014; Chow et al., 2007). Although its universal importance, service quality is commonly perceived as an intangible and abstract phenomenon whose form is largely determined by the consumer's experiences and perceptions (Lehtinen & Lehtinen, 1991).

Patients play the role of consumers in the healthcare setting, while service providers are physicians, nurses, and other health professionals. Patients exhibit varied cognitive capacity, emotions, and medical expertise, which impact their expectations and perceptions of service quality in ways that differ from usual consumer settings. Healthcare services involve tangible and intangible factors — from physical facilities, cleanliness, and equipment to the interpersonal behavior, skills, and compassion of medical personnel.

As discussed in Table 1, SERVQUAL dimensions continue to be core to assessing patient perceptions of service quality within telemedicine, especially responsiveness, empathy, and reliability. With the COVID-19 pandemic's pivot toward digital consultations, where tangibility is minimized, these dimensions underscore the significance of communication quality, trust, and timely follow-up. Overall perceptions by patients are thus determined not just by clinical outcomes but also the extent to which providers can transform their communication and relational strategies in virtual care.

Service Quality in the Health Sector

The rapid expansion of telehealth services has compelled the healthcare sector to adapt quickly and confront emerging challenges. In response, researchers, policymakers, healthcare professionals, and decision-makers have developed various frameworks to evaluate and ensure service quality (Naidu, 2009;

Andaleeb, 2001). According to Grönroos (1984), healthcare service quality can be divided into two key dimensions: technical quality and functional quality. While technical quality refers to the clinical accuracy and the appropriateness of medical procedures and diagnoses, functional quality emphasizes how care is delivered, focusing on aspects such as communication, empathy, and patient interaction (Lam, 1997).

In many cases, patients may not be able to distinguish between a physician's clinical expertise (curing) and their interpersonal skills (caring). Thus, while technical quality involves what is delivered, functional quality reflects how the service is experienced by the patient (Lam, 1997).

Despite the growing emphasis on service quality, many health systems continue to prioritize technical performance and clinical outcomes, often overlooking patient feedback (Alaloola & Albedaiwi, 2008). From this technical standpoint, the success of procedures, diagnostic precision, and adherence to professional standards are key indicators of quality (Rashid & Jusoff, 2009). However, patients — who typically lack in-depth knowledge of medical procedures — tend to evaluate care based on observable and experiential factors. As such, patient expectations, perceptions, and personal experiences can offer valuable insight into both technical and non-technical aspects of healthcare delivery (Wysong & Driver, 2009). Gathering patient feedback is therefore essential for quality improvement, with the aim of enhancing satisfaction without attributing blame or judgment (Mpinganjira, 2011).

Patient satisfaction plays a crucial role in shaping the public image and credibility of healthcare institutions (Donabedian, 1980). It also influences patient loyalty and the likelihood of recommending services to others, commonly referred to as word-of-mouth promotion (Andaleeb, 2001). As patient expectations continue to rise, healthcare providers are increasingly challenged to identify and address key service quality factors that directly contribute to satisfaction. Doing so not only improves care outcomes but also promotes cost and time efficiency for healthcare facilities (Pakdil & Harwood, 2005).

To systematically assess service quality, the SERVQUAL model has been widely applied in healthcare settings. Numerous studies have validated its utility for evaluating healthcare service performance, including those by Babakus & Mangold (1992), Reidenbach & Sandifer (1992), Lam (1997), Kilbourne et al. (2004), Wong (2002), Scardina (1994), Vandamme & Leunis (1993), and Taylor & Cronin (1993), as summarized in Table 3.

Objectives

This paper will first review studies that assess the effect of service quality on patient satisfaction when using telemedicine in healthcare settings, and then it will analyze the findings of studies related to patient satisfaction in telemedicine applications to ascertain whether telemedicine and patient satisfaction are correlated.

There are multiple research questions to be resolved.

R1. Which SERVQUAL dimensions most strongly shape patient satisfaction in telemedicine-based healthcare?

R2. What is the strength and nature of the relationship between telehealth use and patient satisfaction?

R3. How do patient satisfaction and perceived service quality differ between telemedicine and face-to-face consultations?

R4. Under what conditions do patients prefer telemedicine over traditional in-person consultations?

METHODS

Sources of Information, The Search Procedure, And The Research Selection

The sources of data were the Embase and EBSCO PubMed (MEDLINE), Embase and Google Scholar. It can also be used to evaluate hospital service quality, but its feasibility must be determined in various circumstances. To combine the expressions, the Boolean operators (AND, OR and NOT) were used. For example, MEDLINE database was searched with (Service quality) [title/abstract] AND (telemedicine) [title/abstract] AND (patient satisfaction) [title/abstract].

The inclusion criteria to choose the articles are: the interviews/survey assessing the patient perception with telemedicine irrespective of disease; only those studies that themed around service quality, telemedicine, and some measurement of patient satisfaction. The exclusion criteria are studies that are not assessing the evaluation of patient satisfaction in telemedicine as well as studies published before December 2000.

Data Collection Process

Figure 1 shows a diagram of the data collecting procedure. The papers that included service quality, measurement of patient perception, and telemedicine were taken before the abstracts were reviewed for applicability to our purpose. The inclusion and exclusion criteria listed above were used to analyze the articles. Since in MEDLINE, research on Service Quality dimensions is limited to less than ten with telemedicine, the articles are referred from Google scholar. Consensus meetings and discussion sessions were conducted to increase the reliability as the screening and analysis is carried out. Both meetings and discussions were used to identify factors and discuss the finding and conclusions. Standard techniques were used to reduce selection bias and ensure that the search was thorough. Notes on service quality, telemedicine, patient satisfaction, in a matrix were compiled.

Summary Measurements And Data Items

Our litmus test was passed by publications that combined telemedicine, patient experience, and service quality with a performance or efficacy indicator. Those who failed to achieve these goals were removed.

Individual Study Bias And Study-Wide Bias Risk

During consensus sessions, the idea of bias was discussed. Bias during data selection was minimized through a multi-step strategy. First, well-defined inclusion and exclusion criteria (telemedicine, service quality, and patient satisfaction focus; exclusion of non-relevant or pre-2000 studies) were applied uniformly. Second, independent screening followed by consensus meetings and discussion sessions helped ensure reliability and reduced subjective bias in article selection. Third, the use of multiple databases (MEDLINE, Embase, EBSCO, Google Scholar) with Boolean operators minimized publication bias and ensured comprehensive coverage. Together, these measures strengthened the objectivity and validity of the selected studies.

The consensus meetings acted as a mechanism to check the authors' selection bias and selective reporting.

Results Synthesis And Summary Measures

The method involves looking at studies that integrate telemedicine intervention service quality with patient happiness, as well as articles that include effectiveness or efficiency. These observations were physically counted. The frequency of each topic was displayed using an affinity matrix once all observations were collated into an Excel file and distilled into themes pertaining to aspects of service quality, effectiveness, or efficiency. The ranking of these was based on frequency.

LIMITATIONS

Even though service quality investigation is done largely based on the SERVQUAL Model., qualitative studies are needed to investigate more refined/modified service quality dimensions, which may be suitable for changing scenario of healthcare diagnosis and delivery using advanced technology. Some studies on telemedicine and patient satisfaction are limited to small sample and some are limited by geography.

RESULTS

Figure 1 illustrates our search procedure. From 323 articles totally, the initial search yielded 412 results, 103 were taken in an abstract and full-text evaluation, 49 papers were selected for inclusion in the study from medical databases.

INDIVIDUAL STUDY SELECTION, STUDY ATTRIBUTES AND FINDINGS

Figure 1 shows how we went about our search. After a preliminary search generated 323, results relating to service quality, tele-health, and service quality, 103 were subjected to an abstract and then full-text evaluation, and finally 49 studies selected for the study. The articles which are not in English and human criteria are been excluded. For Service quality dimensions and models papers were retrieved from Google scholar not only in healthcare but other from service industries too.

Figure 1. Literature search process with inclusion and exclusion criteria

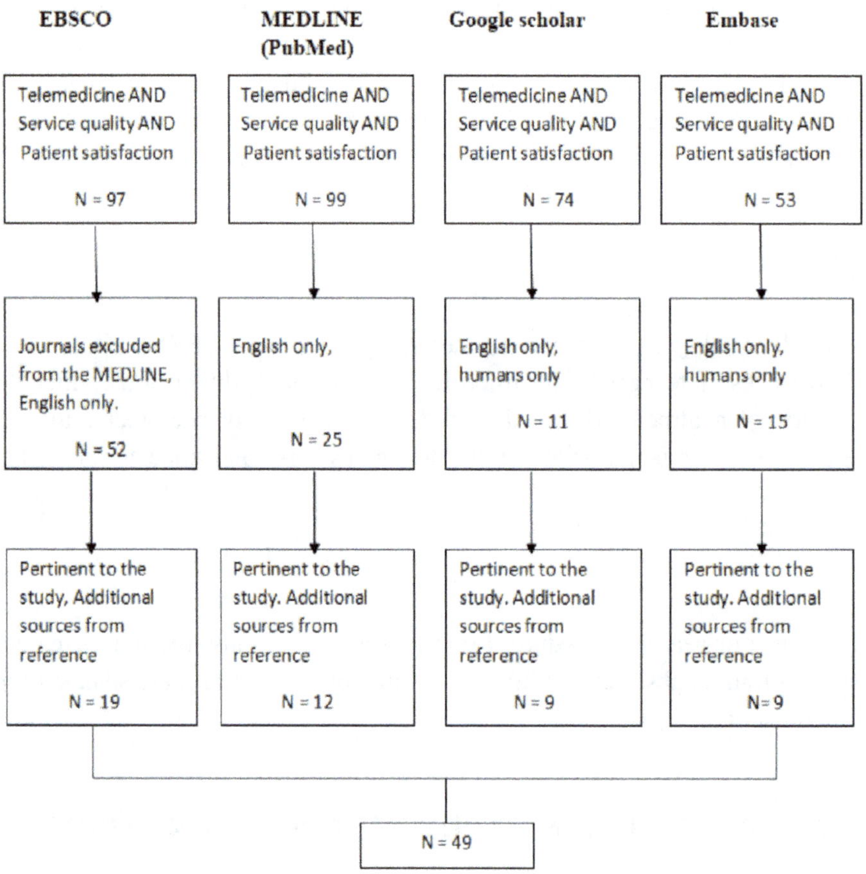

Table 2. Service Quality Models

Author	Title	Model	Sample audience	Service quality addressed through
Grönroos, 1984	"A service quality model and its marketing implications".	"Technical and functional quality model"	219 - service sector companies (bank, insurance, restaurants, shipping, airline companies, etc.,)	"Functional and technical quality"
Parasuraman et al., 1985	"A conceptual model of service quality and its implications for future research".	"Gap model"	Ranged from 298-487 -service companies viz. telephone, securities brokerage, insurance, banks, etc.,	Ten dimensions ("reliability, security, responsiveness, access, communication, tangibles, credibility, courtesy, competence, and understanding/knowing")
Haywood-Farmer, 1988	"A service quality model and its marketing implications".	"Attribute service quality model"		"Physical facilities and processes, behavior of people and conviviality, and professional judgment"
Brogowicz et al., 1990	"A synthesised service quality model with managerial implications".	"Synthesized model of service quality"		"Technical and functional quality outlining planning, implementation, and control tasks"
Cronin and Taylor, 1994	"Measuring service quality: a reexamination and extension".	"Performance-only model"	660 -banking, dry cleaning, pest control, and fast food	Confirmatory 22 items, same as "SERVQUAL but with performance-only statements"
Mattsson, 1992	"A service quality model based on an ideal value standard".	"Ideal value model"	40 guests as they check in and check out/2 large luxury hotels	18 elements of value and 9 elements of customer satisfaction
Teas, 1993	"Expectations, performance evaluation, and consumers' perceptions of quality".	"Normed quality and evaluated performance model"	120 - selected randomly from discount stores	Limited subset of "SERVQUAL" items (2 items for each of 5 dimensions)
Berkley and Gupta, 1994	"Improving service quality with information technology"	"IT alignment model"		The model doesn't cover the service quality measurement
Dabholkar et al., 1996	"Measure of service quality for retail stores: scale development and validation".	"Attribute and overall affect model"	505- undergraduate students/fast food setting	3 items measuring expected service quality, specifically of ordering situation
Spreng and Mackoy, 1996	"An empirical examination of a model of perceived service quality and satisfaction".	"Perceived quality and satisfaction model"	273- undergraduate students	"Desires, expectations, perceived performance, and desired congruency" (comprising 10 attributes each)
Philip and Hazlett, 1997	"The measurement of service quality: a new P-C-P attributes model".	"Pivotal, Core, and Peripheral attribute model"		"Pivotal attributes, core attributes, and peripheral attributes".
Sweeney et al., 1997	"Retail service quality and perceived value".	"Retail service quality and perceived value model"	1016- electrical appliances stores	"Functional quality" through 5 SERVQUAL items and "technical quality" through 1 item

continued on following page

Table 2. Continued

Author	Title	Model	Sample audience	Service quality addressed through
Oh, 1999	"Service quality, customer satisfaction, and customer value: a holistic perspective".	"Service quality, customer value, and customer satisfaction model"	545 -two luxury hotels survey	8 items for perceptions of hotel settings and one item for perceived price and
Dabholkar et al., 2000	"A comprehensive framework for service quality: an investigation of critical conceptual and measurement issues through a longitudinal study".	"Antecedent mediator model"	397 - undergraduate and postgraduate students	SERVQUAL element through measurement of "reliability, comforts, personal attention, and features".
Frost and Kumar, 2000	"INTSERVQUAL: an internal adaptation of the GAP model in a large service organisation".	"Internal service quality model"	724 -Singapore airline staff at different levels	"SERVQUAL" dimensions
Soteriou and Stavrinides, 1997	"An internal customer service quality data envelopment analysis model for bank branches".	"Internal service quality Data Envelope Analysis model"	194 - 26 bank branches	Measurement of customers' perceptions using "SERVQUAL"-based instrument
Broderick and Vachirapornpuk, 2002	"Service quality in internet banking: the importance of customer role".	"Internet banking model"	160 incidents on 55 topic episodes posted in UK Internet website community	"Service encounters, service setting, customer expectation, and image"
Zhu et al., 2002	"IT-based services and service quality in consumer banking".	"IT-based model"	185 - bank customers with experience of using IT-based service options viz. ATM and 24-hr call line	"SERVQUAL items with perception"-only statements
Santos, 2003	"E-service quality: a model of virtual service quality dimensions".	"E-service quality model"	30 focus groups - 6 to 10 members	"Incubative and active dimensions"
Dagger et al., 2007	"A hierarchical model of health service quality".	"Model of health service quality"	28 participants - 7 per focus group from medical centers	"Interpersonal quality, technical quality, administrative quality environmental quality"
Rakhmawati et al., 2013	"Developing a service quality measurement model of public health center in Indonesia".	"Service quality model for Public Health Center"	800/patients	"Quality of - health care delivery, health care personnel, administration process, and the adequacy of health care resources".
Lee, 2017	"HEALTHQUAL: a multi-item scale for assessing healthcare service quality".	"HEALTHQUAL"	368 patients and 389 public	"Empathy, efficiency, tangibles, safety, and degree of improvements in care service".

Table 3. Research that has assessed hospital service quality using SERVQUAL dimensions.

Dimension	Studies
Assurance	"Aghamolaei et al., 2014", "Babakus and Boller,1992", "Chakravarty, 2011", "Babakus and Mangold,1992", "Anderson, 1996", "Curry, 1999", "Curry and Stark, 2000", "Andaleeb, 2000", Andaleeb, 2001 "Curry and Sinclair, 2002", "Kazemi et al., 2013", "Islam et al., 2016", "Al Fraihi et al., 2016".
Empathy	"Curry and Stark, 2000", "Babakus and Boller,1992"-"Anderson, 1996", "Curry, 1999", "Curry and Sinclair, 2002", "Jabnoun and Chaker, 2003", "Kilbourne et al"- "Arasli et al., 2008"- "Chakravarty, 2011", "Kazemi et al., 2013", "Aghamolaei et al., 2014", "Islam et al., 2016", "Al Fraihi et al., 2016".
Reliability	"Dabholkar et al", "Babakus and Boller, 1992", "Babakus and Mangold, 1992", "Anderson, 1996", "Curry, 1999", "Curry and Stark, 2000", "Curry and Sinclair, 2002", "Kilbourne et al", "Chakravarty, 2011"- "Kazemi et al., 2013"- "Aghamolaei et al., 2014", "Islam et al., 2016", "Al Fraihi et al., 2016 and Jabnoun and Chaker, 2003".
Responsiveness	"Kilbourne et al", "Babakus and Boller, 1992", "Babakus and Mangold", "Curry", "Curry and Stark, 2000"- "Andaleeb, 2001", "Andaleeb, 2000", "Curry and Sinclair", "Jabnoun and Chaker, 2003", "Chakravarty, 2011", "Kazemi et al., 2013", "Aghamolaei et al., 2014", "Islam et al., 2016", "Anderson, 1996", "Al Fraihi et al., 2016".
Tangibles	"Babakus and Mangold, 1992", "Babakus and Boller", "Anderson, 1996", "Curry", "Curry and Stark, 2000", "Curry and Sinclair", "Kilbourne et al", "Chakravarty, 2011", "Kazemi et al., 2013", "Aghamolaei et al., 2014", "Islam et al., 2016", "Al Fraihi et al., 2016", "Jabnoun and Chaker, 2003".

The research conducted for telemedicine, service quality, and patient satisfaction are listed in Table 4. (n = 27). We observed telemedicine and satisfaction, a screening criterion, for each article or research in the sample. The most current studies are at the top of the list, which is arranged by publication date.

Table 4. Compilation of observations for the sample

Author	Title	Journal	Summary/relevance	SampleSize, Miscellaneouscomments
Kopel et al., 2001	"Evaluating satisfaction with a child and adolescent psychological telemedicine outreach service".	J Telemed Telecare	"A child and adolescent telepsychiatry service with the videoconferencing in rural New South Wales was evaluated. Patients and their and rural clinicians, conveyed high satisfaction with the telepsychiatry service".	218 - patients and 337 - health officials were interviewed
Cariello, 2003	"Computerized telephone nurse triage. An evaluation of service quality and cost".	Ambul Care Manage	"The study examined service quality from the perception of callers using the system for pediatric client. A revised form of the SERVQUAL was administered to members who used nurse triage services. Majority of callers rated the level of service quality very highly. Education, employment status, age of the caller, child gender, birth order, and age of child did not affect the rating of service quality".	314 - respondents
Smith et al., 2004	"Diagnostic accuracy and patient satisfaction with telemedicine for the follow-up of paediatric burns patients".	J Telemed Telecare	"Videoconferencing technique offered for the post-acute burns care in Queensland for children was studied. The agreement between clinical assessments conducted via conventional, face-to-face manner conducted and videoconference assessments the were compared This study endorses that the quality of information collected by a videoconference appointment is comparable to that collected by traditional method for a follow-up burns consultation".	of 35 - children with a previous burn injury were studied
Finkelstein et al., 2004	"Tele-homecare_ quality, perception, satisfaction".	Mary Ann	"The study aimed to show that telehomecare linking homebound patients with their home health-care nurses provides high-quality, clinically beneficial, and patient satisfactory interactions over telephone system. All the patients were satisfied with the health care facility and increasing level of telehomecare intervention increases the satisfaction".	567 - virtual visits conducted for the 53 subjects completing the study.

continued on following page

Table 4. Continued

Author	Title	Journal	Summary/relevance	SampleSize, Miscellaneouscomments
Klaz et al., 2005	"Teledermatology_ quality assessment by user satisfaction and clinical efficiency".	Isr Med Assoc J	"The study evaluated patients' satisfaction and effectiveness of a computerized store forwarding teledermatology service referred by primary care physicians to a certified dermatologist using email with digital photographs. The level of the service and satisfaction and was high among patients in both rural and urban areas, with notably higher scores in rural units".	508 - patients, both rural and urban.
Edgar Rodas et al., 2005	"Low-bandwidth telemedicine for pre- and postoperative evaluation in mobile surgical services".	J Telemed Telecare	"The effectiveness of low-bandwidth telemedicine used for the pre- and postoperative assessment of patients treated through mobile surgery service in remote Ecuador. It is concluded that telemedicine reduces the time required on spot for preoperative planning, and provides consistent postoperative surveillance, resulting in improving the effectiveness of mobile surgery services".	Out of 194 - patients, 144 - were studied preoperatively and 50 postoperatively
Jacobs et al., 2016	"Patient satisfaction with a teleradiology service in general practice".	BMC Family Practice	"A cross-sectional study investigated the satisfaction of patients about a new teleradiology facility was which is offered in an island in the Netherlands. Patients in the island experienced high satisfaction levels with the teleradiology service provided in primary care".	587 - patients between June 2007 and June 2009
Mulgrew et al., 2011	"Comparison of parent satisfaction with care for childhood obesity delivered face-to-face and by telemedicine".	Telemed J E Health	"The study is conducted to establish whether a significant difference in quality of care existed between consultations for childhood obesity delivered by face to face and by telemedicine, as measured by parent satisfaction, and found that there was no significant difference between consultations for childhood obesity delivered face to face and by telemedicine in parent satisfaction".	Parents of 54 -children under 12 years. The sample size was not large enough to determine if the satisfaction in the telemedicine group

continued on following page

Table 4. Continued

Author	Title	Journal	Summary/relevance	SampleSize, Miscellaneouscomments
Constantinescu et al., 2012	"Satisfaction with telemedicine for teaching listening and spoken language to children with hearing loss".	J Telemed Telecare	"The Hear and Say Centre in Brisbane offers AVT sessions to families after diagnosis. Satisfaction of parent and therapist with the telemedicine was examined by questionnaire. All parents felt comfortable as face-to-face when discussing matters with the therapist online, and were satisfied or as satisfied as face-to-face with their level and their child's level of interaction/rapport with the therapist. Also the therapists were satisfied with the telemedicine AVT programme".	13 of the 17 parents and five therapists. Small sample may not be enough
Amjeriya et al., 2012	"Measurement of service quality in healthcare organization".	International Journal of Engineering Research & Technology (IJERT)	"The purpose is to determine the use of SERVQUAL to evaluate patients' perceptions about health care quality in XY Hospital. Result revealed that hospital service attributes have positive effect and are important to build patient satisfaction".	62 patients of the hospital are surveyed to find out the service quality perceived by them.
LeRouge et al., 2015	"Patient perspectives of telemedicine quality".	Patient Prefer Adherence.	"The study explored the quality attributes needed for effective telemedicine consultations from the patient's viewpoint. This result of the analysis reveals that quality attributes such as instructions and guidance regarding the health and peripheral sophistication were ranked high".	32 members with six focus group
XinyuanWu, BA et al., 2015	"Feasibility and Efficacy of Patient-Initiated Mobile Teledermoscopy for Short-term Monitoring of Clinically A typical Nevi".	JAMA Dermatol	"The examined the feasibility, patient receptivity and efficacy of teledermoscopy for monitoring of clinically atypical nevi. Results from this study recommend that teledermoscopy is effective and feasible method for short-term examination of clinically atypical nevi".	34 patients with 1 or more clinically atypical nevi at an institutional referral center
Aliman and Mohamad, 2016.	"Linking Service Quality, Patients' Satisfaction and Behavioral Intentions: An investigation on Private Healthcare in Malaysia".	6th International Research Symposium in Ser. Mgt., IRSSM-6 UiTM Malaysia	"Service quality dimensions affected the intention behaviors positively. Every service factor had positive relationships with patients' satisfaction".	300 hospital outpatients who were treated at the private hospitals

continued on following page

Table 4. Continued

Author	Title	Journal	Summary/relevance	SampleSize, Miscellaneouscomments
Wootton et al., 2015	"Relationship between the quality of service provided through store-and-forward telemedicine consultations and the difficulty of the cases – implications for long-term quality assurance".	Front. Public Health	"The difficulty of telemedicine cases and the quality of the resulting consultation in a telemedicine network is examined. There was a weak negative relation between case difficulty and output quality, i.e., the more challenging cases tended to result in lower quality consultations. However, the effect was non-significant. Larger study might be effective".	10 telemedicine cases was selected over a 3-month period
Poulsen et al., 2015	"Satisfaction with rural rheumatology telemedicine service".	International Journal of Rheumatic Diseases	"Patient satisfaction with the rheumatology telemedicine service offered to a rural place in northern Australia is assessed. Patients are satisfied with the rheumatology telemedicine service, and may prefer the service to extensive travelling".	The study assessed 107 rheumatology outpatients
Polinski et al., 2016	"Patients' Satisfaction with and Preference for Telehealth Visits".	J Gen Intern Med	"The study aimed at assessing satisfaction levels in using telemedicine using SERVQUAL. Patient-centered communication, such as having an empathetic and caring attitude, showing responsiveness to the emotional needs of the patient, and providing assurance to the patient are the dimensions identified".	1734 patients completed the surve at Minute Clinic offering telehealth in January–September 2014
Jennifer L Fang et al., 2016	"Emergency Video Telemedicine Consultation for Newborn Resuscitations_ The Mayo Clinic Experience".	Mayo Clin Proc.	"The study brought out the experience with emergency video telemedicine consultations for newborn deliveries at Mayo Clinic with high-risk. Despite technical issues related to quality audio and video the telemedicine consult improved patient safety, quality of care, or both and prevented unnecessary transfers to a higher level of care".	64 surveys were completed offering newborn telemedicine consultations to 6 health system sites.

continued on following page

Table 4. Continued

Author	Title	Journal	Summary/relevance	SampleSize, Miscellaneouscomments
Shafiq et al., 2017	"Service Quality Assessment of Hospitals in Asian Context: An Empirical Evidence From Pakistan".	The Journal of Health Care Organization, Provision, and Financing	"The study adapted the SERVQUAL instrument to develop a service quality measurement scale. The findings indicated that all five dimensions of SERVQUAL are found suitable in Asian countries with 13 items are relevant. Reliability, tangibility, responsiveness, empathy, and assurance were ranked in order with respect to the quality gap".	Data were collected from 9 different hospitals inpatients and outpatients, and the scale was
Yan Qiu et al., 2018	"Internet-Based and Mobile-Based General Practice_ Cross-Sectional Survey".	J Med Internet Res	"The study was to explore the features of outpatients' satisfaction the internet hospital of the First Affiliated Hospital, Zhejiang University, China. The internet hospital is suitable for all health seekers ranging from surgery, gynecology and obstetrics, internal medicine, dermatology, pediatrics, ophthalmology, stomatology to emergency".	715 patients with 365 health-related problems who visited Web-based clinic via a computer or smartphone.
Burns et al., 2019	"Implementation of speech pathology telepractice services for clinical swallowing assessment - An evaluation of service outcomes, costs and consumer satisfaction".	J Telemed Telecare	"This study examined the service outcomes, costs and patient satisfaction involved in organizing adult clinical swallowing assessments using telepractice. High patient and clinician satisfaction was reported with cost benefits".	Five hub-spoke telepractice services, encompassing 18 facilities offering speech pathology.
Verma et al., 2020	"e-Healthcare service quality_ consumer satisfaction and its association with demographic characteristics".	Int J Health Care Qual Assur	"The purpose of the study is to identify the important elements of quality with e-Healthcare services by means of Zineldin's 5Qs model. The analysis recognized quality of hospital atmosphere, quality of interaction, and quality of object as the main predictors of consumer satisfaction with e-Healthcare services".	252 respondents in a private hospital in Punjab, India, from February 2018 to March 2019

continued on following page

Table 4. Continued

Author	Title	Journal	Summary/relevance	SampleSize, Miscellaneouscomments
Eva Serhal et al., 2020	"Client Satisfaction and Experience With Telepsychiatry_ Development and Validation of a Survey Using Clinical Quality Domains".	J Med Internet Res.	"This study aims to form a validated survey tool to measure satisfaction and patient experience with telepsychiatry based on the quality of healthcare domains in the context of telepsychiatry across 4 domains viz. access and timeliness, appropriateness, effectiveness, and safety. Result shows that safety and access and timeliness domains were found to be statistically significant predictors of satisfaction".	274 patients who received clinical consultations through the TeleMental Health Program at the Centre for Addiction and Mental Health
Ramaswamy et al., 2020	"Patient Satisfaction With Telemedicine During the COVID-19 Pandemic_ Retrospective Cohort Study".	J Med Internet Res.	"The study analyzed patient satisfaction toward Telemedicine during pre–COVID-19 and COVID-19 (before vs after March 4, 2020) period. Video visit utilization increased by 8729%during the COVID-19 pandemic compared to the same period last year".	analyzed 38,609 Press Ganey patient satisfaction survey
Sultan et al., 2020	"Utilization of Telemedicine Virtual Visits in Pediatric Spin... _ Journal of Pediatric Orthopaedics".	Journal of Pediatric Orthopaedics: Sept	"This study aimed to estimate the feasibility and patient satisfaction related with virtual visit (VV) utilization in PSD patients. The results shows that telemedicine VVs offered an alternative to traditional in-office visits for PSD patients with patients receiving faster care with comparable satisfaction".	Of the 189 VVs offered to pediatric orthopaedic patients at a large academic health care system, January 1, 2017 - December 31, 2018
Wang Binliang, 2021	"A study of patient satisfaction based on general hospitals in Taizhou, Zhejiang province, China".	International Journal of Science Arts and Commerce	"In this study, a model with perceived value and patient satisfaction as the intermediate variables is constructed. The quality of telemedicine service directly impacts behavioural intention and patient satisfaction. The quality of telecommunication service comprises five dimensions: tangibility, reliability, responsibility, assurance and emergency. Patients of different age, education and distance differ in the perception and the influence of different dimension of quality of telemedicine service is quite different".	371 were patients who received the remote consultation service offered by the Zhejiang telemedicine centre.

continued on following page

Table 4. Continued

Author	Title	Journal	Summary/relevance	SampleSize, Miscellaneouscomments
Andrew N Mason., 2022	"The Most Important Telemedicine Patient Satisfaction Dimension: Patient-Centered Care".	Telemed J E Health	"Satisfaction levels of telemedicine patients was examined using SERVQUAL model. Four dimensions of satisfaction were identified, and patient-centered care was shown to be the most significant dimension. Patient perceptions of benefits received from the telemedicine service have an effect on patient satisfaction".	surveyed 440 telemedicine patients
Almutairi et al., 2021	"Kuwaiti hospital patients' continuance intention to use telemedical systems in the wake of the COVID19 pandemic".	Healthc Technol Lett.	"The study investigated factors influencing patients' intention to use telemedicine continuously after the COVID-19 pandemic in Kuwait. The findings revealed that information and system quality have a positive influence on patient's satisfaction. Patients' continuance intention of using telemedicine is found to be impacted by their satisfaction."	290 patients availing telemedical services from a private hospital in Kuwait
Ganguly et al., 2024	"Telemedicine Use Among Caregivers of Pediatric Cancer Patients in India: A Mixed-Methods Study"	JCO Global Oncology Abstracts (2024)	"The study explored caregiver satisfaction with telemedicine in pediatric oncology during and after the pandemic. "	Over 90% of caregivers reported telemedicine was convenient, time- and cost-saving, and would recommend its use. However, some highlighted challenges with communication and rapport compared to in-person visits.
Fadaizadeh et al. (2024)	"Patient and Physician Satisfaction With Telehealth During and After COVID-19: A Meta-Analysis"	Healthcare Informatics Research	Meta-analysis confirmed high satisfaction among patients and physicians during/ after COVID-19. Telehealth was seen as effective and acceptable, but technical barriers and training gaps remain significant.	Meta-analysis of multiple studies (2020–2023), covering thousands of patients and providers.
Khairat et al. (2023)	"Patient and Provider Perspectives on Improving Telemedicine User Experience in Primary Care"	Telemedicine Reports	A qualitative study exploring patient and provider perspectives on telemedicine. Key satisfaction factors included technical reliability, clear communication, and integration with EHR systems.	40 participants (patients and providers) interviewed; qualitative thematic analysis.

Patient Satisfaction

Patient satisfaction in telemedicine is a multidimensional construct that extends beyond convenience. Literature consistently demonstrates that satisfaction depends not only on accessibility and reduced travel but also on trust, perceptions of provider attentiveness, and the emotional quality of interaction.

Studies in tele-audiology (Constantinescu, 2012) and tele-psychiatry show that empathetic engagement and clear communication allow patients to feel as comfortable as in traditional face-to-face care, suggesting that trust and emotional reassurance are central to positive experiences. Research in tele-dermatology and radiology (Klaz et al., 2005; Jacobs et al., 2016) similarly highlights that satisfaction is mediated by providers' ability to adapt their consultation style to overcome the absence of physical presence. These findings indicate that patient perceptions of being "heard" and supported are key determinants of satisfaction, not just the efficiency of the digital platform.

National-level studies reinforce these relational insights. In China, internet hospital surveys revealed that education and distance influenced satisfaction, with patients reporting higher comfort when providers communicated clearly and instilled confidence (Qiu et al., 2018; Wang Binliang, 2021). In India, evaluations of the eSanjeevani platform during COVID-19 found that patients valued not only timely access but also the reassurance and attentiveness of providers, which enhanced trust in digital consultations.

Across contexts, determinants of satisfaction therefore include:

- Functional factors such as accessibility, responsiveness, and reliability.
- Relational factors such as empathy, clarity of communication, and emotional reassurance.
- Trust-related factors including confidence in both the provider's competence and the platform's data security.

These insights reveal that patient satisfaction with telemedicine is not superficial but deeply rooted in human perceptions and emotions. Frameworks such as SERVQUAL must therefore be expanded to capture these human aspects, ensuring that evaluations of digital care reflect both efficiency and relational quality.

SYNTHESIS OF RESULTS

The 27 articles reported patient satisfaction, telemedicine and quality factors, the following frequency of occurrence of the factors is identified in Table 5. Common factors are grouped out of 18 factors. The frequency doesn't signify the strength of the factor but its use in literature is identified.

Table 5. Factor Matrix

Factor	Frequency
Better communication, service	18
Preferred Mode	13
Accessibility	10

continued on following page

Table 5. Continued

Factor	Frequency
Wait time reduction	8
Cost saving	7
Decrease clinic visits	5
Time saving	3

The findings collectively demonstrate that patient satisfaction with telemedicine is influenced by key factors such as effective communication, high service quality, perceived usefulness, accessibility, reduced wait times, and cost savings. A notable observation across the literature is that interpretations of satisfaction can vary depending on whether single-item measures or multi-dimensional approaches are used. Studies consistently report high levels of patient satisfaction with telemedicine services across a wide range of specialties, including psychiatry, pediatrics, dermatology, radiology, surgery, and obstetrics, among others, despite occasional technical issues.

Importantly, demographic variables such as education, employment status, age of the caller, child's gender, birth order, and age did not significantly affect perceptions of service quality. Both patients and therapists reported satisfaction with telemedicine, with patients indicating comfort levels and rapport comparable to face-to-face interactions. Satisfaction was notably high in both urban and rural settings, with rural populations often reporting even higher satisfaction levels.

Comparative studies found no significant difference in satisfaction between in-person and telemedicine consultations. Additionally, telemedicine was found to enhance patient safety and quality of care, particularly in emergency settings, by preventing unnecessary transfers to higher levels of care. Service quality dimensions were positively associated with behavioral intentions and patient satisfaction, which also correlated with cost-effectiveness.

Research during the COVID-19 pandemic revealed a significant increase in telemedicine utilization, with a reported 87.29% rise in video visits compared to the previous year. Studies also indicate that information quality and system quality strongly influence patient satisfaction and their intention to continue using telemedicine post-pandemic. In some cases, patients expressed a preference for telemedicine over traditional in-person visits due to its convenience and timely access to care.

Statistical validation and contrasting evidence

Across the 49 included studies, statistical validation commonly comprised descriptive summaries, association tests (e.g., correlations, regressions) linking SERVQUAL dimensions to satisfaction, group comparisons between telemedicine and in-person consultations, and reliability testing of adapted SERVQUAL instruments. A consistent pattern shows responsiveness, empathy, and assurance as significant positive predictors of telemedicine satisfaction, supported by acceptable-to-high internal consistency of measurement scales.

Conversely, several studies reported null or mixed effects, particularly for tangibility (perceived limitations of physical examination, device/internet issues) and continuity/coordination (fragmented follow-up pathways). Differences frequently depended on context (clinical specialty, patient demographics, rural vs. urban connectivity, and post-pandemic normalization). We therefore interpret the evidence as directionally positive but heterogenous, with technology-mediated factors moderating SERVQUAL's impact.

To enhance transparency, we summarize the contrasting evidence below and indicate implications for interpretation:

Table 6.

Aspect	Evidence typically reported	Limitations noted	Implication for synthesis
Responsiveness / Empathy / Assurance	Significant positive associations with satisfaction; reliable multi-item scales	Cross-sectional designs; potential self-selection of digitally capable users	Strongest, most consistent drivers of telemedicine satisfaction
Tangibility	Lower or mixed ratings vs. in-person; tech quality influences perceptions	Measurement mismatch (physical cues vs. digital cues); device/connectivity variance	Interpret cautiously; prioritize "digital tangibility" indicators (AV quality, UI, environment)
Comparative satisfaction (TM vs. F2F)	Often comparable; sometimes higher for access/time	Case-mix differences; follow-up rates confound satisfaction	Use adjusted comparisons; consider specialty-specific analyses
Scale reliability	Cronbach's α commonly ≥0.80 reported	Heterogeneous item adaptations; limited validation for tele-contexts in some studies	Report α where available; recommend **measurement-invariance** checks in future work

Planned analytic clarifications in text. We now: (1) identify where statistical significance was reported; (2) report scale reliability when provided; (3) apply a vote-counting/effect-direction summary to distinguish convergent vs. divergent results; and (4) discuss moderators (specialty, tech quality, timeframe) that explain heterogeneity. We also outline future needs for measurement-invariance testing of adapted SERVQUAL, meta-regression by context, and longitudinal designs to address causality.

PRACTICAL EVIDENCE: PLATFORM USAGE, PATIENT OUTCOMES, AND IMPLEMENTATION CHALLENGES

Platform Usage

Telemedicine uptake has spread quickly in various contexts. India's government-funded eSanjeevani platform, for instance, crossed 100 million consultations as of 2024, one of the world's largest digital health endeavors. In China, "Internet Hospitals" have rapidly expanded to cover both acute and chronic care demands, whereas in high-income nations, services like Teladoc and Amwell are reporting high utilization, especially in mental health, dermatology, and primary care. These data show that telemedicine has transitioned from being an add-on service to becoming a component of healthcare provision.

Patient Outcomes

Beyond satisfaction, telemedicine has demonstrated robust results in various specialties. Diabetes and hypertension chronic disease programs exhibit increased treatment compliance and decreased hospital readmission when telemedicine follow-up is included. Tele-psychiatry has revealed therapy adherence levels of or greater than in-person treatment, and tele-dermatology shows high concordance with office-based consultations. Patient-reported outcomes also identify decreases in stress, travel burden, and expense, in addition to increased continuity of care.

Implementation Challenges

Despite its potential, there are several challenges in the way. Digital literacy skills deficiencies, in particular among older adults and socioeconomically disadvantaged populations, limit access. Infrastructure issues—unbalanced internet coverage and device availability—hinder balanced participation, especially in rural and low-resource environments. Provider concerns on the other end include workload burden, medico-legal risk, and virtual diagnostic limitations. System-level issues like confusing reimbursement practices and absence of standardized training add to barriers to long-term sustainability.

DISCUSSION

This review underscores that patient satisfaction with telemedicine is repeatedly influenced by dimensions of service quality such as communication, accessibility, responsiveness, empathy, and reliability. From the studies reviewed, successful provider–patient interaction was the most commonly mentioned determinant of satisfaction, emphasizing the need for clear instructions, active listening, and reassurance in virtual care. Telemedicine has also been found useful in shortening waiting times, decreasing expenses, and reducing the necessity for travel, especially among patients in remote and underserved areas.

Comparative data indicates that telemedicine consultations can achieve satisfaction levels similar to traditional in-person encounters, provided that technical reliability is ensured. Notably, patients and caregivers tended to report developing rapport and comfort with clinicians during video consultations, refuting earlier assumptions that digital interfaces necessarily weaken therapeutic relationships. Furthermore, the evidence suggests that demographic variables such as age, education, or socioeconomic status exert limited influence on service quality perceptions, although digital literacy and infrastructure remain essential drivers.

Linking Findings to Research Questions through SERVQUAL

The findings can be critically interpreted using the SERVQUAL framework and aligned with the study's research questions.

- **R1 (important service quality dimensions):** Of SERVQUAL's five dimensions, responsiveness, empathy, and reliability were consistently identified as the most critical for patient satisfaction in telemedicine. Tangibility, however, had limited relevance in digital contexts, reflecting the need for adaptation.
- **R2 (association between patient satisfaction and telehealth):** The evidence showed that assurance (confidence in providers) and responsiveness were closely linked to higher satisfaction, confirming SERVQUAL's core proposition that service quality drives satisfaction.
- **R3 (differences between telemedicine and face-to-face care):** Satisfaction levels were broadly comparable across modalities when empathy and assurance were maintained. Yet, technological

reliability—outside the original SERVQUAL dimensions—proved decisive for positive patient experiences.

- **R4 (preference for telemedicine):** Patients often favored telemedicine for its responsiveness and convenience, but reduced tangibility and occasional technical challenges tempered this preference.

Thus, while SERVQUAL provides a valuable framework for evaluating telemedicine service quality, it requires extension to include digital-specific elements such as system usability, technological trust, and continuity of care.

Ethical, Behavioral, and Equity Issues in Digital Care

The expansion of telemedicine brings ethical, behavioral, and equity issues that are as significant as technical reliability and patient satisfaction.

- **Ethical issues** concern safeguarding patient confidentiality and securely managing sensitive health information. Some studies observed that while telemedicine enhanced efficiency, technical glitches raised concerns about safety and quality (Fang et al., 2016). This underscores the ethical responsibility of providers to ensure robust data protection and transparent communication about risks. Informed consent in digital environments should also clarify privacy safeguards, technological limitations, and alternative options.
- **Behavioral factors** highlight how patients and providers adapt to digital interactions. Parents in tele-audiology programs in Brisbane reported being as comfortable online as in person, showing that empathetic communication can sustain trust even virtually (Constantinescu, 2012). Conversely, dermatology and radiology studies found that rapport sometimes depended on providers' ability to adjust their consultation styles to compensate for the lack of physical presence (Klaz et al., 2005; Jacobs et al., 2016). Patient willingness to continue telemedicine is thus shaped not only by system performance but also by provider attentiveness and professionalism in virtual settings.
- **Equity issues** remain central. Rural patients in Australia reported greater satisfaction with tele-rheumatology than with long-distance travel (Poulsen et al., 2015), while China's nationwide internet hospital survey showed that satisfaction varied by education and distance, pointing to unequal access (Qiu et al., 2018; Wang Binliang, 2021).

In India, the government's eSanjeevani platform expanded access during COVID-19, especially in rural areas, but gaps in digital literacy and internet connectivity still restricted universal uptake. These examples illustrate that telemedicine can both reduce and reinforce healthcare inequalities depending on infrastructure and policy.

In total, ethical safeguards, adaptive behavioral practices, and equity-focused strategies must complement technological development. Otherwise, satisfaction metrics may obscure hidden disparities. Incorporating strong data protection mechanisms, training providers in digital communication, and investing in inclusive infrastructure are essential to ensuring that telemedicine evolves as an equitable, trusted, and patient-centered form of healthcare delivery.

LIMITATIONS

Even though the SERVQUAL Model serves as the foundation for service quality research, qualitative studies are still required to examine more complex or altered aspects of service quality that could be appropriate for the evolving landscape of healthcare diagnosis and delivery through the use of cutting-edge technology.Some studies on telemedicine and patient satisfaction are limited to small sample and some are limited by geography.

CONCLUSIONS

The service quality dimensions are influenced by many factors like reliability, responsiveness, security, access, communication, courtesy, credibility, competence, tangibles, and understanding. Patient satisfaction is complex in nature as the experience encountered by the patients affects not only the satisfaction but also cognitive factors influencing the satisfaction. The users are satisfied with the telemedicine facilities provided.

While researchers have examined the Quality dimensions in different models for healthcare sector, the factors contributing to patient satisfaction is dynamic and remains to be clearly defined. Attempts have been made to improve the factors and metrics used to measure satisfaction. While studies have highlighted and urged for greater research into several dimensions, the quality of their use in telemedicine must be validated, since it is uncertain to what degree this will be relevant in the current pandemic crisis. Research indicates that hospital service characteristics positively affect telemedicine-using patients' satisfaction. The idea of telemedicine depends largely on technology. As a result, it may not rely on technology to provide a service, which sets it apart from standard medical processes. The global COVID-19 health crisis has provided a rare opportunity for health systems to learn from and build on previous global experiences. There are problems encountered by the patients such as accessibility, cost, time, social distancing and travel restrictions which have made telemedicine a reliable and preferred mode for patients.

Like other services in the healthcare industry, telemedicine applications can benefit from the validity and applicability of quality characteristics such as tangibility, responsiveness, assurance, empathy, and dependability.

This review reveals that patient satisfaction in telemedicine is influenced by factors such as convenience, responsiveness to patients' emotional needs and queries (communication), accessibility to technology, time and cost. The intention to use telemedicine in future is determined by patient satisfaction. The quality parameters examined in this study are based on a thorough literature assessment, with a particular emphasis on the telemedicine and patient satisfaction domains. Therefore, more research is needed to find more important quality elements and their overall impact on patient happiness and loyalty in order to broaden the influence of the components that have been established.

FUTURE STUDIES

Although this research yields important information about the extension of SERVQUAL to telemedicine, various research paths continue to be available for future studies. Refinement and validation of telemedicine-tailored SERVQUAL dimensions such as platform usability, data protection, and digital trust are needed, for instance. More sophisticated validation techniques, such as longitudinal, multi-site, and cross-cultural designs, must be used by future research to test causality and measure invariance across telemedicine and traditional care. Furthermore, future studies must investigate concerns of equity and access through a focus on underserved groups like rural patients, elderly individuals, and digitally excluded users. Studies of hybrid models that merge telemedicine with face-to-face consultations are also crucial, particularly for chronic disease management and care continuity. Last but not least, the incorporation of emerging technologies like AI-driven decision support systems, wearable devices, and remote monitoring tools should be reviewed in order to further learn about their influence on patient satisfaction and perceived service quality.

REFERENCES

Aghamolaei, T., Eftekhaari, T. E., Rafati, S., Kahnouji, K., Ahangari, S., Shahrzad, M. E., Kahnouji, A., & Hoseini, S. H. (2014). 'Service quality assessment of a referral hospital in Southern Iran with SERVQUAL technique: Patients' perspective'. *BMC Health Services Research, 14*(1), 1–5.

Al Fraihi, K.J., FAMCO, D. & Latif, S.A. (2016). Evaluation of outpatient service quality in Eastern Saudi Arabia: Patient's expectations and perceptions. *Saudi Medical Journal, 37*(4), 420.

Alaloola, N.A. and Albedaiwi, W.A. (2008) 'Patient satisfaction in a Riyadh tertiary care centre', *International journal of health care quality*.

Aliman, N. K., & Mohamad, W. N. (2016). 'Linking service quality, patients' satisfaction and behavioral intentions: An investigation on private healthcare in Malaysia'. *Procedia: Social and Behavioral Sciences, 224*, 141–148.

Almutairi, I. L., Alazemi, B. F., & Almutairi, F. L. (2021). 'Kuwaiti hospital patients' continuance intention to use telemedical systems in the wake of the COVID19 pandemic'. *Healthcare Technology Letters, 8*(6), 159–168.

Amjeriya, D & Malviya, R.K (2012) 'Measurement of service quality in healthcare organization. *International Journal of Engineering Research and Technology',* Oct;1(8):1-7.

Andaleeb, S. S. (2000). Service quality in public and private hospitals in urban Bangladesh: A comparative study. *Health Policy (Amsterdam), 53*(1), 25–37.

Andaleeb, S. S. (2001). Service quality perceptions and patient satisfaction: A study of hospitals in a developing country. *Social Science & Medicine, 52*(9), 1359–1370.

Anderson, E. A. (1996). Measuring service quality at the university of Texas MD Anderson cancer center. *International Journal of Health Care Quality Assurance*.

Arasli, H., Ekiz, E. H., & Katircioglu, S. T. (2008). Gearing service quality into public and private hospitals in small islands: Empirical evidence from Cyprus. *International Journal of Health Care Quality Assurance, 21*(1), 8–23.

Babakus, E., & Boller, G. W. (1992). An empirical assessment of the SERVQUAL scale. *Journal of Business Research, 24*(3), 253–268.

Babakus, E., & Mangold, W. G. (1992). Adapting the SERVQUAL scale to hospital services: An empirical investigation. *Health Services Research, 26*(6), 767.

Berkley, B. J., & Gupta, A. (1994). Improving service quality with information technology. *International Journal of Information Management, 14*(2), 109–121.

Bitar, H., & Alismail, S. (2021). The role of eHealth, telehealth, and telemedicine for chronic disease patients during COVID-19 pandemic: A rapid systematic review. *Digital Health, 7*, 20552076211009396.

Broderick, A. J., & Vachirapornpuk, S. (2002). Service quality in internet banking: The importance of customer role. *Marketing Intelligence & Planning*.

Brogowicz, A.A. Delene, L.M. and Lyth, D.M. (1990) 'A synthesised service quality model with managerial implications', *International journal of service industry management, 1*(1), pp.0-0.

Burns, C. L., Ward, E. C., Gray, A., Baker, L., Cowie, B., Winter, N., Rusch, R., Saxon, R., Barnes, S., & Turvey, J. (2019). Implementation of speech pathology telepractice services for clinical swallowing assessment: An evaluation of service outcomes, costs and consumer satisfaction. *Journal of Telemedicine and Telecare*, *25*(9), 545–551.

Butt, M. M., & De Run, E. C. (2008). 'Measuring Pakistani Mobile Cellular Customer Satisfaction', *Icfai. Journal of Services Marketing*, *6*(1).

Cao, Y., & Kim, K. (2015). How do customers perceive service quality in differently structured fast food restaurants? *Journal of Hospitality Marketing & Management*, *24*(1), 99–117.

Cariello, F. P. (2003). Computerized telephone nurse triage: An evaluation of service quality and cost. *The Journal of Ambulatory Care Management*, *26*(2), 124–137.

Chakravarty, A. (2011). Evaluation of service quality of hospital outpatient department services. *Medical Journal, Armed Forces India*, *67*(3), 221–224.

Chow, I. H. S., Lau, V. P., Lo, T. W. C., Sha, Z., & Yun, H. (2007). Service quality in restaurant operations in China: Decision-and experiential-oriented perspectives. *International Journal of Hospitality Management*, *26*(3), 698–710.

Chowdhary, N. and Prakash, M. (2007) 'Prioritizing service quality dimensions. *Managing Service-Quality:AnInternationalJournal*

Constantinescu, G. (2012). Satisfaction with telemedicine for teaching listening and spoken language to children with hearing loss. *Journal of Telemedicine and Telecare*, *18*(5), 267–27.

Cronin, J. J.Jr, & Taylor, S. A. (1992). Measuring service quality: A reexamination and extension. *Journal of Marketing*, *56*(3), 55–68.

Curry, A. (1999). Innovation in public service management. *Managing Service Quality*.

Curry, A., & Sinclair, E. (2002). Assessing the quality of physiotherapy services using SERVQUAL. *International Journal of Health Care Quality Assurance*.

Curry, A., & Stark, S. (2000). 'Quality of service in nursing homes. *Health Services Management Research*, *13*, 205–215.

Dabholkar, P. A., Shepherd, C. D., & Thorpe, D. I. (2000). A comprehensive framework for service quality: An investigation of critical conceptual and measurement issues through a longitudinal study. *Journal of Retailing*, *76*(2), 139–173.

Dabholkar, P. A., Thorpe, D. I., & Rentz, J. O. (1996). A measure of service quality for retail stores: Scale development and validation. *Journal of the Academy of Marketing Science*, *24*(1), 3–16.

Dagger, T. S., Sweeney, J. C., & Johnson, L. W. (2007). A hierarchical model of health service quality: Scale development and investigation of an integrated model. *Journal of Service Research*, *10*(2), 123–142.

eSanjeevani (2021), Porecha M and Singh PV—The government-owned dark horse in India's telemedicinerace. The Ken. https:// the- ken. com/ story/ esanjeevani- the- government- owned- dark- horse-inindias-telemedicine- race/? utm_ source= daily_story&utm_ medium= email &utm_campaign= daily_newsletter (Accessed 18 March 2021).

Fadaizadeh, H., Ahmadi, S., & Sabouri, S. (2024). Patient and physician satisfaction with telehealth during and after COVID-19: A meta-analysis. *Healthcare Informatics Research*, *30*(3), 206–215.

Fang, J. L., Collura, C. A., Johnson, R. V., Asay, G. F., Carey, W. A., Derleth, D. P., Lang, T. R., Kreofsky, B. L., & Colby, C. E. (2016). Emergency video telemedicine consultation for newborn resuscitations: The Mayo Clinic experience [). Elsevier.]. *Mayo Clinic Proceedings*, *91*(12), 1735–1743.

Fatima, T., Malik, S. A., & Shabbir, A. (2018). Hospital healthcare service quality, patient satisfaction and loyalty: An investigation in context of private healthcare systems. *International Journal of Quality & Reliability Management*.

Finkelstein, S. M., Speedie, S. M., Demiris, G., Veen, M., Lundgren, J. M., & Potthoff, S. (2004). Telehomecare: Quality, perception, satisfaction. *Telemedicine Journal and e-Health*, *10*(2), 122–128.

Frost, F. A., & Kumar, M. (2000). INTSERVQUAL–an internal adaptation of the GAP model in a large service organisation. *Journal of Services Marketing*.

Ganguly, S., Saha, S., Roy, A., & Basu, S. (2024). Telemedicine use among caregivers of pediatric cancer patients in India: A mixed-methods study. *JCO Global Oncology*, *10*(Suppl. 16), 1549.

Grönroos, C. A. (1984). service quality model and its marketing implications. *European Journal of Marketing*, *18*, 36–44.

Haywood-Farmer, J. (1988). A conceptual model of service quality [health care quality assurance.]. *International Journal of Operations & Production Management*, *8*(6), 19–29.

Islam, R., Ahmed, S., & Tarique, K. M. (2016). Prioritisation of service quality dimensions for healthcare secto. *International Journal of Medical Engineering and Informatics*, *8*(2), 108–123.

Jabnoun, N., & Chaker, M. (2003). Comparing the quality of private and public hospitals. *Managing Service Quality*.

Jacobs, J. J., Ekkelboom, R., Jacobs, J. P., Van Der Molen, T., & Sanderman, R. (2016). Patient satisfaction with a teleradiology service in general practice. *BMC Family Practice*, *17*(1), 1–8.

Johns, N. (1999). What is this thing called service? *European Journal of Marketing*, *33*, 958–974.

Kazemi, N., Ehsani, P., Abdi, F., & Bighami, M. (2013). Measuring hospital service quality and its influence on patient satisfaction: An empirical study using structural equation modeling. *Management Science Letters*, *3*(7), 2125–2136.

Khairat, S., Xie, B., & Liu, S. (2023). Patient and provider perspectives on improving telemedicine user experience in primary care. *Telemedicine Reports*, *4*(1), 1–10.

Kilbourne, W. E., Duffy, J. A., Duffy, M., & Giarchi, G. (2004). The applicability of SERVQUAL in cross-national measurements of health-care quality. *Journal of Services Marketing*.

Klaz, I., Wohl, Y., Nathansohn, N., Yerushalmi, N., Sharvit, S., Kochba, I., & Brenner, S. (2005). Teledermatology: Quality assessment by user satisfaction and clinical efficiency. *Sat*, *13*, 21.

Kopel, H., Nunn, K., & Dossetor, D. (2001). Evaluating satisfaction with a child and adolescent psychological telemedicine outreach service. *Journal of Telemedicine and Telecare*, *7*(2, suppl), 35–40.

Ladhari, R. (2009). A review of twenty years of SERVQUAL research. *International Journal of Quality and Service Sciences*.

Lam, S. S. (1997). 'SERVQUAL: A tool for measuring patients' opinions of hospital service quality in Hong Kong'. *Total Quality Management*, *8*(4), 145–152.

Lee, D. (2017). HEALTHQUAL: A multi-item scale for assessing healthcare service quality. *Service Business*, *11*(3), 491–516.

Lehtinen, U., & Lehtinen, J. R. (1991). Two approaches to service quality dimensions. *Service Industries Journal*, *11*(3), 287–303.

LeRouge, C. M., Garfield, M. J., & Hevner, A. R. (2015). Patient perspectives of telemedicine quality. *Patient Preference and Adherence*, *9*, 25.

Mason, A. N. (2022). The most important telemedicine patient satisfaction dimension: Patient-centered care. *Telemedicine Journal and e-Health*, *28*(8), 1206–1214.

Mattsson, J. (1992). A service quality model based on an ideal value standard. *International Journal of Service Industry Management*, *3*(3), 0-0.

Mekoth, N., George, B. P., Dalvi, V., Rajanala, N., & Nizomadinov, K. (2012). Service quality in the public sector hospitals: A study in India. *Hospital Topics*, *90*(1), 16–22.

Mohammed, P., & Mercy, M. (2011). 'Understanding service quality and patient satisfaction in private medical practice: A case study. *African Journal of Business Management*, *5*(9), 3690–3698.

Monaghesh, E., & Hajizadeh, A. (2020). The role of telehealth during COVID-19 outbreak: A systematic review based on current evidence. *BMC Public Health*, *20*(1), 1–9.

Mosadeghrad, A. M. (2014). Factors affecting medical service quality. *Iranian Journal of Public Health*, *43*(2), 210.

Mulgrew, K. W., Shaikh, U., & Nettiksimmons, J. (2011). Comparison of parent satisfaction with care for childhood obesity delivered face-to-face and by telemedicine. *Telemedicine Journal and e-Health*, *17*(5), 383–387.

Naidu, A. (2009). Factors affecting patient satisfaction and healthcare quality. *International Journal (Toronto, Ont.)*.

Niranjan, T. T., & Metri, B. A. (2008). client-vendor-end user triad: A service quality model for is/ites outsourcing. *Journal of Services Research*, *8*(1).

Oh, H. (1999). Service quality, customer satisfaction, and customer value: A holistic perspective. *International Journal of Hospitality Management*, *18*(1), 67–82.

Pakdil, F., & Harwood, T. N. (2005). Patient satisfaction in a preoperative assessment clinic: An analysis using SERVQUAL dimensions. *Total Quality Management & Business Excellence*, *16*(1), 15–30.

Parasuraman, A., Zeithaml, V. A., & Berry, L. L. (1985). A conceptual model of service quality and its implications for future research. *Journal of Marketing*, *49*(4), 41–50.

Philip, G., & Hazlett, S. A. (1997). The measurement of service quality: A new P-C-P attributes model. *International Journal of Quality & Reliability Management*.

Polinski, J. M., Barker, T., Gagliano, N., Sussman, A., Brennan, T. A., & Shrank, W. H. (2016). 'Patients' satisfaction with and preference for telehealth visits'. *Journal of General Internal Medicine*, *31*(3), 269–275.

Poulsen, K. A., Millen, C. M., Lakshman, U. I., Buttner, P. G., & Roberts, L. J. (2015). Satisfaction with rural rheumatology telemedicine service. *International Journal of Rheumatic Diseases*, *18*(3), 304–314.

Qiu, Y., Liu, Y., Ren, W., Qiu, Y., & Ren, J. (2018). Internet-based and mobile-based general practice: Cross-sectional survey. *Journal of Medical Internet Research*, *20*(9), e8378.

Rakhmawati, T., Sumaedi, S., Bakti, I. G. M. Y., Astrini, N. J., Widianti, M. Y. T., Sekar, D. C., & Vebriyanti, D. I. (2013). Developing a service quality measurement model of public health center in Indonesia. *Management Science and Engineering*, *7*(2), 1–15.

Ramaswamy, A., Yu, M., Drangsholt, S., Ng, E., Culligan, P. J., Schlegel, P. N., & Hu, J. C. (2020). Patient satisfaction with telemedicine during the COVID-19 pandemic: Retrospective cohort study. *Journal of Medical Internet Research*, *22*(9), e20786.

Rashid, W. E. W., & Jusoff, K. (2009). Service quality in health care setting. *International Journal of Health Care Quality Assurance*.

Reidenbach, R. E., & Sandifer-Smallwood, B. (1990). Exploring perceptions of hospital operations by a modified SERVQUAL approach. *Marketing Health Services*, *10*(4), 47.

Rodas, E., Mora, F., Tamariz, F., Cone, S. W., & Merrell, R. C. (2005). Low-bandwidth telemedicine for pre-and postoperative evaluation in mobile surgical services. *Journal of Telemedicine and Telecare*, *11*(4), 191–193.

Santos, J. (2003). E-service quality: A model of virtual service quality dimensions. *Managing Service Quality*.

Scardina, S. A. (1994). SERVQUAL: A tool for evaluating patient satisfaction with nursing care. *Journal of Nursing Care Quality*, *8*(2), 38–46.

Serhal, E., Kirvan, A., Sanches, M., & Crawford, A. (2020). Client satisfaction and experience with telepsychiatry: Development and validation of a survey using clinical quality domains. *Journal of Medical Internet Research*, *22*(9), e19198.

Seth, N., Deshmukh, S. G., & Vrat, P. (2005). Service quality models: A review. *International Journal of Quality & Reliability Management*.

Shafiq, M., Naeem, M. A., Munawar, Z., & Fatima, I. (2017). Service quality assessment of hospitals in Asian context: An empirical evidence from Pakistan. *INQUIRY: The Journal of Health Care Organization, Provision, and Financing*, *54*, 0046958017714664.

Smith, A. C., Kimble, R., Mill, J., Bailey, D., O'Rourke, P., & Wootton, R. (2004). Diagnostic accuracy of and patient satisfaction with telemedicine for the follow-up of paediatric burns patients. *Journal of Telemedicine and Telecare*, *10*(4), 193–198.

Sohail, M. S., Royal, M., Saeed, M., & Ahmed, Z. (2007). Determinants of service quality in the hospitality industry: The case of Malaysian hotels. *Journal of Accounting–Business & Management*, *14*, 64–74.

Soteriou, A. C., & Stavrinides, Y. (1997). An internal customer service quality data envelopment analysis model for bank branches. *International Journal of Operations & Production Management*, *17*(8), 780–789.

Spreng, R. A., & Mackoy, R. D. (1996). An empirical examination of a model of perceived service quality and satisfaction. *Journal of Retailing*, *72*(2), 201–214.

Sritharan, V. (2013). Service quality: An empirical analysis of national saving banks in Northern Province in Srilanka. *Int. J. Adv. Res. Manag. Soc. Sci*, *2*, 134–147.

Sultan, A. A., Acuña, A. J., Samuel, L. T., Rabin, J. M., Grits, D., Gurd, D. P., ... & Goodwin, R. C. (2020). Utilization of telemedicine virtual visits in pediatric spinal deformity patients: a comparison of feasibility and patient satisfaction at a large academic center. Journal of Pediatric Orthopaedics, 40(8), e712-e715.

Sweency, J. C., Soutar, G. N., & Johnson, L. W. (1997). Retail service quality and perceived value: A comparison of two models. *Journal of Retailing and Consumer Services*, *4*(1), 39–48.

Taylor, S. A., & Cronin, J. J.Jr. (1994). Modeling patient satisfaction and service quality. *Journal of Health Care Marketing*, *14*(1).

Teas, R. K. (1993). 'Expectations, performance evaluation, and consumers' perceptions of quality'. *Journal of Marketing*, *57*(4), 18–34.

Telemedicine Society of India. (2020), Tamil Nadu Chapter. TeleHealth Newsletter. https:// tsitn. org/ enewsletter-nov- 2020/. (Accessed 04 December 2020).

Vandamme, R. and Leunis, J. (1993) 'Development of a multiple-item scale for measuring hospital service quality', *International Journal of Service Industry Management, 4*(3), pp.0-0.

Verma, P., Kumar, S., & Sharma, S. K. (2020). e-Healthcare service quality: Consumer satisfaction and its association with demographic characteristics. *International Journal of Health Care Quality Assurance*, *33*(6), 413–428.

Wang, B. (2021). A study of patient satisfaction based on general hospitals in Taizhou, Zhejiang province, China. *International Journal of Science Arts and Commerce*, *6*(6).

Wong, J. C. (2002). Service quality measurement in a medical imaging department. *International Journal of Health Care Quality Assurance*.

Wootton, R., Liu, J., & Bonnardot, L. (2015). Relationship between the quality of service provided through store-and-forward telemedicine consultations and the difficulty of the cases–implications for long-term quality assurance. *Frontiers in Public Health, 3*, 217.

Wu, X., Oliveria, S. A., Yagerman, S., Chen, L., DeFazio, J., Braun, R., & Marghoob, A. A. (2015). Feasibility and efficacy of patient-initiated mobile teledermoscopy for short-term monitoring of clinically atypical nevi. *JAMA Dermatology, 151*(5), 489–496.

Wysong, P. R., & Driver, E. (2009). 'Patients' perceptions of nurses' skill'. *Critical Care Nurse, 29*(4), 24–37.

Zaibaf, M., Taherikia, F., & Fakharian, M. (2013). 'Effect of perceived service quality on customer satisfaction in hospitality industry: Gronroos' service quality model development'. *Journal of Hospitality Marketing & Management, 22*(5), 490–504.

Zhu, F. X., Wymer, W., & Chen, I. (2002). IT-based services and service quality in consumer banking. *International Journal of Service Industry Management.*

KEY TERMS AND DEFINITIONS

Assurance: Assurance refers to the confidence and trust that healthcare providers instill in patients through their competence, knowledge, and respectful communication during telemedicine consultations.

Empathy: Empathy is the ability of healthcare professionals to understand and respond to patients' emotional needs, showing genuine care and personalized attention in virtual healthcare settings.

Patient Satisfaction: Patient satisfaction is a measure of how well the expectations and experiences of patients are met by the quality of telemedicine services, including communication, accessibility, and outcomes.

Reliability: Reliability in telemedicine describes the consistency and dependability of healthcare services, ensuring that promised care and follow-up are delivered as expected.

Responsiveness: Responsiveness is the promptness and willingness of healthcare providers to address patient inquiries, resolve issues, and provide timely support during telemedicine interactions.

Service Quality: Service quality in telemedicine encompasses all aspects of care delivery, including technical performance, interpersonal skills, and the overall patient experience, which collectively determine the value of healthcare services.

Tangibility: Tangibility refers to the visible and physical elements of telemedicine, such as the clarity of audiovisual communication, the professional appearance of providers on screen, and the ease of using digital platforms.

Telemedicine: Telemedicine is the use of digital technologies, such as video conferencing and secure messaging, to deliver healthcare services remotely, allowing patients to access medical consultations and support without needing to visit a physical clinic.

Chapter 12
Predictive Analytics in Personalized Medical Care:
Early Risk Assessment and Management

Pooja Dehankar
Ajeenkya D.Y. Patil School of Engineering, India

Susanta Das
https://orcid.org/0000-0002-9314-3988
Ajeenkya D.Y. Patil University, India

ABSTRACT

The widespread implementation and utilization of electronic health records has resulted in technological advancements in computers and data, which have enabled the creation of patient care models that are automated, personalized, and instantaneous. Artificial intelligence (AI), machine learning (ML), reinforcement learning (RL), and deep learning, are well adapted to use such data. This chapter examines how AI-driven solutions can revolutionize the healthcare industry, with emphasis on how ML techniques can be used to provide personalized medical interventions. The chapter covers ethical frameworks that must be in place in order to guarantee the proper application of AI-driven medical solutions. The chapter also addresses issues with data privacy, algorithm bias, and integration difficulties with current healthcare infrastructures. In order to fully utilize ML while maintaining patient safety, privacy, and equity in the delivery of healthcare, it highlights the significance of cooperative efforts between healthcare practitioners, technology specialists, legislators, and ethicists.

1. INTRODUCTION

Artificial intelligence has completely changed the way that medical practice, research, and policy are conducted, revolutionizing the field of healthcare. AI is now able to analyze data, generate predictions, and help decision-making thanks to advancements in machine learning and deep learning. This could significantly improve patient outcomes, diagnosis, and treatment across several medical specialties. Diagnostic AI algorithms are quite good at finding anomalies in medical imaging; in certain cases, they even outperform human scientists in this regard. By enabling medical personnel to diagnose patients

DOI: 10.4018/979-8-3373-3531-5.ch012

more quickly and accurately, artificial intelligence (AI) is completely changing the healthcare industry. It makes it possible to detect cancer early on in X-rays and assists in identifying minute neurological abnormalities in MRIs. AI-driven predictive analytics are revolutionising the healthcare business by precisely predicting disease progression, pinpointing at-risk populations, and improving the allocation of resources. AI models that analyze large amounts of patient data can predict the probability of contracting specific diseases. This enables health care providers to design individualized treatment plans and put into practice targeted preventive actions. AI algorithms are essential in the drug development sector because they speed up the process of finding therapeutic targets, drug candidates, and repurposing molecules. Biological data analysis, drug interaction prediction, and molecular dynamics simulation are all done with machine learning. This expedites the drug development process and expedites the release of life-saving drugs. However, there are still challenges to face (Singh et al., 2024).

The application of AI in healthcare has attracted a lot of interest from academic writers, indicating how quickly this topic at the nexus of technology and medicine is developing. Several facets of AI-driven healthcare solutions have been the subject of research investigations, from the use of machine learning algorithms in diagnostics to the prejudice and data privacy as ethical issues. Interestingly, an increasing amount of writing highlights the potential of AI to transform healthcare processes, improve patient outcomes, and aid in the creation of personalized strategies for therapy. Using machine learning algorithms in medical imaging is one important topic of interest in the literature for improved analysis. Research have shown that AI is effective in identifying abnormalities like cancer and anomalies, with astonishing precision. The use of AI in diagnostic procedures not only speeds up the analysis of large datasets but also enhances the accuracy and consistency of medical diagnoses, which has a positive effect on treatment choices and patient outcomes. The ethical ramifications of AI in healthcare are a crucial topic that has been extensively studied in the literature. There has been much discussion about privacy, security, and potential biases in algorithms because AI systems rely on large volumes of sensitive medical data. Academics stress that in order to guarantee responsible AI application and build confidence among patients, healthcare professionals, and legislators, strong ethical frameworks and regulatory requirements are essential (Johnson, 2018).

Precision medicine represents a significant advancement in healthcare that has the potential to enhance the current symptom-driven approach to medicine by enabling early interventions through enhanced diagnostics and customizing more effective and cost-effective therapies. The ability to analyze extensive patient data along with more general aspects to track and differentiate between ill and relatively healthy individuals is necessary to determine the optimal course for personalized and population medicine. This will improve our understanding of the biological markers that can indicate changes in health. While using healthcare data in clinical decision-making has proven challenging due to the complexity of disease at the individual level, technological improvements have significantly reduced some of the existing barriers (Ahmed et al., 2020).

In the broad healthcare setting, where the complexities of human biology meet the intricacies of medical practice, artificial intelligence and increased data intelligence are powerful catalysts for change. AI-driven medical solutions are changing the way we detect, treat, and understand diseases, thereby significantly and fundamentally changing the heart of healthcare every day. The new era of healthcare is driven by data-driven intelligence and machine learning, and it promises to revolutionize patient care as well as the entire healthcare ecosystem. The use of AI in healthcare is not just a small update, but a significant revolution. It was a long time ago when the main foundations of medicine were empirical study and the wisdom of seasoned practitioners (Ahmadi & Rabie Nezhad Ganji, 2023).

The National Institute of Mental Health and the Agency for Healthcare Research and Quality organized a technical expert panel tasked with assessing the current level of research on behavioral intervention technologies (BITs) in mental health and determining the most important areas for future study. Behavioral and psychological interventions that target behavioral and mental health outcomes by utilizing information and communication technology elements are referred to as BITs. Videoconferencing and ordinary telephone technology to offer psychotherapy have been well validated. A wide range of mental health outcomes have been demonstrated by the effectiveness of web-based therapies. When utilized in isolation, social media platforms like online support groups have yielded unsatisfactory results. The effects of mobile technologies on mental health have not gotten much attention. Virtual reality has demonstrated good efficacy in treating pediatric illnesses and anxiety (Mohr et al., 2013).

2. PREDICTIVE ANALYTICS FOR HEALTHCARE

Predictive analytics can identify people who are highly susceptible to contracting specific diseases by analyzing patient data, including genetic information, lifestyle factors, and medical history. Healthcare professionals can take immediate action, put preventive measures in place, and enhance patient outcomes by issuing early warnings. Treatment regimens can be customized with the use of predictive analytics to meet the needs of each patient. Healthcare providers can forecast patient response, identify the most effective treatments, and optimize pharmaceutical dosages to maximize treatment efficacy and reduce side effects by reviewing patient data. Healthcare organizations can detect and manage people at risk for particular health disorders with the use of predictive analytics. Healthcare professionals can create focused interventions, manage resources efficiently, and enhance population health outcomes by examining data at the community level. Healthcare systems can allocate resources more efficiently when predictive analytics is used. Healthcare providers may effectively manage inventory, staffing levels, and resource utilization to fulfill patient needs by projecting demand for their services. Patterns of fictitious or abusive medical claims can be found using predictive analytics. Healthcare providers can identify trends in claims data, look into questionable actions, and shield healthcare systems from fraud and financial losses by using this analysis (Cohen et al., 2014).

3. ML IN PERSONALIZED MEDICAL INTERVENTIONS

The game of checkers has been used to thoroughly examine two machine-learning techniques. Sufficient research has been conducted to confirm that it is possible to design a computer to learn to play checkers more effectively than the programmer. Furthermore, when given only the game's rules, a sense of direction, and a redundant and incomplete list of parameters that are assumed to be related to the game but whose correct signs and relative weights are unknown and unspecified, it can learn to do this in an incredibly short amount of time. These tests validate some machine learning ideas that apply to a wide range of additional scenarios (Samuel, 1959).

The growing AI revolution offers some incredibly exciting prospects, and we can only hope that machine learning—among other applications of AI—will have a significant, beneficial, and enduring impact on medicine. But in order to do this, it will be critical to set realistic expectations and begin closing the gap as quickly as possible between the world of AI and the practicalities of clinical practice.

This is the only way to keep artificial intelligence (AI) from turning into just another exaggerated trend that fades away after a few years due to inflated expectations (Manlhiot, 2018).

Personalized medicine is a paradigm that exists more in theory than in practice. However, due to growing awareness of the shortcomings in providing patients with drugs that are both beneficial and risk-free, improved molecular understanding of how to optimize drug selection and dosing, and growing demand for incorporating more clinically relevant genetic information into the drug development process to increase both productivity and innovation, personalized medicine is becoming a reality. Clinical pharmacologists can ensure that "good therapeutics follow good diagnostics" by using their expertise in therapeutics. They are well-suited to analyze genetic data and promptly educate others about genetics so that clinical practice can make useful decisions, particularly on medicine dosage for specific patients (Lesko, 2007).

While the uniform approaches of traditional healthcare frameworks are praiseworthy, they frequently encounter difficulties in catering to the distinct and varied demands of patients. The comprehensive complexity of each person's health profile are not taken into consideration by the one-size-fits-all model, which frequently leads to less than ideal results and a dearth of focused interventions. This restriction emphasizes how urgently we need to move toward tailored treatment approaches. The ability of machine learning to analyze vast amounts of patient data and identify trends presents once-in-a-lifetime chance to explore the field of personalized medicine. By examining a variety of datasets including genetic data, health history, and lifestyle variables, with diagnostic imaging, ML algorithms can reveal subtle relationships, enabling the finding prognostic signs and subtle illness markers as well as individualized care routes (Kasula, 2023).

With personalized medicine, there is no longer a "one-size-fits-all" approach to healthcare; instead, treatments are tailored to the unique needs of each patient. As epidemiological datasets continue to burgeon in quantity and complexity, advanced technologies such as statistical machine learning and artificial intelligence (AI) become necessary to evaluate and construct prognostic models from underlying data. By using this kind of data, machine learning can help with tailored treatment because of its accurate predictions. Personalized treatment for patients with spine diseases can also be greatly aided by other AI technologies, such as computer vision and natural language processing (Khan et al., 2020).

The most prevalent disease in humans, skin cancer, is mostly diagnosed visually. A clinical screening is done first, and then a dermoscopic study, biopsy, and histological examination may be necessary. Because skin lesions can vary widely in their appearance, automatically classifying them from photographs is a difficult challenge. Deep convolutional neural networks (CNNs) 4, 5 have been shown to be promising for a wide range of fine-grained object categories 6, 7, 8, 9, 10, and 11 in general and highly variable tasks (Esteva et al., 2017).

An increasing number of people are worried that algorithms could perpetuate gender and racial inequalities through the data used to train them or the people who create them (Angwin et al., 2016).

The argument put up by proponents of algorithmic methods such as data mining is that they remove human prejudice from the decision-making process. That being said, an algorithm is only as good as the data it uses. The biases of previous decision makers can be passed down to these algorithms due to the frequent imperfections in data. In such instances, data might merely be a reflection of the pervasive prejudices that exist in society as a whole. In still other cases, exclusion and inequality patterns already present can be found through data mining, which can reveal very beneficial regularities. Inconsiderate dependence on data mining can prevent historically marginalized and vulnerable populations from fully engaging in society (Barocas & Selbst, 2016).

Healthcare is going to change as a result of AI. The accountability and transparency of judgments made by AI-based systems, the possibility of collective damages resulting from algorithmic bias, and the duties and integrity of physicians are the main ethical challenges that may arise with this revolution. These worries must be weighed against the need to use AI's far greater and more precise computational capability to improve healthcare systems for the general public (Lysaght et al., 2019).

4. ETHICAL FRAMEWORKS

The emerging discipline of public health ethics is experiencing exciting times. Both individuals tackling these topics from a more theoretical and those from a more practical or practitioner point of view tend to share this sentiment. We are all connected by the feeling that conventional medical ethics are lacking something. There are three plausible explanations for this emotion in turn. First, the list of topics covered by orthodox medical ethics omits many important public health topics. Second, there are questions regarding whether the theoretical framework or underlying presumptions utilized in medical ethics are sufficient when applied to instances in public health. Third, either or both of these could be accurate (Dawson, 2009).

The ethical issues surrounding health informatics are becoming increasingly significant as it becomes more widely used in healthcare, especially in the setting of biomedical informatics (Séroussi et al., 2020). The development of AI-powered decision support tools, the growth of care teams, the necessity of data sharing to assist research and guarantee continuity of care, and EHRs are all factors pushing the need for new standards of reliability. These guidelines need to cover things like protecting patient privacy and confidentiality, stopping security lapses, guaranteeing correct patient data, balancing data sharing and reuse regulations, and enhancing app efficacy transparency. Prioritizing data security, data privacy, and social acceptance of the data-driven decision-making process is crucial for ensuring the long-term sustainability of the healthcare industry (Rahman et al., 2021).

Approaches to clinical ethical conundrums that depend on fundamental laws or guidelines are challenging to implement due to their ambiguity and incompatibility with fundamental morals. In reaction, the usage of fundamental values is rejected by the judiciary, and specification results in a vast collection of well-defined regulations that are probably simple to apply. Weighing the relative importance of disparate and conflicting values in an application is done through balancing. We argue against both specification and casuistry, arguing that balancing is better since it best demonstrates the logic underlying moral judgment. Therefore, teaching medical professionals about ethical may be best accomplished through balancing (DeMarco & Ford, 2006).

The use of personal data, function automation, and dependence on assistive medical equipment all create ethical and societal concerns that are echoed by AI in healthcare. Many legal and ethical issues may surface during the implementation phase of AI in healthcare if there are no well-founded ethical norms or even regulatory framework in place (Palkova, 2021).

5. DATA PRIVACY

Patient health information is kept confidential and isn't disclosed to unauthorized individuals or businesses thanks to data privacy and protection laws. A fundamental ethical principle in healthcare is patient confidentiality. Violating patient anonymity can have serious repercussions, including diminished trust in medical professionals and institutions, financial and legal penalties, and unfavorable press. Strict laws and regulations that guarantee the protection of patients' sensitive data are in place, and the healthcare sector is under constant regulatory supervision. For example, the Health Insurance Portability and Accountability Act (HIPAA) in the US requires healthcare providers to protect patients' private health information. Patients are also empowered by data privacy and protection to manage their own health information and make knowledgeable decisions about how to use it. People are required to give consent for medical facilities to use their personal information, as well as to be informed about how that information is collected, used, and decided upon. In order to protect patients' rights and foster confidence in healthcare systems, it is imperative that patient autonomy be respected and that data management procedures be transparent. Ethical considerations in healthcare are closely linked to data privacy and protection. The ethical requirements for the development and application of AI technologies in healthcare contexts include ensuring the responsible use of data, safeguarding vulnerable populations, fostering justice and transparency in AI-driven healthcare, and reducing bias and discrimination (Gautam & Sharma, 2024).

6. BIAS

Invalid and unreliable predictive methodologies can have major implications when it comes to hospital death prediction. To guarantee the accuracy and efficacy of the predictive techniques employed, quality assessment is essential. Errors can be avoided and patient outcomes can be enhanced in this way (Nicora et al., 2022). Another crucial factor to take into account is bias risk. Predictive algorithms may produce biased results if specific populations are over- or underrepresented in the data used to create them. It is critical to evaluate the bias risk and create countermeasures. Lastly, data fusion can raise the precision and dependability of hospital death prediction models (Shi et al., 2019). Data fusion strategies can assist overcome constraints in individual data sources and increase the overall accuracy of forecasting approaches by merging numerous sources of information.

The three types of bias in the medical industry are algorithmic, human, and data-driven. By fostering deeply ingrained cultural biases, bias in AI algorithms for health care can have disastrous effects. By misdiagnosing patient groups who have a history of being underrepresented in current databases, such as gender and ethnic minorities, this can exacerbate already-existing disparities.

The development of equitable AI for healthcare can be aided by open science methodologies. Developing AI algorithms and participatory science with a focus on the user is one of these; sharing code, especially AI algorithms that can synthesize underrepresented data to remove bias, is another; ethical data sharing and inclusive data standards are other ways to encourage interoperability (Norori et al., 2021).

7. INTEGRATION DIFFICULTIES WITH CURRENT HEALTHCARE INFRASTRUCTURES

Those who supply basic and secondary healthcare make up the healthcare industry. Information sharing between providers is required. To address this demand, information systems (IS) built on various hardware and software platforms are available. Information and communication technology (ICT) in the healthcare sector is varied and distributed, making data exchange a problem. The integration of many distributed IS is desperately needed. Though many attempts have been made, integration issues can only be partially resolved by using conventional techniques. To meet the requirements of healthcare information systems integration, enterprise application integration, or EAI, presents an additional approach (Khoumbati & Themistocleous, 2006).

Digital technologies are becoming essential in today's business environment for establishing operations in any firm, including the healthcare sector. Smart devices and IT infrastructure can be used to gather, process, analyze, and send data using the newest technology. This allows for the implementation of trends in medicine, such as personalization, participation, predictability, and value approach. In light of these tendencies, a methodology for developing a medical organization's management system that can thoroughly and cohesively develop the system's numerous components must be developed. Hardware, information systems, application architectures, business process systems, and "smart" medical devices that are fully capable of engaging in hospital information exchange are all included in this. It is best to construct these components inside of a single model. A medical organization model can be built using an architectural method (Levina et al., 2024).

Strengthening the four primary pillars of the health care system—public health, health care delivery, personal health management, and health-related research—is necessary to improve health in our country. Lack of access to data, information, and knowledge is the cause of many preventable errors in the health sector that lead to subpar quality. To address these issues, a national health information infrastructure (NHII) provides the knowledge management and connectivity required. We can achieve improved health and a more effective healthcare system. The requirements of public health, research, health care delivery, and individual health management should all be taken care of by the US government's national health information infrastructure. Additionally, pertinent global aspects should be covered (e.g., standards for sharing data and knowledge across national boundaries). To create a strong national health information infrastructure for the United States—basically, a "paperless" health care system—public and commercial sectors will need to work together. As advised by the President's Information Technology Advisory Committee and the National Committee on Vital and Health Statistics, the federal government should take the lead in ensuring a national health information infrastructure. To enable personal identification for health purposes, advancements in financing, incentives, standards, and ongoing privacy framework refinement are required (Detmer, 2003).

8. EQUITY IN HEALTH CARE

"Equity in Health Care" refers to the distribution of medical resources and the receipt of care services based on need. The amount paid is determined on the payer's capacity. It emphasizes a dedication to guaranteeing everyone's access to high-quality, acceptable healthcare services. Even while the evidence shows significant health gaps between social groups within countries, international efforts to achieve health equity have concentrated on addressing the enormous health disparities between wealthier and poorer off nations (Braveman, 1998).

The lack of unfair inequities in health could be characterized as equity in health. Social justice and equity require quantifiable functional criteria in order to be defined because various people will perceive them in different ways. Equity in health can be described as the lack of systematic biases or inequities across social groups with different levels of social entitlement or deprivation in the social hierarchy, or in the most significant social determinants of health, for the sake of measurement and functionality.

Socially disadvantaged populations are routinely exposed by health disparities to health-related issues in the future. People are categorized in the social hierarchy according to their income, power, and status, which is a result of social entitlement or deprivation. Another way to conceptualize deprivation is as being either absolute or relative. The process of delivering health interventions by combining resources including cash, personnel, supplies, and medications is known as health care provision. One of the main equity challenges, particularly in developing nations, was the unequal distribution of resources and access to health services between the urban and rural populations. A nation's decision about its health finance system is influenced by equity concerns in addition to other factors. Taxes, out-of-pocket expenses, social insurance, and private health insurance are some of the sources of funding for healthcare. When it comes to the use of health care services, equity should examine how people actually use the system and how disparities in need and demand exist between various groups. Privatizing health care services carries the risk of substituting a financial motivation for a service ethic, which would lead to unequal access and additional obstacles for the underprivileged and those living in remote areas to receive healthcare. Unquestionably, throughout the past few decades, health care systems have undergone significant change in many nations. This has led to a multitude of duties that the state must do in order to attain equity (Arinah et al., 2016).

Understanding how health disparities arise, identifying the key contributors to their creation, and selecting the most modifiable elements are necessary before devising methods to lessen them. Selecting tactics might be aided by acknowledging a number of concepts pertaining to the causes and expressions of injustices. It's crucial to take into account whether the goal is to lessen differences in the incidence of illness or in the severity of illness (including co-morbidity, disability, dysfunction, and death) while making judgments. The robustness of primary care resources and services in communities and nations is found to have a significant impact on health service equity, especially with regard to their potential to lessen severity (Starfield, 2004).

9. PERSONALIZED MEDICINE

The idea of personalized medicine, which holds that a patient's treatment may be customized based on their unique genetic and molecular profile, has far-reaching effects that go well beyond the technology enabling it. The implementation of personalized medicine will necessitate modifications to the healthcare system's infrastructure, the business models for diagnostics and treatments, government and commercial payer payment policies, and the way regulations are overseen. With the help of personalized medicine, medical procedures will move away from the reactive management of illness and toward proactive healthcare management that includes screening, early detection, and prevention. It will also change the roles that patients and doctors play in the healthcare system. In an industry that has historically resisted information technology, it will lead to a higher reliance on electronic medical records and decision support tools. A systems approach to implementation is necessary for personalized medicine. Nonetheless, it is the responsibility of the stakeholders themselves to push for a uniform set of laws and regulations that open the door for the implementation of customized medicine in a highly decentralized and market-driven healthcare sector. The pharmaceutical, biotechnology, diagnostic, and information technology industries, healthcare providers and payers, patient advocacy groups, industry policy organizations, significant academic institutions, and government agencies came together to form the Personalized Medicine Coalition (PMC), a nonprofit umbrella organization, to meet this need. In order to bring personalized medicine into mainstream clinical practice, the PMC offers a framework for these stakeholders to come to consensus positions on important public policy problems (Abrahams et al., 2005).

10. APPLICATION OF AI-DRIVEN MEDICAL SOLUTIONS

The advent of communication technology has had a significant impact on healthcare today. At a reasonable cost, real-time remote patient monitoring of health indicators and disease symptoms is made possible by communication technology. These communication technologies also make it feasible to monitor health at the community level, which saves time and allows us to serve more patients. In the healthcare sector, consistency in communication is essential, and artificial intelligence (AI)-based communication guarantees this. AI with the Internet of Things (IoT) in healthcare makes self-diagnosing capacity via wireless body area networks (WBANs), which uses wearable sensing devices. Because wearable WBANs require transmission of electromagnetic waves onto the human body, they are difficult to implement. With the use of specialized communication protocols and a mobile application, mHealth is an additional technology that makes it possible to get healthcare services whenever and wherever needed. With the use of real-time digital visual assistance, augmented and virtual reality facilitates more precise surgery and quick diagnostics. Specialized wireless communication is needed for all those technologies (Ponnusamy et al., 2022).

Healthcare process optimization with artificial intelligence (AI) is still in its early stages. The primary source of problems in a doctor's job is scheduling. In addition to offering data for quicker and more precise diagnosis, an AI-driven chatbot might help to maximize wait times. When a human doctor, not a virtual one, is involved in the diagnosis process, patients are more likely to trust AI-driven solutions. Chatbots powered by AI could in fact aid in the improvement of diagnostic procedures. Nonetheless, to build patient confidence in the diagnosis, doctors must continue to be involved in the procedure. The authors' analysis of the benefits of a diagnostic procedure for doctors and patients demonstrates that, whereas scheduling may lower the process's overall usefulness, AI-based solutions may raise it (Lyon et al., 2021).

Medical imaging analysis diagnosis accuracy was greatly enhanced by AI.

High accuracy in early disease identification was demonstrated by AI predictive models.

Patient outcomes were improved by AI-based technologies that improved individualized treatment strategies. AI algorithms are used to successfully extract and analyze clinical insights from unstructured EHR data (Kasula, 2021).

The environment is changing as a result of the integration of artificial intelligence (AI) into smart city healthcare systems, which promises more effective, accessible, and individualized medical care. AI algorithms that use health data from linked devices allow for early diagnosis and customized treatment plans. However, there exist obstacles in the form of technical difficulties and ethical issues that demand the use of responsible AI. In order to create reliable AI, the recommendations emphasize a move toward patient-centered care and call for rapid technological development, interdisciplinary cooperation, and strong ethical frameworks. Smart cities are leading the way in transforming urban well-being by utilizing AI-powered, networked healthcare ecosystems (Katal, 2024).

Empirical research on AI applications in healthcare that were found were methodically examined in accordance with preset inclusion criteria. These included studies that presented quantitative results about the diagnosis, treatment, distribution of resources, and accessibility to healthcare.

To summarize and understand the effects of AI-driven interventions on the development of sustainable healthcare, quantitative data taken from specific research were subjected to statistical methodologies such as meta-analysis and descriptive statistics (Kasula & Whig, 2023).

11. SPECIFIC MEDICAL SCENARIOS

11.1. Oncology

In oncology, predictive analytics enables personalized cancer treatments through the use of large data sets, including both genomic and medical image data (Ahmed et al., 2025). Systems like IBM Watson for Oncology analyze data on medical history, lab results, and genetics of a patient to present to the oncologist evidence-based treatment options tailored for the individual. Recommendations are categorized in this system as "recommended," "for consideration," and "not recommended," helping doctors make informed decisions to avoid ineffective or toxic therapies (Mohanty & Mohanty, 2025). Machine learning models analyze tumor genomics and clinical data to predict cancer recurrence and survival rates. This helps in the determination of the need for aggressive treatments, such as chemotherapy in early-stage breast cancer patients (Chen et al., 2022). Cancer-related symptoms, such as pain or fatigue, can be predicted using EHRs to enable proactive management in a personalized way that improves quality of life (Zeinali, 2025).

11.2. Cardiology

Predictive analytics for cardiology addresses the identification of high-risk patients for cardiovascular events and the personalization of management plans (Ekundayo & Nyavor, 2024).

Cardiovascular Risk Prediction: AI models analyze ECG data, patient history, and lab results to predict the likelihood of a heart attack or stroke more accurately than traditional risk scores, such as the Framingham score. This allows for early, preventive interventions and lifestyle modifications (Akbilgic et al., 2021).

Kaiser Permanente uses wearable devices and remote monitoring platforms that track vital signs, including heart rate and blood pressure, in real time. Predictive algorithms analyze this data to detect early warning signs of deterioration, for example, in heart failure patients, and alert clinicians for timely intervention, thus reducing emergency visits and hospitalizations (Kakria et al., 2015). Machine learning for monitoring a patient's progress regarding cardiac rehabilitation provides personalized programs on exercise, diet, and stress management, based on recovery speed and activity levels, which results in improved functional outcomes (Zaree et al., 2023)

11.3. Neurology

Predictive analytics in neurology aids the physician in the early detection and management of neurodegenerative diseases and acute conditions (Pal et al., 2025). AI models analyze a combination of MRI scans, genetic markers, and behavioral data, including speech patterns and linguistic clarity, to identify neurodegenerative diseases at an early stage even before clinical symptoms have been clearly apparent. This early detection allows for interventions that can potentially slow the disease's progression (Ali, 2022).

Viz.ai is an example AI tool that analyzes CT scans in stroke patients for large vessel occlusion. The stroke team receives immediate notification of their findings to initiate appropriate treatment, which greatly decreases the "door-to-needle" time and thus improves outcomes (Karamchandani et al., 2023). A research team at Vanderbilt University Medical Center (VUMC) developed a model using EHR data to predict the likelihood of suicide attempts in at-risk individuals, prompting timely outreach and proactive intervention by clinical teams (Walsh et al., 2021).

12. CRITICAL DISCUSSIONS AND CHALLENGES

There is a growing concern that models trained on non-representative historical data could perpetuate or even worsen existing health disparities. For instance, an algorithm developed to manage high-risk patients was found to favor white patients disproportionately because it used historical healthcare spending as a proxy for need and thereby underestimated the needs of Black patients who had received less care (Paulus & Kent, 2020).

The use of large volumes of sensitive patient data-genomic profiles, EHRs, and lifestyle information-raises serious concerns about privacy and security. Strong anonymization of data and secure management practices are vital to prevent misuse and maintain patient trust (Van Duc et al., 2024).

Most of the advanced models in machine learning are considered to be "black boxes" because their decision-making processes cannot be easily understood either by a clinician or a patient. The lack of explainability makes it difficult to establish accountability if a model's prediction leads to some adverse outcome, raising legal and ethical questions (McDermid et al., 2021).

Predictive models require high-quality, comprehensive data. The health data is invariably fragmented, incomplete, or inconsistent between systems and institutions. It can become a limiting factor in the model's general performance and generalization across very diverse populations (Olalekan Kehinde, 2025).

One of the main challenges in effectively integrating predictive analytics into existing clinical workflows includes the need for infrastructural support, health professional training, and overcoming physician skepticism about relying on AI-based recommendations over and above clinical judgment (Elhaddad & Hamam, 2024).

13. INTERDISCIPLINARY PERSPECTIVES

Data Science & Statistics to develop and validate powerful machine learning algorithms and statistical models that can handle a wide range of complicated and heterogeneous data (Fan et al., 2020). Clinicians provide the necessary context for data interpretation and model validation that makes the tools clinically relevant and useful. Public health professionals help to address population-level trends and health disparities (Reps et al., 2018). Researchers and experts in these fields formulate regulatory frameworks and develop guidelines on ethics to deal with issues such as informed consent, data ownership, algorithmic fairness, and liability (Bodo et al., 2017). Computer Science & Engineering emphasize developing infrastructure necessary to store data that needs real-time processing and seamless integration into EHRs and CDSS (Rolla, 2023). Public and patient involvement in design can help make sure tools are practical, trustworthy, and respect the patient's autonomy and social determinants of health (Williamson, 2014).

Sepsis Prediction at Johns Hopkins Hospital is a centralized command center uses AI to analyze real-time patient data taken from EHRs. This enables the early detection of sepsis and thus reduces mortality rates (Liu et al., 2021). Parkland Health & Hospital System's Suicide Prevention is an initiative uses data from universal suicide risk screenings to identify high-risk patients and link them with additional care (Roaten et al., 2018). Kaiser Permanente launched a predictive analytics system to identify high-risk patients for various conditions so that early and personalized interventions can be performed (Kanter et al., 2013). Predicting Readmission Predictive modeling, which many health organizations use, identifies patients who have high probabilities of hospital readmissions. These models help them provide targeted support after discharge (Yu et al., 2015).

14. RISKS OF DIGITAL EXCLUSION

Some of the major risks related to digital exclusion in predictive analytics for personalized medical care include algorithmic bias, increasing health disparities, misdiagnosis, loss of patient trust, and misallocation of resources (Paccoud et al., 2024). The majority of predictive models are trained on historical data. If this data is not representative of the population at large-that is, if it mostly reflects data from white, urban, or high-income patients-the algorithms will adopt and even exacerbate pre-existing cultural bias. Eventually, this can lead to poor or biased predictions for a variety of underrepresented groups, such as racial and ethnic minorities, older individuals, those with disabilities, and rural populations, causing inequity in healthcare outcomes (Kleinberg et al., 2022).

Given the "digital divide" or disparities in technology access and use of the internet, those who are already socially and economically disadvantaged will be less likely to benefit from AI-driven healthcare. This could lead to a situation where advanced, personalized care is concentrated in well-off populations while leaving marginalized groups behind and thus further exacerbating existing health inequalities (Ono et al., 2024).

The biases in the models, along with the lack of access to needed digital tools, could lead to misdiagnosis, delayed or ineffective treatment, and could pose harm to patients. For example, several studies have shown that algorithms for the detection of skin cancer or the prediction of cardiovascular risk perform worse in people with darker skin tones or from non-European descent (Alharbi et al., 2025).

When patients experience errors from AI tools, or when processes are perceived as opaque and unfair, it has the potential to erode their trust-not just in the technology, but in the healthcare system as a whole. Trust is foundational to the patient-provider relationship; its loss can contribute to lower engagement with services and poor adherence to medical advice (Pozzi, 2024). Biased AI systems can misallocate health resources by prioritizing certain groups over others due to flawed risk assessments. This can result in inefficient resource allocation, increasing wait times for some individuals and failing to provide necessary care for those who need it (Abràmoff et al., 2023).

For many individuals, including older adults and those living in rural areas, access to reliable internet, the requisite digital devices, or even the skills to use these digital health tools remains very difficult. The result is an inability to take part in telemedicine, contribute through portals, or share their data to inform their personalized care (Magdalena et al., 2015). Predictive models are informed by large amounts of high-quality data. Digital exclusion contributes to data "missingness" for some populations, leading to incomplete or unrepresentative data that further compromises the accuracy and generalizability of models (Boyd, 2021).

15. FUTURE PERSPECTIVES

Further advances in deep learning and more advanced AI techniques will enable much higher prediction accuracy for challenging applications, including analyzing medical imaging and genomic data (Sharma et al., 2024). Future models will integrate data from a wider range of sources, including social determinants of health, real-time data from wearable devices, and genomic information, for a more holistic patient view (Ali & Shah, 2025). Wearables and continuous monitoring will enable real-time data analysis, allowing for immediate alerts and proactive interventions before health crises set in. Examples include predicting fluctuations in the level of blood sugar in diabetic patients (Balasooriya & Nanayakkara, 2020). A growing emphasis on the development of more transparent and interpretable AI models will instill confidence among clinicians and patients and help with regulatory compliance (Barnes & Hutson, 2024).

Federated Learning approach enables models to be trained across decentralized datasets in different institutions without sensitive data ever leaving its source. This addresses privacy concerns while leveraging diverse data (Aouedi et al., 2022). Predictive analytics will also fundamentally alter the healthcare paradigm from reactive treatment to proactive prevention by identifying high-risk individuals early for targeted lifestyle changes or interventions (Rahman et al., 2024).

16. CONCLUSION

The future toolkit for data-driven analytics of genomic large data includes advanced machine learning techniques like deep learning and artificial intelligence. Future innovations in healthcare and customized medicine will be dependent on the forthcoming advancements in these fields.

Predictive analytics and machine learning have shown to be effective techniques for improving healthcare's ability to prevent disease. With the promise for more successful preventative measures and better healthcare outcomes, these technologies have completely changed how diseases are found, diagnosed, and treated. The potential of machine learning and predictive analytics to support early diagnosis and detection is one of their major effects. These algorithms can spot minor trends and signs that human clinicians would miss by examining large amounts of patient data. In cases like cancer, heart disease, diabetes, and neurological illnesses, early detection can result in prompt therapies and enhance the prognosis for patients.When it comes to determining a person's likelihood of contracting particular diseases, predictive analytics is essential.

In the healthcare sector, big data plays a crucial role. For patient monitoring and other healthcare services, healthcare practitioners rely on the data collected via Big Data. Individualized strategies for curing persons of ailments could be developed using the data. Big Data has also completely changed the fields of diagnosis, treatment, and evaluation in healthcare. Various regions of the world develop treatment programs based on Big Data. Information about health is to be modeled and analyzed with the use of big data.

In order to improve patient outcomes and care, predictive analytics is utilized in the healthcare industry to assess patient risk, offer tailored treatment, and boost operational effectiveness. Supply chain risk management, predictive maintenance, and quality control in manufacturing can all benefit from predictive models that maximize productivity and minimize downtime. The energy and utilities sector uses predictive analytics in asset performance management, demand forecasting, and regulatory compliance to ensure consistent and effective service delivery.

It assists with inventory management, customer satisfaction, and competitive analysis to help merchants satisfy customer expectations and stay ahead of the competition. Predictive analytics significantly enhances marketing strategies through customer segmentation, personalized marketing, campaign optimization, sales forecasting, CLV prediction, churn prediction, market trend analysis, and sentiment analysis.

The integration of research and actual data demonstrated the significant influence of AI on many aspects of healthcare delivery, highlighting its potential to transform procedures and aid in the accomplishment of sustainable development objectives.

REFERENCES

Abrahams, E., Ginsburg, G. S., & Silver, M. (2005). The personalized medicine coalition: Goals and strategies. *American Journal of Pharmacogenomics, 5*, 345–355. DOI: 10.2165/00129785-200505060-00002

Abràmoff, M. D., Tarver, M. E., Loyo-Berrios, N., Trujillo, S., Char, D., Obermeyer, Z., & Maisel, W. H. (2023). Considerations for addressing bias in artificial intelligence for health equity. *NPJ Digital Medicine, 6*(1), 170. DOI: 10.1038/s41746-023-00913-9

Ahmadi, A., & RabieNezhad Ganji, N. (2023). AI-driven medical innovations: Transforming healthcare through data intelligence. [IJBLS]. *International Journal of BioLife Sciences, 2*(2), 132–142. DOI: 10.22034/ijbls.2023.185475

Ahmed, M. K., Rozario, E., Mohonta, S. C., Ferdousmou, J., Saimon, A. S. M., Moniruzzaman, M., & Hasan, R. (2025). Leveraging big data analytics for personalized cancer treatment: An overview of current approaches and future directions. *Journal of Engineering, 2025*(1), 9928467. DOI: 10.1155/je/9928467

Ahmed, Z., Mohamed, K., Zeeshan, S., & Dong, X. (2020). Artificial intelligence with multi-functional machine learning platform development for better healthcare and precision medicine. *Database : The Journal of Biological Databases and Curation, 2020*, baaa010. Advance online publication. DOI: 10.1093/database/baaa010

Akbilgic, O., Butler, L., Karabayir, I., Chang, P. P., Kitzman, D. W., Alonso, A., & Soliman, E. Z. (2021). ECG-AI: Electrocardiographic artificial intelligence model for prediction of heart failure. *European Heart Journal. Digital Health, 2*(4), 626–634. DOI: 10.1093/ehjdh/ztab080

Alharbi, T. A. F., Rababa, M., Alsuwayl, H., Alsubail, A., & Alenizi, W. S. (2025). Diagnostic Challenges and Patient Safety: The Critical Role of Accuracy–A Systematic Review. *Journal of Multidisciplinary Healthcare, 18*, 3051–3064. DOI: 10.2147/JMDH.S512254

Ali, H. (2022). AI in neurodegenerative disease research: Early detection, cognitive decline prediction, and brain imaging biomarker identification. *Int J Eng Technol Res Manag, 6*(10), 71. DOI: 10.5281/zenodo.14890442

Ali, N., & Shah, W. (2025). Integrative Systems and Holistic Health Records: A New Paradigm in Personalized Medicine.

Angwin, J., Larson, J., Mattu, S., & Kirchner, L. (2016). Machine bias risk assessments in criminal sentencing. *ProPublica*, (May), 23.

Aouedi, O., Sacco, A., Piamrat, K., & Marchetto, G. (2022). Handling privacy-sensitive medical data with federated learning: Challenges and future directions. *IEEE Journal of Biomedical and Health Informatics, 27*(2), 790–803. DOI: 10.1109/JBHI.2022.3185673

Arinah, W. D. S., Musheer, J., & Juni, M. H. (2016). Health care provision and equity. *International Journal of Public Health and Clinical Sciences, 3*(4).

Balasooriya, K., & Nanayakkara, N. D. (2020, November). Predicting short-term changing blood glucose level of diabetes patients using noninvasive data. In *2020 IEEE REGION 10 CONFERENCE (TENCON)* (pp. 31-36). IEEE. DOI: DOI: 10.1109/TENCON50793.2020.9293823

Barnes, E., & Hutson, J. (2024). Navigating the complexities of ai: The critical role of interpretability and explainability in ensuring transparency and trust. *International Journal of Multidisciplinary and Current Educational Research*, *6*(3).

Barocas, S., & Selbst, A. D. (2016). Big data's disparate impact. *California Law Review*, *104*, 671. DOI: 10.2139/ssrn.2477899

Bodo, B., Helberger, N., Irion, K., Zuiderveen Borgesius, F., Moller, J., van de Velde, B., . . . de Vreese, C. (2017). Tackling the algorithmic control crisis-the technical, legal, and ethical challenges of research into algorithmic agents. *Yale JL & Tech., 19*, 133. /arXiv.2510.25337DOI: 10.48550

Boyd, A. (2021). *Understanding Population Data for Inclusive Longitudinal Research.* University of Bristol.

Braveman, P. (1998). Monitoring equity in health: a policy-oriented approach in low-and middle-income countries. In *Monitoring equity in health: a policy-oriented approach in low-and middle-income countries.*

Chen, P. C., Yeh, Y. M., Lin, B. W., Chan, R. H., Su, P. F., Liu, Y. C., Lee, C. T., Chen, S. H., & Lin, P. C. (2022). A prediction model for tumor recurrence in stage II–III colorectal cancer patients: From a machine learning model to genomic profiling. *Biomedicines*, *10*(2), 340. DOI: 10.3390/biomedicines10020340

Cohen, I. G., Amarasingham, R., Shah, A., Xie, B., & Lo, B. (2014). The legal and ethical concerns that arise from using complex predictive analytics in health care. *Health Affairs*, *33*(7), 1139–1147. DOI: 10.1377/hlthaff.2014.0048

Dawson, A. (2009). Theory and practice in public health ethics: a complex relationship. In *Public health ethics and practice* (pp. 191–210). Policy Press., DOI: 10.46692/9781847421043.012

DeMarco, J. P., & Ford, P. J. (2006). Balancing in ethical deliberation: Superior to specification and casuistry. *The Journal of Medicine and Philosophy*, *31*(5), 483–497. DOI: 10.1080/03605310600912675

Detmer, D. E. (2003). Building the national health information infrastructure for personal health, health care services, public health, and research. *BMC Medical Informatics and Decision Making*, *3*, 1–12. DOI: 10.1186/1472-6947-3-1

Ekundayo, F., & Nyavor, H. (2024). AI-driven predictive analytics in cardiovascular diseases: Integrating big data and machine learning for early diagnosis and risk prediction. *International Journal of Research Publication and Reviews*, *5*(12), 1240–1256. DOI: 10.55248/gengpi.5.1224.3437

Elhaddad, M., & Hamam, S. (2024). AI-driven clinical decision support systems: An ongoing pursuit of potential. *Cureus*, *16*(4). Advance online publication. DOI: 10.7759/cureus.57728

Esteva, A., Kuprel, B., Novoa, R. A., Ko, J., Swetter, S. M., Blau, H. M., & Thrun, S. (2017). Dermatologist-level classification of skin cancer with deep neural networks. *nature, 542*(7639), 115-118. DOI: DOI: 10.1038/nature21056

Fan, J., Li, R., Zhang, C. H., & Zou, H. (2020). *Statistical foundations of data science*. Chapman and Hall/CRC., DOI: 10.1201/9780429096280

Gautam, P., & Sharma, R. (2024). Legal And Ethical Concerns In AI Driven Healthcare-A Study Of Legal Approaches. *Educational Administration: Theory and Practice*, *30*(5), 11781–11788. DOI: 10.53555/kuey.v29i3.5026

Johnson, S. (2018). AI-driven healthcare solutions worldwide. *Int. J. Transcontinental Discoveries*, *5*, 1–6.

Kakria, P., Tripathi, N. K., & Kitipawang, P. (2015). A real-time health monitoring system for remote cardiac patients using smartphone and wearable sensors. *International Journal of Telemedicine and Applications*, *2015*(1), 373474. DOI: 10.1155/2015/373474

Kanter, M. H., Lindsay, G., Bellows, J., & Chase, A. (2013). Complete care at Kaiser Permanente: Transforming chronic and preventive care. *Joint Commission Journal on Quality and Patient Safety*, *39*(11), 484–494. DOI: 10.1016/s1553-7250(13)39064-3

Karamchandani, R. R., Helms, A. M., Satyanarayana, S., Yang, H., Clemente, J. D., Defilipp, G., Strong, D., Rhoten, J. B., & Asimos, A. W. (2023). Automated detection of intracranial large vessel occlusions using Viz. ai software: Experience in a large, integrated stroke network. *Brain and Behavior*, *13*(1), e2808. DOI: 10.1002/brb3.2808

Kasula, B. Y. (2021). AI-Driven Innovations in Healthcare: Improving Diagnostics and Patient Care. *International Journal of Machine Learning and Artificial Intelligence*, *2*(2), 1–8.

Kasula, B. Y. (2023). Harnessing Machine Learning for Personalized Patient Care. *Transactions on Latest Trends in Artificial Intelligence, 4*(4).

Kasula, B. Y., & Whig, P. (2023). AI-driven machine learning solutions for sustainable development in healthcare—Pioneering efficient, equitable, and innovative health service. *International Journal of Sustainable Development Through AI, ML and IoT*, *2*(2), 1–7.

Katal, N. (2024). AI-Driven Healthcare Services and Infrastructure in Smart Cities. In *Smart Cities* (pp. 150–170). CRC Press.

Khan, O., Badhiwala, J. H., Grasso, G., & Fehlings, M. G. (2020). Use of machine learning and artificial intelligence to drive personalized medicine approaches for spine care. *World Neurosurgery*, *140*, 512–518. DOI: 10.1016/j.wneu.2020.04.022

Khoumbati, K., & Themistocleous, M. (2006). Integrating the IT infrastructures in healthcare organisations: A proposition of influential factors. *Electronic. Journal of E-Government*, *4*(1), 27–36.

Kleinberg, G., Diaz, M. J., Batchu, S., & Lucke-Wold, B. (2022). Racial underrepresentation in dermatological datasets leads to biased machine learning models and inequitable healthcare. *Journal of Biomed Research*, *3*(1), 42.

Lesko, L. J. (2007). Personalized medicine: Elusive dream or imminent reality? *Clinical Pharmacology and Therapeutics*, *81*(6), 807–816. DOI: 10.1038/sj.clpt.6100204

Levina, A., Ilin, I., Gugutishvili, D., Kochetkova, K., & Tick, A. (2024). Towards a smart hospital: Smart infrastructure integration. *Journal of Open Innovation, 10*(3), 100339. DOI: 10.1016/j.joitmc.2024.100339

Liu, R., Greenstein, J. L., Fackler, J. C., Bergmann, J., Bembea, M. M., & Winslow, R. L. (2021). Prediction of impending septic shock in children with sepsis. *Critical Care Explorations, 3*(6), e0442. DOI: 10.1097/CCE.0000000000000442

Lyon, J. Y., Bogodistov, Y., & Moormann, J. (2021). AI-driven optimization in healthcare: The diagnostic process. *European Journal of Management Issues, 29*(4), 218–231. DOI: 10.15421/192121

Lysaght, T., Lim, H. Y., Xafis, V., & Ngiam, K. Y. (2019). AI-assisted decision-making in healthcare: The application of an ethics framework for big data in health and research. *Asian Bioethics Review, 11*, 299–314. DOI: 10.1007/s41649-019-00096-0

Magdalena, M., Bujnowska-Fedak, & Grata-Borkowska, U. (2015). Use of telemedicine-based care for the aging and elderly: Promises and pitfalls. *Smart Homecare Technology and Telehealth, 3*, 91–105. DOI: 10.2147/SHTT.S59498

Manlhiot, C. (2018). Machine learning for predictive analytics in medicine: Real opportunity or overblown hype? *European Heart Journal Cardiovascular Imaging, 19*(7), 727–728. DOI: 10.1093/ehjci/jey041

McDermid, J. A., Jia, Y., Porter, Z., & Habli, I. (2021). Artificial intelligence explainability: The technical and ethical dimensions. *Philosophical Transactions of the Royal Society A, 379*(2207), 20200363. DOI: 10.1098/rsta.2020.0363

Mohanty, M., & Mohanty, A. (2025). Machine Learning-Based Recommender Systems for Cancer Patients. In *Artificial Intelligence in Oncology: Cancer Diagnosis and Treatment, Medical Imaging, and Personalized Medicine* (pp. 101-114). Cham: Springer Nature Switzerland. DOI:DOI: 10.1007/978-3-031-94302-7_7

Mohr, D. C., Burns, M. N., Schueller, S. M., Clarke, G., & Klinkman, M. (2013). Behavioral intervention technologies: Evidence review and recommendations for future research in mental health. *General Hospital Psychiatry, 35*(4), 332–338. DOI: 10.1016/j.genhosppsych.2013.03.008

Nicora, G., Rios, M., Abu-Hanna, A., & Bellazzi, R. (2022). Evaluating pointwise reliability of machine learning prediction. *Journal of Biomedical Informatics, 127*, 103996. DOI: 10.1016/j.jbi.2022.103996

Norori, N., Hu, Q., Aellen, F. M., Faraci, F. D., & Tzovara, A. (2021). Addressing bias in big data and AI for health care: A call for open science. *Patterns (New York, N.Y.), 2*(10). Advance online publication. DOI: 10.1016/j.patter.2021.100347

Olalekan Kehinde, A. (2025). Leveraging machine learning for predictive models in healthcare to enhance patient outcome management. *Int Res J Mod Eng Technol Sci, 7*(1), 1465. DOI: https://www.doi .org/10.56726/IRJMETS66198

Ono, G. N., Obi, E. C., Chiaghana, C., & Ezegwu, D. (2024). Digital divide and access: Addressing disparities in Artificial Intelligence (AI) health information for Nigerian rural communities. *Social Science Research, 10*(3).

Paccoud, I., Leist, A. K., Schwaninger, I., van Kessel, R., & Klucken, J. (2024). Socio-ethical challenges and opportunities for advancing diversity, equity, and inclusion in digital medicine. *Digital Health, 10*, 20552076241277705. DOI: 10.1177/20552076241277705

Pal, S., Kaushik, A., Goel, F., Pal, A., & Garg, V. K. (2025). Revolutionizing Early Diagnosis: The Role of Artificial Intelligence in Neurodegenerative Disorders. *International Journal of Advances in Scientific Research, 16*(03), 31–37. DOI: 10.55218/JASR.2025160306

Palkova, K. (2021). Ethical guidelines for artificial intelligence in healthcare from the sustainable development perspective. *European Journal of Sustainable Development, 10*(1), 90–90. DOI: 10.14207/ejsd.2021.v10n1p90

Paulus, J. K., & Kent, D. M. (2020). Predictably unequal: Understanding and addressing concerns that algorithmic clinical prediction may increase health disparities. *NPJ Digital Medicine, 3*(1), 99. DOI: 10.1038/s41746-020-0304-9

Ponnusamy, V., Vasuki, A., Clement, J. C., & Eswaran, P. (2022). AI-Driven Information and Communication Technologies, Services, and Applications for Next-Generation Healthcare System. *Smart Systems for Industrial Applications*, 1-32. https://doi.org/DOI: 10.1002/9781119762010.ch1

Pozzi, G. (2024). Machine Learning-Induced Epistemic Injustice in Medicine and Healthcare. DOI DOI: 10.4233/uuid:78be5850-2df9-40fe-973d-e537d0d172c0

Rahman, M. A., Hossain, M. S., Showail, A. J., Alrajeh, N. A., & Alhamid, M. F. (2021). A secure, private, and explainable IoHT framework to support sustainable health monitoring in a smart city. *Sustainable Cities and Society, 72*, 103083. DOI: 10.1016/j.scs.2021.103083

Rahman, M. H., Uddinb, M. K. S., Hossanc, K. M. R., & Hossaind, M. D. (2024). The role of predictive analytics in early disease detection: A data-driven approach to preventive healthcare. *Journal of the Learning Sciences, 32*(2), 2024. DOI: 10.70937/faet.v1i01.22

Reps, J. M., Schuemie, M. J., Suchard, M. A., Ryan, P. B., & Rijnbeek, P. R. (2018). Design and implementation of a standardized framework to generate and evaluate patient-level prediction models using observational healthcare data. *Journal of the American Medical Informatics Association : JAMIA, 25*(8), 969–975. DOI: 10.1093/jamia/ocy032

Roaten, K., Johnson, C., Genzel, R., Khan, F., & North, C. S. (2018). Development and implementation of a universal suicide risk screening program in a safety-net hospital system. *Joint Commission Journal on Quality and Patient Safety, 44*(1), 4–11. DOI: 10.1016/j.jcjq.2017.07.006

Rolla, K. J. (2023). Trends and Futuristic Applications of Big Data and Electronic Health Record Data in Empowering Constructive Clinical Decision Support Systems. *Bio Science Research Bulletin-Biological Sciences, 39*(2). Advance online publication. DOI: 10.48165/bpas.2023.39.2.6

Samuel, A. L. (1959). Some studies in machine learning using the game of checkers. *IBM Journal of Research and Development, 3*(3), 210–229. DOI: 10.1147/rd.33.0210

Séroussi, B., Hollis, K. F., & Soualmia, L. F. (2020). Transparency of health informatics processes as the condition of healthcare professionals' and patients' trust and adoption: the rise of ethical requirements. *Yearbook of medical informatics, 29*(01), 007-010. DOI: DOI: 10.1055/s-0040-1702029

Sharma, A., Lysenko, A., Jia, S., Boroevich, K. A., & Tsunoda, T. (2024). Advances in AI and machine learning for predictive medicine. *Journal of Human Genetics*, *69*(10), 487–497. DOI: 10.1038/s10038-024-01231-y

Shi, Z., Chen, W., Liang, S., Zuo, W., Yue, L., & Wang, S. (2019). Deep interpretable mortality model for intensive care unit risk prediction. In *Advanced Data Mining and Applications: 15th International Conference, ADMA 2019, Dalian, China, November 21–23, 2019, Proceedings 15* (pp. 617-631). Springer International Publishing. DOI:DOI: 10.1007/978-3-030-35231-8_45

Singh, A. P., Saxena, R., Saxena, S., & Maurya, N. K. (2024). Artificial Intelligence Revolution in Healthcare: Transforming Diagnosis, Treatment, and Patient Care. *Asian Journal of Advances in Research*, *7*(1), 241–263.

Starfield, B. (2004). Promoting equity in health through research and understanding. *Developing World Bioethics*, *4*(1), 76–95. DOI: 10.1111/j.1471-8731.2004.00068.x

Van Duc, N., Chau, T. T. M., Long, P. H., Nhung, L. T. C., Huy, B. Q., Bin, Z., & Yusof, Hassan, A.F.B. (2024). The Role of Big Data in Assessing the Impact of Nutrition and Lifestyle Modifications on Gastrointestinal Disorder Prevention and Management. QuestSquare, 7, 55–66.

Walsh, C. G., Johnson, K. B., Ripperger, M., Sperry, S., Harris, J., Clark, N., Fielstein, E., Novak, L., Robinson, K., & Stead, W. W. (2021). Prospective validation of an electronic health record–based, real-time suicide risk model. *JAMA Network Open*, *4*(3), e211428–e211428. DOI: 10.1001/jamanetworkopen.2021.1428

Williamson, L. (2014). Patient and citizen participation in health: The need for improved ethical support. *The American Journal of Bioethics*, *14*(6), 4–16. DOI: 10.1080/15265161.2014.900139

Yu, S., Farooq, F., Van Esbroeck, A., Fung, G., Anand, V., & Krishnapuram, B. (2015). Predicting readmission risk with institution-specific prediction models. *Artificial Intelligence in Medicine*, *65*(2), 89–96. DOI: 10.1016/j.artmed.2015.08.005

Zaree, A., Dev, S., Yaseen Khan, I., Arain, M., Rasool, S., Khalid Rana, M. A., Kanwal, K., Bhagat, R., Prachi, F. N. U., Puri, P., & Mohamad, T. (2023). Cardiac rehabilitation in the modern era: Optimizing recovery and reducing recurrence. *Cureus*, *15*(9), e46006. DOI: 10.7759/cureus.46006

Zeinali, N. (2025). *Enhancing Cancer Symptom Detection in Electronic Health Records Using Artificial Intelligence* (Doctoral dissertation, The University of Iowa). DOI: DOI: 10.25820/etd.008020

KEY TERMS AND DEFINITIONS

Big Data Analytics: The use of advanced computers that can process large volumes of heterogeneous healthcare data from various sources, such as EHRs and wearables, to extract meaningful insights and provide valid predictions.

Care Management: Using data insights to optimize and streamline health care delivery, including developing targeted interventions, strategies to promote prevention, and personalized care plans that improve patient outcomes and operational efficiency.

EHR: EHRs are the digital version of a patient's paper chart; they contain comprehensive medical history, diagnoses, lab results, medications, and treatment plans. EHRs are one of the major data sources for predictive analytics in healthcare.

Genetic Information: Data obtained from the analysis of an individual's genome, used in predictive models to determine susceptibility to hereditary diseases and personalized treatment regimens.

Personalized Medicine: A model of care that targets treatment, management, and plans of care that meet the individual patient's specific needs, taking into consideration their unique characteristics, such as their genetic profile, lifestyle, environmental factors, and preferences.

Predictive Analytics: The use of data, statistical algorithms, Artificial Intelligence (AI), and machine learning techniques to analyze current and historical facts to identify patterns and forecast future outcomes such as disease progression or treatment responses.

Risk Stratification: A process of systematically classifying patients into categories based on their levels of risk, which will enable healthcare providers to effectively allocate resources and target specific interventions.

Chapter 13
Before the Interface: Designing User Research Instruments and Methods to Enable Digital Health Innovation for ALS Patients With Partial Locked-In Syndrome

Bruno Giesteira
https://orcid.org/0000-0003-4896-6659
Universidade do Porto, Portugal

Eliana Santiago
University of Porto, Portugal

Andreia Sousa
https://orcid.org/0000-0001-8070-8970
Lusófona University, Portugal

Pedro Amado
https://orcid.org/0000-0002-6934-144X
University of Porto, Portugal

Filipe Gonçalves
https://orcid.org/0000-0002-4423-7443
Faculty of Health Sciences, University of A Coruña, Spain

ABSTRACT

This chapter explores the innovative development and integration of tailored user research instruments to inform digital health solutions for People Living with Amyotrophic Lateral Sclerosis (PALS) exhibiting characteristics of partial Locked-In Syndrome (LIS). Addressing the complex interplay of motor, cognitive, and emotional impairments typical of this population, the study proposes a synergistic framework combining three adapted instruments: the ALS Functional Rating Scale-Revised (ALSFRS-R/EX), the User Experience Questionnaire Plus (UEQ+), and a bespoke Cognitive-Motor-Emotional (CME) Observation Grid. These instruments were tailored to detect subtle variations in user function, affect, and interaction. Results show how embodied and sensory drawing participatory methods and customis-

DOI: 10.4018/979-8-3373-3531-5.ch013

ation of instruments, along with semi-structured questionnaire and interviews with caregivers, can yield actionable insights for designing a model for solutions in neurodegenerative or communication-limiting contexts beyond Augmentative and Alternative Communication (AAC).

INTRODUCTION

Digital technologies now play a central role in how individuals with complex health conditions access communication, care, and social participation. Designing effective systems requires a grounded understanding of users' lived experiences, particularly when supporting populations with progressive neuromotor disorders. This chapter therefore introduces the rationale for a pre-digital, observational approach to understanding expressive, functional, and emotional needs before interface development.

Within this context, digital health innovation has been recognised as a transformative force in health promotion and disease prevention (Topol, 2019). However, its success depends on a profound understanding of users' specific needs, especially when working with individuals experiencing progressive neuromotor disorders. This chapter argues that tailored pre-digital fieldwork, involving carefully designed cognitive, motor, functional, and emotional observation instruments, is indispensable for developing affective and empathetic digital communication solutions for ALS patients in early or partial LIS stages, as well as for other phenotypically similar individuals (Schnetzer et al., 2023).

A personalised patient-centred approach that integrates biomedical care, technological and digital health innovation, social stimulation, and existential dimensions is essential to address the multifaceted challenges posed by ALS and to support individuals in achieving their fullest potential at all stages of the disease.

We need to expand in digital solutions for ALS patients, moving beyond functional communication to embrace a more holistic, non-verbal approach that restores agency and emotional expression through embodied, sensory drawing.

This work is situated within the SiX project—Drawing for Social Re-connectivity—which investigates the potential of embodied, sensory, and collaborative drawing as a foundation for future Extended Reality (XR) tools designed for individuals with partial to complete LIS. By adopting multimodal evaluation instruments and integrating perspectives from patients, caregivers, and therapists, this chapter aims to articulate how empathic, evidence-based insights generated in pre-interface settings can contribute to the development of digital health solutions that respect users' autonomy, emotional expression, and relational presence.

LITERATURE REVIEW

1. ALS Clinical and Psychosocial Context

Amyotrophic Lateral Sclerosis (ALS) is a progressive, incurable, and clinically heterogeneous neurodegenerative disease, either sporadic or inherited, characterised by the degeneration of both upper and lower motor neurons (Hardiman et al, 2017), that often leads to significant motor impairment and communication barriers.

In ALS, symptom onset is typically anatomically localised; however, the disease often progresses asymmetrically across body regions, potentially resulting in a condition that may be described as partial Locked-In Syndrome (LIS) (Schnetzer et al., 2005). In such cases, individuals retain some voluntary control—such as limited speech, handwriting ability, or use of Augmentative and Alternative Communication (AAC) tools—but remain profoundly affected in their ability to interact socially and emotionally.

The clinical trajectory of ALS is highly variable—not only in terms of symptom progression and response to interventions, but also in how individuals and families experience and adapt to the illness. Currently, there is no cure for ALS, and pharmacological options are limited, offering only modest effects without halting disease progression. The median survival is 3–5 years from symptom onset, although 5–10% of patients may live beyond a decade (Hardiman et al., 2017). Neuropsychological manifestations, alongside physical deterioration, contribute to significant reductions in functional ability and quality of life (QoL). Beyond motor decline, 5–15% of patients present with comorbid frontotemporal dementia (FTD), and up to 50% develop cognitive and/or behavioural impairments during the disease course (Masrori & Van Damme, 2020). These impairments may be exacerbated by a lack of social and cognitive stimulation, as well as barriers to participation, routine, and interaction (Gonçalves & Magalhães, 2022), especially considering that non-motor brain functions, such as oculomotor and sphincter control, tend to remain relatively preserved until advanced stages.

Cultural background, family dynamics, gender, and personal beliefs play a critical role in shaping coping strategies, care preferences, and psychosocial resilience. Patients often perceive ALS as a profound interruption in life, marked by uncertainty, loss of autonomy, and existential distress. Participation and stimulation strategies across all domains—physical, psychosocial, emotional, and spiritual—encompassing intrapersonal, interpersonal, and transpersonal dimensions, emerge as vital resources for meaning-making, emotional comfort, and purpose. Yet, these remain among the most neglected components of palliative care and therapeutic planning (Gonçalves et al. 2025). Given the multifactorial nature of ALS, multidisciplinary care is widely recognised as the gold standard, associated with improved QoL and, in some cases, extended survival (Shoesmith et al., 2020). In addition to clinical manifestations, biochemical markers, and therapeutic interventions, demographic, environmental, and lifestyle factors also play a critical and independent role in influencing disease prognosis (Su et al., 2021). The continuum of care should include not only healthcare and community support but also functional optimisation that goes beyond clinical interventions, aiming to enhance participation and humanise care. To achieve truly humanised care, it is essential to move beyond assumptions of a homogeneous user profile. Research must acknowledge the diversity and complexity of motor and communication abilities within this population, as well as their preferences, proxies for care and communication, needs, and available resources. Contemporary research and clinical practice must embrace the full spectrum of motor, cognitive, communicative, and psychosocial abilities within the ALS population.

2. From Functional AAC to Holistic Expressive Approaches

Traditional non-invasive AAC systems, while indispensable for individuals with LIS, typically rely on textual matrices, symbol boards, or scanning-based interfaces that prioritise basic functional outputs, such as letter selection or binary responses. Although these tools significantly enhance fundamental communication capabilities, they frequently fall short in addressing full communication and human expression dimensions—qualities vital for long-term care and psychological well-being, including joy, personal meaning, and creative flow. This focus on utilitarian communication, such as answering questions or spelling, often overlooks the crucial aspects of emotional expression and relational presence, such as creative expression. (Amado et al., 2026) While essential for functional communication, this can limit the richness and nuance of expression, particularly for emotional or abstract concepts. Drawing offers a powerful non-verbal language that can convey emotions, abstract ideas, and complex scenarios in a way that words or pre-set symbols often cannot (Muenssinger et al., 2010; Vanutelli et al., 2023). Traditional AAC typically lacks this direct, intuitive, and highly personal expressive channel. Also, relying solely on pre-programmed phrases or structured communication can diminish a patient's sense of agency and autonomy, as patients often report preferring active over reactive control strategies (Branco et al., 2021).

Research by Larradet et al. (2020) explicitly reviews the scope and limitations of these tools, highlighting their deficiency in emotional expression capabilities and emphasising the importance of non-verbal cues in communication (Amado et al., 2026). Typically, structured interfaces often underprioritize the crucial emotional, affective, hedonic (pleasure), and eudaimonic (meaning and self-realisation) dimensions of human expression. By fundamentally concentrating on utilitarian communication, traditional AAC, despite its practical utility, establishes a fundamental gap in addressing the holistic human needs of the patient. This is not merely a missing feature; it represents a detriment to their psychological health, potentially leading to feelings of isolation, frustration, and a diminished sense of self. The unintended consequence of a purely functional design is the under-support of critical emotional and existential needs, contributing to a communication deficit that impacts overall QoL.

A novel non-verbal, non-invasive approach using embodied, sensory drawing is proposed as a more holistic means of communication for patients and their caregivers. The proposal for a customizable system aims to unlock the potential for affect acknowledgement and relational presence, offering a vital alternative to conventional linguistic or symbolic interfaces (Amado et al., 2025). Drawing, as a truly generative creative expression, empowers patients to create something unique and entirely their own. And, as a form of communication, it can provide an assorted array of strategies — generative, interactive, and body extensions, customizable to each patient's needs or specific requirements (Aparicio, 2015).

3. Systemic Design Biases and the Need for a Paradigm Shift

The design choice for pre-programmed or structured communication in traditional AAC reflects a pervasive design philosophy that prioritises efficiency, predictability, and — despite recent efforts in expanding patients' communication with EEG and BCI implants (Caiado & Ukolov, 2025; Khan et al., 2025; Lavazza et al., 2025; Liu et al., 2025; Wang et al., 2025) — ease of implementation over generative expression and individual agency. This trend warrants critical re-evaluation, especially in the context of severe disability. The preference for pre-defined communication elements in assistive technology is often rooted in engineering efficiency and the desire for predictable outcomes. However, in the highly personal and dynamic context of human expression, particularly for individuals with severe physical limitations, this efficiency comes at the cost of authentic self-expression and personal control. This highlights a systemic design bias within AAC technology towards discrete, quantifiable communication, which can inadvertently reinforce the patient's passive role. It suggests a need for a fundamental paradigm shift in design thinking, as illustrated in Table 1 below, moving from "what can be efficiently transmitted" to "how can the richness and uniqueness of human expression be enabled".

Table 1. Provides a comparative overview of AAC technologies for traditional verbal or symbolic communication and embodied drawing to highlight their distinct capabilities and limitations in addressing the communication needs of ALS patients.

AAC Category	Verbal Communication	Embodied Drawing
Primary Focus	Functional needs (spelling, basic responses)	Holistic communication (emotional, relational, creative, hedonic, eudaimonic)
Expressive Range	Limited (discrete, predefined)	Rich and nuanced (abstract, complex)
Modality	Linguistic/Symbolic	Non-verbal, embodied, sensory
Emotional/Affective Dimension	Users must explicitly verbalize them, or match symbolic features	Users choose or create the *representamen* to match their needs (affect acknowledgment, relational presence, well-being)
Agency/Autonomy	Pre-set/available options	Creative/generative options [within the available options: System designers must balance the complexity of the interface with the capabilities]
Generative Capacity	Low (selection-based)	High (creation-based, co-authored)
Key Limitations	Lacks nuance, emotional depth, and personal agency; can feel impersonal	Requires custom development, technical hurdles, and specialized adaptation; still emerging
Key Strengths	Essential for basic needs; widely available; established	Offers deep psychological benefits (agency, identity, anxiety reduction); fosters emotional connection; provides a richer palette for expression

4. XR, HCD, Participatory Design, and Digital Empathy

Extended Reality (XR) presents a powerful opportunity to move beyond the limitations of traditional AAC for ALS patients, offering a new frontier for emotional and embodied communication through immersive and customizable experiences.

For individuals with complex needs like LIS, a Human-Centred Design (HCD) through Co-Design and Participatory Design approach is paramount (Penedos-Santiago et al., 2025) as it moves beyond generic solutions to create highly personalized and accessible tools, ensuring solutions that are not only functional, but also encompass the diversity and complexity of motor and communication abilities within this population, that improve QoL. This iterative approach typically involves stages such as empathising with users, defining their needs, ideating solutions, prototyping, and testing, thereby ensuring that the resulting technology is genuinely tailored to the human experience it seeks to enhance.

This approach is aligned with the Digital Empathy Theory (Rachmad, 2017), which posits that the working principle for fostering empathy in mediated interactions is the integration of technology with human empathic capabilities. The theory promotes communication practices that emphasise genuine emotional understanding and response, even though digital media enables individuals to build deeper and more meaningful relationships in digital contexts. Key indicators of digital empathy include the ability to read and interpret emotions via digital media, providing empathic responses, and building genuine emotional connections through technology, further evidenced by the frequency and quality of interactions demonstrating understanding and emotional support in online communication.

Drawing as a tool can adapt to any communicative goal, regardless of complexity, and takes on different forms and modes of operation depending on its context (Penedos-Santiago et al., 2025). Also, by deploying it in a customizable Extended Reality (XR) solution, it may provide a powerful opportunity to extend beyond the limited to in-person settings or narrowly tailored interventions (Barchielli et al., 2025). By exploring drawing as a non-verbal communication form, the research addresses the need for more holistic and emotionally resonant communication methods in assistive technology. It is our objective to establish collaborative virtual communication spaces where stakeholders can interact, establishing a dialogue through a shared form of expression and vocabulary.

5. User Research and Instrumentation

The goal is to develop an expressive drawing system for individuals with partial to complete Locked-in Syndrome (LIS), the first phase of the HCD methodology — user research — becomes fundamental for achieving an empathic understanding. To grasp the complex world of these patients, it's essential to delve into both their external circumstances and their internal experiences (Surma-aho et al. 2022). This requires a robust research methodology that allows us to comprehend the profound physical limitations, the communication barriers, and the emotional and cognitive landscapes of LIS patients, along with the perspectives of their caregivers and medical professionals. By establishing this deep empathetic foundation through comprehensive user research, we aim to ensure the technology we design is not only functional but also deeply resonant with their unique needs and aspirations.

Conventional clinical tools, such as the ALS Functional Rating Scale-Revised (ALSFRS-R/EX), measure patient functionality but lack the capacity to evaluate emotional engagement or the usability of technological aids (Cedarbaum et al., 1999). Meanwhile, the User Experience Questionnaire Plus (UEQ+) is a modular UX evaluation tool designed to assess system experience across tailored dimensions (UEQ+, 2024); its broad applicability does not fully capture the nuanced needs of our project.

To bridge this gap, our methodology required more than just reported functional assessments (ALSFRS-R/EX) and experience (UEQ+). It was imperative to concurrently understand the patient's dynamic mood and overall well-being, as directly impacted by the drawing activity. This comprehensive approach also necessitated exploring any motor, cognitive, or emotional impairments that the drawing process might elicit.

METHODOLOGY

This research was conducted in the context of the SiX Project — 'Drawing for Social Re-connectivity. Exploring Inclusive, Collaborative and Digital Environments for Patients with Partial to Complete Locked-In Syndrome" — an interdisciplinary initiative aimed at developing expressive, embodied, and socially connected Extended Reality (XR) platforms. This chapter focused on pre-interface, paper-based drawing sessions to test a synergistic evaluation framework and build an empathetic understanding of the context of PALS.

Acknowledging the complex interplay of motor, cognitive, and emotional impairments typical of this population, this study proposes a novel evaluation framework, grounded in a Human-Centred Design (HCD) philosophy, with elements of Participatory Design and Co-Design practices. Our approach triangulates data from five instruments: the ALS Functional Rating Scale-Revised (ALSFRS-R/EX), the User Experience Questionnaire Plus (UEQ+), a bespoke Cognitive-Motor-Emotional (CME) Observation Grid, a Semi-Structured Questionnaire, and Semi-Structured Interviews with Caregivers integrated. ALSFRS-R/EX /EX, UEQ+, CME Observation Grid, and Semi-Structured Questionnaire were applied during participatory drawing workshops. Semi-structured interviews with Caregivers were conducted after these sessions.

Preliminary workshop: Conceptual and Ergonomic Grounding

Prior to engaging with ALS patients, we conducted a preliminary workshop with a control group, comprising voluntary able-bodied master's students in Product and Industrial Design at the Faculty of Engineering, University of Porto, in December 2024. The session aimed to simulate motor and perceptual constraints characteristic of ALS and partial LIS using low-tech prosthetics and physical limitations (e.g., restricting neck movement, applying elastic bands to simulate spasticity, altering writing angles) (Figure 1).

Participants engaged in the same structured drawing-based tasks later applied in clinical settings, including name writing, shape drawing, music interpretation, and haptic tracing. This workshop generated detailed ergonomic and affective feedback, highlighting patterns of frustration, compensatory strategies, and perceptual confusion. These insights informed adjustments to our cognitive-motor-emotional (CME) observation grid and framed our expectations for user behaviours in real-world contexts. The simulation also played a crucial role in empirical grounding for the conceptual values we aimed to embed in our system, such as dignity, self-expression, and participation — consistent with the early stages of Value Sensitive Design (VSD) (Friedman, Kahn, & Borning, 2002; Winkler & Spiekermann, 2021).

Figure 1. Preliminary workshop with a control group comprising Master's students in Product and Industrial Design at the Faculty of Engineering, University of Porto, in December 2024. The aim was to reproduce the motor constraints of the upper limbs and hands. ©Cláudia Lima.

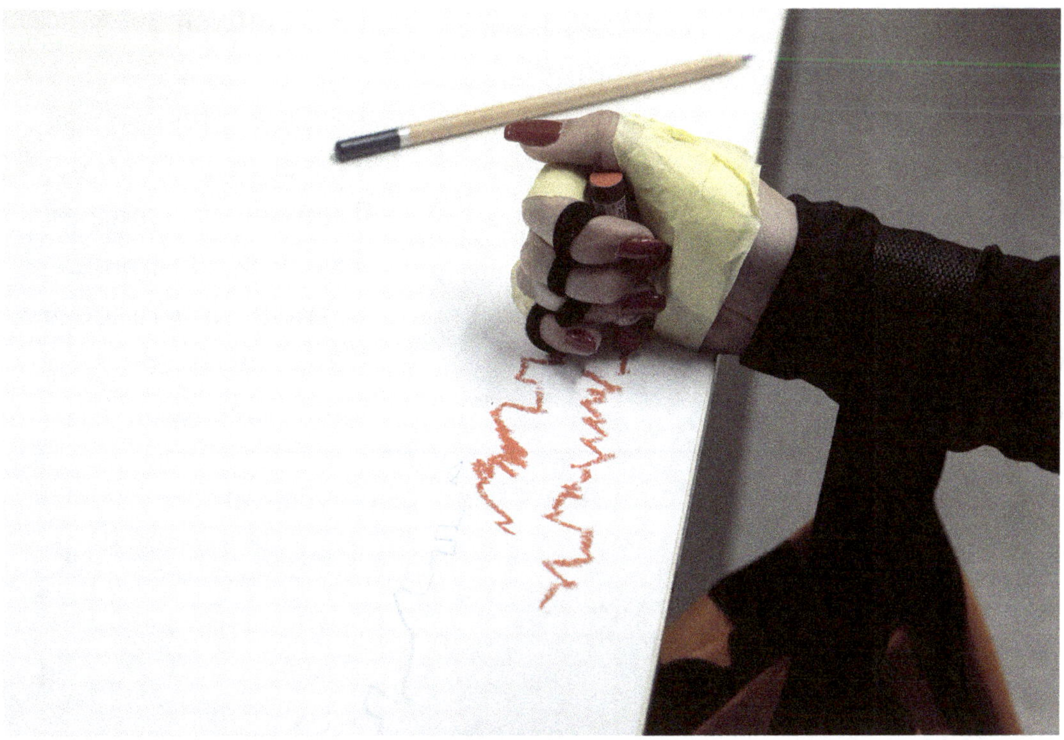

MULTIMODAL EVALUATION FRAMEWORK

1. ALSFRS-R/EX quantified patients' motor impairments, guiding interaction design.

The ALSFRS-R/EX (*Figure 2*) is a validated, clinical questionnaire developed to assess the functional status of ALS patients across four domains: bulbar, fine motor, gross motor, and respiratory. In this study, it helped profile participants' levels of motor control and inform the feasibility of the interface. Scores were collected by therapists and used to notify the feasibility of drawing activities and physical access to interaction materials (Brooks et al., 2000). In this study, scores collected by therapists will guide the feasibility of drawing activities and inform interface accessibility and help to understand the disease progression.

Figure 2. ALSFRS-R/EX: Successive functional domains across scale version (Wicks et al., 2009)

ALSFRS (original) 1996	ALSFRS-R (revised) 1999 additional items	ALSFRS-EX (extension) 2008 pilot items
Speech	Dyspnea	Ventilator use
Saliva	Orthopnea	Fingers/button pressing
Swallowing	Respiratory support	Head movement
Handwriting		Facial expressiveness
Cutting food/utensils		Travel outside home
Dressing/hygiene		Transfer to/from bed
Turning in bed		Travel inside home
Walking		Participation in leisure
Climbing stairs		Care management
Breathing		Computer use

Successive versions include all items from prior version.

2. Customised UEQ+ evaluated patient perception of the drawing experience.

The User Experience Questionnaire Plus (UEQ+) (*Figure 3*), a modular evaluation instrument which was customised for this study (Giesteira et al., 2025) to include emotional resonance, novelty, social connectedness, and stimulation. It was administered to PALS after each session, supporting a comparative understanding of subjective perceptions of expressiveness and interaction quality (Laugwitz, Held, & Schrepp, 2008). Although the UEQ+ is primarily designed to assess digital user experiences, its modular structure and customisable nature make it suitable for evaluating pre-interface interactions — such as paper-based activities— especially when those activities are part of a design process aiming toward future digital development.

Figure 3. UEQ+: Modular items for evaluating emotional and cognitive experience.

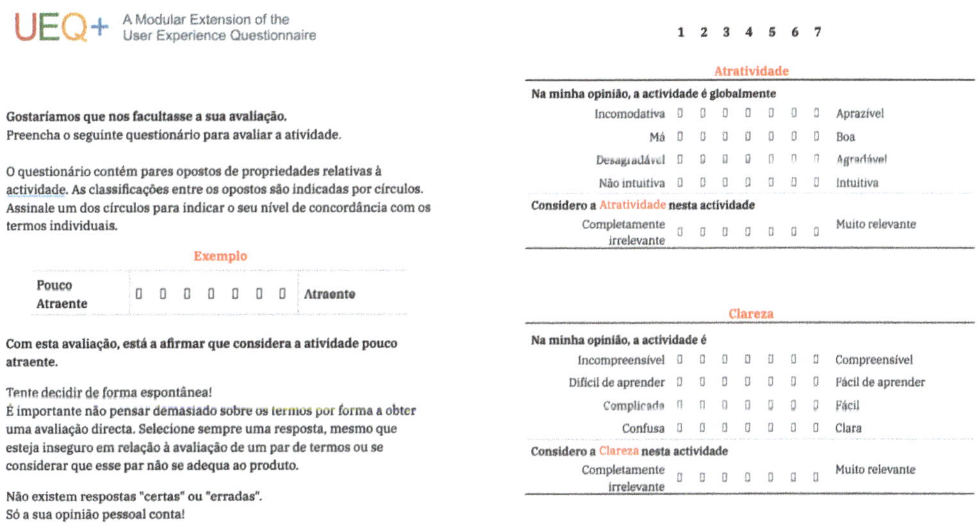
UEQ+ A Modular Extension of the User Experience Questionnaire

Gostaríamos que nos facultasse a sua avaliação.
Preencha o seguinte questionário para avaliar a atividade.

O questionário contém pares opostos de propriedades relativas à actividade. As classificações entre os opostos são indicadas por círculos. Assinale um dos círculos para indicar o seu nível de concordância com os termos individuais.

Exemplo

Pouco Atraente	▯ ▯ ▯ ▯ ▯ ▯ ▯	Atraente

Com esta avaliação, está a afirmar que considera a atividade pouco atraente.

Tente decidir de forma espontânea!
É importante não pensar demasiado sobre os termos por forma a obter uma avaliação directa. Selecione sempre uma resposta, mesmo que esteja inseguro em relação à avaliação de um par de termos ou se considerar que esse par não se adequa ao produto.

Não existem respostas "certas" ou "erradas".
Só a sua opinião pessoal conta!

Atratividade

	1	2	3	4	5	6	7	
Na minha opinião, a actividade é globalmente								
Incomodativa	▯	▯	▯	▯	▯	▯	▯	Aprazível
Má	▯	▯	▯	▯	▯	▯	▯	Boa
Desagradável	▯	▯	▯	▯	▯	▯	▯	Agradável
Não intuitiva	▯	▯	▯	▯	▯	▯	▯	Intuitiva
Considero a Atratividade nesta actividade								
Completamente irrelevante	▯	▯	▯	▯	▯	▯	▯	Muito relevante

Clareza

Na minha opinião, a actividade é								
Incompreensível	▯	▯	▯	▯	▯	▯	▯	Compreensível
Difícil de aprender	▯	▯	▯	▯	▯	▯	▯	Fácil de aprender
Complicada	▯	▯	▯	▯	▯	▯	▯	Fácil
Confusa	▯	▯	▯	▯	▯	▯	▯	Clara
Considero a Clareza nesta actividade								
Completamente irrelevante	▯	▯	▯	▯	▯	▯	▯	Muito relevante

3. Participatory Design (PD) involved patients and caregivers in the iterative design process.

A bespoke Cognitive Motor Emotional (CME) Observation Grid was developed in-house specifically for this research context. It provided real-time observation metrics of cognitive engagement, motor effort, emotional reaction, and fatigue (Figure 4, with the first three dimensions of the metrics visible). Researchers coded observable events, including gaze direction, posture change, vocal reaction, and pauses, using a protocol to align behaviours with potential UX states. Observations were documented in situ and video-recorded for further coding.

Figure 4. CME Grid: Example of observational UX validation procedure in the digital adaptation phases.

Grelha de Observação CME

COGNITIVO

Esforço e Fadiga: Sinais de exaustão cognitiva (perda de foco, respostas lentas).
POUCO MUITO
0 1 2 3 4 5 6 7 8 9 10

OBSERVAÇÕES

Decisão e controlo: na seleção de cores formas e posicionamento na folha.
POUCO MUITO
0 1 2 3 4 5 6 7 8 9 10

OBSERVAÇÕES

Atenção e foco: compreensão da tarefa
POUCO MUITO
0 1 2 3 4 5 6 7 8 9 10

OBSERVAÇÕES

MOTOR

Velocidade e precisão: no manuseamento e troca dos materiais
POUCO MUITO
0 1 2 3 4 5 6 7 8 9 10

OBSERVAÇÕES

Fadiga e esforço repetitivo: sinais de exaustão ou precisão reduzida ao longo da tarefa
POUCO MUITO
0 1 2 3 4 5 6 7 8 9 10

OBSERVAÇÕES

Alcance do movimento: amplo ou reduzido, altera de acordo com a tarefa (ritmo) demonstra dificuldade na execução
POUCO MUITO
0 1 2 3 4 5 6 7 8 9 10

OBSERVAÇÕES

EMOCIONAL

Frustração e autonomia: há sinais de frustração/control
POUCO MUITO
0 1 2 3 4 5 6 7 8 9 10

OBSERVAÇÕES

Prazer e autoexpressão: nível de envolvimento e expressão na tarefa
POUCO MUITO
0 1 2 3 4 5 6 7 8 9 10

OBSERVAÇÕES

Motivação e confiança: sinais de motivação/ desmotivação e confiança na tarefa
POUCO MUITO
0 1 2 3 4 5 6 7 8 9 10

OBSERVAÇÕES

4. Semi-Structured Questionnaire

To complement observational and functional data, the research team developed a semi-structured feedback instrument, designed to elicit both pre- and post-session insights from participants. This tool combines quantitative self-assessments—such as fatigue, anxiety, well-being, and motivation rated on a 10-point Likert scale—with a series of open-ended exploratory prompts aimed at capturing users' affective responses, imaginative engagement, and interpersonal dynamics during the drawing-based activities (figure 5). Questions invited reflection on the novelty of the experience ("Have you ever drawn music before?"), the sense of embodied engagement ("Did you feel like you were dancing?"), and the potential for emotional and social connection ("Would you like to draw/dance with someone else?"). Participants were also asked to speculate on meaningful themes they would like to express through drawing and whether customisation (e.g., choosing the music) might enhance the experience. This instrument supported the emergence of subjective, emotionally charged insights often absent from standard UX evaluations, aligning with participatory design principles and enabling deeper understanding of users' values, preferences, and relational contexts.

Figure 5. Semi-Structured Questionnaire

Questionário semi-aberto

Pré avaliação

Fadiga

POUCO										MUITO
0	1	2	3	4	5	6	7	8	9	10

Ansiedade

POUCO										MUITO
0	1	2	3	4	5	6	7	8	9	10

Bem Estar Geral

POUCO										MUITO
0	1	2	3	4	5	6	7	8	9	10

Motivação

POUCO										MUITO
0	1	2	3	4	5	6	7	8	9	10

NOVIDADE

Alguma vez tinha experimentado desenhar o som?

EMBODIMENT

Sentiu que dançava?

PERSONALIZAÇÃO

Faria diferença se pudesse escolher a música que irá "dançar" / desenhar? Nesta forma alternativa de encarar o desenho, que outras situações gostaria de desenhar?

COMUNICAÇÃO / EMPATIA

Gostaria de "dançar" / desenhar uma música a dois?

[mesmo em caso negativo] Em que outras situações se vê a precisar, mas acima de tudo a querer desenhar a dois?

Sente que esta forma de desenhar pode ajudar a compreender o que o outro sente? [de que forma? Ou qual a forma mais eficaz (p. Ex. procurar saber se pelos materiais ou cor dos riscadores, pelas formas ou objetos desenhados, pela posição ou o tamanho, a rapidez ou expressão,...)]

Como descreveria os momentos partilhados com outra pessoa? Neste caso a atividade com o cuidador ou a atividade em que dá continuidade ao desenho de outra pessoa?

Avaliação pós sessão

Fadiga

POUCO										MUITO
0	1	2	3	4	5	6	7	8	9	10

Ansiedade

POUCO										MUITO
0	1	2	3	4	5	6	7	8	9	10

Bem Estar Geral

POUCO										MUITO
0	1	2	3	4	5	6	7	8	9	10

Motivação

POUCO										MUITO
0	1	2	3	4	5	6	7	8	9	10

5. Semi-Structured Interviews with Caregivers

Additionally, a total of five semi-structured interviews (Figure 5) with caregivers were conducted: one formal caregiver and four informal caregivers, all of whom are directly related to the PALS participating in the study. The interview protocol explored two main dimensions: (i) the caregiver's perception of the field session experience and the patient's engagement during drawing activities, and (ii) the broader family and emotional dynamics surrounding daily life, communication, affection, and co-creative rituals.

Questions were designed to elicit not just factual feedback, but relational values such as mutual empathy, dignity, cognitive engagement, and emotional synchrony. For example, caregivers were asked how they interpreted the patient's motivation, whether the activity had been discussed afterward, and how such interactions intersected with existing family rituals (e.g., storytelling, shared games, or memory-sharing practices).

FIELDWORK: PARTICIPANTS AND SETTING

Fieldwork was conducted with six PALS exhibiting partial LIS symptoms, recruited through APELA – Portuguese Association for Amyotrophic Lateral Sclerosis, a non-profit organization that provides support and follow-up therapies for PALS and their caregivers. The participatory drawing workshops took place in a care centre and were supported by therapists and caregivers. All participants provided informed consent after receiving detailed information about the nature, objectives, and procedures of the study. They were explicitly told that participation would not affect the progression of their medical condition (positively or negatively), and that the research had no therapeutic or medical intervention goals — it was solely observational, exploratory, and aimed at informing future design possibilities. Ethical considerations were addressed in accordance with the principles of informed consent, data anonymization, and responsible reporting, as outlined in the Declaration of Helsinki (World Medical Association, 2013). Caregivers were also engaged as collaborators, not just informants.

This study was conducted at the northern delegation of the APELA. At the time of the study, this delegation was offering monthly follow-up sessions to 104 PALS (this number only accounts for those who had completed one or more in-person visits to the facility) from whom sociodemographic and clinical data were collected. The male population represented 58% of PALS (*n*=60), with a global mean age of 61.9 years (±11.9, SD). Regarding the disease onset, it was predominantly medullary (63.5%), followed by bulbar (33.7%), axial (1.9%), and respiratory (1.0%). Participants were distributed across different cities in northern Portugal, with the furthest individual residing 235 km from the delegation (despite the geographical distance, this person received bimonthly in-person visits and participated in remote follow-up sessions via online platforms, covering areas such as advanced technology, nutrition, and psychological support, complementary to local support). In terms of caregiving, 24 participants reported having formal caregivers, while the remaining relied on informal support. Marital status indicated that 71.2% (n=74) were married, 21.2% (n=22) were single or divorced, and 7.7% (n=8) were widowed. Functional dependency levels were classified as follows: 6.7% (n=7) were independent, 16.3% (n=17) had mild dependency, 32.7% (n=34) moderate, and 34.6% (n=36) severe, and 9.6% total dependent (this means 24h of daily care and supervision).

For this study, individuals with diverse profiles were invited to participate voluntarily, with no institutional obligation or external pressure, including people living with ALS (PALS) and their formal or informal caregivers. Eligibility was limited to PALS in moderate or lower stages of dependency. Exclusion criteria comprised PALS presenting with severe secondary comorbidities, including marked cognitive or behavioural impairments, a diagnosis of frontotemporal dementia, or an inability to comprehend and respond to subjective assessment tools.

Figure 6. Participatory drawing workshops (A) - Field Sessions at APELA April 2025. A. performing the motor warm-up activity (writing their name, testing drawing tools). Due to his gradual loss of motor skills in his arms and hands, A. has developed a physically accessible signature that allows him to retain control over his identity. ©Cláudia Lima.

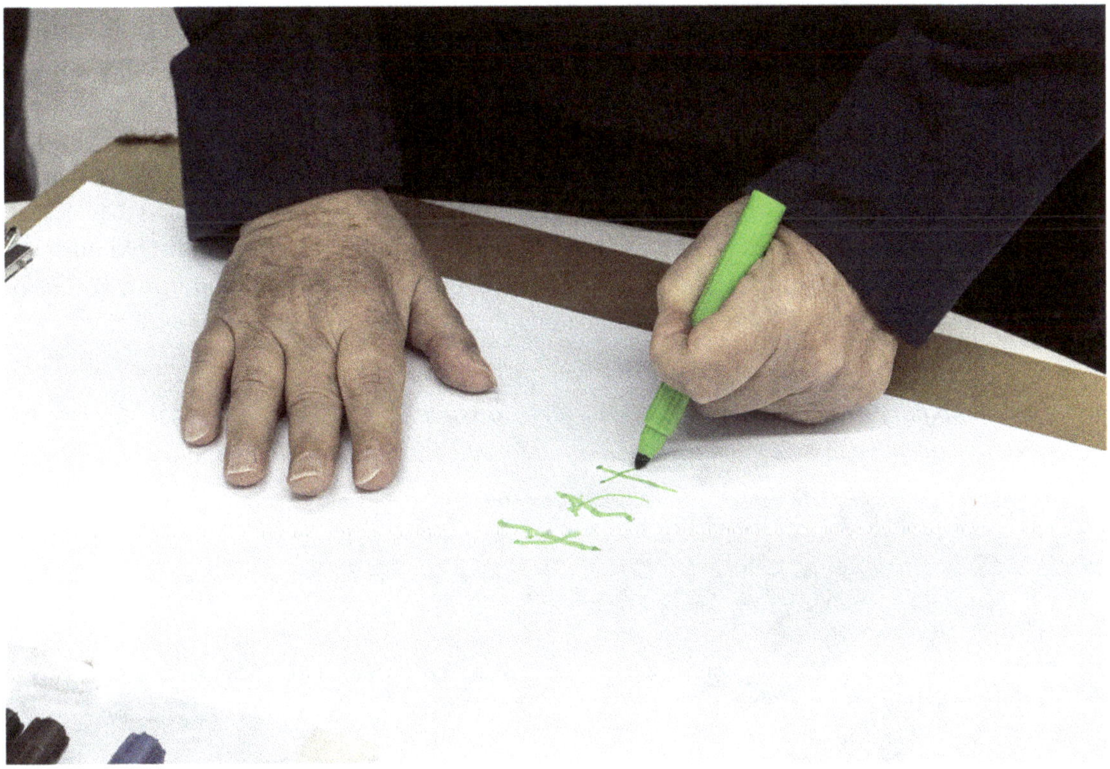

Between 7 and 11 April 2025, we conducted the first round of field sessions with PALS at APELA (Figure 6). These sessions were designed to collect functional, affective, cognitive, and experiential data from individuals with partial LIS manifestations. All six participants (5 male, 1 female, aged between 49 and 68, at different stages of disease progression and with varying, emotional, and social profiles) took part. Their clinical profiles varied in terms of motor and bulbar impairments: two individuals presented with severe motor loss in the upper limbs; two were non-verbal at symptom onset; and one experienced respiratory limitations and fatigue as the most restricting factors. Despite these conditions, all participants demonstrated an effective communication capability. Of these, three retained oral communicative abilities without any loss of speech intelligibility, while the remaining two communicated daily using low-tech solutions, such as LCD letter boards or mobile text-to-speak apps. Each participant engaged in a 45-minute structured protocol including:

- A **motor warm-up activity** (writing their name, testing drawing tools) (Fig.2);
- A **haptic-proprioceptive task**, conducted by a formal or informal caregiver (drawing symbols on the participant's back for visual interpretation);

- A **sound-interpretation drawing activity**, using music (The Beatles' *Twist and Shout* and Debussy's *Clair de Lune*), exploring the connection between embodied movement, emotion, and expression.

Haptic drawing *(Figure 7)* was integrated as a pre-digital activity to access embodied, co-creative forms of expression—essential in conditions such as partial Locked-In Syndrome (LIS), where verbal or gestural language is often limited. This strategy draws on practices in art and performance that regard touch and motion as cognitive and relational tools. Artist Morgan O'Hara's *Live Transmission* series captures the micro-movements of hands during daily acts, framing drawing as "embodied listening" and translating presence into visible traces (O'Hara, 2024). Similarly, Dennis Oppenheim's *Two Stage Transfer Drawing* (1971) staged drawing as a tactile, relational event: a child drawing on the back of an adult, whose own motor responses were transferred onto paper. These practices informed our tactile-back-drawing task, which required participants to interpret touch-based stimuli through mark-making, promoting both focus and trust in the caregiver–patient dyad *(Figure 7).*

Figure 7. Participatory drawing workshops (M) - Field Sessions at APELA April 2025. M. performing the haptic-proprioceptive task, conducted by G., an informal caregiver. ©Silvia Simões.

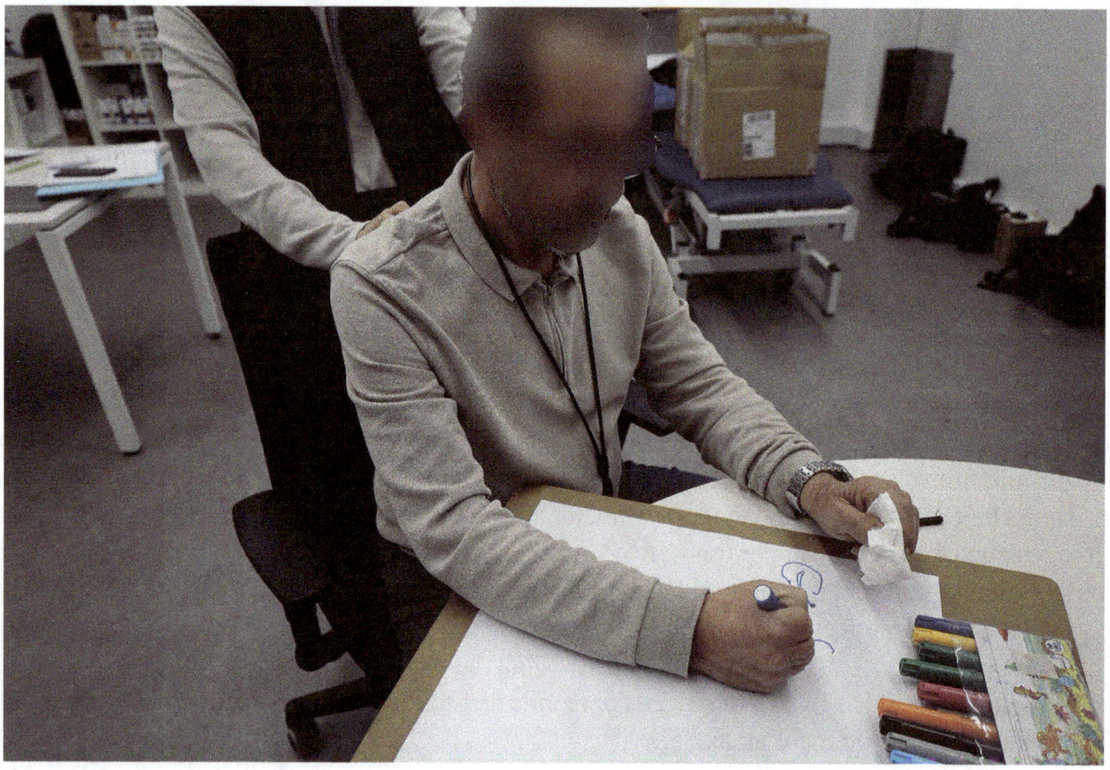

Sound-interpretation drawing leveraged music as a temporal, emotional, and spatial stimulus, enabling participants to explore memory, rhythm, and emotional valence through embodied motion. This draws on therapeutic practices where music stimulates autobiographical memory and sensorimotor pathways

(Czamanski-Cohen & Weihs, 2016), and on embodied cognition frameworks that interpret gesture and affect as interlinked (Wilson & Golonka, 2013). Our sessions combined structured musical contrasts—e.g., *The Beatles' Twist and Shout* vs. *Debussy's Clair de Lune*—to examine shifts in gesture, rhythm, and emotional tone, while prompting spontaneous visual responses (*Figure 8*).

Figure 8. Participatory drawing workshops (I) - Field Sessions at APELA April 2025. I. performing the sound-interpretation drawing activity, along with the music Twist and Shout by The Beatles, exploring the connection between embodied movement, emotion, and expression. ©Silvia Simões.

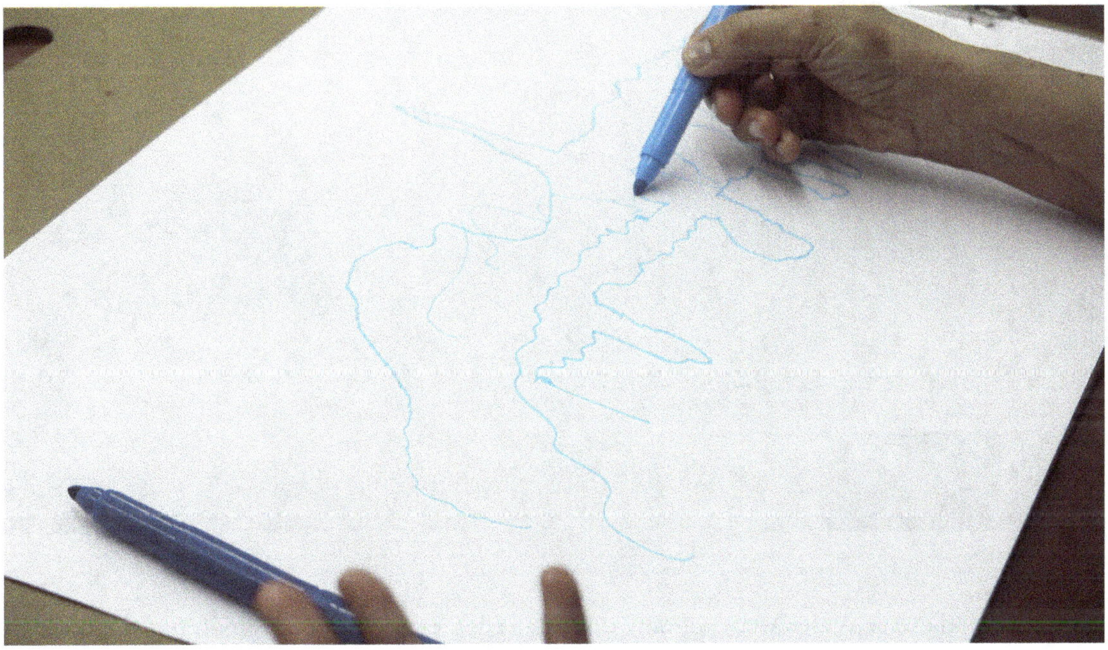

These embodied activities served not only as expressive tools, but also as frictional moments that surfaced both capacity and constraint (Baumer & Brubaker, 2017). They generated essential data for designing adaptive digital systems and contributed to conceptual and empirical layers of the Value Sensitive Design process. Beyond utility, they allowed users to inhabit moments of shared creativity, revealing values such as autonomy, agency, playfulness, and relational meaning. This aligns with the project's broader ambition: to move digital health innovation toward emotionally literate, ethically grounded, and sensorimotor-aware interaction design.

The structure was designed to address four VSD-relevant dimensions: fine and gross motor control, emotional and motivational engagement, interpersonal bonding, and subjective perception of usability.

The UEQ+ questionnaire was administered using a hybrid method appropriate to the patients' physical capabilities. Some participants, who retained minimal hand mobility, were able to respond directly (*Figure 9*). For others, whose motor impairments were more severe, responses were from caregivers and therapists present during the sessions. This hybrid approach allowed for the collection of subjective UX data while maintaining inclusivity and respecting individual limitations.

Figure 9. Participatory drawing workshops (M) - Field Sessions at APELA April 2025. Once the activities were completed, M was able to respond directly to our questionnaires. ©Cláudia Lima.

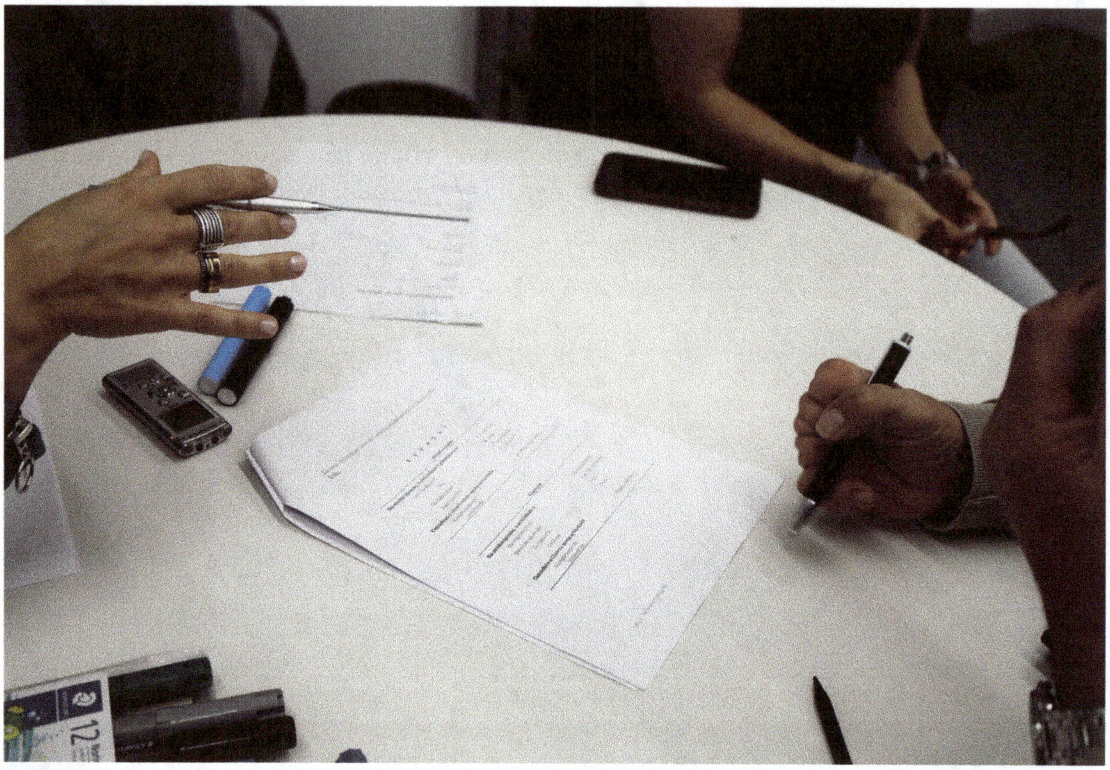

Importantly, these activities were not only data-gathering exercises but also intervention moments, aimed at fostering empowerment, playfulness, and social engagement through drawing. This aligns with a Value Sensitive Design approach, which integrates not only users' needs but also their personal values, frustrations, and modes of expression, in the early pre-digital stages of technological development.

FINDINGS

The triangulated use of ALSFRS-R/EX, UEQ+, and the CME Grid provided a dynamic, multi-perspective view. The data were coded and analysed qualitatively to identify recurring themes and patterns surrounding interaction breakdowns, affective states, and accessible sensory strategies.

This triangulated approach aligns with principles of Value Sensitive Design (VSD) (Friedman, Kahn, & Borning, 2002), particularly in its early commitment to surfacing users' emotional well-being, social identity, and dignity through co-created inquiry tools. By involving patients, carers, and therapists not merely as subjects but as epistemic contributors, the research situates user values at the foundation of the design process.

This approach is consistent with the tripartite model proposed in VSD literature, which includes conceptual, empirical, and technical investigations (Friedman, 2004; Friedman et al., 2013; Winkler &

Spiekermann, 2021). In this phase of the project (WP2 - Exploratory Analysis through field work), we focused primarily on the conceptual and empirical dimensions: identifying stakeholders' values (e.g., autonomy, emotional safety, expressiveness) and systematically observing their responses to co-creative, paper-based sessions. An additional layer — technical research and development, where these values are encoded in the features and constraints of the digital artefact — remains a future task. This layered approach ensures values are not post-rationalised but progressively embedded throughout the design process.

While the technological artefact itself has not yet been implemented, the methodology corresponds to what Poel and Kroes (2014) define as the intended value (designers' aspirations) and contributes to shaping the embodied value (those embedded in the future system). The realised value, in contrast, will only emerge through real-world use in future project phases. By recognising this temporal layering of value expression, the approach maintains methodological integrity while anchoring design in value-sensitive foresight. However, despite the availability of ICT devices and accessibility features, awareness and literacy in using ICT devices remain significant barriers to improving patients' QoL. A study found that awareness of these features is particularly low among older patients (Hirayama et al., 2025). Proactive support and early education on ICT accessibility are necessary, especially for older patients and those with milder symptoms, as existing support for this group is often insufficient. Extended Reality (XR) offers a new frontier for emotional and embodied communication, moving beyond the limitations of traditional AAC for ALS patients. While XR has the potential to enhance satisfaction and communication through immersive experiences, its successful adoption is influenced by critical factors like digital health literacy, socioeconomic status, and generational differences. A user-centred design approach is essential, as patient characteristics and a lack of involvement in the design process can be significant barriers to adoption and lead to user dissatisfaction and abandonment (Curran & Hollett, 2024). These gaps in awareness and support must be addressed to ensure that digital health solutions can effectively enhance a patient's QoL in collaboration with their caregivers.

The integration of the ALSFRS-R/EX, UEQ+, and CME Grid generated a layered and complementary set of findings that reflect both the functional limitations and lived experiences of PALS with partial LIS. These preliminary analyses were organised into four key thematic insights:

THEMATIC INSIGHTS

1. Diverse Emotional Responses and Personal Preferences

Participants (henceforth coded as A, I, J, M, and U for the patients and JC for one of the caregivers) expressed a wide range of emotional reactions to the drawing-based activities, shaped by their personal histories, emotional states, and disease progression.

- **A** displayed profound emotional investment, reporting reduced fatigue after a 90-minute session and expressing a desire to represent intimate, sensory memories— "the path of water during a shower."
- **J,** initially anxious and hesitant, responded well to social scaffolding and metaphorical framing (e.g., "drawing music"), gradually building confidence.

- **M,** whose session was marked by silence and limited expression, revealed through his caregiver's feedback a heightened sense of proprioception —his drawings, described as "the most meaningful" by his partner, appeared as symbolic expressions of withheld emotion, particularly around themes of abandonment and dignity.
- **U**, though physically constrained, showed motivation and curiosity. His caregiver noted the novelty and "controlled freedom" of the drawing experience as a rare opportunity for expressive agency.
- **I**, the only female participant, responded with sustained attention and humour. Despite respiratory and postural limitations, she remained focused and contributed actively, showing notable affective uplift and communicative desire, particularly when given space for visual storytelling.

2. Motor-Cognitive Imbalance

Data from the CME Observation Grid reinforced a consistent gap between cognitive clarity and motor ability across all five participants.

- While **A** exemplified this with visible frustration caused by motor delay, both **I** and **M** demonstrated strategic compensations—adjusting posture or gesture rhythm to maintain control, even if visually subtle.
- **U**, despite his curiosity, encountered barriers in the physical translation of mental imagery, requiring continuous framing and support.

This imbalance confirms the need for low barriers of adoption, latency-compensating digital systems that accommodate intentional delay and micro-movement variability.

3. The Value of Framing and Onboarding

All participants benefited from explicit instruction, metaphorical cues, and structured introductions to tasks.

- **J's** response to musical metaphor underscores the power **of framing techniques** in activating emotional and cognitive engagement.
- **I**, who began her session with uncertainty, quickly attuned to metaphorical prompts, demonstrating that onboarding is not merely functional but emotionally enabling.

This finding suggests that adaptive onboarding, including demonstrations, metaphors, and co-narration, should be embedded within digital systems targeting ALS users.

4. Empowerment Through Embodiment

Despite severe physical limitations, participants experienced moments of embodied empowerment during drawing.

- Observers noted postural shifts, eye-brightening, and affective signals (smiles, deep breaths, laughter) at key moments of expression or recognition.

- The UEQ+ scores across all users increased in metrics related to stimulation, novelty, and perceived control, particularly after the second and third tasks.

These findings support the notion that minimal embodied gestures, when anchored in meaning and responsiveness, can produce emotional and psychological benefits, including a reduction in communicative anxiety.

IMPLICATIONS FOR ADAPTIVE DESIGN

The variability in physical, emotional, and communicative capacity among participants highlights the need for highly adaptive digital tools that reflect the progressive nature of ALS.

- **Early-stage users** (e.g., I, J) showed engagement with paper-based and gesture-based interfaces.
- **Later-stage profiles** (e.g., M) may require interfaces that support non-traditional inputs—like slow tracking, eye gaze, or assisted motion.
- Caregivers also provided feedback about comfort, headset weight, and fatigue, emphasising that adaptability must include not only input modalities but also ergonomic and sensory dimensions.

Together, these findings reinforce the value of ethically grounded, user-centred design strategies that go beyond accessibility to account for emotional, cognitive, and interpersonal needs in evolving health conditions.

PERSONAS AND USER SCENARIOS: ENRICHING DESIGN FORESIGHT

Based on the specific and highly individual needs of each patient, our tailored persona approach was developed to achieve truly humanised care by moving beyond assumptions of a homogeneous user profile. By creating individual representations of our participants, we acknowledge the diversity and complexity of their motor and communication abilities, as well as their unique preferences, communication, needs, and available resources. This method directly informs our Tailored Design approach, ensuring that our solutions are as distinct as the individuals they are meant to serve.

Even though our approach differs from the traditional methodology, we believe that creating individualised personas achieves all the advantages championed by Lene Nielsen (2019). By creating empathetic and detailed descriptions of our participants, the method breaks away from the automated and individual perception of each team member. Instead, the project team shares a common and aligned understanding of the users, which allows for more effective communication and more informed decision-making.

As an output, a set of five detailed Personas was constructed to encapsulate the diversity of PALS participating in the study. These included A, I, J, M, and U— 5 males, one female, aged between 49 and 68, at different stages of disease progression and with varying emotional and social profiles. These Personas were developed iteratively, combining observational data, semi-structured interviews, field session reports, and caregiver feedback.

Each Persona integrates functional characteristics (ALSFRS-R/EX scoring), emotional and motivational cues, personal narratives, and interaction patterns with technology.

Table 2. M. Persona (PALS)

<table>
<tr><td colspan="4">PERSONA M. — Age 59</td></tr>
<tr><td colspan="4">Biographical Snapshot</td></tr>
<tr><td colspan="4">Manuel is a resilient and deeply expressive man whose laughter continues to fill the room despite having lost his voice to ALS. His communication now takes place through a combination of gestures, facial cues, and screen-based text—yet he retains a strong presence and emotional expressiveness. His relationship with his wife is marked by affection, silent understanding, and mutual respect. Even though he experiences swallowing difficulties and requires a PEG, he maintains a sense of agency and independence, driving himself to therapies and engaging socially with warmth and humour.</td></tr>
<tr><td colspan="4">Affectionate, emotionally warm, empathetic and values mutual care.
Independent, determined, and methodical in adapting to his condition.
Emotionally stable; displays resilience and humour in the face of adversity.
Shows reflective and creative coping strategies, but no clear evidence of imaginative or artistic pursuits beyond emotional engagement</td></tr>
<tr><td>Occupation</td><td>Residence</td><td>Marital status</td><td>ALS diagnosis</td></tr>
<tr><td>On medical leave (employed at an automotive mirror manufacturing company)</td><td>Carregosa, Aveiro (Portugal)</td><td>Married (to Graça), two children – a daughter (Cátia) and a son (Pedro)</td><td>First symptoms appeared in December 2023; formal diagnosis in August 2024</td></tr>
<tr><td>Follow-up at APELA</td><td>Disease progression</td><td colspan="2">Therapy routine at APELA</td></tr>
<tr><td>Since December 2023 (diagnosis confirmed August 2024)</td><td>Moderate (neither slow nor rapidly progressing)</td><td colspan="2">Weekly sessions – 1x Speech Therapy (ST) and 1x Physiotherapy (PT); also attended therapy locally, currently on hold due to renewal of the first prescription cycle (P1)</td></tr>
<tr><td colspan="4">Five-Factor Personality Profile</td></tr>
<tr><td>Trait</td><td>Level</td><td colspan="2">Justification</td></tr>
<tr><td>Extraversion</td><td>Moderate to High</td><td colspan="2">Communicates expressively despite being non-verbal; enjoys social engagement</td></tr>
<tr><td>Agreeableness</td><td>Very High</td><td colspan="2">Affectionate, emotionally warm, empathetic and values mutual care</td></tr>
<tr><td>Conscientiousness</td><td>High</td><td colspan="2">Independent, determined, and methodical in adapting to his condition</td></tr>
<tr><td>Neuroticism</td><td>Low to Moderate</td><td colspan="2">Emotionally stable; displays resilience and humour in the face of adversity</td></tr>
<tr><td>Openness</td><td>Moderate</td><td colspan="2">Shows reflective and creative coping strategies, but no clear evidence of imaginative or artistic pursuits beyond emotional engagement</td></tr>
</table>

BIOGRAPHY

Manuel enters the room with a firm stride. He carries a wide smile and a laugh that fills the space before any words are spoken. He no longer speaks—Amyotrophic Lateral Sclerosis (ALS) has taken his voice—but his laughter remains. And what laughter it is! Loud, vibrant, irresistible. A smile that shakes his shoulders and wrinkles his eyes until they nearly close. The kind of laugh that draws another out of you, as if it were an invitation.

He is married, and it only takes a glance at him with his wife to sense the affection that binds them. No need for words or touch—there is tenderness in their exchanged looks, in their knowing smiles, and in the small, silent gestures. Graça understands him with a glance, anticipates his needs, laughs with him—and at times, for him. They are two bodies deeply familiar with one another, two presences that remain connected even in silence.

Manuel refuses to be treated as dependent. He drives himself to therapy, hands steady on the wheel, with a determination no one dares challenge. He arrives, switches off the car, and picks up his communication device, skilfully manoeuvring it with the fingers he still controls. He greets others with a wave, a playful grimace, or a raised eyebrow. He speaks with his body, with his face, and with his hands. He needs no sound to make himself seen or felt.

His arms move well, as do his hands. At first glance, ALS does not seem to have taken much from him—but it's during meals that his body resists. Eating causes him to choke easily; sometimes, even a sip is enough. In those moments, everything stops—he focuses, breathes carefully. There's a tense silence, as though each meal requires delicate vigilance. Because of this, and the anxiety it caused, he had to undergo a Percutaneous Endoscopic Gastrostomy (PEG). When he was told, he didn't reply. There was no joke, just silence and a long pause. It was as if—for the first time—the illness had won a small battle within him. He didn't want it, but it had to be done. And it hurts.

Today, he lives with the PEG as though it were part of him—accepted but never forgotten. Moments of hidden sadness still surface now and then, but then the laughter returns. A laugh that is not silent and never has been.

Outside of mealtimes, saliva often escapes, especially when he laughs. It doesn't seem to bother him much—or if it does, he doesn't show it. He picks up a tissue, wipes it away with a calm, almost automatic motion, and quickly resumes smiling.

Communication happens through a small screen, where he writes patiently and persistently. He points with what he has, improvises with gestures. Manuel lives this way—with the body he has, with what life still allows, and with all that his gestures can say. His language is made of laughter, of glances, of presence. And in the shared understanding with his wife, he finds the strength that keeps him upright—and smiling—every day.

Goals

- To continue living with quality, dignity, and joy
- To communicate effectively
- To maintain independence
- To feel included, not pitied
- To nurture meaningful relationships (with spouse, children, friends, therapists)
- To manage and minimise uncomfortable situations

Needs

- A simple, fast, and intuitive expression device, with shortcut functions
- Accessible and cognitively friendly environments for social interaction
- Privacy and respect in both personal and care-related interactions

Opportunities

- Silent, discreet interfaces for quick communication

- Integration of humour and personality within the communication device
- Personalised products for oral hygiene with inclusive design
- Interfaces that respect the user's pace and value non-verbal communication
- Inclusive social experiences, such as companion apps that do not rely on speech

To complement the ALS patient Personas, we developed Caregiver Personas. For the caregiver personas, we followed a more traditional approach; they were developed based on semi-structured interviews and participatory observation of both formal and informal caregivers. These Personas extend the project's commitment to relational design by capturing the emotional, physical, and ethical labour performed by caregivers within the Six ecosystem. For example, AC, a professional caregiver, embodies values such as dignity through humour, empathic boundaries, and presence-as-support, while JC, a full-time informal caregiver, illustrates the tensions between emotional proximity, anticipatory grief, and motivational resilience. These profiles were essential in shaping the relational use scenarios, and in imagining how future digital tools could act not only as assistive systems but also as relational interfaces, designed to work *with*, *through*, and *for* both patients and caregivers.

Crucially, these Personas served not only as narrative artefacts but as design probes—allowing the team to simulate user interaction with future digital tools, anticipate friction points, and foreground values such as dignity, autonomy, humour, resilience, and expressivity. In alignment with Value Sensitive Design, these Personas enabled the identification of *value tensions*, for instance: A's need for expressivity vs. his growing motor fatigue; J's preference for clarity and control vs. the ambiguity of open-ended drawing tasks; or Us' attachment to family rituals vs. his fear of losing non-verbal communication.

By articulating these lived contradictions, the Personas reinforced the need for adaptive, emotionally responsive, and ethically embedded interfaces. They also served as communication tools across the interdisciplinary team, ensuring that design choices remained grounded in user diversity, rather than a universalised patient ideal.

In addition to Personas, we developed User Scenarios to represent the relational use dynamics between patients and their formal or informal caregivers. The engaging perspective championed by Nielsen (Nielsen, 2019) posits that stories are the most effective tool for creating deep empathy and insight. Our user scenario for M aligns perfectly with this philosophy, as it constructs a vivid and humanised narrative of his daily life instead of focusing on static data or isolated behaviours. This approach allows the project team to move away from a stereotypical view of a user with ALS—one centred solely on functional limitations—and to actively immerse themselves in his complete experience, which includes his dignity, humour, and interpersonal relationships. In this way, the scenario not only informs the team about M.'s needs but also enables designers to emotionally engage with his journey, ensuring that the technological solutions developed are genuinely resonant and person-centred.

This narrative technique enabled us to anticipate interaction flows, emotional turning points, and ergonomic friction points during envisioned XR/VR drawing sessions. For example, J, a formal caregiver for A, is portrayed not only as a physical and technical aide but also as an emotional interpreter and facilitator of dignity during co-creative experiences. His scenario highlights needs such as preventing neck fatigue, establishing trust through onboarding, and utilising humour as a design ally.

The development of our personas and scenarios was guided by the principle that these methods provide designers with a deeper understanding of users and their specific use situations. By employing engaging personas and narrative scenarios, the project team was able to place the user at the very centre of the design process, ensuring that the focus remained on their needs and experiences rather than on the system itself. This approach proved instrumental in influencing our design solutions, as a greater understanding of the users' lives and challenges led to more empathetic and user-centred outcomes.

Table 3. M. User Scenario (PALS)

User Scenario: Manuel in the SiX Project
Communicating with the World: A Wordless XR Expression Session
Persona
Manuel (63 years old, married, father of two, diagnosed with ALS for 3 years, moderate progression, ALSFRS-R score: 32/48. Communicates via writing device. Has a PEG. Maintains arm and hand mobility. Informal caregiver: his wife, Maria da Graça.)
Scenario
Manuel wakes around 7:30 a.m. He stays in bed a few more minutes, listening to the morning activity in the house. Graça is already up, and he hears familiar kitchen sounds—the yoghurt being stirred, the supplement being prepared, the clink of pills. She enters the room with everything ready, as always: practical and attentive. He thanks her with a smile and starts the day slowly. Still having strength in his arms, he administers his PEG supplement himself using the syringes Graça has set aside. He showers calmly, taking particular care around the PEG site, as he was taught. He gets dressed with some help from Graça but insists on doing what he can himself—he dislikes being over-assisted. Once ready, they have breakfast together at the table. Few words are spoken, yet much is communicated. Their humour is ever-present—even if it's just a raised eyebrow or a playful grimace. Today is activity day at the APELA centre. Manuel drives carefully with Graça beside him. Upon arrival, he greets everyone with a cheeky expression—already well known for his dry humour and animated expressions. The XR session begins with setting up the equipment. He adjusts his communication device and prepares his humorous shortcuts. He wants to show who he is—without needing words. The session's task is to create a digital mural using shapes and colours. Manuel thrives—he chooses extravagant elements, adds short phrases, and sparks laughter in the group. Mid-session, he pauses to wipe saliva naturally. It doesn't bother him. At the end, he feels proud. On his screen, he types: "I felt like an artist!" On the drive home, he's already thinking about what to create next time. That evening, they have an early dinner, watch a film, or simply sit on the sofa. At 10 p.m., he heads to bed and sleeps with his ventilator. But he goes to sleep feeling that—even without a voice—he had plenty to say.
Manuel's Goals in the Scenario
To take part in a co-creative XR art session using gestures and expressions as tools for communication and creation. He aims to: ● Express himself without words ● Share his humour and imagination with others ● Feel productive and acknowledged ● Engage in something creative and light-hearted that does not reduce him to his condition.
Context
Location: APELA activity room or adapted home environment **Activity**: Collaborative art session in XR — participants create "digital murals" using shapes, colours, and text, with simple gestures or personalised shortcuts **Device**: Manual adapted controller or eye-tracking system to select shapes, emojis, and short pre-set phrases **Support**: Graça is present, but steps back; a SiX team facilitator provides technical support as needed
Steps Taken by Manuel During the Session

continued on following page

Table 3. Continued

User Scenario: Manuel in the SiX Project

Arrival and Preparation
● Enters with a wide smile and playful expression
● Graça helps with equipment setup but allows him space to act independently
● Adjusts his communication device and sets up quick-access phrases like:
  ● *"More colour!"*
  ● *"This is a mess"*
  ● *"What do you think of this?"*
 	
Introduction and Reassurance
● The facilitator explains the activity:
"Let's build an XR mural together that shows who we are—without words."
● Manuel responds with a winking emoji and points at the screen:
"Let's go!"
 	
Creative Interaction
● Selects vibrant colours and unexpected shapes, combining them with humour
● Adds short phrases to the mural, such as:
  ● *"Looks like an '80s rug"*
  ● *"I need a unicorn here!"*
● Laughs at others' creations, wiping saliva casually in between
● Uses expressive gestures to engage—raising eyebrows, making approving faces, and joking playfully
 	
Social Dynamics
● Graça watches proudly and joins in briefly when invited
● Manuel feels included, generates laughter, and contributes "visual jokes" to the mural
● His non-verbal communication is acknowledged and valued, despite his lack of speech
 	
Closing the Session
● The facilitator asks how he felt. He types:
"I felt like an artist!"
● He offers feedback on the system:
  ● Faster access to humorous expressions
  ● Improved device responsiveness
● He thanks the team via screen:
"That was fun. I'd love to do it again!"

Expected Outcomes
● Manuel feels like an active participant, not infantilised ● He communicates effectively and expressively ● He laughs, creates, and feels understood ● Graça is reassured by seeing him included and respected
What the SiX Team Learns
● Insights into how non-verbal communication can be amplified ● Understanding of interaction pacing for users with drooling challenges ● How to design visual communication tools infused with humour and personality
Key Design Considerations for the SiX Team
● Customisable shortcuts for phrases and emotions (with icons, colour, and sound) ● Touch or gesture-based interface for users with limited but functional hand mobility ● Integration of humour and expressiveness into the creative process ● Tolerance for user-paced interaction—no pressure for immediate responses ● Visual elements that enable wordless creation (emojis, symbols, dynamic colours)
Notes for the SiX Team
● Manuel values experiences that let him be himself—playful, provocative, expressive. ● Activities that place him on equal footing with others, even without speech, are essential. ● His communication is more emotional than literal—the system must reflect this. ● Laughter and lightness are his forms of resistance and connection—they matter deeply.

FUTURE USER JOURNEY MAPS

As part of the future work, the team plans to co-develop Journey Maps with informal caregivers, such as JC, to identify key moments of emotional alignment, confusion, and mutual creativity. These mapped experiences will inform interface features, including visual/sonic feedback, pause scaffolding, and headset weight distribution. These contributions will align with Value Sensitive Design's empirical layer, while extending it into the ethics of co-dependence, embodied friction, and shared expressivity in degenerative contexts.

This qualitative input enriched our understanding, grounding it not only in clinical observation but also in lived, intimate relational patterns. The interview data directly supported the conceptual and empirical layers of VSD, helping the team surface not only what patients do but also *why they do it*, *with whom*, and *what it means* to them.

DISCUSSION

The insights generated from this study resonate with broader debates in human-computer interaction and assistive technology, particularly around the ethics and efficacy of designing with — rather than for — users with severe neuromotor impairments. Building on frameworks such as participatory sense-making and embodied interaction, the findings support the view that co-designed methods yield more than usability insights: they illuminate the tacit, affective, and embodied dimensions of communication.

This approach aligns with and extends insights from Casal-Moldes et al. (2024), who explored affective interfaces for non-verbal users through creative, embodied co-design. Their study emphasised the value of low-threshold creative activities in capturing self-expression among ALS patients with minimal voluntary control. The current chapter builds on this by showing how even limited movement — when framed through affectively rich and sensorily engaging activities — can produce valuable cues about user intentionality, motivation, and emotional state.

Notably, the discussion highlights a methodological contribution: tailoring assessment tools better to reflect the evolving agency of users with progressive conditions. The dynamic interplay between ALSFRS-R/EX (physical thresholds), UEQ+ (subjective-experiential reporting), and CME (real-time behavioural indicators) generates a multi-modal perspective that is essential when users face fluctuating or diminishing capabilities. While traditional UX evaluation often prioritises performance metrics, our approach emphasises human factors, emotional resonance, and engagement as essential criteria for assistive design.

These findings affirm that value-sensitive approaches are essential when designing technologies for neurodegenerative conditions such as ALS. Rather than seeking to normalise experience across users, this work reflects the VSD emphasis on contextual specificity and longitudinal adaptability. Participants' cultural, educational, and familial dynamics shaped not only how they engaged with the drawing tasks, but how they interpreted the act of participation itself. Incorporating these differences systematically into the design process advances VSD's goal of embedding core human values—autonomy, expressiveness, and relationality—into both process and outcome.

Moreover, the data underscore the necessity for anticipatory design — systems that evolve with the user's progression. From an interaction design standpoint, this reinforces the need for XR environments that are modular, reconfigurable, and sensitive to embodied variability. The use of metaphor, sensory scaffolding, and emotionally relevant content proved especially effective for onboarding and sustained engagement.

The participatory drawing workshops also revealed the role of friction — physical, cognitive, and emotional — as a site of both disruption and meaning. While conventional usability frameworks tend to minimise friction, recent perspectives in VSD and critical HCI suggest that designed friction can illuminate user values and foster more deliberate, reflective interaction (Baumer & Brubaker, 2017; Shilton, 2012). In both workshops, the control group and ALS field sessions, moments of frustration often coincided with creative re-routing, emotional articulation, or user-led adaptation. Rather than viewing these solely as deficits, we interpret friction as ethically and affectively generative — a force that deepens understanding of the user's relationship with their condition, their agency, and the system itself.

These results underscore the importance of grounding design in embodied engagement and residual motor capacities. Case studies using immersive XR with ALS patients highlight how virtual environments can scaffold both expressive agency and therapeutic stimulation, particularly when aligned with patients' affective and sensorimotor profiles (Hernández et al., 2022; Barchielli et al., 2025).

Rather than treating user feedback as passive data, participatory frameworks recognise that meaning emerges through embodied interaction and shared interpretation. This is particularly relevant in neuro-degenerative contexts, where non-verbal communication, gesture, and social co-regulation play critical roles in shaping technological engagement (van der Linden & Wright, 2021).

Ultimately, this chapter argues that designing for ALS patients — particularly those on the LIS spectrum — demands an expanded understanding of relational, emotional, and imaginative aspects of user experience. These insights contribute to a growing recognition that digital health innovation must move beyond accessibility checklists and toward ethically grounded, aesthetically sensitive, and progressively adaptive systems.

CONCLUSION

This chapter has demonstrated a novel methodological framework for designing assistive technologies for individuals with ALS, particularly those in the early stages of Locked-In Syndrome. Developed within the SiX Project, this approach successfully moves beyond traditional functional assessments by combining a holistic triangulation of data from a suite of key instruments: the ALS Functional Rating Scale-Revised (ALSFRS-R/EX), a customized User Experience Questionnaire Plus (UEQ+), a bespoke Cognitive-Motor-Emotional (CME) Observation Grid, a Semi-Structured Participatory Questionnaire, and Semi-Structured Interviews with Caregivers. This multi-instrument, empathetic approach provides a robust and replicable model for researchers and designers, yielding both practical insights and theoretical advancements in the domain of digital health.

A significant strength of this methodology lies in its foundation in Human-Centred Design (HCD), Participatory Design, and Co-Design practices, which ensured that users were active participants in creating solutions that are not only functional but also emotionally resonant and dignifying. By integrating the conceptual, empirical, and technical components of Value Sensitive Design (VSD) (Friedman, Kahn, & Borning, 2002), the project demonstrates how pre-interface, paper-based participatory methods can yield actionable insights for designing adaptive and inclusive assistive technologies.

Ultimately, the findings advocate for an experience-centred design philosophy that foregrounds the affective and relational dimensions of the user experience. Rather than viewing technology in purely functional terms, the design process must engage with users' personal narratives, identities, and emotional landscapes. As Wright and McCarthy (2010) argue, technologies must be situated within the lived realities and evolving stories of their users, emphasising embodied experience and the social dimensions, especially when addressing conditions that challenge expressive agency.

The collaborative protocols and real-time observational methods developed in this research are highly adaptable and can be replicated in a wide range of assistive technology projects, particularly those involving progressive neuromotor conditions. Future research should build on this foundation with longitudinal evaluations of digital systems, ensuring that adaptive solutions remain relevant as users' conditions change. Ultimately, our work calls for strengthening participatory frameworks by involving users not only as test subjects but as co-creators in the shaping of their technological futures, thereby ensuring that digital health innovation is truly rooted in dignity, creativity, and human connection.

ACKNOWLEDGMENTS

Research has been conducted within the ambit of the project "Drawing for Social Re-connectivity. Exploring Inclusive, Collaborative and Digital Environments for Patients with Partial to Complete Locked-In Syndrome." DOI https://doi.org/10.54499/2023.11224.PEX

This work was funded by Fundação para a Ciência e Tecnologia (FCT), under HEI-Lab R&D Unit (UIDB/05380/2020, https://doi.org/10.54499/UIDB/05380/2020).

The authors acknowledge the use of OpenAI's ChatGPT-4 (March 14 version) and Google's Gemini for assistance with refining the language and grammar of this manuscript. The authors reviewed and edited the content as needed and took full responsibility for the final publication.

REFERENCES

Amado, P., Penedos-Santiago, E., Giesteira, B., de Sousa, A., Lima, C., & Simões, S. (2025). Drawing closer: Designing haptic mixed reality interfaces for individuals with incomplete locked-in syndrome to enhance expression and communication. In Blashki, K., & Xiao, Y. (Eds.), *Proceedings of the IHCI 2025 + GET 2025 + CGVCVIP 2025.*, https://www.ihci-conf.org/

Amado, P., Penedos-Santiago, E., Lima, C., Simões, S., Giesteira, B., & Peçaibes, V. (2026). Challenges and opportunities for designing digital communication interfaces for persons with partial locked-in syndrome. In Brooks, A. L., Banakou, D., & Ceperkovic, S. (Eds.), *ArtsIT, Interactivity and Game Creation. ArtsIT 2024. Lecture Notes of the Institute for Computer Sciences, Social Informatics and Telecommunications Engineering* (Vol. 651). Springer., DOI: 10.1007/978-3-031-97257-7_9

Aparicio, A. (2015). Immobilis in mobili: Performing arts, BCI, and locked-in syndrome. *Brain-Computer Interfaces*, *2*(2–3), 150–159. DOI: 10.1080/2326263X.2015.1100366

Barchielli, C., Jayousi, S., & Guarducci, S.. (2025). Extended reality and information and communications technology in therapy: Enhancing remote artistic and recreational engagement for physically impaired and socially isolated patients. *Digital Health*, *11*. Advance online publication. DOI: 10.1177/20552076251350440

Baumer, E. P. S., & Brubaker, J. R. (2017). Post-userism. In *Proceedings of the ACM Conference on Human Factors in Computing Systems (CHI 2017)* (pp. 6291–6303). https://doi.org/DOI: 10.1145/3025453.3025740

Branco, M. P., Pels, E. G. M., & Sars, R. H.. (2021). Brain–computer interfaces for communication: Preferences of individuals with locked-in syndrome. *Neurorehabilitation and Neural Repair*, *35*(3), 267–279. DOI: 10.1177/1545968321989331

Brooks, B. R., Miller, R. G., Swash, M., & Munsat, T. L. (2000). El Escorial revisited: Revised criteria for the diagnosis of amyotrophic lateral sclerosis. *Amyotrophic Lateral Sclerosis and Other Motor Neuron Disorders*, *1*(5), 293–299.

Caiado, F., & Ukolov, A. (2025). The history, current state and future possibilities of non-invasive brain–computer interfaces. *Medicine in Novel Technology and Devices*, *25*, 100353. DOI: 10.1016/j.medntd.2025.100353

Casal-Moldes, Á., Campo-Prieto, P., Rodríguez-Fuentes, G., & Cancela-Carral, J. M. (2024). Multisensory stimulation in amyotrophic lateral sclerosis disease: Case report of an innovative proposal through immersive virtual reality. *Applied Sciences (Basel, Switzerland)*, *14*(20), 9238. DOI: 10.3390/app14209238

Cedarbaum, J. M., Stambler, N., Malta, E., Fuller, C., Hilt, D., Thurmond, B., & Nakanishi, A. (1999). The ALSFRS-R: A revised ALS functional rating scale that incorporates assessments of respiratory function. *Journal of the Neurological Sciences*, *169*(1–2), 13–21. DOI: 10.1016/S0022-510X(99)00210-5

Curran, V. R., & Hollett, A. (2024). The use of extended reality (XR) in patient education: A critical perspective. *Health Education Journal*, *83*(4), 338–351. DOI: 10.1177/00178969231198955

Czamanski-Cohen, J., & Weihs, K. L. (2016). The bodymind model: A platform for studying the mechanisms of change induced by art therapy. *The Arts in Psychotherapy*, *51*, 63–71. DOI: 10.1016/j.aip.2016.09.005

Friedman, B. (2004). Value-sensitive design. In Bainbridge, W. S. (Ed.), *Encyclopedia of Human–Computer Interaction* (pp. 769–774). Berkshire Publishing.

Friedman, B., Kahn, P. H., & Borning, A. (2002). Value sensitive design: Theory and methods. *University of Washington Technical Report*. https://www.researchgate.net/publication/228970457

Friedman, B., Kahn, P. H., & Borning, A. (2013). Value sensitive design and information systems. In *Early Engagement and New Technologies: Opening Up the Laboratory* (pp. 55–95). Springer. https://doi.org/DOI: 10.1007/978-94-007-7844-3_4

Gonçalves, F., & Magalhães, B. (2022). Effects of prolonged interruption of rehabilitation routines in amyotrophic lateral sclerosis patients. *Palliative & Supportive Care*, *20*(3), 369–374. DOI: 10.1017/S1478951521000584

Gonçalves, F., Teixeira, M. I., Rego, F., & Magalhães, B. (2025). The role of spiritual care management: Needs and resources in people with amyotrophic lateral sclerosis. *Palliative & Supportive Care*, *23*, e111. DOI: 10.1017/S1478951525000495

Hardiman, O., Al-Chalabi, A., Chio, A., Corr, E. M., Logroscino, G., Robberecht, W., Shaw, P. J., Simmons, Z., & van den Berg, L. H. (2017). Amyotrophic lateral sclerosis. *Nature Reviews. Disease Primers*, *3*, 17071. DOI: 10.1038/nrdp.2017.7

Hirayama, T., Nagasawa, J., & Shibukawa, M.. (2025). Survey research on the awareness and usage of accessibility features of ICT devices among patients with amyotrophic lateral sclerosis. *Journal of Clinical Neuroscience*, *139*, 111434. DOI: 10.1016/j.jocn.2025.111434

Khan, S., Kallis, L., & Mee, H.. (2025). Invasive brain–computer interface for communication: A scoping review. *Brain Sciences*, *15*(4), 336. DOI: 10.3390/brainsci15040336

Larradet, F., Barresi, G., & Mattos, L. S. (2020). Affective communication enhancement system for locked-in syndrome patients. In M. Antona & C. Stephanidis (Eds.), *Universal Access in Human–Computer Interaction. Design Approaches and Supporting Technologies*. HCII 2020. Lecture Notes in Computer Science (Vol. 12188). Springer. https://doi.org/DOI: 10.1007/978-3-030-49282-3_10

Laugwitz, B., Held, T., & Schrepp, M. (2008). Construction and evaluation of a user experience questionnaire. In *Symposium of the Austrian HCI and Usability Engineering Group* (pp. 63–76). Springer.

Lavazza, A., Balconi, M., & Ienca, M.. (2025). Neuralink's brain–computer interfaces: Medical innovations and ethical challenges. *Frontiers in Human Dynamics, 7*. Advance online publication. DOI: 10.3389/fhumd.2025.1553905

Liu, X.-Y., Wang, W.-L., & Liu, M.. (2025). Recent applications of EEG-based brain–computer interface in the medical field. *Military Medical Research, 12*(1), 14. DOI: 10.1186/s40779-025-00598-z

Masrori, P., & Van Damme, P. (2020). Amyotrophic lateral sclerosis: A clinical review. *European Journal of Neurology, 27*(10), 1918–1929. DOI: 10.1111/ene.14393

Muenssinger, J. I., Halder, S., & Kleih, S. C.. (2010). Brain painting: First evaluation of a new brain–computer interface application with ALS-patients and healthy volunteers. *Frontiers in Neuroscience, 4*. Advance online publication. DOI: 10.3389/fnins.2010.00182

Nielsen, L. (2019). *Personas – User Focused Design* (2nd ed.). Springer.

O'Hara, M. (2024). Live transmission drawing as embodied presence. https://www.morganohara.art

Oppenheim, D. (1971). *Two Stage Transfer Drawing*. [Performance and photographic documentation].

Penedos-Santiago, E., Simões, S., Amado, P., & Giesteira, B. (2025). Drawing for social re-connectivity through collaborative and digital environments: Preliminary drawing activities. In A. Abreu, J. V. Carvalho, A. Mesquita, A. Sousa Pinto, & M. Mendonça Teixeira (Eds.), *Perspectives and Trends in Education and Technology. ICITED 2024*. Lecture Notes in Networks and Systems (Vol. 859). Springer. https://doi.org/DOI: 10.1007/978-3-031-78155-1_23

Poel, I., & Kroes, P. (2014). Can technology embody values? In Kroes, P., & Verbeek, P.-P. (Eds.), *The Moral Status of Technical Artefacts* (pp. 103–124). Springer., DOI: 10.1007/978-94-007-7914-3_7

Rachmad, Y. E. (2017). Digital empathy theory. *Σπάρτη Διεθνής Έκδοση Βιβλίων*, 14(8). https://doi.org/DOI: 10.17605/OSF.IO/9D8NQ

Schnetzer, L., McCoy, M., Bergmann, J., Kunz, A., Leis, S., & Trinka, E. (2023). Locked-in syndrome revisited. *Therapeutic Advances in Neurological Disorders, 16*. Advance online publication. DOI: 10.1177/17562864231160873

Shilton, K. (2012). Values levers: Building ethics into design. *Science, Technology & Human Values, 38*(3), 374–397. DOI: 10.1177/0162243912436985

Shoesmith, C., Abrahao, A., & Benstead, T.. (2020). Canadian best practice recommendations for the management of amyotrophic lateral sclerosis. *Canadian Medical Association Journal, 192*(46), E1453–E1468. DOI: 10.1503/cmaj.191721

Su, W. M., Cheng, Y. F., & Jiang, Z.. (2021). Predictors of survival in patients with amyotrophic lateral sclerosis: A large meta-analysis. *EBioMedicine, 74*, 103732. DOI: 10.1016/j.ebiom.2021.103732

Surma-aho, A., & Hölttä-Otto, K. (2022). Conceptualization and operationalization of empathy in design research. *Design Studies, 78*, 101075. DOI: 10.1016/j.destud.2021.101075

Topol, E. (2019). *Deep medicine: How artificial intelligence can make healthcare human again*. Basic Books.

van der Linden, J., & Wright, P. (2021). Participatory sense-making in human–computer interaction. *ACM Transactions on Computer-Human Interaction*, *28*(5), 1–33.

Vanutelli, M. E., Salvadore, M., & Lucchiari, C. (2023). BCI applications to creativity: Review and future directions, from little-c to C2. *Brain Sciences*, *13*(4). Advance online publication. DOI: 10.3390/brainsci13040665

Wang, Y., Tang, Y., & Wang, Q.. (2025). Advances in brain–computer interface for amyotrophic lateral sclerosis communication. *Brain-X*, *3*(1), e70023. DOI: 10.1002/brx2.70023

Wicks, P., Massagli, M. P., Wolf, C., & Heywood, J. (2009). Measuring function in advanced ALS: Validation of ALSFRS-EX extension items. *European Journal of Neurology*, *16*(3), 353–359. DOI: 10.1111/j.1468-1331.2008.02434.x

Wilson, A. D., & Golonka, S. (2013). Embodied cognition is not what you think it is. *Frontiers in Psychology*, *4*, 58. DOI: 10.3389/fpsyg.2013.00058

Winkler, T., & Spiekermann, S. (2021). Twenty years of value sensitive design: A review of methodological practices in VSD projects. *Ethics and Information Technology*, *23*(1), 17–31. DOI: 10.1007/s10676-020-09545-2

World Medical Association. (2013). World Medical Association Declaration of Helsinki: Ethical principles for medical research involving human subjects. *Journal of the American Medical Association*, *310*(20), 2191–2194. DOI: 10.1001/jama.2013.281053

Wright, P., & McCarthy, J. (2010). *Experience-centered design: Designers, users, and communities in dialogue*. Morgan & Claypool.

KEY TERMS AND DEFINITIONS

Amyotrophic Lateral Sclerosis (ALS): A progressive neurodegenerative disease that affects upper and lower motor neurons, leading to motor impairment, communication challenges, and, in some cases, cognitive and behavioural changes.

Augmentative and Alternative Communication (AAC): Technologies and strategies that support or replace speech for individuals with communication impairments; typically text- or symbol-based, prioritising functional communication but often limited in expressive depth.

Digital Empathy: The capacity of digital systems to mediate, support, or enhance empathic understanding by facilitating emotional expression, recognition, and relational connection within mediated interactions.

Extended Reality (XR): An umbrella term covering immersive technologies such as Virtual Reality (VR), Augmented Reality (AR), and Mixed Reality (MR), used to create interactive environments that enhance communication, engagement, and presence.

Locked-In Syndrome (LIS): A condition characterised by severe motor paralysis with preserved consciousness and cognitive function; in partial LIS, individuals retain limited voluntary control such as minimal speech or eye movement.

Quality of Life (QoL): Refers to an individual's overall perception of well-being, encompassing physical, psychological, social, and functional dimensions as they relate to their health condition, personal goals, and daily activities. In clinical and rehabilitative contexts such as ALS, QoL reflects not only symptom burden and functional capacity but also emotional fulfilment, autonomy, participation, and the ability to derive meaning and connection in everyday life.

Value-Sensitive Design (VSD): A design approach that integrates human values—such as dignity, autonomy, and agency—into technological development through conceptual, empirical, and technical investigations.

Chapter 14

Digital Technology Supporting Medication Adherence:

The Mobili® Automatic Dose Dispenser in Portugal

João Gregório
https://orcid.org/0000-0002-6130-9453
CBIOS, Universidade Lusófona, Portugal

Marta B. Martins
https://orcid.org/0009-0007-2171-7296
CBIOS, Universidade Lusófona, Portugal

Marta de Oliveira Rodrigues
https://orcid.org/0000-0002-6373-092X
CIDESD - Research Center in Sports Sciences, Health Sciences and Human Development, University of Trás-os-Montes and Alto-Douro, Vila Real, Portugal

Lígia Reis
https://orcid.org/0000-0002-5736-3481
CBIOS, Universidade Lusófona, Portugal & Universidad de Alcalá de Henares, Madrid, Spain

Paulo A. S. Moreira
https://orcid.org/0000-0002-5454-7971
CIDESD - Research Center in Sports Sciences, Health Sciences and Human Development, University of Trás-os-Montes and Alto-Douro, Vila Real, Portugal

António Teixeira Rodrigues
Centre for Health Evaluation and Research, National Association of Pharmacies, Lisbon, Portugal & Life and Health Sciences Research Institute, School of Medicine, University of Minho, Braga, Portugal

Melanie Maia
WHO Collaborating Center on Health Workforce Policy and Planning, Global Health and Tropical Medicine, Universidade NOVA de Lisboa, Portugal

Anne-Gerd Granas
University of Oslo, Oslo, Norway

ABSTRACT

This chapter explores the complex relationship between medication adherence, digital health, and patient-centred care (PCC), with a focus on chronic multimorbidity and polypharmacy. It begins by addressing the conceptual evolution of adherence and its determinants, followed by a discussion of how digital technologies can support person-centred approaches to improve therapeutic outcomes. The chapter presents Mobili®, an innovative portable automated dispenser, and outlines the design and implementation of the MobiMAd@PT project in Portugal. Drawing on international evidence and implementation science

DOI: 10.4018/979-8-3373-3531-5.ch014

frameworks, it analyses the usability, effectiveness, and scalability of such interventions. Emphasis is placed on co-design, contextual adaptation, and integrated care models involving community pharmacies. The chapter concludes by outlining best practices for future digital adherence strategies, highlighting the importance of collaborative, user-driven approaches to enhance healthcare quality and sustainability.

INTRODUCTION

The global demographic transition has significantly reshaped public health priorities, with population aging emerging as a defining challenge of the 21st century. As life expectancy increases, healthcare systems face a sharp rise in the prevalence of chronic conditions and multimorbidity—the co-occurrence of two or more chronic illnesses in the same individual (Navickas et al., 2016). This epidemiological shift has profound implications for clinical management and health service delivery, particularly in terms of medication use. In older adults, multimorbidity often leads to complex therapeutic regimens and, consequently, to polypharmacy, typically defined as the concurrent use of five or more medications (Bricca et al., 2023; Masnoon et al., 2017). While clinically justified in many cases, polypharmacy presents significant risks, including drug-drug interactions, adverse events, and, most importantly, poor therapeutic adherence.

Medication adherence—broadly understood as the extent to which patients take medications as prescribed—is a cornerstone of chronic disease management and a key determinant of health outcomes. However, non-adherence remains alarmingly prevalent, especially among individuals managing complex regimens (Foley et al., 2021). In the context of polypharmacy, the barriers to adherence multiply: from forgetfulness and adverse events to low health literacy, demotivation, and inadequate follow-up (Pantuzza et al., 2017; Religioni et al., 2025). As a result, improving medication adherence has become a major public health goal, demanding both multifaceted, multidisciplinary approaches and person-centered strategies.

In recent years, digital health has emerged as a promising frontier to address these challenges. Technologies such as mobile health (mHealth) applications, telemedicine platforms, and smart medication dispensers offer new ways to support patients in managing their treatments, monitor therapeutic behaviors in real-time, and facilitate communication with healthcare providers. These tools align with the broader shift toward patient-centered care (PCC), which emphasizes individual needs, preferences, and active involvement in health decisions. Digital solutions—when well-designed and integrated—can enhance PCC by increasing access to services, personalizing interventions, and enabling continuous support beyond traditional clinical encounters.

This book chapter explores the intersection of polypharmacy, medication adherence, and digital health through a patient-centered lens. It begins by examining the conceptual foundations of therapeutic adherence and the multifactorial determinants that influence it. Building on this, the chapter discusses digital health as a facilitator of adherence, highlighting the technological, behavioural, and organizational aspects of its implementation. Special attention is given to automated dose dispensing technologies, such as Mobili®, and their role in community-based interventions to support medication adherence for older adults with multimorbidity.

Drawing on international evidence and implementation science frameworks, the chapter also presents the case of the MobiMAd@PT project—an initiative which is piloting digital adherence support systems in Portuguese community pharmacies. By situating this intervention within the broader landscape of healthcare innovation, this chapter offers insights into best practices, potential pitfalls, and pathways for scaling patient-centered digital solutions in chronic care. Ultimately, it argues that addressing the polypharmacy–adherence nexus requires not only technological tools, but a fundamental reorientation of care toward the needs, contexts, and voices of patients.

MULTIMORBIDITY, POLYPHARMACY AND MEDICATION ADHERENCE

The demographic transition is increasingly evident across societies and is primarily driven by the aging of the population (Fernandes et al., 2023). As a result of an ever-growing decreased birth rate, aligned with progress in various aspects, such as healthcare, sanitation and living standards, life expectancy has increased worldwide, with those 65 and older being the population segments with the fastest growth rate (Jarzebski et al., 2021; United Nations, 2019). However, as longevity is a significant public health achievement, it also poses an additional challenge: with people living longer, the probability of health problems occurring rises, and chronic issues become more common (Gianfredi et al., 2025).

The advancing of age has been considered the most consistent risk factor for the phenomenon of multimorbidity (Navickas et al., 2016; Nguyen et al., 2019). Estimates suggest that up to 95% of primary care patients aged 65 and older have multimorbidity (Nicholson et al., 2024). However, this is not an issue exclusive to older adults—numerous studies have documented significant prevalence rates among working-age populations, although its frequency increases markedly with age (Ahmed et al., 2025; Bell & Saraf, 2016; Vargese et al., 2020). The consequences of multimorbidity are wide-ranging, encompassing decreased functional capacity, diminished quality of life, increased utilization of healthcare services, and higher mortality rates (Arokiasamy et al., 2015; Koné Pefoyo et al., 2015; Soley-Bori et al., 2021). These impacts underscore the importance of understanding its epidemiology, as doing so is essential for the development of effective strategies and tools aimed at prevention and burden reduction (Head et al., 2021). In this context, the progression from multimorbidity to polypharmacy is often straightforward, as polypharmacy is frequently employed to manage symptoms and prevent complications associated with the coexistence of multiple chronic conditions in a single patient (Schiøtz et al., 2017). The most widely accepted definition describes polypharmacy as the daily use of five or more medications (Bricca et al., 2023) and although it frequently refers to prescription drugs, it also considers over-the-counter medications, dietary supplements and other health products (Masnoon et al., 2017). Although polypharmacy is often a clinical necessity to manage multiple coexisting health conditions, helping to alleviate symptoms and slow disease progression (Delara et al., 2022; Nicholson et al., 2024; Skou et al., 2022), growing concerns have been raised regarding the excessive number of medications prescribed to patients with multimorbidity. Since most patients in a multimorbidity situation are medicated in a single-disease based approach, a number of interrelated issues can arise from polypharmacy, including an increased risk of inappropriate prescriptions, adverse medication events and reactions, prescribing cascades, drug–drug interactions, unplanned hospitalization (Davies et al., 2020; Petrovic et al., 2022; Tommelein et al., 2015), over or under dosage, inadequate patient monitoring and poor adherence (Davies et al., 2020). In such cases, the cumulative burden of treatment may outweigh the intended medication benefits, leading to increased risks of harm (Daunt et al., 2023; Guthrie et al., 2015; Mangin et al., 2018; Nicholson et al., 2024; Pazan & Wehling, 2021).

As the global patient population with polypharmacy is increasing, addressing medication adherence becomes a growing concern (Daunt et al., 2023). Clinical guidelines emphasize that medication adherence is essential for both managing and preventing the long-term consequences associated with multimorbidity (Kernick et al., 2017). However, treatment efficacy remains significantly limited by poor adherence, particularly in the context of chronic disease management (Sendekie et al., 2022). This issue is influenced by multiple factors, among which the complexity of medication regimens plays a central role (Sánchez-Fidalgo et al., 2017). Such complexity—stemming not only from the number of medications prescribed, but also from the diversity of pharmaceutical forms, dosing frequencies, and routes of administration—constitutes a major barrier to consistent adherence (Foley et al., 2021; Pantuzza et al., 2017).

The complexity of the medication regimen a patient is presented with refers to a multitude of aspects of the regimen itself, not merely the quantity of medications; it covers elements like how many doses are taken each day, how many units are in each dose, dosage formats, and other recommendations (Cobretti et al., 2017). Moreover, pharmacotherapeutic features including the quantity of drugs taken at a time and the required schedules, determine how complicated a patient's medication regimen can be (Kassaw et al., 2024). All these factors, besides being frequently overlooked by physicians, increase the likelihood of medical errors, contributing to a greater risk of poor treatment outcomes (Wimmer et al., 2016). Effective strategies to address this issue rely on a collaborative approach between patients and healthcare providers, and include simplifying treatment regimens, enhancing communication, promoting patient education and tailored information, and implementing regular medication adherence monitoring interventions (Pattani et al., 2024).

UNDERSTANDING MEDICATION ADHERENCE: DEFINITIONS, TAXONOMIES, AND CONTRIBUTING FACTORS

Adherence to medication is a multifaceted phenomenon, encompassing a broad range of health-related behaviors that go beyond simply taking prescribed drugs. It reflects the extent to which patients follow medical recommendations regarding medication intake, lifestyle adjustments, and dietary modifications (Sabaté, 2003; World Health Organization, 2003). According to the WHO, adherence is defined as "the extent to which a person's behavior—taking medication, following a diet, and/or executing lifestyle changes—corresponds with agreed recommendations from a healthcare provider" (Sabaté, 2003). It adopts a definition of adherence to chronic disease treatment that results from the integration of the concepts proposed by Haynes, 1979 and Rand, 1993. These authors define adherence as the degree to which an individual's behavior—including medication intake, adherence to a diet, and adoption of lifestyle changes—is in accordance with and consistent with the recommendations provided by healthcare professionals. This definition emphasizes the importance of a collaborative relationship between patients and healthcare professionals, highlighting the central role of communication and shared decision-making (Zelko et al., 2016). Complementing this perspective, (Maffoni et al., 2020) consider treatment adherence not as an end goal in itself, but as a means to achieve a greater goal: maintaining or improving health by reducing the signs and symptoms associated with a particular clinical condition. Adherence to treatment is one of the main challenges in the management of multimorbidity and is influenced by a multitude of interrelated factors. As evidenced by (Maffoni et al., 2020), patients' beliefs and concerns regarding prescribed therapies—namely, how they perceive polypharmacy and how they prioritize different medications—contribute to the complexity of the medication management process. This scenario can intensify the physical and emotional effort required of patients (Valderas et al., 2009).

Although *adherence* is a widely used term in both clinical practice and academic literature, several others—such as *compliance* and *concordance*—have been employed interchangeably over time, often leading to conceptual ambiguity. *Compliance* typically suggests a passive, almost obedient behavior on the part of the patient, implying adherence to taking a medication or using a medical advice without questioning. *Concordance*, on the other hand, emphasizes the negotiation and agreement between the patient and healthcare provider, highlighting shared decision-making. While each term reflects different historical and philosophical perspectives on the patient-provider relationship, their inconsistent usage has contributed to confusion in research and practice.

To address this issue and promote conceptual clarity, a standardized taxonomy of adherence was proposed by (Vrijens et al., 2012) and later expanded by (Bernardo et al., 2023). This comprehensive framework distinguishes three interconnected but conceptually distinct domains:

1. **Adherence to medications**
2. **Management of adherence**
3. **Adherence-related sciences**

The first domain, *adherence to medications*, is process-oriented and can be further subdivided into three key phases:

- **Initiation** refers to the point at which the patient takes the first dose of a prescribed medication.
- **Implementation** reflects the extent to which a patient's actual dosing regimen corresponds with the prescribed regimen, from initiation up to the final dose.
- **Discontinuation** occurs when the patient intentionally or unintentionally ceases the medication before the planned end of therapy.

In addition to these three stages, an important complementary construct is **persistence**, which denotes the duration of time from the first dose to the last dose taken, regardless of whether doses were missed intermittently. Persistence provides a temporal lens to adherence, distinguishing between patients who take medications continuously and those who prematurely interrupt their treatment.

The second domain, **management of adherence**, refers to the set of structured activities undertaken by healthcare systems, professionals, or caregivers to monitor, support, and optimize patients' adherence to prescribed regimens. This may include technological tools (e.g., electronic monitoring), personalized counseling, and systems-level interventions aimed at reducing barriers or enhancing engagement. Importantly, this domain reinforces that adherence is not solely the responsibility of the patient but is influenced by the quality and organization of care delivery.

The third domain, **adherence-related sciences**, encompasses the research fields dedicated to understanding the causes, mechanisms, and consequences of discrepancies between prescribed and actual medication use. This includes disciplines such as behavioral medicine, health psychology, implementation science, and pharmacoepidemiology. By studying these gaps, adherence-related sciences contribute to the development of targeted interventions, health policy, and educational strategies.

Together, these three domains form a robust and operational framework for conceptualizing and analyzing adherence in both clinical and research settings. Their application helps clarify terminology, align multidisciplinary efforts, and ultimately improve patient outcomes by addressing the complexity of real-world medication-taking behavior.

Despite the recognition of adherence as critical to effective treatment outcomes, global rates remain suboptimal. While optimal adherence is estimated around 80% (Parikh et al., 2025), actual adherence in developed countries averages around 50%, and is even lower in underdeveloped settings (Camarneiro, 2021). This gap translates into substantial clinical, economic, and even environmental consequences (Kini & Ho, 2018), reinforcing the urgency of addressing medication non-adherence (MNA) as a global public health priority (World Health Organization, 2003). These percentages are merely a rough estimate because adherence is influenced by a complex array of interrelated factors, which span multiple dimensions of the patient's experience and the healthcare system. These factors are commonly categorized into five key domains: patient-related, therapy-related, condition-related, healthcare system-related, and socioeconomic (Cramer, 1991; Ulley et al., 2019):

- **Patient-related factors** involve a combination of psychological, cognitive, and demographic elements. A patient's mental health status, including the presence of anxiety or depression, can significantly affect their capacity to engage in consistent medication-taking behaviors, especially in the context of chronic illness (Hyvert et al., 2023). Low health literacy and limited understanding of one's condition or prescribed treatments are also strongly associated with poor adherence (Ricke et al., 2023). Inadequate comprehension may lead to incorrect dosing, unintentional non-adherence, or premature treatment discontinuation. Furthermore, demographic characteristics such as age, gender, ethnicity, marital status, and educational background influence medication behaviors through pathways related to access, beliefs, and social roles (Cramer, 1991). Patients with lower levels of self-efficacy or negative beliefs about medication efficacy or safety may also demonstrate lower adherence.
- **Therapy-related factors** primarily concern the nature and complexity of the prescribed treatment regimen. Regimens that require multiple medications—particularly with varying dosing schedules, administration routes, or special storage or timing instructions—impose a significant burden on patients. Elderly individuals, who are frequently subjected to polypharmacy due to multimorbidity, are especially vulnerable to adherence difficulties and prescription errors (Pantuzza et al., 2017; Turgeon et al., 2017). Additionally, adverse drug reactions can be particularly discouraging in long-term therapies, leading patients to discontinue medication independently without medical consultation. The perception of adverse events may outweigh perceived benefits, especially in conditions that are asymptomatic or slowly progressing.
- **Condition-related factors** refer to the characteristics of the illness itself. Chronic diseases that are asymptomatic for long periods or have delayed consequences may be perceived as less urgent by patients, reducing their motivation to adhere strictly to treatment regimens (Cramer, 1991). Diseases requiring lifelong management without immediate symptomatic relief also contribute to treatment fatigue and reduced adherence over time. Moreover, patients with multiple coexisting conditions may struggle to prioritize among medications, particularly if no clear rationale is provided for each therapy, as suggested by (Maffoni et al., 2020).
- **Healthcare system-related factors** encompass the structure, accessibility, and quality of healthcare services. Poor communication between healthcare providers and patients is a well-documented barrier to adherence, as is the lack of clear instructions or follow-up mechanisms. Inadequate consultation time, fragmented care, and the absence of continuity in provider-patient relation-

ships further undermine trust and therapeutic engagement (Areej Bayatra, 2024). In many health systems, logistical barriers such as long waiting times, limited geographic availability of services, and medication shortages can significantly compromise adherence. Structural inequities—such as high out-of-pocket costs or administrative complexity in accessing therapies—exacerbate these challenges, particularly in under-resourced settings.

- **Socioeconomic factors** are among the most consistent and powerful predictors of adherence behavior. Low-income patients are often forced to choose between competing financial demands, leading to medication rationing, dose skipping, or non-initiation of therapies altogether (Cutler et al., 2018). Employment status, housing instability, and educational attainment are closely linked to the capacity to adhere. Importantly, social support networks—whether familial, community-based, or institutional—play a critical role in mediating these effects. The presence of a supportive caregiver or peer can facilitate adherence through reminders, encouragement, and assistance with logistics. Conversely, social isolation is associated with poorer health outcomes and increased rates of non-adherence (Maffoni et al., 2020).

Moreover, different typologies of non-adherence have been described. *Primary non-adherence* occurs when a patient does not fill a new prescription, whereas *secondary non-adherence* refers to the failure to take medication as prescribed despite obtaining it (Jayasree et al., 2024). Furthermore, non-adherence can be intentional—driven by beliefs, adverse events concerns, or mistrust—or unintentional, resulting from forgetfulness, cognitive limitations, or financial constraints (Ricke et al., 2023). In addition to these categories, health system policies, availability of health services, and the overall quality of care delivery—including the nature of the provider-patient relationship—play a crucial role in shaping adherence patterns (Cramer, 1991; Midão et al., 2018). Family and community support may help mitigate individual challenges, fostering proactive engagement with treatment plans. As highlighted by Maffoni et al., 2020, adherence in patients with multimorbidity is particularly challenging, as it often involves prioritizing medications, managing physical and emotional burden, and navigating complex regimens. In this context, non-adherence to medication regimens is associated with worsening clinical conditions, an increase in adverse events, and decreased treatment efficacy, resulting in significant impacts on health and quality of life, especially among the elderly population (Maffoni et al., 2020; Yarnall et al., 2017). In such cases, adherence is not merely a behavioral issue but a systemic one, requiring personalized, patient-centered interventions that consider the full context of the individual's life.

Understanding the interplay between these domains and typologies of adherence is essential for developing effective, patient-centered strategies to improve adherence, in particular if taking medicines correctly (many times daily, before or after food, through many routes such as orally, dermatologically, subcutaneously), is too disrupting to the other daily activities. Addressing them requires a comprehensive, context-sensitive approach that integrates behavioral, structural, and systemic interventions.

Digital Health as an Emerging Solution for Medication Adherence

As described, the complexity of medication regimens due to rising rates of multimorbidity and polypharmacy presents enduring challenges for medication adherence. Digital health interventions have thus emerged as a promising solution (Islam et al., 2024; Miao et al., 2024) encompassing tools like smart dispensers (Foglia et al., 2024; Hänninen et al., 2023), telemonitoring (Miao et al., 2024), apps (Ngo et al., 2022), and remote care platforms (Dang et al., 2024), or even Artificial Intelligence and Chatbots.

AI-driven support tools and chatbots have shown good potential to be of added-value in maintaining adherence, providing real-time behavioral feedback and tailored advice, although robust evidence of its clinical impact is still developing (Z. S. N. Reis et al., 2025).

The use of technology is increasingly playing a significant role in promoting medication adherence, particularly in rural areas, where access to health services and care is often compromised. In this context, Maita et al., 2024 highlight the potential of digital interventions, such as teleconsultations and remote treatment monitoring, as effective solutions to mitigate geographic disparities, promoting continuity and treatment effectiveness. Furthermore, features such as medication reminders and symptom tracking facilitate adherence and enable better communication with healthcare professionals (Jiang et al., 2024).. However, persistent barriers, as poor internet coverage and low digital literacy, point to the need for digital training programs (Maita et al., 2024). Such initiatives can reduce inequalities in access to information and promote more autonomous and confident use of technological tools (Gregório et al., 2023; Norman & Skinner, 2006).

Older adults and disadvantaged groups often struggle with digital tools due to limited technological proficiency and access. Studies emphasize the need for user-centered design and ongoing support to bridge these gaps (Gandapur et al., 2016). Ageing presents an additional barrier, as elderly individuals (often on multiple medications) face cognitive decline and mobility limitations, which hinder adherence. Although technological advances offer promising solutions, like mobile apps with reminders, dosage tracking, and data sharing with healthcare professionals, these depend on the patient's motivation and the active involvement of professionals. Limitations in access and digital literacy reduce the feasibility of these approaches (Christie et al., 2021).

Despite the potential of digital health to improve the management of chronic conditions, its effective implementation requires adaptation to local settings, with a focus on simplicity, accessibility, and the credibility of information (Scott & Mars, 2015). Operational simplicity, advocated by (Trinh et al., 2023), is seen as a critical success factor, especially among populations with lower digital literacy. Developing certified, accessible digital health strategies that are coordinated with traditional care represents a promising path to strengthening medication adherence and improving health outcomes in communities. Some studies reveal that many users, particularly older individuals or those less familiar with technology, express fears about using electronic devices. Additionally, many users find high-pitched or excessively loud sounds uncomfortable, especially in public spaces, leading to devices being turned off or abandoned (Thomas et al., 2021). While some participants feel embarrassed about needing assistance, others show insecurity and fear of making mistakes, which leads them to reject the use of these technologies (Chen & Chan, 2013). Moreover, cognitive barriers, such as memory or comprehension difficulties, and the absence of social support (e.g. family members not properly explaining how devices work) make adoption even more difficult (Holden, 2011; van Westrenen, 2011).

It is also important to recognise that, in cases of greater emotional vulnerability, continuous monitoring of clinical conditions may paradoxically heighten users' anxiety or insecurity. Studies show that dependence on data provided by devices can lead to excessive concern, thereby compromising emotional well-being (Choudhury & Asan, 2021; Etkin, 2016; O'Kane et al., 2008; Simpson & Mazzeo, 2017). On the other hand, some users value symptom monitoring and reminders as facilitators of adherence, especially during periods of low motivation or forgetfulness (Patoz et al., 2021). The key seems to lie in the technologies' ability to adapt to users' real needs—being intuitive, reliable, and integrated into clinical follow-up without replacing it (S. Reis et al., 2024). Effective solutions need user-centered interfaces and clear integration into clinical workflows to ensure acceptability among patients and providers (Islam et al., 2024; Miao et al., 2024). This need for human involvement is also reinforced by concerns about technical reliability: potential failures or misinformation undermine users' trust and reduce adherence (Hartch et al., 2025). Successful digital adherence interventions are often anchored in participatory co-design and robust implementation frameworks, addressing both technical and real-world contextual challenges by providing tailored solutions that take into account systemic and cultural factors (Gregório et al., 2021; Miao et al., 2024).

The Interplay of Digital Health and Patient-Centered Care Approaches

Patient-centered care (PCC) is a philosophy of healthcare that empowers individuals by respecting their preferences, needs, and values, and by actively involving them in all decisions about their health. Originating conceptually in the 1970s, PCC gained prominence when the Institute of Medicine identified it as one of six key dimensions of high-quality care (Alkhaibari et al., 2023). There is no single universal definition of PCC, but common themes include forming a partnership between providers and patients (and often families), treating patients with respect and empathy, individualizing care to patients' values and circumstances, and ensuring patients are well-informed and involved in decision-making (Jo Delaney, 2018). Epstein & Street's influential definition, for example, describes PCC as an approach that "treats patients with respect, recognizes their preferences, engages and involves them, and provides them with knowledge about their illness and care" (Epstein & Street, 2011)In practical terms, PCC is often summarized by the motto "nothing about me, without me," underscoring that healthcare should not occur without the patient's active participation (Backman et al., 2020; Delbanco et al., 2001).

Modern digital health tools have immense potential to support patient-centered care by enhancing access, information-sharing, and patient engagement. Indeed, many digital health solutions are explicitly designed with patient empowerment in mind. For example, patient-facing health records and portals give individuals immediate access to their medical information and test results, enable secure messaging with providers, and offer educational resources. A 2022 systematic review defined such "patient-centered digital health records" as tools that enable two-way information exchange between patients and the health system (e.g. portals tethered to electronic records or personal health record apps). It showed that highly engaged patients using portals/PHRs tend to have better disease knowledge, treatment adherence, and use of preventive services (Brands et al., 2022). Digital health enhances patient-centered care by improving access and convenience, particularly through telehealth and mobile health (mHealth) platforms. Telemedicine enables care delivery at home, benefiting patients in remote or underserved areas, while maintaining care quality and communication. Similarly, mHealth interventions show promise in expanding mental health services in low-resource settings, though their success depends on addressing barriers such as digital literacy, access, and user engagement (Ambalavanan et al., 2025; Kengne Talla et al., 2024). These findings illustrate a key theme: digital health can amplify PCC by breaking down barriers of distance and information asymmetry, thereby bringing patients and providers closer together.

Many digital tools are intentionally built to promote patient self-management and empowerment, aligning with PCC's goal of active patient participation. For instance, mobile apps for chronic disease management often incorporate educational content, symptom tracking, reminders, and feedback loops that help patients take charge of daily decisions (Kitsiou et al., 2025). Crucially, digital health can also facilitate shared decision-making, a core component of patient-centered care. Decision aids delivered via technology have proven effective in engaging patients. A meta-analysis of technology-based contraceptive decision aids, found that such tools improved users' knowledge and led to higher contraceptive uptake and continuation rates compared to usual care (Goueth et al., 2022). By structuring complex information and guiding patients through preference-sensitive decisions, digital aids exemplify how technology can support patients as partners in care decisions, ensuring treatments align with their goals.

Digital innovation is even influencing how we define "value" in healthcare. Value-based care frameworks increasingly incorporate patient-centered metrics – and digital health is seen as a vehicle to achieve those outcomes. A digital health intervention is considered valuable not just for its clinical efficacy or cost-effectiveness, but for how well it engages and benefits the patient from their perspective. This reinforces the idea that PCC and digital health are synergistic: technology should not be adopted for its own sake, but rather as a mean to achieve patient-centered value (better experiences, better engagement, better outcomes). One systematic review of digital maturity frameworks in hospitals identified patient-centered care as a critical dimension, encompassing how well technology enables patients and families to actively participate in their care decisions (Miller & Reihlen, 2023).

While digital tools can enhance patient-centered care, they can also introduce new challenges or even undermine PCC if implemented poorly. One concern is that technology might inadvertently depersonalize the care experience. For example, clinicians worry that excessive screen time (documenting in Electronic Health Records) or algorithmic decision support could reduce face-to-face interaction and empathy (Efthymiou, 2025). This concern highlights the importance of incorporating narrative practices (attention to patient stories, reflective listening) into digital health education can nurture empathy and communication skills in providers. The technology per se isn't the enemy of compassion – but healthcare must deliberately design digital workflows that preserve room for empathy and personal connection.

Another challenge is ensuring equity and access in the digital age. If digital health is to strengthen PCC, it must be accessible to all patients, including those with limited technology access or skills. Patients are more likely to engage with digital tools that feel tailored to them and that respect their privacy and cultural context. Factors like patients' digital literacy, trust in technology, and the perceived personalization of the interaction heavily influence engagement (Ambalavanan et al., 2025). Thus, designers of these tools are now focusing on features like empathetic chatbot dialogue, personalized content, and easy-to-use interfaces to mirror the personal touch of a human caregiver. When these factors are neglected, there's a risk that some patients – particularly those who are older, less tech-savvy, or from marginalized communities – could be left behind, widening disparities (Gregório et al., 2023). PCC demands meeting patients where they are, so digital solutions must be adaptable to different patient needs (e.g. offering multilingual support, low-bandwidth options, or caregiver-mediated use).

In a final analysis, digital health should be seen as an enabler, not a replacement, of patient-centered care. The vision is a healthcare system where a patient can easily access their information, communicate with their caregivers, receive tailored support via apps or telehealth, and know that all these digital touchpoints are coordinated and attuned to their individual needs. Achieving this will require ongoing effort – careful implementation, evaluation, and refinement – but the path is clear. By thoughtfully integrating digital health and PCC, we can move closer to the holy grail of healthcare: not only better outcomes, but also better experiences and partnerships that honor the humanity of every patient.

The Mobili® Automatic Dose Dispenser

Considering the complexity inherent in therapeutic management in contexts of multimorbidity and polypharmacy, and the multiple factors that negatively influence treatment adherence, it is imperative to develop innovative strategies that promote sustainable adherence behaviors. In this context, digital innovation has emerged as a promising resource in promoting therapeutic self-management, particularly in aging and vulnerable populations, by enabling personalized interventions, strengthening communication between users and healthcare professionals, and mitigating behavioral and structural barriers (Batson, 2021). In response to these challenges, a promising example is Mobili®, a portable automatic dose dispensing system (ADD) developed by the Norwegian company MedThings®, which combines dispensing, monitoring, and remote support features in a single device, designed to be easily integrated into patients' daily lives (MedThings, 2024).

Figure 1.

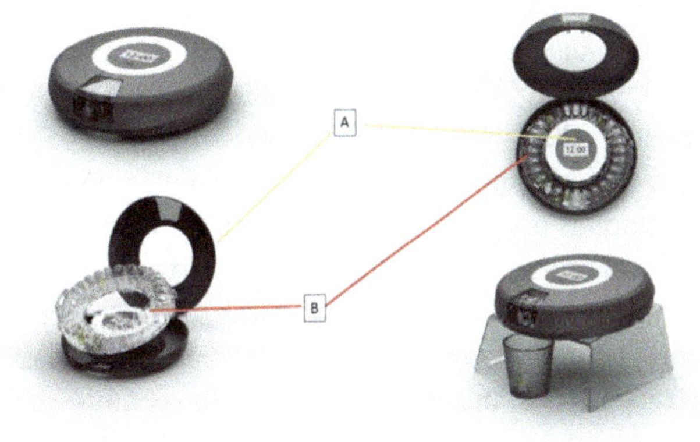

Mobili® is a digital health device designed to support medication adherence by automating the dispensing of pre-packaged doses according to a scheduled treatment plan. It integrates four central components: (1) portability, enabling patients to carry the device independently—unlike many existing automatic dose dispensers (ADDs) that are bulky and poorly suited for everyday use; (2) a reusable eDosette, equipped with a Radio Frequency Identification (RFID) chip, where medications are inserted into designated compartments, allowing for up to 28 scheduled administrations, depending on the complexity of the pharmacological regimen; (3) a real-time monitoring system of adherence, which records every use and enables remote intervention by healthcare professionals, in the event of missed doses or detectable non-adherence patterns;and (4) remote dispensing of extra doses, eliminating the need for healthcare professionals to drive to patients' homes, thereby saving time and fuel. This is in line with the UN Sustainable Development Goals (SDGs), particularly Goal 7 (Affordable and Clean Energy) and Goal 13 (Climate Action) (MedThings, 2024).

The eDosette is a key feature of Mobili®'s design. It functions as a smart, closed medication cassette that prevents unintended use and cross-contamination. Each cassette has 28 compartments which can be pre-filled with the correct medicines for any dose and managed by healthcare personnel in community pharmacies, hospitals, or nursing homes, or even by trained caregivers in coordination with healthcare services in a municipality. The unique RFID system ensures that the correct cassette is inserted every time, reinforcing safety and traceability in medication administration and preventing medication errors, such as medicines being given to the wrong patient. In addition to its physical components, Mobili® includes audible and visual alerts, which serve as behavioral prompts to remind patients to take their medications at the appropriate times. This functionality directly addresses common adherence barriers such as forgetfulness and demotivation. Moreover, the device's digital connectivity and tracking capabilities allow for seamless communication between the patient and healthcare providers, promoting timely adjustments and support. Future solutions will include seamless transfer of information and cassettes when patients move between primary and secondary care facilities.

Compared to more traditional medication administration systems—such as manual pillboxes or stationary automatic dispensers—Mobili® represents a substantial advancement in both technological design and clinical applicability. While older systems may offer partial solutions, they often lack flexibility, real-time monitoring, and user-centered design features that accommodate mobile and active lifestyles (Aldeer et al., 2018). By integrating dose dispensing, portability, remote monitoring and remote dispensing of extra doses of medication into a single solution, Mobili® provides an integrated response to several key adherence barriers, including treatment complexity, lack of supervision, and emotional disengagement often experienced by patients with multimorbidity. Importantly, this system fosters greater self-efficacy and autonomy, enabling early professional intervention when needed, while preserving patient mobility and independence (Aldeer et al., 2018; MedThings, 2024).

When using Mobili®, medicines are dispensed based on a plan determined by the physicians' last prescription. The entire solution is managed from MedThings' cloud solution – Mobili® App - from a PC or a mobile phone. All dispensers are connected to a 4G network so that plans can be easily changed and updated. It is typically used in conjunction with a centralized system and is supervised by healthcare professionals or caregivers. The system not only supports the physical act of medication dispensing but also includes monitoring features that can alert caregivers in cases of missed doses or errors, contributing to early intervention and continuous care support.

Mobili® strengths are:

- **Innovative and User-Friendly Design**: Created by the designer Bjørn Toreid, Mobili® features an appealing and functional design, paired with intuitive technology that ensures ease of use for patients and caregivers alike.
- **Remote Dispensing Capability**: Mobili® enables timely, autonomous medication intake while allowing healthcare professionals to monitor adherence remotely, bridging the gap between patients and care teams—especially in underserved or rural areas.
- **Sustainable Materials:** The device is made from in common materials that are easy to recycle, making it environmentally friendly and aligned with sustainability goals.
- **Advanced Technology Integration:** An in-built RFID chip allows secure and precise communication between the medication cassette and the dispenser, ensuring accurate identification and reducing the risk of errors.

Designed for multiple use cases, Mobili® is particularly effective for managing chronic diseases, making it relevant to a broad spectrum of patients. Its appeal spans a wide age range, from younger individuals requiring medication support to the growing and often socially and physically active population of elderly, whose increasing home dwelling numbers highlight a rising demand for more flexible medication adherence solutions. Moreover, there is growing interest from hospitals, primary care systems and municipalities for systems that are flexible and traceable, recognizing the value of such digital tools in improving healthcare outcomes and system efficiency.

Initial studies and real-world applications suggest that devices like *Mobili®* can significantly improve adherence, especially among older adults and patients with complex treatment regimens. Furthermore, the use of such technology may reduce medication errors and relieve caregiver burden, reinforcing its potential both clinically and economically. While further large-scale randomized controlled trials are needed to validate long-term effectiveness and adaptability across healthcare systems, *Mobili®* represents a promising step forward in the digitalization of adherence enhancing technologies to support chronic disease management. Its user-centered design and integration into multidisciplinary care pathways position it as a valuable tool in promoting safe, effective, and patient-centered care.

Case Study: The MobiMAd@PT Project

The MobiMad@PT project is a research initiative aimed at evaluating the effectiveness of Mobili®, a portable, automated dose dispensing system developed by the Norwegian start-up Medthings described above, in improving medication adherence among patients with multimorbidity in Portugal. Rooted in principles of proximity, continuity of care, and user-centred approaches, the project integrates digital health technologies into community pharmacy services to address one of the most persistent challenges in chronic disease management: non-adherence to prescribed medication regimens.

The project is informed by the growing investment in Individualized Medication Preparation (IMP) services by Portuguese pharmacies. According to the Centre for Health Evaluation & Research of the National Association of Pharmacies (CEFAR, ANF), as of 2020, 366 pharmacies in Portugal were delivering this service, marking a 47% increase over four years. These services vary in terms of equipment and preparation methods, ranging from manual to fully automated systems that produce blister packs or sachets weekly, fortnightly, or monthly.

In this context, the MobiMad@PT project builds upon pharmacists' experience with IMP and aims to assess the real-world impact of deploying Mobili® in community settings. The general objective is to evaluate Mobili®'s effectiveness in improving pharmacological adherence. Specific goals include: (1) assessing its effectiveness compared to current systems and practices; (2) evaluating its usability by both patients and healthcare professionals; (3) characterizing its adaptability to the Portuguese healthcare system; and (4) developing a protocol for a large-scale, multicentre study assessing clinical, economic, and humanistic outcomes.

The methodology is structured across four main phases. Phase one establishes operational and ethical foundations, including project governance, ethical approvals, data protection planning, internal communication strategies, and stakeholder engagement.

Phase two focuses on local adaptation of the Mobili® intervention. Participating pharmacists undergo three structured training sessions covering the dispenser, mobile app, and study protocol. Several focus groups with pharmacists are planned—one during training, one at study onset, and one at the end—to explore perceptions of Mobili®'s compatibility with workflows, perceived benefits, and potential barriers (Cyr, 2015). These qualitative insights help tailor the intervention to the local context and inform resource preparation.

In phase three, a crossover pilot randomized controlled trial (RCT) evaluates usability and effectiveness. The study will involve 6 to 8 experienced pharmacies offering IMP services, recruiting 72 to 96 eligible patients with chronic multimorbidity. Patients are randomized into two sequences:

- Sequence A: Mobili® use for 6 weeks, optional washout, then IMP (usual practice) for 6 weeks.

- Sequence B: IMP for 6 weeks, optional washout, then Mobili® for 6 weeks.

Recruitment is scheduled to restart three months after the first cohort. Pharmacists are responsible for preparing the personalized eDosette/Mobili® in line with national guidelines, ensuring delivery and correct use. While Mobili® is designed for autonomous use, pharmacists provide regular contact during scheduled pharmacy visits.

Quantitative data is collected at baseline, during intervention, and at follow-up. Primary outcomes include medication adherence; secondary outcomes include user satisfaction and quality of life. Validated tools are used to ensure consistency and reliability. Medication reviews are also conducted to identify medication-related problems.

Parallel to the RCT, a qualitative component provides additional insights. Semi-structured post-intervention interviews with pharmacists (Ferreira, 2014) explore their experiences, feasibility of service delivery, and perceived patient engagement impact. Patients also complete structured satisfaction surveys. This mixed-methods design offers a comprehensive view of both outcomes and implementation processes.

Phase four culminates in the development of a research protocol for a future multicenter trial. Informed by pilot data, this protocol will outline methodological and analytical strategies for a robust evaluation of Mobili®. National and international stakeholders—including pharmacy associations, health authorities, and patient organisations—are consulted in this phase to ensure alignment with policy priorities and system needs.

The project is theoretically anchored in the Consolidated Framework for Implementation Research (CFIR 2.0), which identifies key factors such as innovation characteristics, participant roles, internal and external environments, and implementation processes that influence success (Damschroder et al., 2022). It also applies Design Science Research Methodology (DSRM), a participatory and iterative approach ideal for co-developing digital health solutions within specific healthcare contexts (Gregório et al., 2021; Lapão et al., 2017, 2021; Simões et al., 2018). Deploying Mobili® in Portugal draws from lessons learned in Norwegian pilots, leveraging DSRM to ensure cultural appropriateness, user-friendliness, and equitable implementation (Plamondon & Bisung, 2019).

The expected outcomes include improved medication adherence, increased user satisfaction, and potential improvements in quality of life. By reinforcing the role of pharmacists in follow-up and therapeutic transitions, the project aims to generate evidence supporting scalable, patient-centered digital health innovations in primary care. Furthermore, findings from the project will offer valuable insights for researchers in medication adherence and implementation science. If proven effective in real-world contexts, Mobili® could foster a community-wide culture of adherence, enhance care quality, and generate substantial economic benefits for both patients and health systems.

Automated multidose dispensing (MDD) systems present compelling opportunities for international scalability, particularly in aging societies grappling with increasing rates of chronic diseases and medication complexity. A growing body of evidence from Northern and Western Europe underscores both the benefits and challenges of implementing these systems in primary care. These findings offer critical insights for countries aiming to replicate MDD systems within their own healthcare structures.

One of the most illustrative examples is Sweden, where by 2011, approximately 180,000 individuals—80% of whom were aged 60 or older—were receiving their medications via automated MDD systems (Bardage et al., 2014). Importantly, 40% of these users lived independently in private homes, while 60% resided in elderly care facilities. Support was provided in both environments, demonstrating the system's flexibility and capacity to reach a wide range of elderly users. These results indicate that, with appropriate infrastructure and support mechanisms, MDD systems can operate effectively across different care contexts and levels of dependency, providing a replicable model for other countries facing similar demographic pressures.

Further supporting its scalability, West et al., 2014 emphasized the value of MDD systems from a community pharmacy perspective, particularly regarding medication waste reduction and operational efficiency. These systems can streamline medication preparation, reduce manual dispensing errors, and support the economic sustainability of healthcare systems. In addition, Bardage et al., 2014 found a predominantly positive perception of MDD systems among healthcare professionals, particularly in cases involving patients with cognitive decline, polypharmacy, poor adherence, and motor function limitations. Such professional endorsement across care settings suggests that, if well-integrated into practice, automated MDD systems can be effectively scaled at the national and international levels.

However, replicating MDD systems internationally is not without complexity. Variations in healthcare organizations can pose substantial barriers. For instance, Sweden's centralized model contrasts with Norway's more decentralized and individualized approach, which can hinder direct transferability (A. V. Jøsendal et al., 2022). In decentralized systems, medication list reconciliation and communication between actors—such as GPs, pharmacists, and home care nurses—becomes more fragmented. This can lead to increased discrepancies in medication records and prescribing errors if coordination is not strengthened (A. Jøsendal & Bergmo, 2019; Wekre et al., 2010).

Cultural and behavioral factors also present challenges. Older adults may be hesitant to adopt unfamiliar technologies, particularly in regions with low digital health literacy. Moreover, risks like improper use of the system, medicine sharing, and misunderstanding device instructions can undermine its intended safety benefits (A. V. Jøsendal et al., 2022). Evidence from multiple studies also highlights the risk of disempowering patients and reducing medication knowledge when MDD replaces manual handling without adequate education and counseling (Holbø et al., 2019; Kwint et al., 2013). These findings underscore the need for culturally adapted training, community engagement, and patient involvement strategies in international implementations.

From a systems-level perspective, successful scaling of MDD requires a strong foundation in regulation, infrastructure, and human resource planning. Regulatory alignment on pharmaceutical dispensing, interoperability, and device certification is essential. Moreover, a trained workforce is critical for managing the setup, monitoring, and adjustment of MDD systems, especially in community settings. Pharmacists, for instance, must be supported with clear guidelines on their roles and responsibilities in both dispensing and patient education (Josendal et al., 2021).

In conclusion, automated MDD systems hold significant potential for global scalability. Their demonstrated ability to improve medication adherence, streamline pharmaceutical services, and enhance patient safety aligns with the goals of person-centered digital health. Nevertheless, successful international replication hinges on locally responsive implementation strategies that address system fragmentation, promote patient engagement, and integrate the technology seamlessly into existing workflows. With thoughtful adaptation, MDD systems can serve as a valuable tool in addressing the medication management needs of complex and aging populations worldwide.

CONCLUSION

The convergence of population aging, the rise of chronic multimorbidity, and the widespread phenomenon of polypharmacy presents a formidable challenge to contemporary health systems. Medication adherence, a critical determinant of effective chronic disease management, continues to be undermined by the complexity of therapeutic regimens, individual and systemic barriers, and the evolving dynamics of patient-provider relationships. This chapter has examined these interconnected themes through the lens of digital health and patient-centred care (PCC), arguing for a more integrated, contextually adapted, and evidence-informed approach to improving medication adherence.

Digital health technologies, when appropriately designed and implemented, offer unprecedented opportunities to support adherence across the continuum of care. From reminders and alerts to real-time usage tracking and remote intervention capabilities, such tools can mitigate common barriers such as forgetfulness, motivational decline, or the absence of structured follow-up. Moreover, as this chapter has discussed, the true promise of digital health lies not in its technological sophistication per se, but in its alignment with the principles of person-centered care. By enhancing communication, personalizing support, and enabling autonomy, digital interventions can extend PCC beyond clinical settings and into the daily routines of patients.

The case of *Mobili®* and the *MobiMAd@PT* project provides a valuable real-world example of how a digital adherence solution can be adapted and implemented within a specific health system—in this case, the Portuguese community pharmacy context. As described, the project's use of implementation science frameworks, particularly CFIR 2.0 and the Design Science Research Methodology (DSRM), ensures that both technological and contextual factors are taken into account. The device's portability, usability, and integration with pharmacy workflows address not only logistical barriers but also support the therapeutic alliance between patients and pharmacists. In this regard, the *MobiMAd@PT* project stands out for its commitment to participatory design and contextual adaptation—key enablers of international replication and long-term sustainability.

From a policy perspective, the integration of digital adherence tools into community-based care models aligns with global and national strategies that promote proximity care and digital transformation. The WHO's Global Strategy on Digital Health (2021) calls for the development of equitable, people-centered digital solutions that address pressing public health needs. Nationally, the growth of Individualized Medication Preparation (IMP) services in Portuguese pharmacies indicates a fertile ground for innovation, with more than 360 pharmacies already investing in automated dose preparation systems. Leveraging this infrastructure while embedding evidence-based digital tools like *Mobili®* can accelerate the transition to more efficient and responsive medication management models.

Nevertheless, several challenges must be acknowledged. First, digital divides—particularly among older adults or those in socioeconomically disadvantaged groups—risk exacerbating health inequalities if not addressed with inclusive design and appropriate support mechanisms. Second, regulatory and ethical frameworks must keep pace with technological advances, ensuring data protection, informed consent, and interoperability across platforms. Third, the long-term cost-effectiveness of such interventions must be demonstrated through robust economic evaluations, particularly in publicly funded systems where resource allocation decisions are tightly scrutinized.

Beyond these challenges, a broader cultural transformation is needed—one that positions adherence not merely as patient compliance, but as a shared goal within a collaborative care process. This requires empowering healthcare providers, particularly pharmacists and primary care professionals, to take on more proactive roles in monitoring, supporting, and educating patients. It also demands that digital health interventions are not seen as stand-alone fixes but are integrated into broader care pathways, supported by training, reimbursement, and continuous evaluation.

Best practices emerging from the literature and the *MobiMAd@PT* experience suggest several guiding principles for future efforts:

1. **Co-design with users**: Involving patients and healthcare providers from the earliest stages of development ensures that digital solutions are usable, acceptable, and aligned with real-world needs.
2. **Contextual adaptation**: Transferring technologies across systems or countries requires careful consideration of cultural, organisational, and infrastructural contexts.
3. **Hybrid evaluation models**: Combining quantitative outcomes (e.g., adherence rates, quality of life) with qualitative insights (e.g., satisfaction, usability) enhances the depth and applicability of findings.
4. **Implementation frameworks**: Using structured methodologies like CFIR 2.0 and DSRM helps navigate complexity and facilitates learning across settings.
5. **Sustainability planning**: From the outset, projects should consider how digital interventions can be financed, maintained, and scaled over time, including engagement with health authorities and industry partners.

In conclusion, the intersection of digital health, therapeutic adherence, and patient-centered care presents both a critical challenge and an exciting opportunity for the future of healthcare (e.g. Andrade et al., 2025; Hu et al., 2024; Victoria-Castro et al., 2024). As populations age and chronic conditions proliferate, health systems must evolve to provide more personalized, integrated, and sustainable solutions. Digital tools offer a promising path forward. However, their success will depend not only on technological innovation but on the collective commitment of researchers, clinicians, policymakers, and patients to reimagine what it means to support adherence in the context of modern care.

AKNOWLEDGMENTS

We would like to thank Catarina Domingos, Sara Sousa, Margarida Rebelo and Patrícia Almeida for their contributions on the project described on this chapter.

REFERENCES

Ahmed, A., Khan, H. T. A., & Lawal, M. (2025). The Prevalence, Pattern, and Burden of Multimorbidity Among Older Adults in Niger State, Northern Nigeria. *Illness, Crises, and Loss*, *33*(3), 684–701. DOI: 10.1177/10541373241268305

Aldeer, M., Javanmard, M., & Martin, R. P. (2018). A review of medication adherence monitoring technologies. In *Applied System Innovation* (Vol. 1, Issue 2, pp. 1–27). MDPI AG. https://doi.org/DOI: 10.3390/asi1020014

Alkhaibari, R. A., Smith-Merry, J., Forsyth, R., & Raymundo, G. M. (2023). Patient-centered care in the Middle East and North African region: A systematic literature review. *BMC Health Services Research*, *23*(1). Advance online publication. DOI: 10.1186/s12913-023-09132-0 PMID: 36759898

Ambalavanan, R., Snead, R. S., Marczika, J., Towett, G., Malioukis, A., & Mbogori-Kairichi, M. (2025). Challenges and strategies in building a foundational digital health data integration ecosystem: A systematic review and thematic synthesis. *Frontiers in Health Services*, *5*. Advance online publication. DOI: 10.3389/frhs.2025.1600689 PMID: 40621432

Andrade, J. B. C. D., Fagundes, T. P., Katsuyama, E., & Silva, G. S. (2025). Digital Health in Low-Resource Settings: Comprehensive Challenges and Opportunities With a Focus on Stroke Care. *Stroke*, *57*(1). Advance online publication. DOI: 10.1161/STROKEAHA.125.05044 PMID: 40905151

Areej Bayatra, R. N. and Y. I. (2024). Overcoming Low Adherence to Chronic Medications by Improving their Effectiveness using a Personalized Second-generation Digital System. *Current Pharmaceutical Biotechnology*, *25*(16), 11. PMID: 38288794

Arokiasamy, P., Uttamacharya, U., Jain, K., Biritwum, R. B., Yawson, A. E., Wu, F., Guo, Y., Maximova, T., Espinoza, B. M., Salinas Rodríguez, A., Afshar, S., Pati, S., Ice, G., Banerjee, S., Liebert, M. A., Snodgrass, J. J., Naidoo, N., Chatterji, S., & Kowal, P. (2015). The impact of multimorbidity on adult physical and mental health in low- and middle-income countries: What does the study on global ageing and adult health (SAGE) reveal? *BMC Medicine*, *13*(1). Advance online publication. DOI: 10.1186/s12916-015-0402-8 PMID: 26239481

Backman, W. D., Levine, S. A., Wenger, N. K., & Harold, J. G. (2020). Shared decision-making for older adults with cardiovascular disease. In *Clinical Cardiology* (Vol. 43, Issue 2, pp. 196–204). John Wiley and Sons Inc. https://doi.org/DOI: 10.1002/clc.23267

Bardage, C., Ekedahl, A., & Ring, L. (2014). Health care professionals' perspectives on automated multi-dose drug dispensing. *Pharmacy Practice*, *12*. Advance online publication. DOI: 10.4321/S1886-36552014000400005 PMID: 25580170

Batson, C. D. (2021). The empathy-altruism hypothesis. In *Positive psychology: An international perspective* (pp. 12–32). Wiley Blackwell.

Bell, S. P., & Saraf, A. A. (2016). Epidemiology of Multimorbidity in Older Adults with Cardiovascular Disease. In *Clinics in Geriatric Medicine* (Vol. 32, Issue 2, pp. 215–226). W.B. Saunders. https://doi .org/DOI: 10.1016/j.cger.2016.01.013

Bernardo, C., Tosin, M. H. de S., Almada, M., Sampaio, R., de Oliveira, B. G. R. B., Costa, E., Vrijens, B., & Alves da Costa, F. (2023). Translation and cross-cultural adaptation of the ABC taxonomy for medication adherence into Portuguese – Updating patients into people. *Research in Social & Administrative Pharmacy*, *19*(4), 653–659. DOI: 10.1016/j.sapharm.2022.12.010 PMID: 36621396

Brands, M. R., Gouw, S. C., Beestrum, M., Cronin, R. M., Fijnvandraat, K., & Badawy, S. M. (2022). Patient-Centered Digital Health Records and Their Effects on Health Outcomes: Systematic Review. In *Journal of Medical Internet Research* (Vol. 24, Issue 12). JMIR Publications Inc. https://doi.org/DOI: 10.2196/43086

Bricca, A., Smith, S. M., & Skou, S. T. (2023). Management of multimorbidity. *Journal of Multimorbidity and Comorbidity*, *13*, 263355652311566. DOI: 10.1177/26335565231156693 PMID: 36911182

Camarneiro, A. P. F. (2021). Therapeutic adherence: Contributions to understanding and intervention. *Revista de Enfermagem Referencia*, *5*(7). Advance online publication. DOI: 10.12707/RV20145

Chen, K., & Chan, A. H. S. (2013). Use or non-use of gerontechnology-A qualitative study. *International Journal of Environmental Research and Public Health*, *10*(10), 4645–4666. DOI: 10.3390/ijerph10104645 PMID: 24084674

Choudhury, A., & Asan, O. (2021). Impact of using wearable devices on psychological Distress: Analysis of the health information national Trends survey. *International Journal of Medical Informatics*, *156*. Advance online publication. DOI: 10.1016/j.ijmedinf.2021.104612 PMID: 34649113

Christie, R. H., Abbas, A., & Koesmahargyo, V. (2021). Technology for Measuring and Monitoring Treatment Compliance Remotely. In *Journal of Parkinson's Disease* (Vol. 11, Issue s1, pp. S77–S81). IOS Press BV. https://doi.org/DOI: 10.3233/JPD-212537

Cobretti, M. R., Page, R. L., Linnebur, S. A., Deininger, K. M., Ambardekar, A. V., Lindenfeld, J. A., & Aquilante, C. L. (2017). Medication regimen complexity in ambulatory older adults with heart failure. *Clinical Interventions in Aging*, *12*, 679–686. DOI: 10.2147/CIA.S130832 PMID: 28442898

Cramer, P. (1991). The development of defense mechanisms: Theory, research, and assessment. In *The development of defense mechanisms: Theory, research, and assessment*. Springer-Verlag Publishing., DOI: 10.1007/978-1-4613-9025-1

Cutler, R. L., Fernandez-Llimos, F., Frommer, M., Benrimoj, C., & Garcia-Cardenas, V. (2018). Economic impact of medication non-adherence by disease groups: A systematic review. In *BMJ Open* (Vol. 8, Issue 1). BMJ Publishing Group. https://doi.org/DOI: 10.1136/bmjopen-2017-016982

Damschroder, L. J., Reardon, C. M., Widerquist, M. A. O., & Lowery, J. (2022). The updated Consolidated Framework for Implementation Research based on user feedback. *Implementation Science : IS, 17*(1). Advance online publication. DOI: 10.1186/s13012-022-01245-0 PMID: 36309746

Dang, T. H., Wickramasinghe, N., Jayaraman, P. P., Burbury, K., Alexander, M., Whitechurch, A., Quinn, S., Rowan, G., Brooks, S. L., & Schofield, P. (2024). Safety and adherence to medications and self-care advice in oncology (SAMSON): Pilot randomised controlled trial protocol. *BMJ Open, 14*(7). Advance online publication. DOI: 10.1136/bmjopen-2023-079122 PMID: 39043598

Daunt, R., Curtin, D., & O'Mahony, D. (2023). Polypharmacy stewardship: a novel approach to tackle a major public health crisis. In *The Lancet Healthy Longevity* (Vol. 4, Issue 5, pp. e228–e235). Elsevier Ltd. https://doi.org/DOI: 10.1016/S2666-7568(23)00036-3

Davies, L., Spiers, G., Kingston, A., Todd, A., Adamson, J., & Hanratty, B. (2020). Adverse Outcomes of Polypharmacy in Older People: Systematic Review of Reviews. *Journal of the American Medical Directors Association, 21*. Advance online publication. DOI: 10.1016/j.jamda.2019.10.022 PMID: 31926797

Delara, M., Murray, L., Jafari, B., Bahji, A., Goodarzi, Z., Kirkham, J., Chowdhury, Z., & Seitz, D. P. (2022). Prevalence and factors associated with polypharmacy: A systematic review and Meta-analysis. *BMC Geriatrics, 22*(1). Advance online publication. DOI: 10.1186/s12877-022-03279-x PMID: 35854209

Delbanco, T., Berwick, D. M., & Boufford, J. I. Edgman-Levitan, Ollenschläger, G., Plamping, D., & Rockefeller, R. G. (2001). Healthcare in a land called PeoplePower: nothing about me without me. *Health Expectations, 4*(3), 144–150. https://doi.org/https://doi.org/10.1046/j.1369-6513.2001.00145.x

Efthymiou, E. (2025). Integrating digital and narrative medicine in modern healthcare: a systematic review. In *Medical Education Online* (Vol. 30, Issue 1). Taylor and Francis Ltd. https://doi.org/DOI: 10.1080/10872981.2025.2475979

Epstein, R. M., & Street, R. L. (2011). The values and value of patient-centered care. In *Annals of Family Medicine* (Vol. 9, Issue 2, pp. 100–103). Annals of Family Medicine, Inc. https://doi.org/DOI: 10.1370/afm.1239

Etkin, J. (2016). The Hidden Cost of Personal Quantification. *The Journal of Consumer Research, 42*(6), 967–984. DOI: 10.1093/jcr/ucv095

Fernandes, F., Rios, L. G., Neto, E., & Turra, C. M. (2023). World population aging as a function of period demographic conditions. *Demographic Research, 48*(13), 353–372. DOI: 10.4054/DemRes.2023.48.13

Ferreira, V. (2014). *Artes de entrevistar: Composição, criatividade e improvisação a duas vozes*. Ed Húmus.

Foglia, E., Asperti, F., Antonacci, G., Jani, Y. H., Garagiola, E., Bellavia, D., & Ferrario, L. (2024). Automated Drugs Dispensing Systems in Hospitals: A Health Technology Assessment (HTA) Study Across Six European Countries. *ClinicoEconomics and Outcomes Research, 16*, 679–696. DOI: 10.2147/CEOR.S468417 PMID: 39319287

Foley, L., Larkin, J., Lombard-Vance, R., Murphy, A. W., Hynes, L., Galvin, E., & Molloy, G. J. (2021). Prevalence and predictors of medication non-Adherence among people living with multimorbidity: A systematic review and meta-Analysis. In *BMJ Open* (Vol. 11, Issue 9). BMJ Publishing Group. https://doi.org/DOI: 10.1136/bmjopen-2020-044987

Gandapur, Y., Kianoush, S., Kelli, H. M., Misra, S., Urrea, B., Blaha, M. J., Graham, G., Marvel, F. A., & Martin, S. S. (2016). The role of mHealth for improving medication adherence in patients with cardiovascular disease: A systematic review. In *European Heart Journal - Quality of Care and Clinical Outcomes* (Vol. 2, Issue 4, pp. 237–244). Oxford University Press. https://doi.org/DOI: 10.1093/ehjqcco/qcw018

Gianfredi, V., Nucci, D., Pennisi, F., Maggi, S., Veronese, N., & Soysal, P. (2025). Aging, longevity, and healthy aging: the public health approach. In *Aging Clinical and Experimental Research* (Vol. 37, Issue 1). Springer Science and Business Media Deutschland GmbH. https://doi.org/DOI: 10.1007/s40520-025-03021-8

Goueth, R. C., Maki, K. G., Babatunde, A., Eden, K. B., & Darney, B. G. (2022). Effects of technology-based contraceptive decision aids: a systematic review and meta-analysis. In *American Journal of Obstetrics and Gynecology* (Vol. 227, Issue 5, pp. 705-713.e9). Elsevier Inc. https://doi.org/DOI: 10.1016/j.ajog.2022.06.050

Grcgório, J., Maricoto, T., Moreira, P. A. S., Roque, F., Correia-De-Sousa, J., Herdeiro, M. T., Almeida, I. F., Tsiligiann, I., Agh, T., & Jácome, C. (2023). Addressing the digital divide: Who is being left behind in the evaluation of e-Health interventions to improve medication adherence? *Biomedical and Biopharmaceutical Research*, *20*(1), 93–105. DOI: 10.19277/bbr.20.1.315

Gregório, J., Reis, L., Peyroteo, M., Maia, M., Mira da Silva, M., & Lapão, L. V. (2021). The role of Design Science Research Methodology in developing pharmacy eHealth services. *Research in Social & Administrative Pharmacy*, *17*(12), 2089–2096. DOI: 10.1016/J.SAPHARM.2021.05.016 PMID: 34119446

Guthrie, B., Makubate, B., Hernandez-Santiago, V., & Dreischulte, T. (2015). The rising tide of polypharmacy and drug-drug interactions: Population database analysis 1995-2010. *BMC Medicine*, *13*(1). Advance online publication. DOI: 10.1186/s12916-015-0322-7 PMID: 25889849

Hänninen, K., Ahtiainen, H. K., Suvikas-Peltonen, E. M., & Tötterman, A. M. (2023). Automated unit dose dispensing systems producing individually packaged and labelled drugs for inpatients: a systematic review. In *European Journal of Hospital Pharmacy* (Vol. 30, Issue 3, pp. 127–135). BMJ Publishing Group. https://doi.org/DOI: 10.1136/ejhpharm-2021-003002

Hartch, C., Dietrich, M. S., Lancaster, B. J., Mulvaney, S. A., & Stolldorf, D. P. (2025). Satisfaction and Usability of a Commercially Available Medication Adherence App (Medisafe) Among Medically Underserved Patients With Chronic Illnesses: Survey Study. *JMIR Human Factors*, *12*. Advance online publication. DOI: 10.2196/63653 PMID: 39773694

Haynes, R. B. (1979). *Determinant of compliance: The disease and the mechanics of treatment*. https://api.semanticscholar.org/CorpusID:208401416

Head, A., Fleming, K., Kypridemos, C., Pearson-Stuttard, J., & O'Flaherty, M. (2021). Multimorbidity: The case for prevention. *Journal of Epidemiology and Community Health, 75*(3), 242–244. DOI: 10.1136/jech-2020-214301 PMID: 33020144

Holbø, K., Das, A., Bøthun, S., Formanek, M. N., & Halvorsen, T. (2019). Multidosetjeneste for hjemmeboende – brukernes erfaringer og behov for nye løsninger. *Nordisk Välfärdsforskning | Nordic Welfare Research, 4*(1), 20–31. https://doi.org/DOI: 10.18261/issn.2464-4161-2019-01-03

Holden, R. J. (2011). Cognitive performance-altering effects of electronic medical records: An application of the human factors paradigm for patient safety. *Cognition Technology and Work, 13*(1), 11–29. DOI: 10.1007/s10111-010-0141-8 PMID: 21479125

Hu, J., Li, C., Ge, Y., Yang, J., Zhu, S., & He, C. (2024). Mapping the evolution of digital health research: Bibliometric overview of research hotspots, trends, and collaboration of publications in JMIR (1999-2024). *Journal of Medical Internet Research, 26*, e58987. PMID: 39419496

Hyvert, S., Yailian, A. L., Haesebaert, J., Vignot, E., Chapurlat, R., Dussart, C., De Freminville, H., & Janoly-Dumenil, A. (2023). Association between health literacy and medication adherence in chronic diseases: a recent systematic review. In *International Journal of Clinical Pharmacy* (Vol. 45, Issue 1, pp. 38–51). Springer Science and Business Media Deutschland GmbH. https://doi.org/DOI: 10.1007/s11096-022-01470-z

Islam, S. M. S., Maddison, R., Karmarkar, C., & Rahman, S. (2024). Can digital health help improve medication adherence in cardiovascular disease? In *Expert Review of Medical Devices* (Vol. 21, Issue 12, pp. 1071–1075). Taylor and Francis Ltd. https://doi.org/DOI: 10.1080/17434440.2024.2441954

Jarzebski, M. P., Elmqvist, T., Gasparatos, A., Fukushi, K., Eckersten, S., Haase, D., Goodness, J., Khoshkar, S., Saito, O., Takeuchi, K., Theorell, T., Dong, N., Kasuga, F., Watanabe, R., Sioen, G. B., Yokohari, M., & Pu, J. (2021). Ageing and population shrinking: Implications for sustainability in the urban century. *NPJ Urban Sustainability, 1*(1). Advance online publication. DOI: 10.1038/s42949-021-00023-z

Jayasree, A., Shanmuganathan, P., Ramamurthy, P., & Alwar, M. C. (2024). Types of Medication Non-adherence & Approaches to Enhance Medication Adherence in Mental Health Disorders: A Narrative Review. In *Indian Journal of Psychological Medicine* (Vol. 46, Issue 6, pp. 503–510). SAGE Publications Ltd. https://doi.org/DOI: 10.1177/02537176241233745

Jiang, M., Zhao, Q., Li, J., Wang, F., Tianyu, H., Cheng, X., Yang, B. X., Ho, G. W. K., & Fu, G. (2024). *A Generic Review of Integrating Artificial Intelligence in Cognitive Behavioral Therapy*. https://doi.org//arXiv.2407.19422DOI: 10.48550

Jo Delaney, L. (2018). Patient-centred care as an approach to improving health care in Australia. *Collegian (Royal College of Nursing, Australia), 25*(1), 119–123. DOI: 10.1016/j.colegn.2017.02.005

Jøsendal, A., & Bergmo, T. (2019). *How Discrepancies in Medication Records Affect the Creation and Trust in a Shared Electronic Medication List in Norway.*

Josendal, A. V., Bergmo, T. S., & Granas, A. G. (2021). The Practice Guidelines for Multidose Drug Dispensing Need Revision—An Investigation of Prescription Problems and Interventions. *Pharmacy (Basel, Switzerland)*, *9*(1), 13. DOI: 10.3390/pharmacy9010013 PMID: 33418861

Jøsendal, A. V., Bergmo, T. S., & Granås, A. G. (2022). Multidose Drug Dispensing in Primary Care: A Review of the Literature. In *Medication Safety in Municipal Health and Care Services* (pp. 321–348). Cappelen Damm Akademisk/NOASP. https://doi.org/DOI: 10.23865/noasp.172.ch15

Kassaw, A. T., Sendekie, A. K., Minyihun, A., & Gebresillassie, B. M. (2024). Medication regimen complexity and its impact on medication adherence in patients with multimorbidity at a comprehensive specialized hospital in Ethiopia. *Frontiers in Medicine*, *11*. Advance online publication. DOI: 10.3389/fmed.2024.1369569 PMID: 38860203

Kengne Talla, P., Allison, P., Bussières, A., Rodrigues, A., Bergeron, F., Giraudeau, N., & Emami, E. (2024). Teledentistry for improving access to, and quality of oral health care: An overview of systematic reviews and meta-analyses (Preprint). *Journal of Medical Internet Research*. Advance online publication. DOI: 10.2196/65211 PMID: 40737673

Kernick, D., Chew-Graham, C. A., & O'Flynn, N. (2017). Clinical assessment and management of multimorbidity: Nice guideline. In *British Journal of General Practice* (Vol. 67, Issue 658, pp. 235–236). Royal College of General Practitioners. https://doi.org/DOI: 10.3399/bjgp17X690857

Kini, V., & Ho, P. M. (2018). Interventions to Improve Medication Adherence: A Review. *Journal of the American Medical Association*, *320*(23), 2461–2473. DOI: 10.1001/jama.2018.19271 PMID: 30561486

Kitsiou, S., Gerber, B. S., Buchholz, S. W., Kansal, M. M., Sun, J., & Pressler, S. J. (2025). Patient-Centered mHealth Intervention to Improve Self-Care in Patients With Chronic Heart Failure: Phase 1 Randomized Controlled Trial. *Journal of Medical Internet Research*, *27*. Advance online publication. DOI: 10.2196/55586 PMID: 39813671

Koné Pefoyo, A. J., Bronskill, S. E., Gruneir, A., Calzavara, A., Thavorn, K., Petrosyan, Y., Maxwell, C. J., Bai, Y. Q., & Wodchis, W. P. (2015). The increasing burden and complexity of multimorbidity disease epidemiology - Chronic. *BMC Public Health*, *15*(1), 1–11. DOI: 10.1186/s12889-015-1733-2

Kwint, H.-F., Stolk, G., Faber, A., Gussekloo, J., & Bouvy, M. L. (2013). Medication adherence and knowledge of older patients with and without multidose drug dispensing. *Age and Ageing*, *42*(5), 620–626. DOI: 10.1093/ageing/aft083 PMID: 23832265

Lapão, L. V., Da Silva, M. M., & Gregório, J. (2017). Implementing an online pharmaceutical service using design science research. *BMC Medical Informatics and Decision Making*, *17*(1). Advance online publication. DOI: 10.1186/s12911-017-0428-2 PMID: 28347304

Lapão, L. V., Peyroteo, M., Maia, M., Seixas, J., Gregório, J., Da Silva, M. M., Heleno, B., & Correia, J. C. (2021). Implementation of digital monitoring services during the COVID-19 pandemic for patients with chronic diseases: Design science approach. *Journal of Medical Internet Research*, *23*(8). Advance online publication. DOI: 10.2196/24181 PMID: 34313591

Maffoni, M., Traversoni, S., Costa, E., Midão, L., Kardas, P., Kurczewska-Michalak, M., & Giardini, A. (2020). Medication adherence in the older adults with chronic multimorbidity: a systematic review of qualitative studies on patient's experience. In *European Geriatric Medicine* (Vol. 11, Issue 3, pp. 369–381). Springer. https://doi.org/DOI: 10.1007/s41999-020-00313-2

Maita, K. C., Maniaci, M. J., Haider, C. R., Avila, F. R., Torres-Guzman, R. A., Borna, S., & Forte, A. J. (2024). The impact of digital health solutions on bridging the health care gap in rural areas: A scoping review. *The Permanente Journal, 28*(3), 130.

Mangin, D., Bahat, G., Golomb, B. A., Mallery, L. H., Moorhouse, P., Onder, G., Petrovic, M., & Garfinkel, D. (2018). International Group for Reducing Inappropriate Medication Use & Polypharmacy (IGRIMUP): Position Statement and 10 Recommendations for Action. *Drugs & Aging, 35*(7), 575–587. DOI: 10.1007/s40266-018-0554-2 PMID: 30006810

Masnoon, N., Shakib, S., Kalisch-Ellett, L., & Caughey, G. E. (2017). What is polypharmacy? A systematic review of definitions. In *BMC Geriatrics* (Vol. 17, Issue 1). BioMed Central Ltd. https://doi.org/DOI: 10.1186/s12877-017-0621-2

MedThings. (2024). *The Mobili e-dosett sets a new standard for medication management*. MedThings.

Miao, Y., Luo, Y., Zhao, Y., Liu, M., Wang, H., & Wu, Y. (2024). Effectiveness of eHealth Interventions in Improving Medication Adherence Among Patients With Cardiovascular Disease: Systematic Review and Meta-Analysis. In *Journal of Medical Internet Research* (Vol. 26, Issue 1). JMIR Publications Inc. https://doi.org/DOI: 10.2196/58013

Midão, L., Giardini, A., Menditto, E., Kardas, P., & Costa, E. (2018). Polypharmacy prevalence among older adults based on the survey of health, ageing and retirement in Europe. *Archives of Gerontology and Geriatrics, 78*, 213–220. DOI: 10.1016/j.archger.2018.06.018 PMID: 30015057

Miller, T., & Reihlen, M. (2023). Assessing the impact of patient-involvement healthcare strategies on patients, providers, and the healthcare system: A systematic review. *Patient Education and Counseling, 110*, 107652. DOI: 10.1016/J.PEC.2023.107652 PMID: 36804578

Navickas, R., Petric, V.-K., Feigl, A. B., & Seychell, M. (2016). Multimorbidity: What Do We Know? What Should We Do? *Journal of Comorbidity, 6*(1), 4–11. DOI: 10.15256/joc.2016.6.72 PMID: 29090166

Ngo, E., Truong, M. B. T., Nordeng, H., & Wright, D. (2022). Impact of a Mobile Application for Tracking Nausea and Vomiting During Pregnancy (NVP) on NVP Symptoms, Quality of Life, and Decisional Conflict Regarding NVP Treatments: MinSafeStart Randomized Controlled Trial. *JMIR mHealth and uHealth, 10*(7). Advance online publication. DOI: 10.2196/36226 PMID: 35787487

Nguyen, H., Manolova, G., Daskalopoulou, C., Vitoratou, S., Prince, M., & Prina, A. M. (2019). Prevalence of multimorbidity in community settings: A systematic review and meta-analysis of observational studies. *Journal of Comorbidity, 9*. Advance online publication. DOI: 10.1177/2235042x19870934 PMID: 31489279

Nicholson, K., Liu, W., Fitzpatrick, D., Hardacre, K. A., Roberts, S., Salerno, J., Stranges, S., Fortin, M., & Mangin, D. (2024). Prevalence of multimorbidity and polypharmacy among adults and older adults: a systematic review. In *The Lancet Healthy Longevity* (Vol. 5, Issue 4, pp. e287–e296). Elsevier Ltd. https://doi.org/DOI: 10.1016/S2666-7568(24)00007-2

Norman, C. D., & Skinner, H. A. (2006). eHealth literacy: Essential skills for consumer health in a networked world. In *Journal of Medical Internet Research* (Vol. 8, Issue 2). JMIR Publications Inc. https://doi.org/DOI: 10.2196/jmir.8.2.e9

O'Kane, G., & Craig, P., & SUTHERLAND, D. (2008). Riverina men's study: An exploration of rural men's attitudes to health and body image. *Nutrition & Dietetics: the Journal of the Dietitians Association of Australia*, *65*, 66–71. DOI: 10.1111/j.1747-0080.2007.00176.x

Pantuzza, L. L., & Ceccato, M. das G. B., Silveira, M. R., Junqueira, L. M. R., & Reis, A. M. M. (2017). Association between medication regimen complexity and pharmacotherapy adherence: A systematic review. *European Journal of Clinical Pharmacology*, *73*(11), 1475–1489. DOI: 10.1007/s00228-017-2315-2 PMID: 28779460

Parikh, M. A., Ramachandran, S., & Nsiah, I. Patrick; Campbell, J., Castora-Binkley, M., Karmakar, T., Black; Heather, & Bentley, J. P. (2025). Author affiliations Estimating optimal thresholds for adherence to RASA medications among older adults with hypertension. In *JMCP.org* (Vol. 31, Issue 1).

Patoz, M. C., Hidalgo-Mazzei, D., Blanc, O., Verdolini, N., Pacchiarotti, I., Murru, A., Zukerwar, L., Vieta, E., Llorca, P. M., & Samalin, L. (2021). Patient and physician perspectives of a smartphone application for depression: A qualitative study. *BMC Psychiatry*, *21*(1). Advance online publication. DOI: 10.1186/s12888-021-03064-x PMID: 33514333

Pazan, F., & Wehling, M. (2021). Polypharmacy in older adults: a narrative review of definitions, epidemiology and consequences. In *European Geriatric Medicine* (Vol. 12, Issue 3, pp. 443–452). Springer Science and Business Media Deutschland GmbH. https://doi.org/DOI: 10.1007/s41999-021-00479-3

Petrovic, M., O'Mahony, D., & Cherubini, A. (2022). Inappropriate prescribing: hazards and solutions. In *Age and Ageing* (Vol. 51, Issue 2). Oxford University Press. https://doi.org/DOI: 10.1093/ageing/afab269

Plamondon, K., & Bisung, E. (2019). The CCGHR Principles for Global Health Research: Centering equity in research, knowledge translation, and practice. *Social Science & Medicine*, *239*, 112530. DOI: 10.1016/j.socscimed.2019.112530 PMID: 31539786

Rand, C. S. (1993). Measuring Adherence with Therapy for Chronic Diseases: Implications for the Treatment of Heterozygous Familial Hyperchoksterolemia. *The American Journal of Cardiology*, •••, 72. PMID: 8213501

Reis, S., Maldonado, E., Matos De Barros, J., Louro, A. A., Guimarães, M., Barroso, B., Fernandes, H., & Novo, A. (2024). Analysis of inequalities in access to healthcare in North-east Portugal Análise das desigualdades no acesso aos cuidados de saúde no nordeste de Portugal. *Cadernos de Saúde 8, 16*, 29–38. https://doi.org/DOI: 10.34632/cadernosdesaude.2024.16020

Reis, Z. S. N., Pereira, G. M. V., Dias, C. dos S., Lage, E. M., de Oliveira, I. J. R., & Pagano, A. S. (2025). Artificial intelligence-based tools for patient support to enhance medication adherence: a focused review. In *Frontiers in Digital Health* (Vol. 7). Frontiers Media SA. https://doi.org/DOI: 10.3389/fdgth.2025.1523070

Religioni, U., Barrios-Rodríguez, R., Requena, P., Borowska, M., & Ostrowski, J. (2025). Enhancing Therapy Adherence: Impact on Clinical Outcomes, Healthcare Costs, and Patient Quality of Life. In *Medicina (Lithuania)* (Vol. 61, Issue 1). Multidisciplinary Digital Publishing Institute (MDPI). https://doi.org/DOI: 10.3390/medicina61010153

Pattani, D., Shirin, S., Safa Basheer, S., & Kasim, V. A. (2025). Adherence and Impact of Medication Regimen Complexity among Geriatric Patients: A Review. *Indian J. Pharm. Pract*, *18*, 28–34.

Ricke, E., Dijkstra, A., & Bakker, E. W. (2023). Prognostic factors of adherence to home-based exercise therapy in patients with chronic diseases: A systematic review and meta-analysis. In *Frontiers in Sports and Active Living* (Vol. 5). Frontiers Media S.A., DOI: 10.3389/fspor.2023.1035023

Sabaté, E. (2003). *Adherence to long-term therapies: evidence for action*. World Health Organization.

Sánchez-Fidalgo, S., Guzmán-Ramos, M. I., Galván-Banqueri, M., Bernabeu-Wittel, M., & Santos-Ramos, B. (2017). Prevalence of drug interactions in elderly patients with multimorbidity in primary care. *International Journal of Clinical Pharmacy*, *39*(2), 343–353. DOI: 10.1007/s11096-017-0439-1 PMID: 28238102

Schiøtz, M. L., Høst, D., Christensen, M. B., Domínguez, H., Hamid, Y., Almind, M., Sørensen, K. L., Saxild, T., Holm, R. H., & Frølich, A. (2017). Quality of care for people with multimorbidity - A case series. *BMC Health Services Research*, *17*(1). Advance online publication. DOI: 10.1186/s12913-017-2724-z PMID: 29151022

Scott, R., & Mars, M. (2015). Telehealth in the developing world: Current status and future prospects. *Smart Homecare Technology and Telehealth*, *25*. Advance online publication. DOI: 10.2147/shtt.s75184

Sendekie, A. K., Netere, A. K., Kasahun, A. E., & Belachew, E. A. (2022). Medication adherence and its impact on glycemic control in type 2 diabetes mellitus patients with comorbidity: A multicenter cross-sectional study in Northwest Ethiopia. *PLoS ONE, 17*(9 September). https://doi.org/DOI: 10.1371/journal.pone.0274971

Simões, A. S., Maia, M. R., Gregório, J., Couto, I., Asfeldt, A. M., Simonsen, G. S., Póvoa, P., Viveiros, M., & Lapão, L. V. (2018). Participatory implementation of an antibiotic stewardship programme supported by an innovative surveillance and clinical decision-support system. *The Journal of Hospital Infection*, *100*(3), 257–264. DOI: 10.1016/j.jhin.2018.07.034 PMID: 30071264

Simpson, C. C., & Mazzeo, S. E. (2017). Calorie counting and fitness tracking technology: Associations with eating disorder symptomatology. *Eating Behaviors*, *26*, 89–92. https://doi.org/https://doi.org/10.1016/j.eatbeh.2017.02.002 PMID: 28214452

Skou, S. T., Mair, F. S., Fortin, M., Guthrie, B., Nunes, B. P., Miranda, J. J., Boyd, C. M., Pati, S., Mtenga, S., & Smith, S. M. (2022). Multimorbidity. *Nature Reviews. Disease Primers*, *8*(1). Advance online publication. DOI: 10.1038/s41572-022-00376-4 PMID: 35835758

Soley-Bori, M., Ashworth, M., Bisquera, A., Dodhia, H., Lynch, R., Wang, Y., & Fox-Rushby, J. (2021). Impact of multimorbidity on healthcare costs and utilisation: A systematic review of the UK literature. *The British Journal of General Practice*, *71*(702), E39–E46. DOI: 10.3399/bjgp20X713897 PMID: 33257463

Thomas, B. E., Kumar, J. V., Periyasamy, M., Khandewale, A. S., Mercy, J. H., Raj, E. M., Kokila, S., Walgude, A. S., Gaurkhede, G. R., Kumbhar, J. D., Ovung, S., Paul, M., Rajkumar, B. S., & Subbaraman, R. (2021). Acceptability of the medication event reminder monitor for promoting adherence to multidrug-resistant tuberculosis therapy in two indian cities: Qualitative study of patients and health care providers. *Journal of Medical Internet Research*, *23*(6). Advance online publication. DOI: 10.2196/23294 PMID: 34110300

Tommelein, E., Mehuys, E., Petrovic, M., Somers, A., Colin, P., & Boussery, K. (2015). Potentially inappropriate prescribing in community-dwelling older people across Europe: A systematic literature review. *European Journal of Clinical Pharmacology*, *71*. Advance online publication. DOI: 10.1007/s00228-015-1954-4 PMID: 26407687

Trinh, M., Harris, M. T., Azevedo, R. F. L., & Rogers, W. A. (2023). Understanding older adults' perceptions of mHealth apps. *Gerontechnology (Valkenswaard)*, *22*(1). Advance online publication. DOI: 10.4017/GT.2023.22.1.841.10

Turgeon, J., Michaud, V., & Steffen, L. (2017). The Dangers of Polypharmacy in Elderly Patients. *JAMA Internal Medicine*, *177*(10), 1544. DOI: 10.1001/jamainternmed.2017.4790 PMID: 28973278

Ulley, J., Harrop, D., Ali, A., Alton, S., & Fowler Davis, S. (2019). Deprescribing interventions and their impact on medication adherence in community-dwelling older adults with polypharmacy: A systematic review. *BMC Geriatrics*, *19*(1). Advance online publication. DOI: 10.1186/s12877-019-1031-4 PMID: 30658576

United Nations. (2019). *World Population Ageing 2019: Highlights*. www.unpopulation.org

Valderas, J. M., Starfield, B., Sibbald, B., Salisbury, C., & Roland, M. (2009). Defining comorbidity: Implications for understanding health and health services. *Annals of Family Medicine*, *7*(4), 357–363. DOI: 10.1370/afm.983 PMID: 19597174

van Westrenen, F. (2011). Cognitive work analysis and the design of user interfaces. *Cognition Technology and Work*, *13*(1), 31–42. DOI: 10.1007/s10111-010-0153-4

Vargese, S. S., Mathew, E., Johny, V., & Kurian, N., V, G. A., & Raju, A. S. (2020). Prevalence and pattern of multimorbidity among adults in a primary care rural setting. *Clinical Epidemiology and Global Health*, *8*(2), 482–485. DOI: 10.1016/j.cegh.2019.10.014

Victoria-Castro, A. M., Martin, M. L., Yamamoto, Y., Melchinger, H., Weinstein, J., Nguyen, A., & Wilson, F. P. (2024). Impact of digital health technology on quality of life in patients with heart failure. *Heart Failure*, *12*(2), 336–348. PMID: 37943227

Vrijens, B., De Geest, S., Hughes, D. A., Przemyslaw, K., Demonceau, J., Ruppar, T., Dobbels, F., Fargher, E., Morrison, V., Lewek, P., Matyjaszczyk, M., Mshelia, C., Clyne, W., Aronson, J. K., & Urquhart, J. (2012). A new taxonomy for describing and defining adherence to medications. *British Journal of Clinical Pharmacology*, *73*(5), 691–705. DOI: 10.1111/j.1365-2125.2012.04167.x PMID: 22486599

Wekre, L. J., Spigset, O., Sletvold, O., Sund, J. K., & Grimsmo, A. (2010). Multidose drug dispensing and discrepancies between medication records. *Quality & Safety in Health Care, 19*(5). Advance online publication. DOI: 10.1136/qshc.2009.038745 PMID: 20688757

West, M., Lyubovnikova, J., Eckert, R., & Denis, J.-L. (2014). Collective leadership for cultures of high quality health care. *Journal of Organizational Effectiveness: People and Performance, 1*, 240–260. DOI: 10.1108/JOEPP-07-2014-0039

Wimmer, B. C., Bell, J. S., Fastbom, J., Wiese, M. D., & Johnell, K. (2016). Medication Regimen Complexity and Polypharmacy as Factors Associated With All-Cause Mortality in Older People: A Population-Based Cohort Study. *The Annals of Pharmacotherapy, 50*(2), 89–95. DOI: 10.1177/1060028015621071 PMID: 26681444

World Health Organization. (2003). *Adherence to long-term therapies: evidence for action* (p. 196 p.). World Health Organization.

Yarnall, A. J., Sayer, A. A., Clegg, A., Rockwood, K., Parker, S., & Hindle, J. V. (2017). New horizons in multimorbidity in older adults. *Age and Ageing, 46*(6), 882–888. DOI: 10.1093/ageing/afx150 PMID: 28985248

Zelko, E., KlemencKetis, Z., & TusekBunc, K. (2016). Medication Adherence in Elderly with Polypharmacy Living at Home: A Systematic Review of Existing Studies. *Materia Socio-Medica, 28*(2), 129. DOI: 10.5455/msm.2016.28.129-132 PMID: 27147920

KEY TERMS AND DEFINITIONS

Medication Adherence: The extent to which a person's medication-taking behavior corresponds with agreed recommendations from a healthcare provider, including initiation, implementation, and discontinuation of treatment.

Polypharmacy: The simultaneous use of multiple medications by a patient—often defined as five or more—which is common in individuals with chronic conditions or multimorbidity and presents challenges in ensuring safe and effective treatment.

Multimorbidity: The co-occurrence of two or more chronic diseases or conditions within a single individual, which complicates treatment regimens and increases the need for integrated and coordinated care.

Patient-Centred Care (PCC): An approach to healthcare that respects and responds to the individual preferences, needs, and values of patients, ensuring that patient values guide all clinical decisions.

Digital Health: The use of digital technologies—including mobile apps, telemedicine, electronic health records, and smart devices—to improve health outcomes, enhance healthcare delivery, and support patient engagement.

Automated Dose Dispensing (ADD): A technological system that prepares and dispenses prescribed medication doses in pre-packaged formats, often integrated with alerts and monitoring tools to support adherence and reduce errors.

Implementation Science: The study of methods and strategies to promote the systematic uptake of evidence-based practices into routine healthcare, aiming to improve the quality and effectiveness of services.

Design Science Research Methodology (DSRM): An iterative and participatory research approach used to develop and evaluate innovative solutions—particularly in complex, real-world healthcare environments—by engaging stakeholders throughout the process.

Chapter 15
Digitalization and Technological Innovations in Surgical Nursing:
Digital Transformation in Surgical Nursing

Dilek Gümüş
https://orcid.org/0000-0002-5338-9377
Bilecik Şeyh Edebali University, Turkey

ABSTRACT

The writers of this chapter claim that in surgical nursing, digitalization and technical developments have drastically changed patient care procedures. Digital tools including electronic health records, artificial intelligence-supported decision systems, wearable devices, simulation technologies and augmented reality have helped nurses to make clinical decisions, guarantee patient safety and raise the quality of treatment. Furthermore underlining the need of digital capabilities in professional growth are redefining nurse roles in robotic surgical applications and supporting nursing education with simulations. Although telehealth technologies provide access and flexibility to help surgery patients follow-up, the ethical and legal aspects of digital applications also provide significant topics of conversation. This chapter explores in a multidimensional sense the consequences of digital change on surgical nursing practices.

INTRODUCTION

The increasing complexity of technological devices requires interdisciplinary cooperation in operating theatres. In this context, surgical nurses play a critical role by observing the patient's care needs and providing adequate care during surgery. Digitalisation helps nurses to fulfil these tasks more effectively, while also increasing communication and collaboration within the team. Especially in stressful and acute situations, effective communication and teamwork are vital to ensure patient safety. At this point, the advantages offered by digitalisation are not only limited to intra-team communication, but also provide an important opportunity to optimise patient safety. Digital systems enable team members to exchange accurate and clear information, so enabling quick and consistent decision-making based on need. Thus, in surgical nursing, digitalisation is absolutely essential to raise patient safety and enhance teamwork (Mattsson, 2020). Digitalisation's inclusion into nursing practice offers both possibilities and difficulties, so transforming healthcare significantly. Digital technologies such as electronic health records (EHR),

DOI: 10.4018/979-8-3373-3531-5.ch015

telehealth, mobile applications and artificial intelligence (AI) enable more patient-centred approaches by increasing the efficiency and accuracy of nursing care (Ganaie & Naz, 2024). However, some barriers need to be overcome for the successful adoption of these technologies. In this context, the efficient application of digital technologies depends much on the digital literacy of nurses. Developing organized training programs and arming nurses with the required technological skills will help them to completely enjoy the advantages of digital systems (Conte, Magon & Caruso, 2024; Wynn et al., 2023a). Nurses with digital skills can use technology more effectively in patient care, which can improve the quality of nursing practice. In this direction, professional development programmes and participation in the design processes of digital systems are among the effective methods to increase the user competence and competence of nurses (Brown et al., 2020). Particularly in fields like clinical decision making, the inclusion of digital health systems into nursing procedures has enormous promise. But problems including not being able to fairly depict the whole spectrum of nursing activity and how it affects patient outcomes arise during the complete deployment of these systems (Hants, Bail & Paterson, 2023). Structured approaches, such the School Education Quality Index (SEQI) educational concept, can now help to guarantee the efficient and suitable use of these tools and help to integrate digital technologies into nursing practice (Hofstetter et al., 2023). Moreover, by streamlining nursing procedures, digitalization could help to raise the quality and efficiency of treatment. By spotting and cutting waste in nursing procedures, one can particularly help to improve patient care. While lowering nurse workload, these improvements can help patient care to be more quality and accessible (Uzun & Cerit, 2023). By allowing creative ideas in nursing, digitalisation presents a strong tool to enhance the experiences of patients and healthcare professionals. While allowing nurses to carry out their responsibilities more efficiently, technological developments have the potential to raise quality and safety in patient care. To make this process successful, though, nurses' digital skills must be developed and reinforced by organized training courses. Therefore, a sustainable change in healthcare services and the best possible benefits of digitalisation in nursing practices can be realised.

Modern technologies like artificial intelligence and augmented reality (AR) have great promise for revolution in nursing. These days, artificial intelligence is applied in nursing mostly to support clinical decision-making procedures, enhance patient monitoring and streamline procedures. While also making nursing operations more efficient, AI-based systems help nurses diagnose and predict patient conditions faster, so improving the quality of care (Martinez-Ortigosa et al., 2023; Ng et al., 2021; O'Connor et al., 2022). Still another significant technology changing the field of nursing is AR. Apart from the ability of artificial intelligence to enhance clinical procedures and operations, AR is a revolutionary tool that especially in the domain of nursing education distinguishes. AR apps give nursing students immersive simulations that not only improve their theoretical knowledge but also give them the chance to hone their communication skills and raise their empathy capacity. This technology increases students' motivation and positively affects their academic performance through interactive learning experiences. Thus, AR, which assumes a complementary role to traditional education methods, makes a valuable contribution to nursing education (Kobayashi et al., 2022; Uymaz & Uymaz, 2022; Wüller et al., 2019). Combining artificial intelligence with augmented reality produces a strong synergy that will help nursing practice and education to be more efficient, creative, patient-centered. Data analytics with AR-based simulations and AI-supported patient monitoring systems together provide students and healthcare professionals the chance to provide better quality treatment and streamline learning processes. These technologies enable digitalization and innovation to find more room in the future of the nursing profession, so accelerating the change of healthcare.

Digital tools and technological innovations are revolutionizing conventional procedures in the field of surgical nursing, so raising efficiency and improving patient outcomes. The inclusion of robotic surgery, which allows minimally invasive treatments, has been one of the most obvious changes of this nature. Through small incisions, remotely controlled robotic systems allow surgeons to execute exact operations; they also help to shorten patients' recovery time, so facilitating the postoperative process. Not only has robotic surgery improved patient care, but it also greatly advanced surgical education. Thanks to simulations including virtual reality platforms and dual console systems, a safe and controlled learning environment is created for surgical assistants and specialists even while robotic surgery training is progressively developing. Thus, novice surgeons and nurses have the opportunity to improve their skills without clinical risk, and as a result, more successful surgical interventions can be performed (Buchs et al., 2013; Chen et al., 2020; Howard et al., 2022). In addition to robotic surgery, another technology that stands out as a major innovation in surgical nursing is wearable devices. By always monitoring patients' vital signs, these devices give doctors real-time data. Particularly in postoperative treatment, real-time monitoring is vital since it enables informed and quick decision-making and helps to avoid complications (Youssef et al., 2024.). Simulation technologies are another crucial invention helping surgical nurses with training and preparation procedures. These realistic simulations let surgeons and nurses learn and execute difficult surgeries free from patient risk. By bridging the gap between theoretical knowledge and practical application, the increasingly ubiquitous use of tools including 3D printed models, telementering and telemetry in training programs offers a complete learning process (Ashrafian et al., 2017; Buchs et al., 2013; Chen et al., 2020). All these technological innovations improve both patient safety and clinical outcomes in the field of surgical nursing, while increasing the competencies of healthcare professionals and supporting their professional development. Robotic surgery, wearable technologies and simulation-based trainings allow nurses to work more effectively, consciously and safely, while providing a significant quality increase in patient care.

DIGITALIZATION PROCESSES IN SURGICAL NURSING

Digitalization is an important transformation process in surgical nursing. Today, emergency general surgical nursing widely employs computer-aided systems to enhance the effectiveness of nurses. According to Lei, He, and Huang (2022), these systems help standardize the way nursing information is managed, make electronic nursing files, better manage nurses' work loads, and make quality control processes smarter. Another important contribution of digitalization is that it facilitates nurses' data management processes. Digital documents allow nurses to collect and analyze data while interacting with the patient, enabling more effective evaluation of nursing interventions. These documents also facilitate the recording of care processes and increase patient follow-up and treatment effectiveness (Nordgård, 2017). Successful application of digitalization in the nursing profession depends critically on the development of digital competencies. Research done in Germany emphasizes the need of including digital skills into nursing education initiatives. Keeping up with the digital transformation process will help nurses to be more effective in clinical practice and in the modernizing of health systems (Tischendorf et al., 2024a). Still, there are certain restrictions on how digitalization might be included into nursing practices. Digital health systems can help nurses' clinical decision-making procedures, but there is not enough data to totally include nursing care into digital systems (Hants et al., 2023). Recall that digital transformation relies on nurses' organizational skills and adaptation as much as technical developments. This process is much enhanced by nursing leadership. Digitalization can inspire nurses and promote the application of current digital tools. Nursing leaders must, however, guide digital strategies and adjust teams to fit this new system if they are to properly manage this transition (Korte & Bohnet-Joschko, 2022). In particular, the digital transformation of perioperative processes is an important step that supports patient-centered improvements. The integration of electronic nursing documents into medical record systems increases patient safety by accelerating data access in surgical processes. Thus, both the quality standards in patient care increase, and the workflow of healthcare professionals becomes more efficient (Ryan et al., 2019). Digitalization processes in surgical nursing encompass various key technologies, including EHR, telehealth applications, and AI-enabled decision support systems. These technologies offer several possibilities and difficulties even if they could maximize patient treatment. Particularly in surgical nursing, EHRs have grown to be essential since they directly influence patient outcomes and job satisfaction of nurses. Although EHRs can raise nurses' degree of professional satisfaction, poorly thought out or ineffective systems can lead to burnout, job discontent, and even professional career departure tendency. Furthermore linked to low EHR usability are higher inpatient mortality rates and 30-day readmission rates for surgical patients (Kademane et al., 2023; Kutney- Lee et al., 2021). Notwithstanding these difficulties, EHRs—when used properly—can significantly help to raise the standard of nursing care. The implementation of even basic systems can increase patient safety by improving care coordination (Kademane et al., 2023). In surgical settings, the presence of standardized nursing diagnoses (NDs) in the content of EHRs may help better measure the impact of nursing care on patient outcomes. Most EHR systems, meanwhile, have only partially linked these diagnosis. This makes it challenging to fully appreciate how nursing care contributes to health outcomes (Cesare et al., 2023). Using integrated EHR systems could cause some operational problems in the first phase. Particularly, we observe negative effects such as longer documentation time and increased nurse turnover. However, in the long term, these systems have the potential to improve certain quality metrics, such as reducing hospital-acquired infection rates (Sanders et al., 2014; Walker-Czyz, 2016). The integration of EHRs into patient care processes affects not only data management and quality standards but also nurse-patient interactions. In most cases, nurses' focus on systems can reduce the quality of communication by making their interactions with the patient more task-oriented. However, some nurses manage to overcome these obstacles and maintain effective patient communication (Forde-Johnston, Butcher & Aveyard, 2022). At this point, the integration of simulated EHRs into nursing education offers a fantastic opportunity. These simulation systems, which better prepare nursing students for real-world clinical settings, fill the gap between theoretical knowledge and practical skills, enabling the training of better-equipped nurses (Sweeney, Morse & Carofiglio, 2019).

In surgical nursing, patient pre- and postoperative management depends much on electronic records. By simplifying procedures, these systems enable nurses to more properly manage patient care processes and raise the quality of treatment. EHR is absolutely essential for standardized framework documentation of patient assessments and surgical preparation processes during the preoperative period. By means of these systems, nurses can arrange patient data and generate more methodically based care plans. But the time spent on EHR chores differs greatly depending on the regional context, which affects the workflow efficiency. Such behavior implies that further standardizing and optimization of EHR systems used in surgical nursing is needed (Zheng et al., 2020). Effective use of electronic records during the perioperative period helps to systematically document nursing diagnoses and treatment plans, so facilitating the patient care process to be executed with a more whole approach. By helping to fully follow the required actions across the surgical process, EHRs help to improve the quality of treatment (Fritzen et al., 2023). EHRs are becoming ever more important in the postoperative period. Improving patient comfort mostly depends on accurate documentation of pain assessments and control of analgesic distribution. Research indicates, however, that pain documentation often falls short of advised guidelines. The state of affairs emphasizes the need of both better training programs and more efficient system support to guarantee accurate and complete records (Erden et al., 2017; Erden et al., 2018). Advanced analysis and prediction systems support EHRs, not only by recording patient information but also by enhancing patient safety. Integrating predictive modeling applications into electronic records facilitates early detection and management of post-surgical complications. By identifying potential risks in advance, we can improve patient outcomes and make more effective interventions (Weller et al., 2018).

In surgical nursing, EHR security and protection of patient privacy are of extreme importance. Nurses have expressed significant concerns about EHR security, pointing out issues such as unauthorized access, inadequate training, and system vulnerabilities among the factors that may threaten patient confidentiality (Issa et al., 2020). Health data is extremely sensitive, thus strict data security policies are absolutely essential. EHR security calls for complete legal compliance with laws including the Health Insurance Portability and Accountability Act (HIPAA), not only protection from individual mistakes. To achieve this compliance, it has become inevitable to implement various security measures at administrative, physical, and technical levels (Kruse et al., 2017; Mbonihankuye, Nkunzimana & Ndagijimana, 2019). At this point, the use of advanced security techniques plays a critical role in making EHR systems more secure. Adoption of technologies like encryption techniques and role-based access control especially helps safeguard patient privacy by ensuring that healthcare professionals only access data for which they are authorized (Fernández-Alemán et al., 2013; Keshta & Odeh, 2020). Protecting patient information, however, calls for a strong culture of privacy awareness among healthcare workers in addition to technical ones. Ensuring data integrity, raising awareness of nurses and other healthcare professionals, and supporting them with training programs are essential steps to maintain trust in digital health systems (Duckert & Barkhuus, 2022; Zhu, Saravanan & Muthu, 2020).

Telehealth applications are an important innovation in surgical nursing. These applications are becoming increasingly important in terms of facilitating access to healthcare services and making care processes more flexible. Telenursing, one of the nursing components of telehealth, is an approach in which nurses provide remote care and nursing services using information and communication technologies. Especially in surgical oncology patients, it is of significant importance to collect and evaluate successful implementation models for the effective implementation of telenursing services (Mozer et al., 2023). The COVID-19 pandemic has caused telehealth applications to be more widely used by surgical patients and clearly demonstrated the potential in this field. This process has developed and drawn attention as a new application area in surgical nursing from a concept known as telesurgery, which offers remote surgical treatment (Yeşilyurt, 2024.). Not only do telehealth tools provide great benefits in areas like teaching surgical patients and tracking postoperative symptoms, but they also limit only treatment delivery. By means of better medication and protocol adherence, mobile health technologies—such as SMS alerts or mobile app-based interventions—improve patients' clinical involvement (Lu et al., 2017). These programs provide solutions for rural and remote areas where access to healthcare services is restricted, so contributing among other things. By saving time and money, telehealth can be as successful as in-person treatments in some areas and help to sustain healthcare services (Speyer et al., 2018). Still, the effective application of telehealth technologies calls for some careful thought regarding several elements. Some of the things that can help or hurt telehealth applications are nurses' digital skills, the usefulness of technology tools, the structure of the organization, and how the healthcare staff feels about these new systems (Koivunen & Saranto, 2018). In light of all these developments, telehealth applications offer important opportunities to improve the quality of care in surgical nursing, strengthen patient follow-up, and reach a wider patient population. Consequently, modern healthcare is including digital health strategies into its surgical nursing practices more and more naturally.

Especially by means of AI-enabled decision support systems, artificial intelligence has become a transforming tool in surgical nursing. These systems provide real-time data analysis and predictive insights, so improving decision-making during surgeries. In this context, surgical environments are including advanced AI technologies including machine learning and understandable artificial intelligence (XAI), so helping to predict and prevent intraoperative adverse events. By analyzing data in the operating room, XAI systems especially can forecast complications like hypoxemia and provide real-time risk scores and justification for these forecasts to doctors. This capacity greatly supports clinical reasoning and decision-making procedures (Gordon, Grantcharov & Rudzicz, 2019; Loftus et al., 2019). Some of the constraints of conventional systems could be eliminated by including artificial intelligence into surgical decision support systems. In particular, problems such as manual data management and limited accuracy can be overcome with faster and more precise solutions thanks to AI models. When fed with live EHR data, AI can provide timely and accurate support to improve the entire process from preoperative planning to postoperative patient management (Hashimoto et al., 2018; Loftus et al., 2019). Still, artificial intelligence supports decisions and helps with operational elements of the surgical process. Procedures are more efficient and effective when AI systems suggest next actions in surgery and speed up intraoperative pathology evaluations, so improving their efficiency (Bouden & Mezioud, 2023; Navarrete-Welton & Hashimoto, 2020). Adoption of artificial intelligence in surgical nursing presents some difficulties notwithstanding all these exciting uses. Carefully addressed and managed should be problems including algorithm bias, the need of data standardizing, and the ethical consequences of artificial intelligence in decision-making procedures. Furthermore, interdisciplinary collaboration is inevitable for the successful implementation of these technologies. Effective collaborations between surgeons and data scientists will ensure the harmonious integration of AI systems into the clinical environment (Hashimoto et al., 2018; Loftus et al., 2023). As AI technologies continue to evolve, they are expected to assume broader roles in surgical nursing and provide improvements in both patient care and surgical outcomes. These developments have the potential to improve the quality of healthcare services by adding an innovative dimension to nursing practice.

Using machine learning (ML) techniques, AI-powered decision support systems project what issues might arise following surgery. This greatly simplifies doctors' decision-making process and helps patients to perform well. In this regard, the application of artificial intelligence in important fields such surgical wound management presents amazing progress. Some machine learning models, such as Support Vector Machine (SVM) and Convolutional Neural Network (CNN), are rather good in forecasting surgical site infections and other issues that might arise during many kinds of surgery (Zhang et al., 2024). Similarly, different AI models are being integrated into clinical decision processes to support perioperative management. For instance, the SUMPOT system, which uses artificial neural network technology, has shown that it could be useful in this area by correctly identifying 90% of patients who are likely to have problems after surgery (Chelazzi et al., 2021). AI systems also offer powerful tools to clinicians in the preoperative planning process. The MySurgeryRisk algorithm developed in this direction improves physicians' risk assessment skills and facilitates more effective planning through real-time analysis of EHR data (Brennan et al., 2019). In addition, XAI techniques bring transparency to AI models, increasing clinical trust and making applications more user-friendly. By explaining the reasons behind predictions, XAI helps surgical teams to predict and mitigate intraoperative adverse events more effectively (Gordon,

Grantcharov & Rudzicz, 2019). By providing a dynamic and unique risk stratification, these AI-driven models not only outperform conventional risk calculators but also allow tailored patient care overall (Hassan et al., 2022).

ROBOTIC SURGERY AND NURSING

The evolution of robotic surgery has been a transforming trip with notable medical technological advancements and innovations. Originally designed for long-distance trauma surgery, robotic systems have developed into flexible and sophisticated instruments extensively applied in minimally invasive surgeries (George et al., 2018). Introduced in 1985, the PUMA 200 was the first significant turn in this technical development. Advanced robotic platforms including the da Vinci Surgical System, which later transformed surgical applications and became global, were made possible by this system (Andreev et al., 2024; Ghezzi & Corleta, 2016). Over the next three decades, the use of robotic surgical systems has not only grown common but also broad their application in surgical disciplines. Robotic surgery is becoming more popular because these systems are very accurate and help patients do better in many areas, like general, oncological, and pediatric surgery (Cundy et al., 2013; Nota et al., 2019). In this process, robotic systems have witnessed innovative developments in many areas, from visualization technologies to surgeon-robot interactions. With each generation, the systems have improved visual quality, enhanced surgical control, and some have added features such as haptic feedback to enhance the user experience (Ashrafian et al., 2017). Even though there isn't a lot of haptic feedback available yet, the benefits of robotic surgery, like 3D vision, motion scaling, and less tremor, have helped get around many of the problems with traditional laparoscopic methods (Enayati, De Momi & Ferrigno, 2016; Ghezzi & Corleta, 2016). Nowadays, the capabilities of robotic surgical systems are not only limited to mechanical elements but are further enhanced by the integration of artificial intelligence and machine learning. This integration supports surgeons' decision-making processes with features such as real-time monitoring, advanced surgical guidance, and personalized interventions (Bellos et al., 2024; Vasey et al., 2022). The evolution of robotic surgery addresses accessibility and efficiency as much as technical advancements. Research and development initiatives nowadays seek to lower the costs of these systems, widen the spectrum of treatments, and raise general system efficiency (Andreev et al., 2024; Peters et al., 2018). However, as important as technological advances are, the human factor is also crucial for the safe and effective use of these systems. As robotic surgery becomes more common, it becomes critical to continuously assess its impact on clinical outcomes and develop comprehensive, standardized training programs for healthcare professionals (Cundy et al., 2013; Ghezzi & Corleta, 2016).

Robotic surgery has significantly impacted nursing care processes, especially in the perioperative setting. Similar to their role in traditional major surgeries, nurses play a critical role in ensuring patient safety during robotic surgeries and focus especially on the intraoperative period when patient positioning is vital (Martins et al., 2019). Nursing roles have also evolved greatly with this new surgical technique. By lowering pre- and postoperative nursing care times, which required the creation of new nursing roles such the specialized robotic nurse (Khalil et al., 2024), the integration of robotic systems into surgical operations has produced a technological transformation and raised operational efficiency. Still, this metamorphosis presents certain difficulties. Robotic-assisted surgeries call for not only technological management but also restructuring of efficient communication among members of different disciplines. Particularly, nurses must get specific instruction to properly apply new systems (Gillespie et al., 2020).

In this context, country-based differences also draw attention. For example, in Turkey, the lack of formal training programs for nurses in robotic surgery settings and the lack of national legislation may negatively affect both the quality of nursing care and patient safety; this situation reveals an urgent need for the development of relevant health policies (Çelik et al., 2024). The effective integration of robotic systems into nursing care is not limited to technical skills but requires a broader understanding and strategic approach. A profound understanding of human-robot interaction, the ability to manage the complexity of robotic-assisted surgeries, and the development of holistic strategies to overcome barriers to implementation are critical to the successful progress of this process (Catchpole et al., 2022; Servaty et al., 2020).

Nurses play a critical role as an integral part of the surgical team in the preparation and management of robotic surgical equipment. In this process, nurses need to have not only technical knowledge but also the ability to manage operational processes. In particular, robotic surgery nurses should have the professional knowledge to manage the complexity of the technology and demonstrate competence in dealing with possible robotic malfunctions (Raheem et al., 2017). This expertise is vital for the uninterrupted progress of surgical procedures and to ensure patient safety. The responsibilities of nurses require a multifaceted contribution to all stages of surgery. Nurses who support the preparation processes before surgery also take an active role during surgery. Especially scrub nurses organize the equipment needed by the surgeon in a timely and accurate manner; at the same time, they ensure the order of the surgical area by strictly following the principles of sterilization (Russell, 2022). The unique structure of the robotic surgery environment makes nurses' communication skills even more important. Strong communication skills provide a significant advantage in collecting and transferring patient information and managing team dynamics, as team interaction in this environment progresses more technically and rapidly (Pograjec & Hubert, 2019). However, in the planning and management of robotic surgery programs, the knowledge and skills of experienced perioperative nurses play a decisive role in the efficient and safe execution of the processes. The presence of such nurses both facilitates team coordination and improves the quality of surgical procedures (Thomas, 2011). Indeed, the active involvement of robotic nurse teams in surgical processes not only enhances patient care but may also increase operational efficiency by shortening surgery times (Khalil et al., 2024). For all these reasons, continuous support for the training and professional development of robotic surgery nurses is a critical requirement for the sustainability of high-quality and safe care delivery (Martins et al., 2019; Raheem et al., 2017).

The training and continuous professional development of robotic surgery nurses have gained immense importance with the increasing use of robotic surgery in healthcare. This new surgical approach demands a high level of technical knowledge and skills from nurses, making their role even more critical to the success of the surgery. Robotic surgery nurses should have not only technical knowledge but also the competence to intervene quickly in problems related to robotic systems. In this context, training processes should be carried out through well-structured programs so that nurses feel safe and can provide high-quality care (Raheem et al., 2017). To meet this demand, particular training courses have been created to help robotic surgery nurses grow professionally. For instance, a program at Polk State College enabled nurses to acquire robotic skills and progress their professions in this field. This training program has a multidimensional structure that includes online modules, theoretical courses, hands-on training, and live surgical experiences (Gudeloglu & Parekattil, 2021). Similarly, other studies in the literature emphasize that such structured programs allow nurses to improve their knowledge and skills. This development directly contributes to both ensuring safe surgical experiences and improving patient outcomes (Sarmanian, 2015). In order for education programs to be effective, it is not only sufficient to transfer basic knowledge; it is also of enormous importance to help nurses adapt to new technologies.

Accordingly, integrating innovative technologies into the training process both improves the quality of learning and contributes to the prevention of complications (Chen et al., 2020). In conclusion, nurses involved in robotic surgery need not only to reinforce their existing skills but also to develop a more profound understanding of their professional role. At this point, the understanding of continuous professional development and lifelong learning supports nurses to follow innovations in the field and develop new practices when necessary (Pinto et al., 2018).

WEARABLE TECHNOLOGIES AND SURGICAL PATIENT MONITORING

Wearable technologies are emerging as an important innovation in the field of surgical patient monitoring. These technologies have the potential to improve early complication detection and patient safety by providing continuous monitoring of patients' vital signs. In this regard, some advanced wearable sensors used in high-risk surgical patients have attracted attention. Developed to continuously monitor heart rate and respiratory rate, devices such as SensiumVitals, HealthPatch, EarlySense, and Masimo Radius-7 stand out with their capacity to detect deterioration in patient condition at an earlier stage. While high accuracy rates are achieved, especially in heart rate measurement, it has also been reported that some sensors are sometimes outside acceptable limits in respiratory rate measurements (Breteler et al., 2019). The use of wearable devices in specific subfields of surgery also increases the importance of these technologies. For particular kinds of surgery, such colorectal surgery, these devices can be used at several phases before and after surgery and are especially useful in tracking postoperative complications and acting quickly (Kavallieros et al., 2024). One of the most important contributions of these devices in the postoperative period is to monitor the physical activity levels of patients. Since a decrease in physical activity can be an early indicator of potential complications, such monitoring allows for earlier detection . Despite these benefits, however, there are still some technical limitations regarding the sensitivity of the devices. False alarms, data transmission problems, and variations in measurement accuracy can prevent the full potential of these technologies from being fully exploited (Wells et al., 2022). Wearable sensors used in surgical departments, however, not only help to monitor patients but also support clinical decision-making and could help to lighten the burden on medical staff members. Including these technologies into systems to replace hand measurements will help to maximize their influence (Van Melzen et al., 2023). These devices also greatly help to involve patients. Particularly by spotting more inactive patients and adjusting treatments, hospitals stays can be shortened and the general recovery process sped up (Edney et al., 2024).

Wearable devices' continuous monitoring of vital signs in the postoperative period helps doctors to identify early on patients' clinical conditions, so allowing them to act quickly. Such devices can continuously monitor key vital signs, especially heart rate, respiratory rate, and body temperature, and support clinical decision-making processes by transmitting these data directly to nurses (Breteler et al., 2019; Weenk et al., 2017; Weller et al., 2024). With these features, wearable technologies offer significant advantages compared to traditional intermittent measurements. The continuous flow of data improves patient safety and enables earlier detection of clinical deterioration (Leenen et al., 2024; Weenk et al., 2019). In particular, algorithm-driven systems make this early detection even more effective. Thanks to integrated algorithms, for instance, advanced devices like the BioIntelliSense BioButton® can identify negative changes in patient condition in advance and notify healthcare teams, so reducing the possible hospital stays (Leenen et al., 2024; Weller et al., 2024). Apart from their technical advantages, the way wearable devices enhance the patient experience is also remarkable. Patients usually find these devices to be comfortable and acceptable, which helps to raise their satisfaction and facilitates simpler technology adaptation (Downey et al., 2018; Leenen et al., 2021). Notwithstanding all these advantages, some technical constraints of wearable devices should also be taken into account. Sometimes the effectiveness and dependability of these technologies are limited by issues including data loss, false alarms, and measurement errors (Breteler et al., 2019; Wells et al., 2022).

Patient safety and hastening of the healing process depend on early identification of postoperative complications. In this regard, especially in the post-discharge process, modern monitoring technologies are rather important. Wearable devices significantly contribute to this process by allowing patients outside of the clinical environment continuous and long-term monitoring. This allows doctors to remotely access patient physiological data and identify early on possible complications. One instance of such technology is the clinical use possibilities of devices like Fitbit. By means of machine learning algorithms, these devices gather diverse biometric data and analyze it, so enabling the detection of problems before they manifest (Beqari et al., 2024). Furthermore, wearable technologies enable postoperative monitoring of not only vital signs but also physical activity and general health state. This multifarious monitoring strategy helps to identify problems early on and supports fast interventions in patient care procedures (Gu et al., 2021; Wells et al., 2022). Not only is this thorough data tracking changing complication management but also the model of treatment. Wearable device data support a more proactive, customized, patient-centered structure of healthcare (Kavallieros et al., 2024). Thus, the early identification of postoperative complications by wearable devices has great potential to raise the efficiency of healthcare services and enhance patient outcomes (Lal, Memon & Khan, 2024).

Wearable devices have a significant impact on patient education and motivation. By recording and reporting individuals' physical activity levels, sleep patterns, and other health behaviors, these devices allow individuals to manage their health more consciously. This helps them develop healthier habits (Patel, Asch, & Volpp, 2015). These effects are limited to general health management and make important contributions to the monitoring and control of chronic diseases. Especially in cases such as diabetes and heart disease, the use of wearable devices in combination with educational support can help improve clinical outcomes (Kamei et al., 2020). However, the psychological and behavioral aspects of wearables are also gaining attention. Such technologies may become more attractive for individuals who are reluctant to use traditional treatment methods or have less health experience. Ease of use and instant feedback features may increase the motivation of individuals (Hunkin, King & Zajac, 2020). However, the impact of these technologies on behavior change is not limited to the digital features they offer. To achieve effective results, it is crucial that these devices are integrated with behavioral change strategies. In other words, the combination of technology and behavioral sciences is the foundation for long-term change (Agarwal & Patel, 2019). This context highlights the potential of wearable devices to enhance individual health motivation. By supporting users' intrinsic motivation to achieve their health goals, these devices also encourage adoption and long-term use (Hayat et al., 2022).

The evaluation of data obtained from wearable devices and their integration into clinical decision-making processes is an important innovation in healthcare. These devices are not only limited to individual health monitoring but are also actively used in medical decision-making processes. Wearable technologies, particularly in areas like heart rhythm analysis, significantly impact doctors' daily clinical decisions. Accordingly, these devices play an important role in the remote screening and diagnosis of cardiovascular diseases, especially heart rhythm disorders (Manninger et al., 2021). Still, there are certain difficulties in including these technologies into clinical practice. Significant obstacles to this integration process are factors including worries about device accuracy, the necessity to preserve patient privacy, and economic sustainability (Bayoumy et al., 2021). In this regard, efficient data collecting and usage depend critically on interaction with health information systems. Real-time patient health status monitoring and analysis of wearable device data combined with the EHR makes possible. Such integration has the possibility to not only track present situation but also offer more precise and customized advice on disease prediction and health management (Karako, 2024).

NURSING EDUCATION WITH SIMULATION TECHNOLOGIES

Simulation technologies are an important innovation in nursing education. These technologies prevent patient harm by providing students with a safe learning environment and also make significant contributions to the development of clinical knowledge and skills (Hanshaw & Dickerson, 2020). Recently, one of the most striking components of simulation technologies has been virtual reality (VR) applications. Particularly, nursing education is increasingly utilizing VR simulations as they provide a risk-free and contact-free learning environment (Plotzky et al., 2021). These virtual simulation environments increase not only students' technical skills but also their learning satisfaction and motivation. Studies have shown that VR-based learning improves knowledge retention and clinical reasoning skills (Padilha et al., 2019; Shin et al., 2019). Similarly, it is generally stated that simulation-based learning methods increase students' self-confidence and contribute to more effective knowledge acquisition. Such experiential learning environments support both students' cognitive levels and affective competencies (Mulyadi et al., 2021). We should emphasize the importance of high-fidelity simulations at this point. These simulations, which are carried out with realistic scenarios and equipment, improve students' thinking skills and carry the acquisition of knowledge and skills to a higher level (Hanshaw & Dickerson, 2020). In addition, web-based simulations, which are included in technological diversity, provide flexibility to nursing education and complement face-to-face education. Interactive learning activities encourage students' active participation and enrich the learning process (Cant & Cooper, 2014). In light of all these developments, it is understood that simulation education is more effective compared to traditional methods and should be increasingly included in the nursing curriculum (Shin, Park & Kim, 2015).

The use of simulation laboratories in surgical nursing has become an important part of nursing education. These laboratories provide students with the opportunity to practice in a safe and controlled environment, allowing them to prepare more effectively for real clinical situations (Hansen & Holz, 2020; Lu, Cuff & Mansour, 2020; Sundler, Pettersson & Berglund, 2015). Especially in high-risk and complex fields such as surgical nursing, simulation laboratories play a critical role in the professional development of students. These environments contribute to the acquisition of the necessary knowledge, skills, and abilities, allowing students to safely develop their clinical competencies (Buckley & Gordon, 2011; Ma et al., 2024). In this framework, the simulation-based learning (SBL) approach stands out as an effective method for developing various professional skills in nursing students. SBL contributes to the multifaceted development of students by supporting clinical performance, critical thinking, professional attitudes, and communication skills (Ma et al., 2024). Another important aspect of simulation applications is the integration of theoretical knowledge with practice. Through scenario-based simulations, students have the opportunity to practice and deepen the learning process by reflecting on their experiences (Sundler et al., 2015). This learning process improves students' technical skills and supports them to become more prepared for real-world nursing practice. Thus, patient safety is increased, and students are enabled to approach situations that may be encountered in clinical settings more consciously (Buckley & Gordon, 2011; Lewis et al., 2019). In conclusion, the integration of simulation laboratories into surgical nursing education not only transforms theoretical knowledge into practice but also increases student satisfaction and self-confidence. This contributes to the training of more competent and equipped health professionals in the long term (Ma et al., 2024; Swenty & Eggleston, 2011).

The effects of simulation on patient safety in surgical nursing have been examined in various studies. Simulation stands out as an effective training and assessment technique that is widely used to improve patient safety in healthcare. These applications allow not only individual clinicians but also teams to improve their technical performance during critical incidents and complex procedures (Schmidt et al., 2013). Thus, safer practice environments can be created at both individual and team levels. Especially in the field of surgical nursing, the importance of simulation-based training becomes more evident. Such trainings strengthen the clinical safety skills of nurses, strengthen the transfer of theoretical knowledge to practice, and ensure the long-term preservation of the skills gained (Peñataro-Pintado et al., 2021). Simulation improves team dynamics and has only limited effect on individual skills. Particularly in operating room teams, simulation training helps to build both technical and non-technical skills, so improving team cohesion, communication, and cooperation (Rathore et al., 2024). Such trainings enable nurses to participate more effectively in safety management processes, support safety culture, and contribute to the development of positive attitudes (Lee & Kim, 2018). However, despite these positive developments, evidence about the direct effects of simulation on patient outcomes is still limited. Consequently, more study is required to more fully show how simulation affects clinical outcomes (Meling & Meling, 2020).

Surgeons' decision-making abilities are being sharpened by VR and AR applications more and more. These technologies provide a creative way for surgical education so that nurses may better execute difficult surgical operations and grasp their knowledge. With realistic and interactive simulations, VR and AR technologies greatly help nurses to develop their clinical skills in surgical education (Ayoub & Pulijala, 2019; Mao et al., 2021; McKnight et al., 2020). These free from real-life hazards virtual environments give nurses a safe learning environment and simultaneously give them the chance to experience and enhance their decision-making process. In particular, VR positively affects the decision-making processes of nurses in terms of both speed and accuracy by providing detailed simulation of surgical procedures (Mao et al., 2021; Mishra et al., 2022). In this respect, VR both accelerates the learning process and contributes to reducing the risk of error in real applications. AR, on the other hand, offers a different learning dimension by integrating digital information into the real world. AR applications help nurses to better visualize the surgical field and make decisions integrated with environmental data (Barsom, Graafland & Schijven, 2016; Sulé et al., 2023). Consequently, by means of the acquired skills, VR and AR technologies enhance the training procedures of nurses and help to raise the quality of patient care (Chen et al., 2020; Hong & Wang, 2023).

ECONOMIC IMPACT OF DIGITALIZATION IN SURGICAL NURSING

Digitalization in surgical nursing has emerged as a transformative force that has significantly impacted economic aspects in healthcare systems. The integration of digital technologies such as telemedicine and electronic medical records has not only improved the efficiency of healthcare delivery but also contributed to significant economic savings. One of the main economic benefits of digitalization in surgical nursing is the reduction in travel and time costs associated with patient follow-up care. A study in

Germany showed that video consultations for follow-up care in orthopedic and trauma surgery resulted in an average cost saving of €76.52 per consultation. This is mainly due to reduced travel and time costs for patients, as well as reduced production losses. By minimizing the need for physical visits, digital health technologies ease the financial burden on patients and health systems and make healthcare more accessible and affordable. Moreover, digitalization indirectly affects economic evaluations by contributing to environmental cost savings. The same study highlighted that video consultations lead to significant reductions in greenhouse gas emissions and other pollutants, resulting in environmental cost savings of between €3.73 and €9.53 per patient (Muschol et al., 2022). These savings are crucial as health systems worldwide strive for carbon neutrality and align economic goals with environmental sustainability.

Digitalization in surgical nursing provides financial efficiency by facilitating administrative processes as well as patient-related savings. As observed in a Turkish hospital, digitization of paper forms in inpatient care has led to significant time and resource savings. For example, the time required to complete patient history forms was reduced from 45 minutes to 12 minutes, saving approximately 27 percent of time. This efficiency translates into more time for direct patient care and reduces operational costs while improving the quality of nursing services. The financial implications of reduced paper and toner consumption are also considerable. In the same study, digitalization saved $1,705.86 in annual paper costs and $283,736 in toner costs in four wards. These savings highlight the potential of digital technologies to contribute to the overall economic efficiency of healthcare institutions by significantly reducing material costs. Furthermore, the wider application of digital technologies in surgical nursing may provide systemic economic benefits. Digitalization enables better allocation of human resources by reducing the time nurses spend on administrative tasks. In Turkey, assuming that 60% of nurses work in inpatient wards, it is estimated that digitization of inpatient forms could save 398 to 559 nursing hours per year (Volkan et al., 2024). This reallocation of time can improve the quality of patient care and reduce labor costs by reducing the need for additional staff.

THE ETHICAL AND LEGAL DIMENSIONS OF DIGITALIZATION IN SURGICAL NURSING

In surgical nursing, digitalization attracts interest in ethical and legal aspects as well as in terms of technical advancements. Several ethical questions are raised by including digital technologies into surgical procedures including data security and protection of patient information as well as guaranteeing privacy. In this framework, the use of surgical robotic systems especially generates fresh ethical and legal obligations concerning the collecting, processing, and storage of patient data. This situation requires surgeons and healthcare professionals to have not only technical knowledge but also knowledge about data management, patient rights, and related legal regulations (Lam, Purkayastha & Kinross, 2021). The effects of digitalization are not only limited to data security but also transform patient-physician interactions. Particularly the use of digital technologies in informed consent procedures helps patients to have a better awareness of the process, so improving their quality of life and lowering their stress levels. Still debatable, though, is the realization of these favorable results for every patient group. More research is needed on the ethical appropriateness and feasibility of digital applications, especially in vulnerable groups such as the elderly, individuals with limited mental capacity, or patients with communication difficulties (Kiernan et al., 2023).

Digital ethical reflection tools are developed to help nurses cope with ethical problems. These tools increase nurses' ethical awareness levels and support their decision-making processes by providing guidance against ethical challenges they face in clinical practice (Jakobsen et al., 2023). Therefore, we can directly link the ethical dimensions of digitalization to both ethical principles and nurses' digital competencies. The basis of an ethically conscious digital practice is nurses' ability to use technology and their ability to evaluate these technologies within the framework of ethical responsibilities. Therefore, nurses need to have not only technical knowledge but also ethical decision-making skills when using digital technologies. The application of ethical decision-making models is critical for both protecting patient rights and fulfilling professional responsibilities, especially in complex clinical scenarios. Moreover, nurses are increasingly expected to act as mediators in such situations (Kraft et al., 2024).

The protection of patient information in digital health applications in surgical nursing is of extreme importance in terms of ensuring patient privacy. The security of health data kept in digital environments is a critical issue in terms of both patient safety and ethical responsibilities. Therefore, various encryption methods have been developed to protect digital health data. In particular, chaos-based encryption systems stand out as an effective solution to prevent unauthorized access and secure patient information (Hamza et al., 2020). At this point, the security of EHR systems is of particular importance. Given the central role of EHRs in storing and managing patient information, multi-layered measures at administrative, physical, and technical levels are required to ensure the security of these systems (Kruse et al., 2017). Data security should not only be limited to technical measures but should also be supported by user awareness and information processes. Both nurses and patients emphasize the importance of protecting patient privacy and express the need for more education and information (Kim, Han & Kim, 2017). Accordingly, it is of extreme importance to raise awareness about the protection of patient data in the design of digital health platforms. Raising users' awareness about digital privacy directly affects the effective and safe use of systems (Duckert & Barkhuus, 2022). In addition, the data protection requirements brought about by digital transformation in the surgical environment make it mandatory for all healthcare professionals to be knowledgeable in this field and to follow best practices (Lam et al., 2021). In this context, it has become a vital necessity to continuously develop and update digital health applications in order to both increase patient safety and protect privacy (Goldenberg & Grantcharov, 2018).

Digital transformation is leading to significant changes in the operating room, and these changes include multi-layered processes such as the creation, management, and utilization of surgical data flow. This digitalization process has made data security more critical due to the increasing volume and variety of data generated during and after surgery. In this regard, one of the main concerns of the digital transformation process is clearly patient data protection. Not only is technological but also ethical and legal obligation design of digital surgical systems to guarantee data security. Accordingly, data protection laws and regulatory frameworks need to adapt to the ever-evolving nature of surgical data. In this process, not only surgeons' expertise in clinical practice, but also their knowledge and responsibilities in data governance, gain importance. Surgeons have a responsibility to protect both their own professional data and that of their patients; therefore, it is crucial that they understand the changing data legislation and best practices in data governance (Lam et al., 2021). The effects of digital transformation are not only limited to surgeons but also manifest themselves in nursing practice. In particular, the integration of AI applications into nursing care raises broader ethical, legal, and social questions such as data privacy, security, access to technology, and user acceptance. Not only are technical solutions insufficient to effectively manage these multidimensional impacts, but we also need to develop a techno-social discourse. This discourse requires the adoption of a holistic approach that integrates patient safety, ethical practices, and legal compliance and requires the active participation of all stakeholders—health professionals, patients, administrators, and technology developers (Seibert et al., 2020).

THE FUTURE OF DIGITALIZATION IN NURSING

Digitalization in nursing has great future potential to revolutionize healthcare delivery and raise the standard of treatment. Since they are at the core of service delivery, nurses are very important in the integration of technologies in the process of digitalization of health systems. As the largest group in the healthcare workforce, nurses can successfully support this transformation process when they have the capacity to use digital technologies effectively and ethically. However, the adoption of these technologies is closely related not only to professional roles and tasks but also to demographic and psychosocial factors such as age, gender, individual attitudes, and willingness to use technology. These variables can facilitate or hinder the acceptance and effective use of digital applications (Wynn et al., 2023a). Therefore, not only the technical dimension but also the theoretical framework of digital nursing practices should be carefully considered. Relevant theories explain how digital technologies play a role as an "agent" in the patient environment and point to the importance of nurses developing their technological competencies to work effectively with these new tools (Wynn et al., 2023b). These theoretical approaches are embodied in nursing practice by the integration of advanced digital technologies like artificial intelligence and robotics, so transforming the field. This integration calls for nurses to develop not only current knowledge and skills but also new digital competencies and adjust to changing roles inside the healthcare ecosystem (Booth et al., 2021; Tischendorf et al., 2024a). However, this digital transformation process brings some important challenges as well as potential benefits. Data security, ethical responsibilities, and the risk of damage to personalized care due to standardization of care are among the key issues that still need to be addressed in the nursing profession (Wong et al., 2023). Only thorough and sustainable educational plans will help one to overcome such difficulties. Therefore, it is of great relevance to create instructional strategies meant to provide nursing professionals with the required digital competencies (Tischendorf et al., 2024a; Tischendorf et al., 2024b). Thus, a comprehensive knowledge of how to include digital tools not only in terms of technological development but also in a way that preserves the fundamental principles of patient-centered care should be developed. This method guarantees the sustainability of person-centered healthcare (Wong et al., 2023) so strengthening nursing practice.

Nurses must adapt to the digitalized character of healthcare while facing different difficulties in the process of the digital transformation. Among these difficulties, elements including adaptation to digital technologies, lack of sufficient digital skills and equipment, lack of institutional support, and growing care burden stand out (Martínez & Leyva-Moral, 2024). In this context, nurses' adaptation to digital technologies requires acquiring technical knowledge and keeping up with rapidly changing systems. However, this may limit the efficiency of nursing practice and the potential benefits from digital tools (Chaharsoughi, Ahmadifaraz & Kahangi, 2022). Furthermore among the significant psychological obstacles preventing the acceptance of digital transformation (Tarsuslu, Agaigl & Bas, 2024) are anxiety, uncertainty, and negative attitudes toward new technologies, particularly artificial intelligence. The literature offers several approaches to meet these complex problems. One of these strategies is nurse-led digital transformation initiatives. This approach aims to improve both the quality of care and patient satisfaction by encouraging nurses to take active leadership in digital health (Martínez & Leyva-Moral, 2024). Moreover, strengthening the perception of digital leadership encourages the effective use of technologies and contributes to the development of more positive attitudes by reducing nurses' anxiety towards systems such as AI (Tarsuslu et al., 2024). In this framework, innovative educational strategies also attract attention. In particular, methods such as digital storytelling increase nurses' empathy skills and allow them to understand technology in a more human framework (Clisbee, Beierwaltes & Eggenberger, 2019). To make all these processes sustainable, it is a critical necessity to provide continuous training and support programs to increase the digital skills of nurses (Chambers et al., 2018).

CONCLUSION

Digitalization and technological innovations in surgical nursing have become an integral part of modern healthcare. This transformation creates radical changes in both clinical practice and nursing education. In particular, the widespread use of EHR systems reduces the workload of nurses and facilitates clinical decision-making by providing fast and secure processing of patient information. By speeding information access, digital record systems improve patient safety and help to more efficiently manage care processes. AI-supported decision systems are another evolution that fits this digital infrastructure. With a more customized and holistic approach, artificial intelligence systems let nurses forecast possible complications and assist them in organizing patient care. Likewise, wearable technologies offer an important innovation in the follow-up of surgical patients. These devices facilitate the early detection of complications by enabling continuous monitoring of vital signs; they also contribute to a more informed care process by encouraging active participation of patients in their health processes. Another vital part of the surgical process, robotic surgical systems redefine the roles of nurses in intraoperative and postoperative operations while raising operational accuracy and efficiency. These systems demand nurses to deepen their technical knowledge and skills while also improving the coordination of surgeons working with nursing teams. These technical developments have completely changed the framework of nursing education and revolutionized clinical practice. Nurses can raise awareness of patient safety, enhance their critical thinking, fast decision-making, and problem-solving ability by means of simulation technologies, AR, and related instructional tools. The economic impact of digitalization in surgical nursing is multifaceted and encompasses direct cost savings for patients, environmental benefits, and operational efficiencies in healthcare systems. Digital technologies improve the economic sustainability of healthcare delivery by reducing travel and time costs, minimizing environmental impacts, and streamlining administrative processes. As healthcare systems continue to embrace digitalization, these economic benefits are likely to expand and further transform the landscape of surgical nursing. However, digitalization also brings with it some basic ethical and legal responsibilities. Particularly, this transformation process must emphasize the critical issues of data security and patient privacy protection. Accordingly, protecting patient information against unauthorized access, continuously strengthening the digital skills of nurses, and ensuring full compliance with legal regulations are vital for both ethical and sustainable implementation of digitalization.

In surgical nursing, digitalization has become a rather effective tool that raises patient outcomes and quality of living. Clinical decision support systems as well as technologies that enable patient follow-up help to make care procedures safer and more successful. We should thus assess this change process not only for its benefits but also for the difficulties it brings about. In particular, factors such as data accuracy, sustainability of costs, and inadequate technological infrastructure are among the important factors that directly affect the success of digital health systems. Therefore, it has become a critical requirement for nurses to adapt to this process in order for future digitalization strategies to be successful. Developing digital skills, using innovative technologies effectively, and strengthening collaboration with health professionals from different disciplines will support better patient outcomes in surgical nursing. When we evaluate all these elements together, we see that digitalization is more than just a tool to enhance current practices. Digitalization now stands out as a dynamic and strategic platform that redefines the understanding of patient-centered care and shapes the future of healthcare.

REFERENCES

Agarwal, A., & Patel, M. (2019). Prescribing Behavior Change: Opportunities and Challenges for Clinicians to Embrace Digital and Mobile Health. *JMIR mHealth and uHealth*, 8. https://doi.org/DOI: 10.2196/preprints.17281

Andreev, A., Glukhov, A., Ostroushko, A., Laptiyova, A., Bokov, D., Mikhailov, N., & Konovalov, P. (2024). *Automated robotic systems in surgical practice*. Science and Innovations in Medicine., DOI: 10.35693/sim540155

Ashrafian, H., Clancy, O., Grover, V., & Darzi, A. (2017). The evolution of robotic surgery: Surgical and anaesthetic aspects. *British Journal of Anaesthesia*, *119*, i72–i84. DOI: 10.1093/bja/aex383

Ayoub, A., & Pulijala, Y. (2019). The application of virtual reality and augmented reality in Oral & Maxillofacial Surgery. *BMC Oral Health*, *19*. Advance online publication. DOI: 10.1186/s12903-019-0937-8

Barsom, E., Graafland, M., & Schijven, M. (2016). Systematic review on the effectiveness of augmented reality applications in medical training. *Surgical Endoscopy*, *30*, 4174–4183. DOI: 10.1007/s00464-016-4800-6

Bayoumy, K., Gaber, M., Elshafeey, A., Mhaimeed, O., Dineen, E., Marvel, F., Martin, S., Muse, E., Turakhia, M., Tarakji, K., & Elshazly, M. (2021). Smart wearable devices in cardiovascular care: Where we are and how to move forward. *Nature Reviews. Cardiology*, *18*, 581–599. DOI: 10.1038/s41569-021-00522-7

Bellos, T., Manolitsis, I., Katsimperis, S., Juliebø-Jones, P., Feretzakis, G., Mitsogiannis, I., Varkarakis, I., Somani, B., & Tzelves, L. (2024). Artificial Intelligence in Urologic Robotic Oncologic Surgery: A Narrative Review. *Cancers (Basel)*, *16*. Advance online publication. DOI: 10.3390/cancers16091775

Beqari, J., Powell, J., Hurd, J., Potter, A., McCarthy, M., Srinivasan, D., Wang, D., Cranor, J., Zhang, L., Webster, K., Kim, J., Rosenstein, A., Zheng, Z., Lin, T., Li, J., Fang, Z., Zhang, Y., Anderson, A., Madsen, J., & Li, X. (2024). A Pilot Study Using Machine Learning Algorithms and Wearable Technology for the Early Detection of Postoperative Complications After Cardiothoracic Surgery. *Annals of Surgery*. Advance online publication. DOI: 10.1097/SLA.0000000000006263

Booth, R., Strudwick, G., McMurray, J., Chan, R., Cotton, K., & Cooke, S. (2021). The Future of Nursing Informatics in a Digitally-Enabled World. *Introduction to Nursing Informatics*, 395 - 417. https://doi .org/.DOI: 10.1007/978-3-030-58740-6_16

Bouden, C., & Mezioud, C. (2023). *Towards an Intelligent Surgical Preoperative Decision Support System: An Approach Based on Decision Trees and the Random Forest*. Intelligent Methods in Engineering Sciences., DOI: 10.58190/imiens.2023.45

Brennan, M., Puri, S., Ozrazgat-Baslanti, T., Feng, Z., Ruppert, M., Hashemighouchani, H., Momcilovic, P., Li, X., Wang, D., & Bihorac, A. (2019). Comparing clinical judgment with the MySurgeryRisk algorithm for preoperative risk assessment: A pilot usability study. *Surgery*, *165*, 1035–1045. DOI: 10.1016/j.surg.2019.01.002

Breteler, M., KleinJan, E., Dohmen, D., Leenen, L., Van Hillegersberg, R., Ruurda, J., Van Loon, K., Blokhuis, T., & Kalkman, C. (2019). Vital Signs Monitoring with Wearable Sensors in High-risk Surgical Patients. *Anesthesiology, 132*, 424–439. DOI: 10.1097/ALN.0000000000003029

Brown, J., Pope, N., Maria, A., Mason, J., & Morgan, A. (2020). Issues affecting nurses' capability to use digital technology at work: An integrative review. *Journal of Clinical Nursing*. Advance online publication. DOI: 10.1111/jocn.15321

Buchs, N., Pugin, F., Volonté, F., & Morel, P. (2013). Learning Tools and Simulation in Robotic Surgery: State of the Art. *World Journal of Surgery, 37*, 2812–2819. DOI: 10.1007/s00268-013-2065-y

Buckley, T., & Gordon, C. (2011). The effectiveness of high fidelity simulation on medical-surgical registered nurses' ability to recognise and respond to clinical emergencies. *Nurse Education Today, 31*(7), 716–721. DOI: 10.1016/j.nedt.2010.04.004

Cant, R., & Cooper, S. (2014). Simulation in the Internet age: The place of web-based simulation in nursing education. An integrative review. *Nurse Education Today, 34*(12), 1435–1442. DOI: 10.1016/j.nedt.2014.08.001

Catchpole, K., Cohen, T., Alfred, M., Lawton, S., Kanji, F., Shouhed, D., Nemeth, L., & Anger, J. (2022). Human Factors Integration in Robotic Surgery. *Human Factors, 66*, 683–700. DOI: 10.1177/00187208211068946

Çelik, S., Tunçbilek, Z., Sarıköse, S., Topaktaş, G., & Canda, A. (2024). Roles, experience and views of nurses working in robotic surgery settings: A mixed-methods study. *Journal of Perioperative Practice, 17504589241231100*. Advance online publication. DOI: 10.1177/17504589241231100

Cesare, M., D'Agostino, F., Maurici, M., Zega, M., Zeffiro, V., & Cocchieri, A. (2023). Standardized Nursing Diagnoses in a Surgical Hospital Setting: A Retrospective Study Based on Electronic Health Data. *SAGE Open Nursing, 9*. Advance online publication. DOI: 10.1177/23779608231158157

Chaharsoughi, N., Ahmadifaraz, M., & Kahangi, L. (2022). The impact of digital technologies in nursing care and their application: A narrative review. *Journal of Multidisciplinary Care*. https://doi.org/.DOI: 10.34172/jmdc.2022.1127

Chambers, R., McKinney, R., Schmid, M., & Beaney, P. (2018). Digital by choice: Becoming part of a digitally ready general practice team. *Primary Health Care*. Advance online publication. DOI: 10.7748/phc.2018.e1502

Chelazzi, C., Villa, G., Manno, A., Ranfagni, V., Gemmi, E., & Romagnoli, S. (2021). The new SUMPOT to predict postoperative complications using an Artificial Neural Network. *Scientific Reports, 11*. Advance online publication. DOI: 10.1038/s41598-021-01913-z

Chen, F., Leng, Y., Ge, J., Wang, D., Li, C., Chen, B., & Sun, Z. (2020). Effectiveness of Virtual Reality in Nursing Education: Meta-Analysis. *Journal of Medical Internet Research, 22*. Advance online publication. DOI: 10.2196/18290

Chen, I., Ghazi, A., Sridhar, A., Stoyanov, D., Slack, M., Kelly, J., & Collins, J. (2020). Evolving robotic surgery training and improving patient safety, with the integration of novel technologies. *World Journal of Urology*, *39*, 2883–2893. DOI: 10.1007/s00345-020-03467-7

Clisbee, D., Beierwaltes, P., & Eggenberger, S. (2019). Reducing Digital Storytelling Implementation Barriers in Nursing Education Workshops. *Journal of Continuing Education in Nursing*, *50*(9), 411–416. DOI: 10.3928/00220124-20190814-07

Conte, G., Magon, A., & Caruso, R. (2024). Digital and technological solutions in cardiovascular nursing and perspectives for a smooth digital shift: A discussion paper. *European Journal of Cardiovascular Nursing*. Advance online publication. DOI: 10.1093/eurjcn/zvae096

Cundy, T., Shetty, K., Clark, J., Chang, T., Sriskandarajah, K., Gattas, N., Najmaldin, A., Yang, G., & Darzi, A. (2013). The first decade of robotic surgery in children. *Journal of Pediatric Surgery*, *48*(4), 858–865. DOI: 10.1016/j.jpedsurg.2013.01.031

Downey, C., Randell, R., Brown, J., & Jayne, D. (2018). Continuous Versus Intermittent Vital Signs Monitoring Using a Wearable, Wireless Patch in Patients Admitted to Surgical Wards: Pilot Cluster Randomized Controlled Trial. *Journal of Medical Internet Research*, *20*. Advance online publication. DOI: 10.2196/10802

Duckert, M., & Barkhuus, L. (2022). Protecting Personal Health Data through Privacy Awareness. *Proceedings of the ACM on Human-Computer Interaction*, *6*, 1–22. DOI: 10.1145/3492830

Duckert, M., & Barkhuus, L. (2022). Protecting Personal Health Data through Privacy Awareness. *Proceedings of the ACM on Human-Computer Interaction*, *6*, 1–22. DOI: 10.1145/3492830

Edney, J., McDonall, J., Khaw, D., & Hutchinson, A. (2024). Use of Wearable Devices to Monitor Postoperative Activity following Cardiac Surgery. A Systematic Scoping Review. *European Journal of Cardiovascular Nursing*. Advance online publication. DOI: 10.1093/eurjcn/zvae054

Enayati, N., De Momi, E., & Ferrigno, G. (2016). Haptics in Robot-Assisted Surgery: Challenges and Benefits. *IEEE Reviews in Biomedical Engineering*, *9*, 49–65. DOI: 10.1109/RBME.2016.2538080

Erden, S., Arslan, S., Deniz, S., Kaya, P., & Gezer, D. (2017). A review of postoperative pain assessment records of nurses. *Applied nursing research. ANR*, *38*, 1–4. DOI: 10.1016/j.apnr.2017.08.003

Erden, S., Arslan, S., Deniz, S., Kaya, P., & Gezer, D. (2018). Corrigendum to "A review of postoperative pain assessment records of nurses☆" [Applied Nursing Research 38C (2017) 1-4]. *Applied nursing research. ANR*, *40*, 162. DOI: 10.1016/j.apnr.2018.01.001

Fernández-Alemán, J., Señor, I., Lozoya, P., & Álvarez, J. (2013). Security and privacy in electronic health records: A systematic literature review. *Journal of Biomedical Informatics*, *46*(3), 541–562. DOI: 10.1016/j.jbi.2012.12.003

Forde-Johnston, C., Butcher, D., & Aveyard, H. (2022). An integrative review exploring the impact of Electronic Health Records (EHR) on the quality of nurse–patient interactions and communication. *Journal of Advanced Nursing*, *79*, 48–67. DOI: 10.1111/jan.15484

Fritzen, A., Santos, D., Da Rocha, B., Jost, M., Caregnato, R., & Linch, G. (2023). Implementation of transoperative and immediate postoperative nursing diagnoses in the computerized management system. *Revista da Escola de Enfermagem da USP*, 57. https://doi.org/DOI: 10.1590/1980-220X-REEUSP-2022-0123en

Ganaie, N., & Naz, H. (2024). Embracing the Digital Shift: Enhancing Nursing Practice in the Digital Age. [IJSR]. *International Journal of Scientific Research*. Advance online publication. DOI: 10.21275/mr24105143930

George, E., Brand, T., LaPorta, A., Marescaux, J., & Satava, R. (2018). Origins of Robotic Surgery: From Skepticism to Standard of Care. *JSLS : Journal of the Society of Laparoendoscopic Surgeons*, *22*. Advance online publication. DOI: 10.4293/JSLS.2018.00039

Ghezzi, T., & Corleta, O. (2016). 30 Years of Robotic Surgery. *World Journal of Surgery*, *40*, 2550–2557. DOI: 10.1007/s00268-016-3543-9

Gillespie, B., Gillespie, J., Boorman, R., Granqvist, K., Stranne, J., & Erichsen-Andersson, A. (2020). The Impact of Robotic-Assisted Surgery on Team Performance: A Systematic Mixed Studies Review. *Human Factors*, *63*, 1352–1379. DOI: 10.1177/0018720820928624

Goldenberg, M., & Grantcharov, T. (2018). Enhancing Clinical Performance and Improving Patient Safety Using Digital Health., 235-248. https://doi.org/.DOI: 10.1007/978-3-319-61446-5_17

Gordon, L., Grantcharov, T., & Rudzicz, F. (2019). Explainable Artificial Intelligence for Safe Intraoperative Decision Support. *JAMA Surgery*. Advance online publication. DOI: 10.1001/jamasurg.2019.2821

Gu, Y., Rasmussen, S., Mølgaard, J., Haahr-Raunkjær, C., Meyhoff, C., Aasvang, E., & Sørensen, H. (2021). Prediction of severe adverse event from vital signs for post-operative patients. *2021 43rd Annual International Conference of the IEEE Engineering in Medicine & Biology Society (EMBC)*, 971-974. https://doi.org/DOI: 10.1109/EMBC46164.2021.9630918

Gudeloglu, A., & Parekattil, S. (2021). A Nurse Training Program for Robotic Skills Acquisition and Career Advancement. *Acta Medica*, *1-4*. Advance online publication. DOI: 10.32552/2021.ACTAMEDICA.511

Hamza, R., Yan, Z., Muhammad, K., Bellavista, P., & Titouna, F. (2020). A privacy-preserving cryptosystem for IoT E-healthcare. *Inf. Sci.*, *527*, 493–510. DOI: 10.1016/J.INS.2019.01.070

Hansen, J., & Holz, M. (2020). Facilitating Multiple Medical-Surgical Nursing Practicum Groups During Simulation Laboratory Days. *Nursing Education Perspectives*. Advance online publication. DOI: 10.1097/01.NEP.0000000000000575

Hanshaw, S., & Dickerson, S. (2020). High fidelity simulation evaluation studies in nursing education: A review of the literature. *Nurse Education in Practice*, *46*, 102818. DOI: 10.1016/j.nepr.2020.102818

Hants, L., Bail, K., & Paterson, C. (2023). Clinical decision-making and the nursing process in digital health systems: An integrated systematic review. *Journal of Clinical Nursing*. Advance online publication. DOI: 10.1111/jocn.16823

Hashimoto, D., Rosman, G., Rus, D., & Meireles, O. (2018). Artificial Intelligence in Surgery: Promises and Perils. *Annals of Surgery*, *268*, 70–76. DOI: 10.1097/SLA.0000000000002693

Hassan, A., Rajesh, A., Asaad, M., Nelson, J., Coert, J., Mehrara, B., & Butler, C. (2022). Artificial Intelligence and Machine Learning in Prediction of Surgical Complications: Current State, Applications, and Implications. *The American Surgeon, 89*, 25–30. DOI: 10.1177/00031348221101488

Hayat, N., Zainol, N., Salameh, A., Mamun, A., Yang, Q., & Salleh, M. (2022). How health motivation moderates the effect of intention and usage of wearable medical devices? An empirical study in Malaysia. *Frontiers in Public Health, 10*. Advance online publication. DOI: 10.3389/fpubh.2022.931557

Hofstetter, S., Zilezinski, M., Behr, D., Kraft, B., Buhtz, C., Paulicke, D., Wolf, A., Klus, C., Stoevesandt, D., Schwarz, K., & Jahn, P. (2023). Integrating Digital Assistive Technologies Into Care Processes: Mixed Methods Study. *JMIR Medical Education, 10*. Advance online publication. DOI: 10.2196/54083

Hong, C., & Wang, L. (2023). Virtual Reality Technology in Nursing Professional Skills Training: Bibliometric Analysis. *JMIR Serious Games, 11*. Advance online publication. DOI: 10.2196/44766

Howard, K., Makki, H., Novotny, N., Mi, M., & Nguyen, N. (2022). Value of robotic surgery simulation for training surgical residents and attendings: A systematic review protocol. *BMJ Open, 12*. Advance online publication. DOI: 10.1136/bmjopen-2021-059439

Hunkin, H., King, D., & Zajac, I. (2020). Perceived acceptability of wearable devices for the treatment of mental health problems. *Journal of Clinical Psychology*. Advance online publication. DOI: 10.1002/jclp.22934

Issa, B., Akour, A., Ibrahim, A., Almarzouqi, A., Abbas, S., Hisham, F., & Griffiths, J. (2020). Privacy, confidentiality, security and patient safety concerns about electronic health records. *International Nursing Review*. Advance online publication. DOI: 10.1111/inr.12585

Jakobsen, L., Olsen, R., Brinchmann, B., & Devik, S. (2023). Developing and Testing Digital Ethical Reflection in Long-Term Care: Nurses' Experiences. *SAGE Open Nursing, 9*. Advance online publication. DOI: 10.1177/23779608221150725

Kademane, A., Kumar, P., Chaudhary, B., & Castillo-González, W. (2023). The Influence of Electronic Health Records on Nursing Practice within Hospital Settings.

Kamei, T., Kanamori, T., Yamamoto, Y., & Edirippulige, S. (2020). The use of wearable devices in chronic disease management to enhance adherence and improve telehealth outcomes: A systematic review and meta-analysis. *Journal of Telemedicine and Telecare, 28*, 342–359. DOI: 10.1177/1357633X20937573

Karako, K. (2024). Integration of wearable devices and deep learning: New possibilities for health management and disease prevention. *Bioscience Trends*. Advance online publication. DOI: 10.5582/bst.2024.01170

Kavallieros, K., Karakozis, L., Hayward, R., Giannas, E., Selvaggi, L., & Kontovounisios, C. (2024). Wearable Devices in Colorectal Surgery: A Scoping Review. *Cancers (Basel), 16*. Advance online publication. DOI: 10.3390/cancers16132303

Keshta, I., & Odeh, A. (2020). *Security and privacy of electronic health records: Concerns and challenges*. Egyptian Informatics Journal., DOI: 10.1016/j.eij.2020.07.003

Khalil, A., Bruno, M., Spano, A., Petrone, F., Ghiani, E., Cosma, G., Chiacchio, G., & Flammia, R. (2024). The pivotal role of the robotic nurse in the management of the robotic urologic surgical environment. *International Journal of Urological Nursing*. Advance online publication. DOI: 10.1111/ijun.12400

Kiernan, A., Fahey, B., Guraya, S., Boland, F., Moneley, D., Doyle, F., & Harkin, D. (2023). Digital technology in informed consent for surgery: Systematic review. *BJS Open, 7*. Advance online publication. DOI: 10.1093/bjsopen/zrac159

Kim, K., Han, Y., & Kim, J. (2017). Nurses' and patients' perceptions of privacy protection behaviours and information provision. *Nursing Ethics, 24*, 598–611. DOI: 10.1177/0969733015622059

Kobayashi, M., Iwamoto, M., Une, S., Kurazume, R., Nakazawa, A., & Honda, M. (2022). THE EFFECT OF COMMUNICATION SKILLS TRAINING FOR NURSING STUDENTS BY AUGMENTED REALITY SIMULATION SYSTEM. *Innovation in Aging*. Advance online publication. DOI: 10.1093/geroni/igac059.1725

Koivunen, M., & Saranto, K. (2018). Nursing professionals' experiences of the facilitators and barriers to the use of telehealth applications: A systematic review of qualitative studies. *Scandinavian Journal of Caring Sciences, 32*, 24–44. DOI: 10.1111/scs.12445

Korte, L., & Bohnet-Joschko, S. (2022). Digitization in Everyday Nursing Care: A Vignette Study in German Hospitals. *International Journal of Environmental Research and Public Health, 19*. Advance online publication. DOI: 10.3390/ijerph191710775

Kraft, B., Kuscher, T., Rothmann, L., Zawatzki, S., Hofstetter, S., Schildmann, J., & Jahn, P. (2024). Exploring digital care: Developing ethical competencies. *Gerontechnology (Valkenswaard)*. Advance online publication. DOI: 10.4017/gt.2024.23.s.1057.opp

Kruse, C., Smith, B., Vanderlinden, H., & Nealand, A. (2017). Security Techniques for the Electronic Health Records. *Journal of Medical Systems, 41*. Advance online publication. DOI: 10.1007/s10916-017-0778-4

Kutney-Lee, A., Carthon, M., Sloane, D., Bowles, K., McHugh, M., & Aiken, L. (2021). Electronic Health Record Usability. *Medical Care, 59*, 625–631. DOI: 10.1097/MLR.0000000000001536

Lal, S., Memon, S., & Khan, E. (2024). Adopting the New Norms of Monitoring Postoperative Patients with Wearable Devices in Ireland - Advantages and Challenges. *Journal of the College of Physicians and Surgeons—Pakistan. Journal of the College of Physicians and Surgeons—Pakistan, 34*(2), 235–237. DOI: 10.29271/jcpsp.2024.02.235

Lam, K., Purkayastha, S., & Kinross, J. (2021). The Ethical Digital Surgeon. *Journal of Medical Internet Research, 23*. Advance online publication. DOI: 10.2196/25849

Lee, M., & Kim, S. (2018). A Safety Simulation Program for Operating Room Nurses. *Clinical Simulation in Nursing, 18*, 6–13. DOI: 10.1016/J.ECNS.2017.12.005

Leenen, J., Ardesch, V., Kalkman, C., Schoonhoven, L., & Patijn, G. (2024). Impact of wearable wireless continuous vital sign monitoring in abdominal surgical patients: Before–after study. *BJS Open, 8*. Advance online publication. DOI: 10.1093/bjsopen/zrad128

Leenen, J., Dijkman, E., Van Dijk, J., Van Westreenen, H., Kalkman, C., Schoonhoven, L., & Patijn, G. (2021). Feasibility of continuous monitoring of vital signs in surgical patients on a general ward: An observational cohort study. *BMJ Open, 11*. Advance online publication. DOI: 10.1136/bmjopen-2020-042735

Lei, Y., He, L., & Huang, H. (2022). Enhancement of Nursing Effect in Emergency General Surgery Based on Computer Aid. *Journal of Healthcare Engineering, 2022*. Advance online publication. DOI: 10.1155/2022/6745993

Lewis, K., Ricks, T., Rowin, A., Ndlovu, C., Goldstein, L., & McElvogue, C. (2019). Does Simulation Training for Acute Care Nurses Improve Patient Safety Outcomes: A Systematic Review to Inform Evidence-Based Practice. *Worldviews on Evidence-Based Nursing*. Advance online publication. DOI: 10.1111/wvn.12396

Loftus, T., Altieri, M., Balch, J., Abbott, K., Choi, J., Marwaha, J., Hashimoto, D., Brat, G., Raftopoulos, Y., Evans, H., Jackson, G., Walsh, D., & Tignanelli, C. (2023). Artificial Intelligence–enabled Decision Support in Surgery. *Annals of Surgery, 278*, 51–58. DOI: 10.1097/SLA.0000000000005853

Loftus, T., Tighe, P., Filiberto, A., Efron, P., Brakenridge, S., Mohr, A., Rashidi, P., Upchurch, G., & Bihorac, A. (2019). Artificial Intelligence and Surgical Decision-Making. *JAMA Surgery*. Advance online publication. DOI: 10.1001/jamasurg.2019.4917

Lu, J., Cuff, R., & Mansour, M. (2020). Simulation in surgical education. *American Journal of Surgery*. Advance online publication. DOI: 10.1016/j.amjsurg.2020.12.016

Lu, K., Marino, N., Russell, D., Singareddy, A., Zhang, D., Hardi, A., Kaar, S., & Puri, V. (2017). Use of Short Message Service and Smartphone Applications in the Management of Surgical Patients: A Systematic Review.. *Telemedicine journal and e-health: the official journal of the American Telemedicine Association*, 24 6, 406-414 . https://doi.org/.DOI: 10.1089/tmj.2017.0123

Ma, L., Yan, R., Wang, X., Gao, X., Fan, N., Liu, L., & Kang, H. (2024). Enhancing Surgical Nursing Student Performance: Comparative Study of Simulation-Based Learning and Problem-Based Learning. *Journal of Multidisciplinary Healthcare, 17*, 991–1005. DOI: 10.2147/JMDH.S440333

Manninger, M., Zweiker, D., Svennberg, E., Chatzikyriakou, S., Pavlović, N., Zaman, J., Kircanski, B., Lenarczyk, R., Vanduynhoven, P., Kosiuk, J., Potpara, T., & Duncker, D. (2021). Current perspectives on wearable rhythm recordings for clinical decision-making: The wEHRAbles 2 survey. *Europace : European Pacing, Arrhythmias, and Cardiac Electrophysiology : Journal of the Working Groups on Cardiac Pacing, Arrhythmias, and Cardiac Cellular Electrophysiology of the European Society of Cardiology*. Advance online publication. DOI: 10.1093/europace/euab064

Mao, R., Lan, L., Kay, J., Lohre, R., Ayeni, O., Goel, D., & Sa, D. (2021). Immersive Virtual Reality for Surgical Training: A Systematic Review. *The Journal of Surgical Research, 268*, 40–58. DOI: 10.1016/j.jss.2021.06.045

Martínez, N., & Leyva-Moral, J. (2024). Digital Transformation Led by Nurses and Nursing Managers' Priorities: A Qualitative Study. *Journal of Nursing Management*. Advance online publication. DOI: 10.1155/2024/8873127

Martinez-Ortigosa, A., Martinez-Granados, A., Gil-Hernández, E., Rodriguez-Arrastia, M., Ropero-Padilla, C., & Román, P. (2023). Applications of Artificial Intelligence in Nursing Care: A Systematic Review. *Journal of Nursing Management*. Advance online publication. DOI: 10.1155/2023/3219127

Martins, R., Trevilato, D., Jost, M., & Caregnato, R. (2019). Nursing performance in robotic surgeries: Integrative review. *Revista Brasileira de Enfermagem, 72*(3), 795–800. DOI: 10.1590/0034-7167-2018-0426

Mattsson, J. (2020). AB024. Digitalization in a technological environment, a pediatric operating theater., 3. https://doi.org/.DOI: 10.21037/pm.2020.ab024

Mbonihankuye, S., Nkunzimana, A., & Ndagijimana, A. (2019). Healthcare Data Security Technology: HIPAA Compliance. *Wirel. Commun. Mob. Comput.*, 2019, 1927495:1-1927495:7. https://doi.org/.DOI: 10.1155/2019/1927495

McKnight, R., Pean, C., Buck, S., Hwang, J., Hsu, J., & Pierrie, S. (2020). Virtual Reality and Augmented Reality—Translating Surgical Training into Surgical Technique. *Current Reviews in Musculoskeletal Medicine, 13*, 663–674. DOI: 10.1007/s12178-020-09667-3

Meling, T., & Meling, T. (2020). The impact of surgical simulation on patient outcomes: A systematic review and meta-analysis. *Neurosurgical Review, 44*, 843–854. DOI: 10.1007/s10143-020-01314-2

Mishra, R., Narayanan, K., Umana, G., Montemurro, N., Chaurasia, B., & Deora, H. (2022). Virtual Reality in Neurosurgery: Beyond Neurosurgical Planning. *International Journal of Environmental Research and Public Health, 19*. Advance online publication. DOI: 10.3390/ijerph19031719

Mozer, C., Gonçalves, J., Santos, L., Furieri, L., & Fioresi, M. (2023). Telenursing practice in the care of surgical cancer patients: A scoping review protocol. *BMJ Open, 13*. Advance online publication. DOI: 10.1136/bmjopen-2023-074502

Mulyadi, M., Tonapa, S., Rompas, S., Wang, R., & Lee, B. (2021). Effects of simulation technology-based learning on nursing students' learning outcomes: A systematic review and meta-analysis of experimental studies. *Nurse Education Today, 107*, 105127. DOI: 10.1016/j.nedt.2021.105127

Muschol, J., Heinrich, M., Heiss, C., Hernández, A., Knapp, G., Repp, H., Schneider, H., Thormann, U., Uhlar, J., Unzeitig, K., & Gissel, C. (2022). Economic and Environmental Impact of Digital Health App Video Consultations in Follow-up Care for Patients in Orthopedic and Trauma Surgery in Germany: Randomized Controlled Trial. *Journal of Medical Internet Research, 24*. Advance online publication. DOI: 10.2196/42839

Navarrete-Welton, A., & Hashimoto, D. (2020). Current applications of artificial intelligence for intraoperative decision support in surgery. *Frontiers of Medicine*, •••, 1–13. DOI: 10.1007/s11684-020-0784-7

Ng, Z., Ling, L., Chew, H., & Lau, Y. (2021). The role of artificial intelligence in enhancing clinical nursing care: A scoping review. *Journal of Nursing Management*. Advance online publication. DOI: 10.1111/jonm.13425

Nordgård, R. (2017). Digital Documentation in Nursing.

Nota, C., Smits, F., Woo, Y., Rinkes, I., Molenaar, I., Hagendoorn, J., & Fong, Y. (2019). Robotic Developments in Cancer Surgery. *Surgical Oncology Clinics of North America, 28*(1), 89–100. DOI: 10.1016/j.soc.2018.07.003

O'Connor, S., Yan, Y., Thilo, F., Felzmann, H., Dowding, D., & Lee, J. (2022). Artificial intelligence in nursing and midwifery: A systematic review. *Journal of Clinical Nursing*. Advance online publication. DOI: 10.1111/jocn.16478

Padilha, J., Machado, P., Ribeiro, A., Ramos, J., & Costa, P. (2019). Clinical Virtual Simulation in Nursing Education: Randomized Controlled Trial. *Journal of Medical Internet Research, 21*. Advance online publication. DOI: 10.2196/11529

Patel, M., Asch, D., & Volpp, K. (2015). Wearable devices as facilitators, not drivers, of health behavior change. *Journal of the American Medical Association, 313*(5), 459–460. DOI: 10.1001/jama.2014.14781

Peñataro-Pintado, E., Díaz-Agea, J., Castillo, I., Leal-Costa, C., Ramos-Morcillo, A., Ruzafa-Martínez, M., & Rodríguez-Higueras, E. (2021). Self-Learning Methodology in Simulated Environments (MAES©) as a Learning Tool in Perioperative Nursing. An Evidence-Based Practice Model for Acquiring Clinical Safety Competencies. *International Journal of Environmental Research and Public Health, 18*. Advance online publication. DOI: 10.3390/ijerph18157893

Peters, B., Armijo, P., Krause, C., Choudhury, S., & Oleynikov, D. (2018). Review of emerging surgical robotic technology. *Surgical Endoscopy, 32*, 1636–1655. DOI: 10.1007/s00464-018-6079-2

Pinto, E., Lunardi, L., Treviso, P., & De Abreu Botene, D. (2018). NuRSe ROle iN ROBOtiC SuRgeRy: challenges and prospects.

Plotzky, C., Lindwedel, U., Sorber, M., Loessl, B., König, P., Kunze, C., Kugler, C., & Meng, M. (2021). Virtual reality simulations in nurse education: A systematic mapping review. *Nurse Education Today, 101*, 104868. DOI: 10.1016/j.nedt.2021.104868

Pograjec, A., & Hubert, J. (2019). [The nurse's role in urologic robotic surgery].. *Progres en urologie: journal de l'Association francaise d'urologie et de la Societe francaise d'urologie*. https://doi.org/.DOI: 10.1016/j.purol.2019.09.004

Raheem, A., Song, H., Chang, K., Choi, Y., & Rha, K. (2017). Robotic nurse duties in the urology operative room: 11 years of experience. *Asian Journal of Urology, 4*, 116–123. DOI: 10.1016/j.ajur.2016.09.012

Rathore, A., Lennox, L., Bickerton, M., Baliga, S., & Gardner, T. (2024). 201 Interdisciplinary Simulation Based Training for the Operating Room Team - a Systematic Review. *British Journal of Surgery*. Advance online publication. DOI: 10.1093/bjs/znae163.612

Russell, B. (2022). Understanding the role of the scrub nurse during robotic surgery. *Nursing standard (Royal College of Nursing (Great Britain): 1987)*. https://doi.org/DOI: 10.7748/ns.2022.e12003

Ryan, J., Doster, B., Daily, S., & Lewis, C. (2019). A Case Study Perspective to the Digital Transformation of a Hospital's Perioperative Process., 1-10. https://doi.org/.DOI: 10.24251/HICSS.2019.491

Sanders, D., Read-Brown, S., Tu, D., Lambert, W., Choi, D., Almario, B., Yackel, T., Brown, A., & Chiang, M. (2014). Impact of an electronic health record operating room management system in ophthalmology on documentation time, surgical volume, and staffing. *JAMA Ophthalmology*, *132*(5), 586–592. DOI: 10.1001/jamaophthalmol.2013.8196

Sarmanian, J. (2015). Robot-Assisted Thoracic Surgery (RATS): Perioperative Nursing Professional Development Program. *AORN Journal*, *102*(3), 241–253. DOI: 10.1016/j.aorn.2015.06.013

Schmidt, E., Goldhaber-Fiebert, S., Ho, L., & McDonald, K. (2013). Simulation Exercises as a Patient Safety Strategy. *Annals of Internal Medicine*, *158*, 426–432. DOI: 10.7326/0003-4819-158-5-201303051-00010

Seibert, K., Domhoff, D., Bruch, D., Schulte-Althoff, M., Fürstenau, D., Biessmann, F., & Wolf-Ostermann, K. (2020). Application Scenarios for Artificial Intelligence in Nursing Care: Rapid Review. *Journal of Medical Internet Research*, *23*. Advance online publication. DOI: 10.2196/26522

Servaty, R., Kersten, A., Brukamp, K., Möhler, R., & Mueller, M. (2020). Implementation of robotic devices in nursing care. Barriers and facilitators: An integrative review. *BMJ Open*, *10*. Advance online publication. DOI: 10.1136/bmjopen-2020-038650

Shin, H., Rim, D., Kim, H., Park, S., & Shon, S. (2019). Educational Characteristics of Virtual Simulation in Nursing: An Integrative Review. *Clinical Simulation in Nursing*, *37*, 18–28. DOI: 10.1016/j.ecns.2019.08.002

Shin, S., Park, J., & Kim, J. (2015). Effectiveness of patient simulation in nursing education: Meta-analysis. *Nurse Education Today*, *35*(1), 176–182. DOI: 10.1016/j.nedt.2014.09.009

Speyer, R., Denman, D., Wilkes-Gillan, S., Chen, Y., Bogaardt, H., Kim, J., Heckathorn, D., & Cordier, R. (2018). Effects of telehealth by allied health professionals and nurses in rural and remote areas: A systematic review and meta-analysis. *Journal of Rehabilitation Medicine*, *50*(3), 225–235. DOI: 10.2340/16501977-2297

Sulé, E., Ghaderi, R., Tariq, S., Kamel, Y., & Maliyil, J. (2023). 1295 To What Extent Would an Augmented Reality Surgical Skills Mobile App Effectively Supplement Surgical Skills Training for UK Medical Students and Foundation Doctors? *British Journal of Surgery*. Advance online publication. DOI: 10.1093/bjs/znad258.618

Sundler, A., Pettersson, A., & Berglund, M. (2015). Undergraduate nursing students' experiences when examining nursing skills in clinical simulation laboratories with high-fidelity patient simulators: A phenomenological research study. *Nurse Education Today*, *35*(12), 1257–1261. DOI: 10.1016/j.nedt.2015.04.008

Sweeney, A., Morse, C., & Carofiglio, C. (2019). Integrating Simulated Electronic Health Record Patients Across Multiple Nursing Courses. *The Journal of Nursing Education*, *58*(8), 495–496. DOI: 10.3928/01484834-20190719-14

Swenty, C., & Eggleston, B. (2011). The Evaluation of Simulation in a Baccalaureate Nursing Program. *Clinical Simulation in Nursing*, *7*. Advance online publication. DOI: 10.1016/J.ECNS.2010.02.006

Tarsuslu, S., Agaoglu, F., & Bas, M. (2024). Can digital leadership transform AI anxiety and attitude in nurses?. *Journal of nursing scholarship: an official publication of Sigma Theta Tau International Honor Society of Nursing*. https://doi.org/.DOI: 10.1111/jnu.13008

Thomas, C. (2011). Role of the Perioperative Nurse in Robotic Surgery. *Perioperative Nursing Clinics, 6*, 227–234. DOI: 10.1016/J.CPEN.2011.06.005

Tischendorf, T., Hasseler, M., Schaal, T., Ruppert, S., Marchwacka, M., Heitmann-Möller, A., & Schaffrin, S. (2024a). Developing digital competencies of nursing professionals in continuing education and training – a scoping review. *Frontiers in Medicine, 11*. Advance online publication. DOI: 10.3389/fmed.2024.1358398

Tischendorf, T., Heitmann-Möller, A., Ruppert, S., Marchwacka, M., Schaffrin, S., Schaal, T., & Hasseler, M. (2024b). Sustainable integration of digitalisation in nursing education—An international scoping review. *Frontiers in Health Services, 4*. Advance online publication. DOI: 10.3389/frhs.2024.1344021

Uymaz, P., & Uymaz, A. (2022). Assessing acceptance of augmented reality in nursing education. *PLoS One, 17*. Advance online publication. DOI: 10.1371/journal.pone.0263937

Uzun, L., & Cerit, B. (2023). *Effect of Digitalization on Nursing Practices using the Lean Approach*. Clinical and Experimental Health Sciences., DOI: 10.33808/clinexphealthsci.904203

Van Melzen, R., Haveman, M., Schuurmann, R., Struys, M., & De Vries, J. (2023). Implementing Wearable Sensors for Clinical Application at a Surgical Ward: Points to Consider before Starting. *Sensors (Basel), 23*. Advance online publication. DOI: 10.3390/s23156736

Vasey, B., Lippert, K., Khan, D., Ibrahim, M., Koh, C., Horsfall, L., Lee, K., Williams, S., Marcus, H., & McCulloch, P. (2022). Intraoperative Applications of Artificial Intelligence in Robotic Surgery: A Scoping Review of Current Development Stages and Levels of Autonomy. *Annals of Surgery, 278*, 896–903. DOI: 10.1097/SLA.0000000000005700

Volkan, E., Köse, İ., Cece, S., & Elmas, Ö. (2024). Analysis of the effect of digital hospital efforts on paper savings in inpatient procedures and on the duration of nursing care services. *Frontiers in Digital Health, 6*. Advance online publication. DOI: 10.3389/fdgth.2024.1367149

Walker-Czyz, A. (2016). The Impact of an Integrated Electronic Health Record Adoption on Nursing Care Quality. *The Journal of Nursing Administration, 46*, 366–372. DOI: 10.1097/NNA.0000000000000360

Weenk, M., Bredie, S., Koeneman, M., Hesselink, G., Van Goor, H., & Van De Belt, T. (2019). Continuous Monitoring of Vital Signs in the General Ward Using Wearable Devices: Randomized Controlled Trial. *Journal of Medical Internet Research*, 22. https://doi.org/DOI: 10.2196/preprints.15471

Weenk, M., Van Goor, H., Frietman, B., Engelen, L., Van Laarhoven, C., Smit, J., Bredie, S., & Van De Belt, T. (2017). Continuous Monitoring of Vital Signs Using Wearable Devices on the General Ward: Pilot Study. *JMIR mHealth and uHealth, 5*. Advance online publication. DOI: 10.2196/mhealth.7208

Weller, G., Lovely, J., Larson, D., Earnshaw, B., & Huebner, M. (2018). Leveraging electronic health records for predictive modeling of post-surgical complications. *Statistical Methods in Medical Research, 27*, 3271–3285. DOI: 10.1177/0962280217696115

Weller, G., Mault, J., Ventura, M., Adams, J., Campbell, F., & Tremper, K. (2024). A Retrospective Observational Study of Continuous Wireless Vital Sign Monitoring via a Medical Grade Wearable Device on Hospitalized Floor Patients. *Journal of Clinical Medicine, 13*. Advance online publication. DOI: 10.3390/jcm13164747

Wells, C., Xu, W., Penfold, J., Keane, C., Gharibans, A., Bissett, I., & O'Grady, G. (2022). Wearable devices to monitor recovery after abdominal surgery: Scoping review. *BJS Open, 6*. Advance online publication. DOI: 10.1093/bjsopen/zrac031

Wong, P., Brand, G., Dix, S., Choo, D., Foley, P., & Lokmic-Tomkins, Z. (2023). Pre-Registration Nursing Students' Perceptions of Digital Health Technology on the Future of Nursing. *Nurse Educator, 49*, E208–E212. DOI: 10.1097/NNE.0000000000001591

Wüller, H., Behrens, J., Garthaus, M., Marquard, S., & Remmers, H. (2019). A scoping review of augmented reality in nursing. *BMC Nursing, 18*. Advance online publication. DOI: 10.1186/s12912-019-0342-2

Wynn, M., Garwood-Cross, L., Vasilica, C., & Davis, D. (2023b). Digital nursing practice theory: A scoping review and thematic analysis. *Journal of Advanced Nursing*. Advance online publication. DOI: 10.1111/jan.15660

Wynn, M., Garwood-Cross, L., Vasilica, C., Griffiths, M., Heaslip, V., & Phillips, N. (2023a). Digitizing nursing: A theoretical and holistic exploration to understand the adoption and use of digital technologies by nurses. *Journal of Advanced Nursing*. Advance online publication. DOI: 10.1111/jan.15810

Yeşilyurt, K. (2024). *The New Dimension of Surgery: Telesurgery and Surgical Nursing*. SDÜ SAĞLIK BİLİMLERİ DERGİSİ., DOI: 10.22312/sdusbed.1423302

Youssef, Y., De Wet, D., Back, D., & Scherer, J. (2024). Digitalization in orthopaedics: A narrative review. *Frontiers in Surgery, 10*. Advance online publication. DOI: 10.3389/fsurg.2023.1325423

Zhang, H., Zhao, J., Farzan, R., & Otaghvar, H. (2024). Risk predictions of surgical wound complications based on a machine learning algorithm: A systematic review. *International Wound Journal, 21*. Advance online publication. DOI: 10.1111/iwj.14665

Zheng, L., Kaufman, D., Duncan, B., Furniss, S., Grando, A., Poterack, K., Miksch, T., Helmers, R., & Doebbeling, B. (2020). A Task-Analytic Framework Comparing Preoperative Electronic Health Record–Mediated Nursing Workflow in Different Settings. *CIN: Computers, Informatics. Nursing, 38*, 294–302. DOI: 10.1097/CIN.0000000000000588

Zhu, S., Saravanan, V., & Muthu, B. (2020). Achieving data security and privacy across healthcare applications using cyber security mechanisms. *The Electronic Library, 38*, 979–995. DOI: 10.1108/el-07-2020-0219

KEY TERMS AND DEFINITIONS

Digitalization: It is the process of transforming analogue data, processes or services using digital technologies.

Surgical Nursing: It is a nursing speciality that provides holistic care of surgical patients throughout the perioperative period.

Technological Innovation: It refers to the improvement of products, services or processes through the development of existing technologies or the introduction of completely new technologies.

Chapter 16
Innovating End-of-Life Psychological Care to Promoting Dignity and Purpose:
A Case Study of Meaning of Life Therapy via Videoconferencing to Promote Dignity and Purpose

Manuela Leite
https://orcid.org/0000-0001-6916-0721
UCIBIO - Applied Molecular Biosciences Unit, Translational Toxicology Research Laboratory, University Institute of Health Sciences (1H-TOXRUN, IUCS-CESPU), Gandra, Portugal & iHealth4Well-being - Innovation in Health and Well-Being – Research Unit, Instituto Politécnico de Saúde do Norte, CESPU, Penafiel, Portugal

Neuza Rocha
https://orcid.org/0009-0003-9049-922X
Clinical and Health Psychology Unit, Psychiatry and Mental Health Service, Hospital da Senhora da Oliveira Guimarães, Portugal

Sónia Remondes-Costa
https://orcid.org/0000-0003-4282-3964
CIDESD - Research Center in Sports Sciences, Health Sciences and Human Development, University of Trás-os-Montes and Alto Douro (UTAD), Vila Real, Portugal

Ricardo João Teixeira
https://orcid.org/0000-0003-3820-1660
University of Coimbra, Center for Research in Neuropsychology and Cognitive Behavioral Intervention (CINEICC), Portugal & REACH - Mental Health Clinic, Portugal

Vera Almeida
UCIBIO - Applied Molecular Biosciences Unit, MedTech-Laboratory of Pharmaceutical Technology, Faculty of Pharmacy, University of Porto, Portugal & UNiPRO-Research Unit in Oral Pathology and Reabilitation, University Institute of Health Sciences (IUCS), CESPU, Gandra, Portugal

José Carlos Rocha
UCIBIO - Applied Molecular Biosciences Unit, Translational Toxicology Research Laboratory, University Institute of Health Sciences (1H-TOXRUN, IUCS-CESPU, Gandra, Portugal & Centro de Psicologia do Trauma e do Luto, Portugal

DOI: 10.4018/979-8-3373-3531-5.ch016

Gerly Macedo
Clinical and Health Psychology Unit, Psychiatry and Mental Health Service, Hospital da Senhora de Oliveira de Guimarães, Guimarães, Portugal

Elisa Veiga
Research Centre for Human Development, Faculty of Education and Psychology, Universidade Católica Portuguesa, Porto, Portugal

ABSTRACT

Meaning of Life Therapy (MLF) has shown to be a promising psychoexistencial intervention for patients receiving palliative care and their caregivers. Even though MLF exhibited utility in promoting meaning in life and dignity, the COVID-19 pandemic made its face-to-face administration unsuitable but also underscored the need to investigate digital alternatives. For this reason, and considering developments in digital mental health interventions, this single case study aims to investigate videoconferencing as an alternative methodology, involving one patient with terminal cancer and his wife. The patient was submitted to MLT through videoconference. Semi-structured interviews post-intervention were also carried out with patient and caregiver. The qualitative analysis underlines the feasibility of videoconferencing in the implementation of the MLT, visible in the psychological adjustment of the patient. It is also important to reflect on the characteristics of the digital therapeutic setting, in terms of establishing the therapeutic relationship and the underlying ethical aspects.

INTRODUCTION

Palliative care and End-of-life Challenges

In the context of palliative care, advanced cancer presents not only as a clinical challenge, but as a deeply human experience that involves multiple dimensions of suffering. At this stage, the priority shifts from cure to promoting quality of life, symptom relief, and emotional and spiritual support, both for the patient and their network of loved ones. The unpredictability of the disease's progression, progressive functional losses, and the psychological impact of confronting finitude require healthcare professionals to listen actively and empathetically and to intervene in ways that promote adaptation to the disease and the development of strategies that sustain dignity and meaning in life until the end. "Palliative care is an approach that improves the quality of life of patients and their families who are facing problems associated with life-threatening illness" (World Health Organization [WHO], 2023). Its main objective is to promote the quality of life of patients (International Association for Hospice and Palliative Care [IAHPC], n.d.; WHO, 2023) through a holistic response, coordinated and carried out by a multidisciplinary team, in order to meet the physical, psychosocial, and spiritual needs of patients (IAHPC, n.d.; Teoli et al., 2025; WHO, 2023).

According to the WHO (2023), "palliative care is explicitly recognized within the human right to health. It should be provided through integrated, person-centered health services that pay special attention to the specific needs and preferences of individuals." Palliative care is intended for all individuals who need it, regardless of age (from childhood to old age) and clinical condition - cardiovascular diseases (38.5%), cancer (34%), chronic respiratory diseases (10.3%), AIDS (5.7%) and diabetes (4.6%)" (WHO, 2023).

Cancer is one of the most complex challenges in the field of health, not only because of its clinical outcomes, but also because of the symbolic weight it carries in the collective imagination. Is strongly associated with one of the most feared and potentially fatal medical conditions, inextricably linking the increased risk of mortality with the perception of intense suffering. The latter stems largely from the aggressiveness of commonly prescribed treatments, such as chemotherapy, and the adverse effects that often compromise the patient's overall well-being.

In this context, the impact on quality of life is profound and multifaceted. The transition to the palliative phase inevitably marks the end of the expectation of a cure, requiring an approach focused on active disease management, with an emphasis on rigorous control (Irwin et al., 2021; Kreitler, 2019).

Covid-19 pandemic, Digital Health and its Impact on Palliative Care and End-of-life

On 30 January 2020 the WHO declared the pandemic caused by the SARS-CoV-2 "(...) a public health emergency of international concern" (WHO, 2020), representing a "major challenging global public health problem" (Phelan et al., 2020).

The COVID-19 pandemic has significantly exacerbated the vulnerabilities inherent to cancer patients, particularly those in palliative care. Since the beginning of the health crisis, this population has been classified as high risk, both because of their greater susceptibility to SARS-CoV-2 infection and because of their increased likelihood of developing serious or fatal complications(Grewal et al., 2020). This finding led to the implementation of particularly restrictive isolation measures, designed to reduce exposure to the virus, but whose side effects had a major impact on the overall well-being of these patients.

In the context of palliative care, such measures intensified dimensions of what is known as "total pain," a concept formulated by Cicely Saunders (Clark, 1999; Richmond, 2005), to describe the simultaneous experience of physical, psychological, social, and spiritual suffering. Prolonged social isolation, resulting from containment strategies, deprived patients of meaningful face-to-face contact and ongoing emotional support, leading to significant psychological consequences, such as feelings of depersonalization and despair (Lourenço et al., 2024). In addition, the high levels of fear and anxiety triggered during the pandemic have aggravated existing symptoms in PC patients(Mistraletti et al., 2024), which highlights the interdependence between the physical and emotional dimensions of suffering in these contexts.

The forced reorganization of health services was another critical factor. The suspension or postponement of treatments, the drastic reduction in face-to-face consultations, and the overload of healthcare teams contributed to an increased perception of insecurity and therapeutic abandonment. This scenario required innovative responses capable of mitigating the fragmentation of care and preserving continuity of care. Thus, the pandemic not only exposed the fragility of palliative care support networks but also highlighted the need for adaptive and integrated models that recognize the centrality of total suffering and the importance of approaches that are both clinical and humanized.

Remotely delivered health interventions in PC, such as telemedicine, are considered a viable resource for improving quality of life, clinical feasibility and acceptability (Mirshahi et al., 2024), as it promotes effective and accessible communication both for the patient and family members (Bentley et al., 2020; Sutherland et al., 2020). The COVID-19 pandemic has exponentially boosted the development and adoption of digital health solutions, expanding their role in healthcare provision in general, with particular relevance to the areas of mental health and palliative care (Dilhani et al., 2024). The term digital health — or eHealth — is a broad concept that integrates the use of digital technologies for communication, information, delivery, and optimization of healthcare. According to the WHO (2019), "digital health, or the use of digital technologies for health, has become a salient field of practice for employing routine and innovative forms of information and communications technology (ICT) to address health needs" and "(...) encompasses a range of related concepts such as telemedicine and telehealth, mobile health (mHealth), health informatics, and wearable devices (...). Among these, the use of videoconferencing to provide care at a distance is becoming more common (Finucane et al., 2021, p. 4).

The effectiveness of digital health interventions has been the subject of increasing research and debate in recent decades, a process that has intensified with the abrupt transition from a predominantly face-to-face care model to digitally mediated approaches. This paradigm shift requires critical analysis that considers, on the one hand, the acceptance and adherence of patients, caregivers, and healthcare professionals and, on the other hand, the advantages, limitations, and risks associated with these practices. In the specific context of palliative care and mental health—where the therapeutic relationship, empathetic communication, and emotional support play a central role—technological mediation takes on special relevance, simultaneously expanding access and challenging the depth of human interaction.

Evidence from systematic reviews demonstrates the feasibility of providing remote emotional and psychosocial support to patients in palliative care (e.g. Wood et al., 2023), highlighting the ability of patients to remain in their homes as one of the main advantages of telehealth (Steindal et al., 2023). Furthermore, according to Keenan et al. (2021), they are "(...) focused more on the ability of telehealth to satisfy autonomy by moving away from a condition-centered life and facilitating opportunities (p. 583).

The reduction in costs and travel time is widely recognized as one of the main benefits of digital health interventions(Jess et al., 2019; Keenan et al., 2021; Wood et al., 2023) especially for patients in rural or remote areas, improving their quality of life(Keenan et al., 2021). In the case of palliative cancer patients, frequent travel for treatments, tests, and consultations, combined with physical frailty and dependence on others, exacerbate barriers to access, which are often intensified by economic difficulties. In this context, telehealth can offer greater flexibility and reduce geographical barriers (Argüero-Fonseca et al., 2021; Perez, 2025).

The therapeutic relationship remains a concern when compared to the traditional face-to-face model. However, videoconferencing can promote the development of interpersonal bonds (Steindal et al., 2023) and, in some cases, be clinically as effective as or more effective than usual practice, asNowels et al. (2024), point out: "this review demonstrates that telehealth can be equivalent or more clinically effective when compared to usual care" (p. 669). In mental health, telepsychology (Haddouk et al., 2025) and telepsychotherapy have expanded significantly during and after the pandemic (Perez, 2025), with increasing adoption by psychologists and psychiatrists. Studies indicate that, especially in the private sector, this modality is perceived as similar to face-to-face care (Azcona et al., 2022).

Nevertheless, technical and access challenges remain, including unstable internet connections (Azcona et al., 2022; Tajan et al., 2023), physical and economic accessibility (Wood et al., 2023), reduced digital competence (Van Goethem et al., 2025), and the need for digital literacy (Altaf Dar et al., 2023), which particularly affect older adults and vulnerable populations. Limitations in reading nonverbal communication (Wood et al., 2023), due to the restricted visual setting, and lack of privacy in the patient's environment (Steindal et al., 2023; Tajan et al., 2023) are additional concerns.

Despite this, patient satisfaction with telehealth during the pandemic was high (Argüero-Fonseca et al., 2021), with video consultations showing promise in supporting palliative care patients and their families (Jess et al., 2019). To fulfill their potential, digital technologies must respond to the holistic needs of patients (Payne et al., 2020), although recent reviews indicate a scarcity of studies that fully integrate emotional and existential aspects (Steindal et al., 2023). The present clinical case, delivered during the COVID-19 pandemic, is situated within this conceptual framework.

Given the COVID-19 pandemic, this single case study is an effort to search for alternatives tailored to meet the needs of PC patients and their families. In this sense, the Meaning of Life Therapy (MLT), developed by Cardoso et al. (2023), appears as an innovative intervention based on the basic principles of psychoexistential interventions. MLT is a brief psychotherapeutic intervention, involving a protocol and questions that will guide the patients through a process of reflection, (re)signification of the meaning of life, and (re)conciliation with the present and past. It attempts to enhance the patients´ psychological adjustment at the end-of-life through the pursuit of meaning and purpose in life, adaptation to the terminal illness and death, and promotion of dignity and peace. At first, MLT was provided face to face (Cardoso et al., 2023) and then adapted to an online intervention due to the pandemic.

The main aim of the present study is to evaluate the effectiveness, acceptability and feasibility of dyadic MLT intervention for a cancer patient and a family member delivered by videoconference, regarding their psychological adjustment in PC. The specific objectives are: (1) to investigate the impact of MLT via videoconference on the psychological adjustment of patient at end-of-life; and (2) to assess the impact of MLT via videoconference on the family member's adjustment to grief and loss; and 3) evaluate the acceptability and feasibility of MLT via videoconference.

METHOD

This research employs a case study approach, which is particularly suited for gaining an in-depth understanding of complex phenomena within their real-life context (Stake, 2005). This methodology is especially valuable due to its unparalleled capacity to generate deep, context-rich insights, when investigating contemporary events (Crowe et al., 2011). The interview is one of the most important data collection strategies in case studies and it was the data collection method chosen in this research. Examining different perspectives in the context of health care practices, case study approach can contribute to reflect the progress and potential relevance of technological mediation toward new policies developments in health care, and the scarcity of research in PC.

Participants

This instrumental single case study involved the participation of a male cancer patient and his wife. The patient was 52 years old, married, Catholic, had complete Basic Education (Grade 9), lived with his wife and stepdaughter, and worked as a warehouse employee. He was diagnosed with prostate adenocarcinoma with bone metastasis in October 2019, and at the time of the intervention, he was receiving palliative care in a PC unit at the hospital, with an ECOG (Eastern Cooperative Oncology Group) score of 2. The patient was recruited by a researcher and a psychologist at the hospital PC unit, after fulfilling the inclusion criteria (assessment carried out in a multidisciplinary consultation - palliative medicine, nursing, and psychology teams). Subsequent meetings were held via videoconference due to the pandemic context. The patient died 14 months after the intervention/investigation protocol.

His wife was 48 years old. She is Catholic, has a university degree and works at a factory.

Materials

Meaning of Life Therapy – MLT

Meaning of Life Therapy (Cardoso et al., 2023) is a brief psychoexistential intervention guided by a 14-question protocol (Table 1) to be carried out in four sessions; in this case, the intervention was implemented in five sessions via videoconference. The questions explore significant life events and experiences for the patients, pieces of advice, words of wisdom for family members, and guidance for future generations. They also enable recollection of past life memories; seek to solve unfinished issues; promote meaning-making and purpose in life; and tackle sensitive areas for PC patients, such as the need for forgiveness, apology and saying goodbye. "The final objective of MLT is the elaboration of a written document - 'Life Letter', allowing for the materialization of a physical legacy, which can be delivered to the patient's relatives or significant others, if this is desired. The focus is on leading the patient to find a sense of meaning and purpose in life and suffering, as well as preserving their dignity and identity" (Freitas et al., 2024, p, 471). The content of the questions is presented to the patients in Session 1, so that they are able to reflect on the answers. In the following two sessions (Session 2 and Session 3) the protocol is administered. The patients´ answers are audio recorded, and their content is transcribed *ipsis verbis*, to produce a legacy letter – the Life Letter (LL). The therapist compiles the responses into a single document, thus drafting the provisional version of the LL. In Session 4, its content is read, and the patients are free to suggest edits, adding or deleting content. In Session 5, the patients are given a copy of the LL, with the modifications suggested, and decide how it should be handled- either keep it or bequeath it to someone (e.g., family member, friends or significant others).

Table 1. Meaning of Life Therapy Intervention Protocol

Part I (Session 2)
1. Which happy events would you like to remember? 2. What are the events in your life that you are grateful for? 3. What do you feel most proud of in life? 4. How would you like to be remembered by your family and friends? 5. What advice would you like to pass along to your family and friends?
Part II (Session 3)
6. Who would you like to ask for forgiveness or who would you like to be forgiven by? 7. Does anyone owe you an apology or do you feel that you owe someone an apology? 8. Is there anyone you would like to give a hug to? 9. Would you like to say goodbye to something or someone? 10. What have you learned about life? 11. What can make you happier now? 12. What can make your life worthwhile and give life a sense of meaning? 13. What do you think you still need to do? 14. How would you like this letter to be handled? Would you like to give it to someone? To whom and why?

Given the pandemic context, some adaptations have been made to the initial protocol, namely changes in the intervention procedures, i.e., face-to-face method to videoconferencing and four to five sessions. The number of sessions was increased to allow for a more pleasant and comfortable environment due to the virtual format.

Semi-structured Interview for the Patient

Considering the main aim of this study – to evaluate the effectiveness and the feasibility of the intervention by videoconference, a Semi-structured Interview was designed (Table 2) to be implemented in two different moments: Part 1 of the interview coincided with Session 5- when the patient was given a copy of the LL - and addressed the following items: preparation of the LL, significant aspects of the intervention, how the LL would be handled, and the patient's perceptions of how the family member would receive the LL.

Part 2 of the Semi-structured Interview took place one month after the LL was bequeathed to the family member (Session 6) and sought to assess the patient's perception of the relative´s reaction after receiving the letter as well as the concept of dignity, focusing on the evaluation of the implementation of MLT by videoconference.

Table 2. Semi-structured Interview for the Patient

Part I (Session 5)
1. Over the past few weeks, we've taken a brief journey through your life, and we concluded it with the creation of this letter. a. How was this process for you? b. What was the most important part for you? c. How did you feel throughout the process? 2. How was the process of creating this letter? 3. Who would you like to give this letter to? How do you think it will be received?
Part II (Session 6)
4. What was your relative's reaction when (s)he received the letter? 5. Do you feel that your relationship with him/her has changed in some way? If so, in which way? In which aspects? 6. In your opinion, what is important to ensure dignity for a person who faces a disease like this? 7. Times have changed and the pandemic forced us to adapt to the new circumstances, including the way we communicate. What was it like for you to write this letter via videoconference? 8. Do you think the result would be different if it were written in a face-to-face intervention, i.e., during a consultation at the hospital? 9. What did you consider the most positive and least positive aspects? 10. In your opinion, would it be important to carry out this project in other hospitals, with patients facing a disease like this?

Semi-structured Interview for the Family Member

The Semi-structured Interview with the family member (Table 3) coincided with the patient's evaluation of the intervention (Session 6), i.e., one month after the intervention ended. In this session, some topics were addressed, such as the family member's perception of the patient's state of mind during the intervention process, possible changes in family relationships, the impact of the LL, and the overall assessment of the intervention. Finally, questions were asked in order to evaluate the procedures applied for the intervention using videoconferencing.

Table 3. Semi-structured Interview for the Family Member: one month after intervention ended

1. How would you describe the patient's state of mind throughout the intervention process? 2. What could have contributed to this? 3. Since the beginning of the intervention, have you noticed any changes in the relationship between the patient and the closest family members? If so, in what sense? 4. How was it for you to receive the letter created by the patient? 5. Did anything change in the way you are experiencing your loved one's illness? 6. How do you evaluate the intervention carried out with the patient? 7. What did you consider the most positive and least positive aspects? 8. Would you recommend this intervention to someone you know who is in the same situation? Why? 9. Times have changed and the pandemic forced us to adapt to the new circumstances, including the way we communicate. How was it for you to participate in this process by videoconference? 10. Do you think it would be different if it were a face-to-face intervention?

Semi-structured Interview for the Patient's Wife after his Death

The follow-up Semi-structured Interview with the patient´s wife took place in two sessions after his death, where the following topics were explored: recollection of the MLT intervention, the role of the LL in the patient´s and family member´s adaptation to end-of-life process and bereavement, and the role of the LL in the family member's grieving process.

Procedures

The first contact with the patient and his wife was at the PC face-to-face consultation. Session 1 with the patient was scheduled by telephone; the subsequent sessions were scheduled at the end of each session, and the access links were sent via e-mail on the same day. Zoom® was the platform used for the videoconferences, using the "Recording" feature for video recording of sessions and "Screen Sharing" for sharing content. The recordings were transcribed *ipsis verbis* into a Word® text. Both participants received detailed explanation on how to use Zoom® and gave permission to record the sessions. Informed consent was also obtained before the participants entered the research.

The MLT intervention with the patient lasted four sessions, fully in compliance with its guidelines. The evaluation of its impact had occurred in two subsequent sessions. Initially weekly sessions were recommended, but it was not always possible due to the patient's clinical state and technological difficulties (Figure 1). The impact assessment of the intervention was complemented by his wife´s testimony at one-month post-intervention and at months 5 and 6 after the patient's death (follow-up sessions). These two follow-up sessions were held in person in the hospital setting (Figure 2).

E-mail was the communication channel used to send the Informed Consent Form, the MLT questions, and the access links. The Informed Consent Form and the two versions of the LL (draft and edited) were shared with the patient through "Screen Sharing".

The final version of the LL was delivered by hand in order to guarantee confidentiality, bearing in mind that the patient´s wife had access to his e-mail account.

During the intervention sessions, the patient showed adequate and cooperative behavior, often establishing eye contact. He was always conscious, showed orientation in time and space, had a logically organized speech, euthymic mood while also demonstrating awareness of his disease and his palliative condition. The reduced privacy and interruptions that occurred during the sessions (e.g., opening the door, wife answering a phone call), led to behaviors of discomfort (pauses in speech, intentional moments of silence) on the part of the patient.

Likewise, the patient´s wife showed adequate and cooperative behavior, maintaining eye contact during the Semi-structured Interview after the end of the MLT intervention. She demonstrated insight into the diagnosis and prognosis of her spouse's illness and emotional lability when addressing significant relational issues. In the follow-up sessions, she maintained her cooperative behavior, showing a low mood and depression and some difficulties in dealing with the loss.

In total, six sessions were held with the patient, and three sessions with his wife - one at the end of the intervention, and two after the patient's death. The Semi-structured Interview lasted an average of 120 minutes.

Figure 1. Flowchart of the Procedures with the Patient

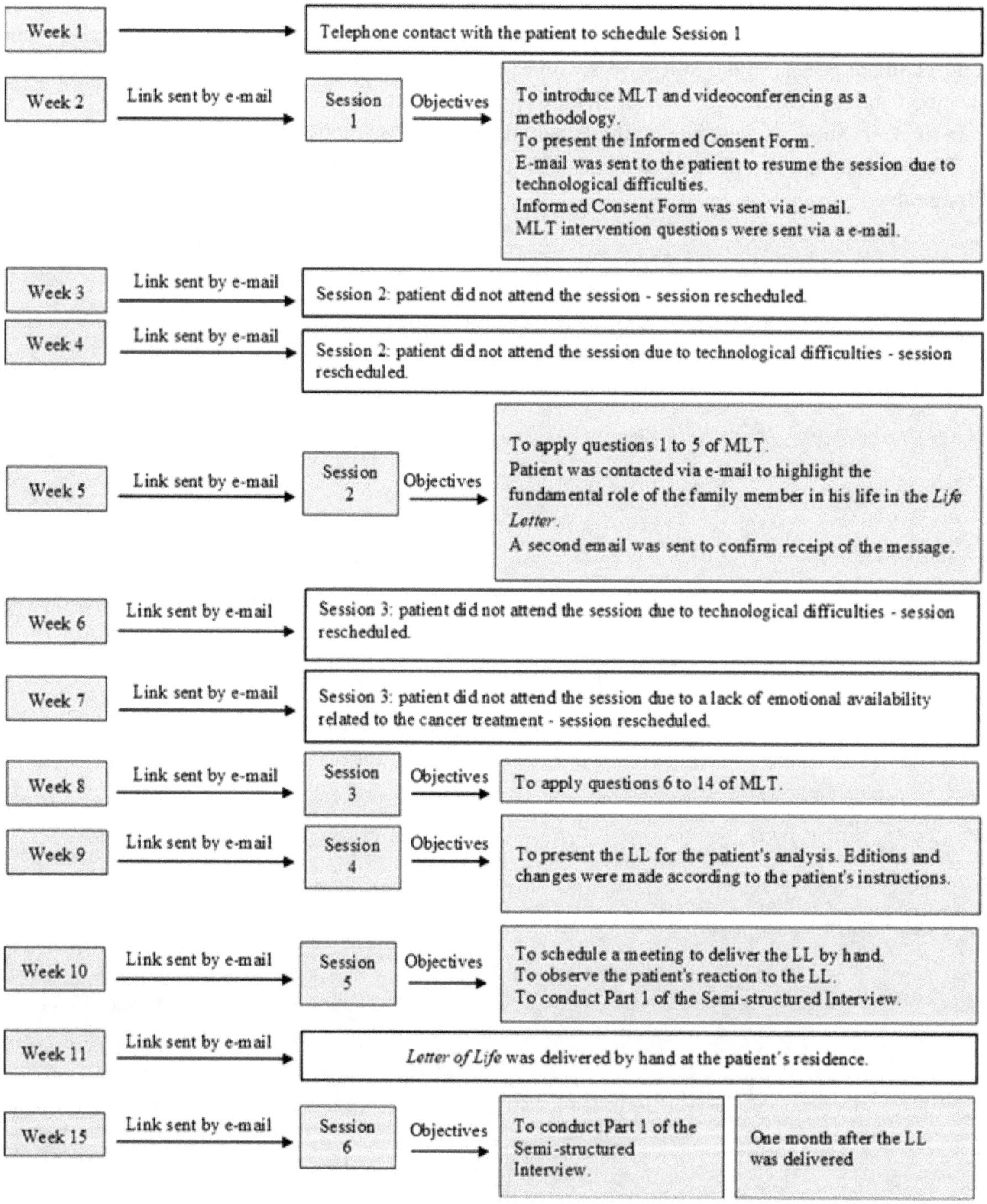

Figure 2. Flowchart of the Procedures with the Patient´s Wife

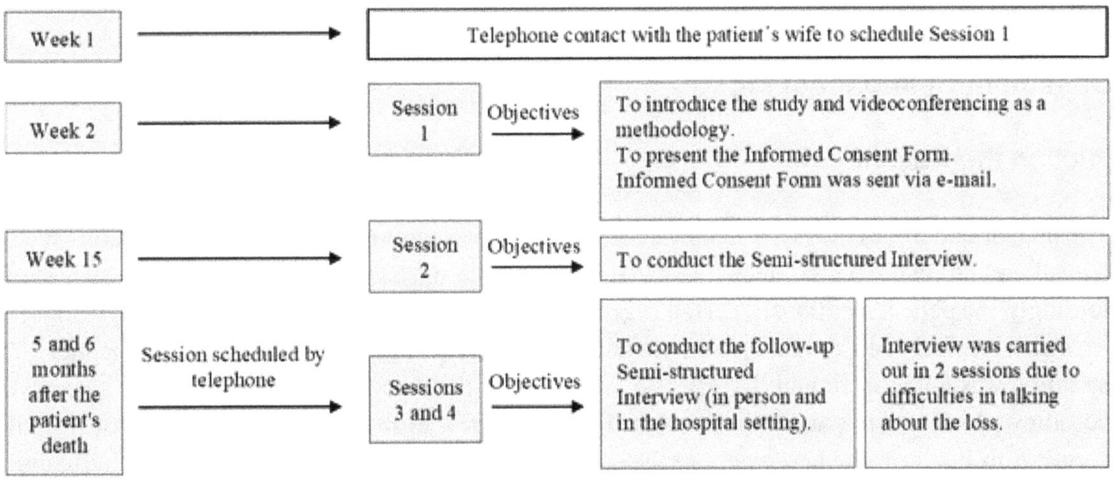

Data Analysis

The patient's answers to the MLT protocol questions and the patient´s and his wife´s evaluation data of the impact of the intervention, collected with the Semi-structured Interviews, were transcribed in full by the researcher. The texts were very carefully analyzed and in a detailed manner to ensure no overlooked. The analysis was of a semi-inductive nature, guided by the objectives of the study. Coding was carried out by segmenting the text into units of meaning, through an open coding process and constant comparison. The codes were progressively grouped into subcategories and broader categories (Saldanha, 2011). The coding process had an iterative approach, where the components and properties of categories were examined progressively. The data coding and analysis process were conducted with the QSR NVivo® 11 software (QSR International, 2012). Three of the research team members participated in this process, thus ensuring triangulation in the data analysis process. The data collection and data analysis involved a reflexive approach that integrates multiple sources of information (e.g., clinical and sociodemographic data, field notes from participant observations), which help to contextualize the patient´s and family member´s experiences and to interpret findings (Stake, 2005).

RESULTS

In order to provide a clearer and complete understanding of this research phenomenon, the results will be displayed in categories and subcategories (Appendix A), marked in bold, with information on the number of references (REFs), indicating their relevance.

Assessment of Impact of MLT

Impact on the Patient

The patient underlines the positive impact of the MLT Intervention (29 REFs) in dimensions such as emotional regulation (7 REFs), since it allowed for recognition, sharing and management of emotions. Accordingly, the patient mentions, "(...) talking about how I feel, talking about my past and also about the future makes me feel good and think, be more coherent and, in a way, see life in a different manner." The intervention was felt as a stimulus to reflection (6 REFs), since, according to the patient, "(...) reviving stories allowed me to think about the problem I have and how to live from day to day, [and] from this perspective, to live it in the best way." At the same time, it constitutes a communication facilitator (6 REFs), in revelations such as "(...) sometimes we cannot say what we really want, or the way we would like to say it. But now I think I've talked about everything, the essentials of my life (...)." During the sessions, it was also possible to verify that, according to the patient's perspective, the therapy promoted the process of disease adaptation (6 REFs), being evident throughout the discourse. According to the patient, "(...) we are aware that our clinical situation facilitates adaptation to the disease and all this is part of dignity, of knowing how to deal [with it], of showing others and saying how we are dealing [with it]."

The Wife's Perception of the Impact of the MLT Intervention on the Patient

The wife's testimony about the impact of the intervention on the patient points to the positive impact (8 REFs) on the patient's well-being and, consequently on herself ("It's good to talk..." 4 REFs), emphasizing that in her opinion, "(...) it is a topic that makes us face a reality that we don't want to [see], but deep down I think that talking about the subject is good for us and that letter will be kept here [pointing to her heart]." For the patient´s wife, the impact of the intervention extended to the level of the relational sphere with the patient's family (3 REFs). In this context, she concluded, "Although he talks to his brothers and nephews on the phone, I honestly think that the ties between him and his own family are stronger." However, she describes her uncertainties regarding the theme of the intervention ("It was difficult"– 2 REFs), highlighting a potential negative impact (3 REFs) of the therapy, which reveals her apprehension about a theme which tends to be avoided/denied, "I confess that I pondered whether I would ask these questions [from the intervention protocol] when you sent them to my e-mail [address], I kept them in the drawer for three days, I didn't know if I should give them to him. I thought I was protecting him."

Impact of Creating and Sharing the LL

As for the creation of the LL, the patient considers the process as a means of facilitating sharing (4 REFs) and mentions, "(...) it is important even for those who have great difficulty in expressing themselves with words, maybe saying and writing a letter that can be read, thought about and corrected; [they] manage to put down on paper what they cannot say in a conversation." Likewise, the patient stresses that during the process, "(...) we are also listening to ourselves and this allows for greater comfort given the situation we are experiencing (...)," considering the process as structuring (6 REFs), for those who, like him, faced a terminal illness.

According to his wife's perspective, the LL is able to facilitate sharing (3 REFs), and notes, "(...) people have to say every day to those we like that we love them and how important they are to us. And this letter translates that." The fact that the LL is a permanent testimony (2 REFs) allowed for emotional comfort for the patient´s wife, contributing to her well-being. Thus, she maintains, "I think that what was written and kept in this letter describes what we are, regardless of the context."

Opinion of the Patient and his Wife about Recommending the Intervention

According to the patient, recommending MLT should be considered on a universal scale (2 REFs), in his opinion, "(...) this is very important and should be carried out in all hospitals."

However, according to the patient´s wife, recommending MLT will vary according to the personality traits ("Perhaps"- 5 REFs) of each individual. In this context, she comments, "(...) it depends whether I know the person well. There are people like me, who like to talk about my problems and talking about them helps to make them smaller, but there are other people who don't like it," and highlights that she would recommend the intervention according to "(...) the person who is on the other side (...)."

Assessment of the Adjustment to the Loss and Grieving Process of the Patient's Wife

During the grieving process, symptomatic control (2 REFs) and COVID-19 contingency measures (1 REF) are categorized as risk indicators, which according to the patient´s wife, led to unconsciousness, "I thought he wasn't ill, he was like when he was at home, he was in pain, but he got over it and then they started of course (...) with medication, medication, medication. Wasn't he conscious? He is no longer conscious." This prevented psychological closeness, which, in her perception, led to the patient´s death, "(…) thinking that I did not want to be in the hospital with him," causing revolt and indignation. These factors made it difficult for the patient´s wife to say goodbye, emphasizing the importance of the LL in the process of adapting to the loss, since it appears as a means of reaching the patient ("hearing his voice" - 1 REF). She mentions, "That letter it's good to (...) recall. Yes, because when I miss him a lot, it's like looking at the photographs, it's like watching the videos that I made and that I keep (...) watching and remembering (...) hearing his voice." In addition, it was perceived as an element of maintenance of interpersonal relationships (2 REFs). She emphasizes, "I want to read it again, but I want to read it with his brothers (…) I will take it to share it with (...) the family." When questioned about the intervention, the patient´s wife reinforces her reluctance towards the questions of the MLT protocol (1 REF), referring that "it was about the end-of-life, patients at the end-of-life (...) maybe I was more disturbed than he was", which reveals her difficulty in dealing/accepting the palliative phase and concomitantly accepting the loss.

Remote Intervention via Videoconference

With regard to the videoconference intervention, the participants highlight its advantages and disadvantages (Figures 3 and 4). For the patient (Figure 3), the advantages of videoconferencing were related to the reduced risks of infection with SARS-CoV-2 (4 REF) noting that "(...) videoconferencing is a way of protecting ourselves," being a relevant method "(...) with regard to individual protection and comfort." Notably, travel reduction (2 REFs) is one of the advantages of this methodology; according to his wife, "The most positive thing was, in fact, not having to travel to the hospital, especially during a pandemic." However, she preferred a face-to-face intervention, since it allowed observing details of non-verbal communication (1 REF), and mentions, "The body helps to understand the message and although this is a videoconference, the details, the expressions are not as clear as in a face-to-face context." She also expressed a preference for an out-of-hospital setting (1 REF), "I would choose face-to-face [interventions], but not in a hospital, if possible."

Reflecting on the reasons for the patient missing one of the therapy sessions, he points to technological difficulties (3 REFs) as a disadvantage of videoconferencing, "The least positive thing was, for example, when my mobile phone broke and I missed the appointment." As for the speech and behavior observed in the patient, he noted that there would be no changes in speech and behavior (3 REFs) if the intervention were held in the hospital setting. In this way, he described he would feel comfortable in both contexts, "(...) I wish all the professionals who take care of me would come to my house, but it is not possible, I know I have to travel [to the hospital], but traveling wouldn't make it different, I would feel equally comfortable."

Figure 3. Impact of Remote Intervention by Videoconference- Patient´s Perspective

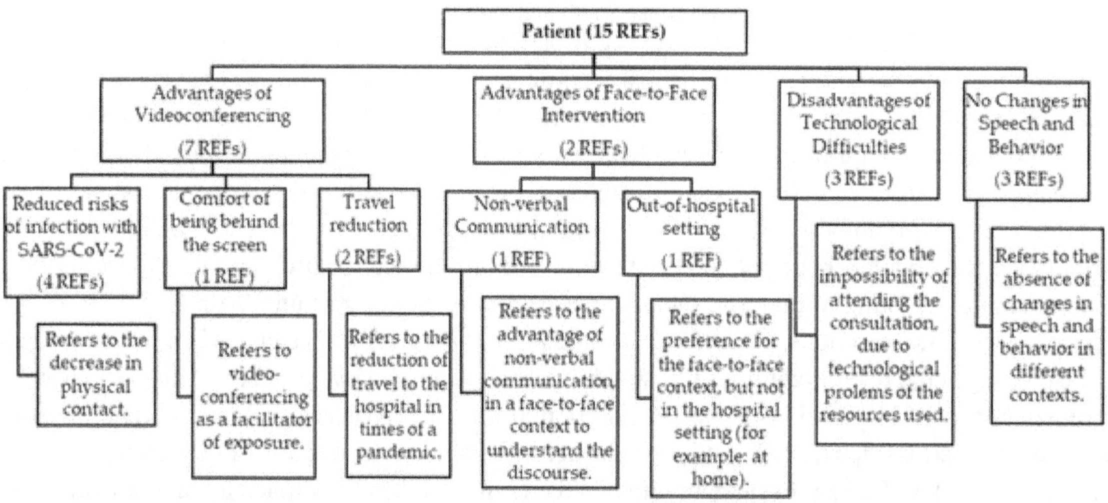

According to the perspective of the patient´s wife (Figure 4), the remote intervention via videoconference poses a barrier to expressing emotions (2 REFs), pondering, " [in] face-to-face [meetings] we can see the emotions at the moment and I think they are different, there are [emotions] here, but it is not the same, something is missing."

Ultimately, taking the above into consideration, the patient´s wife would choose the face-to-face intervention (2 REFs), explaining that, in the method under study "(...) the emotion, the warmth of [a person´s] presence is not the same".

Figure 4. Impact of remote Intervention by Videoconference- Wife´s Perspective

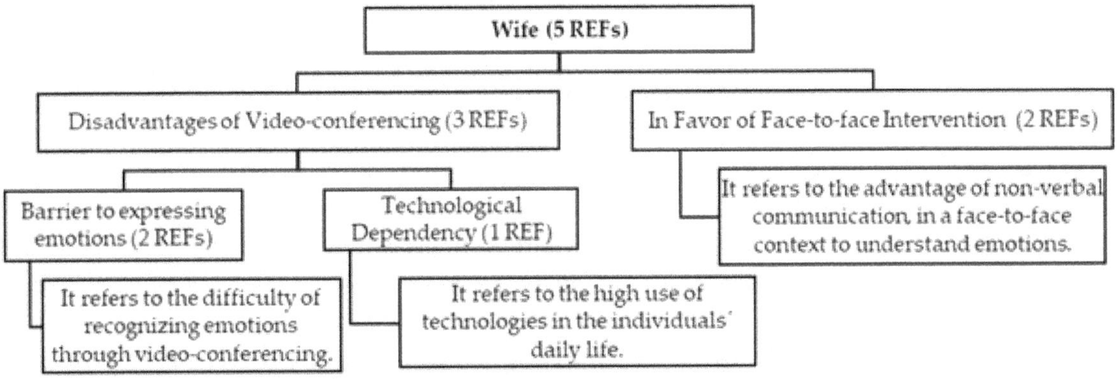

DISCUSSION

Our main objective was to evaluate the effectiveness, acceptability and feasibility of MLT by videoconference, regarding the patient and his wife psychological adjustment at the end-of-life, adopting an instrumental single case study approach (Stake, 2005). Given the scarcity of studies in this field (Steindal et al., 2023), the need for continuous research to evaluate the effectiveness and safety of digital interventions (Arogundade et al., 2024) and qualitative research as well, are fundamental (Payne et al., 2020).

Our results demonstrate that globally the positive aspects of videoconferencing mentioned by the couple outweigh the negative ones, being the reduced travel (and associated costs) and risk of COVID-19 infection the greatest benefits of this intervention methodology. In addition, it enabled the implementation of MLT in the middle of a pandemic, in a period marked by the "distraction effect" in the continuous care of cancer patients (Cortiula et al., 2020; Denys et al., 2020) given the risk of infection.

The cost-benefit issue is consistent with literature, with digital interventions being considered one of the greatest benefits (Arogundade et al., 2024; Jess et al., 2019; Keenan et al., 2021; Stoll et al., 2020; Wood et al., 2023). As a results, appears as an accessible and low-cost methodology (Sutherland et al., 2020), "(…) as a means of making palliative care more widely accessible" (Dilhani et al., 2024, p. 1), useful and viable with the potential to improve the quality of life of patients and their family members (Mirshahi et al., 2024).

Despite the visual contact promoted by videoconferencing, the patient and his wife identify the screen as a barrier to non-verbal communication, considering that a face-to-face approach enables body language analysis - in most interventions the image of the patient shows only the patient´s head and upper chest, which may limit the observation of details of nonverbal behavior. Although the patient's preference for a face-to-face approach, apparently the use of videoconferencing for the implementation of MLT did not change the intervention process, maintaining the use of this method as an alternative form of intervention. In the patient's opinion, the "comfort of being behind the screen" facilitated emotional expression.

This perception is supported by the study carried out by van Gurp et al. (2015), using teleconsultation with patients undergoing PC, which revealed that physical distance offered by videoconferencing was a liberating experience and promoted story sharing. The same was verified with the implementation of online Dignity Therapy (DT), proving to be an effective method to engage patients who would not be involved in an in-person intervention (Bentley et al., 2020). The physical distance promoted by new technologies is also associated with the reduction of stigma, especially in the context of psychotherapeutic interventions (Adjei-Boateng & Ikoh Rph, 2025).

Technological difficulties emerge as one of the negative aspects of this type of intervention, with frequent audio/video errors or interruptions of internet connection. The relative lack of privacy at home and occasional interruptions led to interruptions in the patient's speech. Furthermore, although the couple found no difficulties in using digital media, we cannot ignore the negative impact of being unable to use technological resources, which is observed in an overwhelming majority of older adults.

Technological problems are typical of this kind of intervention (Sutherland et al., 2020), with instability of Internet connection (Azcona et al., 2022; Tajan et al., 2023) and accessibility (Wood et al., 2023) being one of the main limitations of digital interventions. Issues related to privacy and confidentiality have been widely discussed in the literature (e.g. Rodrigues-Ribeiro et al., 2024; Stoll et al., 2020), in order to minimize the impact of lack of privacy in the clients' environments, identified by Tajan et al. (2023). In this sense, it's important to increase digital literacy among potential users (e.g., healthcare professionals, patients, caregivers), raising their awareness of data protection. However, it is also important to promote digital competence, since a lack of digital competence (Van Goethem et al., 2025) effectively hinders the use of digital technologies in healthcare.

As for the impact of MLT, the patient's testimony regarding increased capacity of emotional regulation is the best sign of a positive impact, considering its relevance in the management of terminal illnesses, influencing psychological functioning and adaptation (Brandão et al., 2017).

The reflection process promoted by MLT is a further indication of its positive impact. Feelings of coherence and "seeing life in a different manner" (REF) resulted from this process, which offered a unique opportunity to reaffirm significant aspects of life for the patient due to their psychological, emotional and interpersonal potential, also observed in DT (Vuksanovic et al., 2017). The journey back in time allows for confrontation and learning, which enables patients to understand their current status, and consequently evoke future behaviors and attitudes according to the stages of the terminal illness (Zhang et al., 2017). Self-reflection is therefore a facilitator of psychological adaptation to the disease (Henry et al., 2010). However, in the absence of meaning (facing a negative perspective), self-reflection may lead to despair or demoralization (Lee et al., 2004, 2006), which was not observed in the present study. By evoking positive feelings about the past and the future, MLT has fulfilled, in this case, the psychosocial needs at the end-of-life advocated by Erikson, promoting a feeling of finitude and acceptance, achieving ego integrity instead of despair, which characterizes the final stage of life (Guo & Jacelon, 2014).

The patient's testimony emphasizes that MLT fostered the construction of a sense of meaning and purpose in life, facilitating his willingness to communicate– which is extremely positive– considering that communication is key for the integration of the disease and death process, as well as for the dialogue among patient, family members and the PC team (Melo et al., 2013). The patient also noted improved information sharing during and after the intervention. This is mentioned as a fundamental strategy, which is characterized as a tool to alleviate suffering and to turn a painful process into an experience of personal and family growth (Salazar & Duarte, 2017), stimulating empathic comprehension in the patient-family dyad (Chan et al., 2012), where patients tend to be more communicative than the others (Dahley & Sanders, 2016).

In line with the patient´s testimony, his wife also mentions the positive effects of MLT on the patient´s and her own well-being, promoted by the experiences shared and stronger emotional bond between patient and his family members, demonstrating greater openness to communication in general. This is further supported by studies that describe the positive effects of these interventions not only on the patient but also on family members (Fitchett et al., 2015).

For the patient, in this case, there is no doubt about the benefits of MLT and its relevance in patients approaching death, and he recommends its implementation for all the patients for promoting well-being and facilitating expression of feelings and emotion. The same is not true for his wife, who expressed some concerns because, like herself, not everybody will be able to easily go through this reflection process promoted by the MLT intervention - she highlights the importance of personal characteristics of each individual. Despite the positive evidence of psychoexistencial interventions in promoting the construction of meaning and purpose in life, (e.g. Donato et al., 2016; Rosenfeld et al., 2017) which enable terminally ill patients to reconcile with the past, to be aware of the present and to accept an uncertain future (Breitbart et al., 2004), not all patients and family members have the necessary resources and/or time to effectively engage in conflicting and potentially traumatic existential aspects. Houmann et al. (2014) draw our attention to this precise fact, when referring to DT (a psychoexistencial intervention) as a motivational intervention for a considerable number of patients, but not beneficial to all terminally ill patients. The very process of creating a legacy document (in DT) can lead to several personal and interpersonal conflicts within the family (Houmann et al., 2014).This was also observed in our study, as the patient´s wife showed reluctance to present the MLT questions to the patient and prepare the LL in a protective move, which reflected, above all, her difficulties in dealing with the finitude of the loved one. After the patient's death, his wife's testimony was congruent with the previous statement, highlighting her unwillingness to get involved in the intervention, as the patient was considered an element of support.

In the present single case study, LL, a key component of MLT, is recognized by the patient as a means of facilitating sharing in an organized and structured manner, enabling clear and fluid communication, which, according to the patient, is not always easy. By including structured and direct messages for the family members to be received and appreciated (Vuksanovic et al., 2017), the LL can be a powerful tool for communication and interpersonal relationships or, conversely, for family conflicts and eventual breakups. In this case study, LL had an extremely positive impact on communication and on the improvement of the marital relationship from the patient's standpoint and could also serve as a communication channel with health professionals.

Along these lines, the patient´s wife also recognizes the importance of the LL to facilitate sharing and engender a permanent testimony. The vital character of the LL may be extremely important in the process of adaptation to bereavement - which is evident in the wife's speech - and her emotional dependence, identifying the patient (spouse) as an element of support. In this context, in the absence of the patient's physical, social and psychological presence, the LL appears to be an important resource to maintain a continuing relationship, as advocated by McClement et al. (2007), making it last forever and be a comfort for those who will remain "in the heart", as the wife says. This was reinforced by patient´s wife in her testimony after his death, where the LL revealed itself as a means to facilitate the grieving process, being characterized as a comfort resource that allows her to recall the patient as if she could "hear his voice", in her words.

The wife's expression of contentment after receiving the LL, the relationship of sincerity, honesty, complicity and friendship (reported by the patient) and of mutual support and balance (reported by his wife) are clear examples of the importance, for her, of the presence and company of the patient in adapting to the terminal disease. The positive perception of patients in the face of social support is crucial for disease adaptation as well as for their psychological well-being and, similarly, for their sense of dignity (Chochinov, 2012). The beneficial effect of MLT, evidenced in the relational sphere, in this case study, is congruent with several studies (Bentley et al., 2020; Chochinov, 2012; Goddard et al., 2013; Hall et al., 2013; McClement et al., 2007). In the follow-up sessions with the patient´s wife, it was possible to observe that MLT, especially, the LL, enabled a better psychological adjustment to the loss and played a key role in the grieving process, being considered a source of comfort, reported in the literature (Grijó et al., 2021), and a means of "hearing his voice". However, it should be noted that in addition to the intervention, several factors contribute to the adaptive grief process, such as the affective relationship (key element highlighted throughout the intervention), idiosyncrasies of the caregiver/family member and the death itself. Accepting participation in the MLT demonstrates a path to eventually create a bereavement "pillow" that could replace the loved one.

Study Limitations

Despite the promising results observed in this case study, some limitations can be pointed out. According to the constructivist paradigm, a single case study (Stake, 2005) seeks to address its particularities and complexity in order to understand its nature in specific circumstances. In this approach, generalization regarding the patients´ and family members´ experiences cannot be made. Another limitation is related to the lack of comparison: without comparison with in-person interventions or control groups, it is difficult to assess the relative effectiveness of the remote approach.

It's important to mention important challenges and considerations that, despite not having been the subject of this case study, are relevant. As referred by Lederman and D'Alfonso, (2021), firstly, there is the therapeutic alliance. Can digital tools replicate the depth of human connection? Second, privacy and ethics. Sensitive existential content requires secure handling. Third, cultural sensitivity. meaning-making varies across cultures and belief systems. Fourth, scalability vs. personalization.

SOLUTIONS AND ETHICAL RECOMMENDATIONS

Considering the results and questions arising from this case study, some issues should be considered in the refinement of the implementation of psychoexistencial intervention in PC mediated by new technologies:

1. Guarantee of privacy and information security

Despite the benefits of digital interventions, it is essential to recognize the risks associated with privacy, confidentiality, and data security. Situations such as the one observed in the study, in which the wife assumed the role of mediator in communication and delivery of protocols, highlight vulnerabilities that can compromise confidentiality and generate constraints in the therapeutic relationship. It is recommended that procedures be implemented to minimize such risks, in line with ethical and legal guidelines (Argüero-Fonseca et al., 2021; Ordem dos Psicólogos Portugueses, 2023; Stoll et al., 2020), ensuring the protection of sensitive existential content and compliance with data protection standards

2. Strengthening the Digital Therapeutic Alliance

Although studies demonstrate the effectiveness of telepsychology in building therapeutic relationships (Azcona et al., 2022), the depth of the connection between therapist and patient in the digital environment is still a matter of debate. The concept of the Digital Therapeutic Alliance (DTA) (Kaveladze & Schueller, 2023) offers a framework that integrates human and technological components, proposing that this alliance be defined as the user's perception of the bond, the agreement on therapeutic tasks and goals, and how these are mediated by technology. Investing in strengthening this alliance is crucial to ensuring the effectiveness of remote psychoexistencial intervention.

3. Adoption of hybrid intervention models

Despite some patients' preference for face-to-face sessions, the literature shows high acceptance of hybrid models - combining face-to-face and remote sessions - by patients and psychotherapists (Tajan et al., 2023). This approach allows for moments of direct contact to be preserved, maximizing the relational potential of Therapeutic Alliance (TA) while simultaneously benefiting from the logistical and accessibility advantages provided by digital technologies.

4. Professional training for digital intervention

Limitations in reading nonverbal cues are often cited as an obstacle in technology-mediated interventions, with a potential impact on assessment and therapeutic planning. Continuous training of healthcare professionals in the competent use of digital resources is recommended to combat the insufficient training identified in this field (Rojas-Jara et al., 2022). This investment contributes to increasing the safety and effectiveness of interventions, ensuring that techniques are adapted to virtual reality.

In summary, the implementation of psychoexistencial interventions via videoconferencing in palliative care requires a careful balance between technological innovation and preserving the essence of person-centered clinical practice. The solutions presented - from protecting privacy and security to strengthening the (DTA, adopting hybrid models, professional training, and creating crisis management protocols - are fundamental pillars for ensuring the quality and ethics of this intervention format. By incorporating these recommendations, professionals will not only be able to expand access and continuity of care, but also ensure that the human and relational dimension, which is at the core of psychoexistential intervention, remains intact and meaningful, even when mediated by technology.

FUTURE RESEARCH DIRECTIONS

The advancement of psychoexistencial intervention via videoconferencing in palliative care requires a research agenda that addresses identified gaps and explores new possibilities. Future research could deepen understanding of the DTA (D'Alfonso et al., 2020; Lederman & D'Alfonso, 2021), analyzing its evolution over time and how it compares to the traditional therapeutic alliance. Comparing hybrid and exclusively digital models, considering clinical efficacy, cost-effectiveness, and patient and caregiver satisfaction, is also relevant.

Another area of research lies in the impact of limited nonverbal reading and the effectiveness of strategies to mitigate this barrier, including technological innovations and specific training for professionals. In addition, the development and validation of robust protocols for crisis management in a remote environment, combined with an in-depth analysis of the ethical and legal implications of sharing sensitive existential content, are priority areas.

Finally, studies dedicated to the patient-caregiver dyad may clarify how technological mediation influences communication, cohesion, and relational resilience, consolidating evidence for the optimization of these interventions in the future.

This study demonstrated the acceptability and the benefits of participating in an online intervention as patient-caregiver dyads, as some others did (e.g., Chen et al., 2022; Kim et al., 2023). Unlike other psychosocial interventions, a technology-based MLT via videoconference is an easy-to-deliver, flexible, low-cost, and non-invasive psychosocial support vehicle. A larger clinical trial is needed to examine effects of the MLT intervention both in the short- and longer-term, as well as mechanisms of change. Furthermore, a longer follow-up of the caregiver could provide additional information, for example, one year after the loss.

Hence, further studies should be carried out to evaluate the effectiveness of MLT, as well as the feasibility of using new technologies to allow for an adequate response to the psychoexistencial needs of PC patients and their families, taking into account their physical and psychological vulnerabilities.

CONCLUSIONS

Psychoexistencial intervention via videoconferencing, applied in the form of Meaning Life Therapy (MLT), has demonstrated its applicability and feasibility in the context of palliative care, proving to be a useful, accessible, and low-cost modality for providing care to terminally ill patients. Digital technologies have shown flexibility and adaptability to different locations, contexts, conditions, and characteristics, responding to the specific needs and convenience of users. This adaptability not only promotes more equitable access to care but also reduces risks associated with pandemics and other contexts of health vulnerability.

In the case presented, the acceptance of the intervention by the patient-caregiver dyad demonstrated the feasibility of this procedure in a period marked by severe restrictions and deeply painful experiences - a time when even a simple hug could be impossible. As the patient summarized: "Everything starts with us, and that is the most important thing" a phrase that reflects the core of the psychoexistencial approach and made this study possible.

Despite its inherent limitations, the qualitative assessment yielded valid conclusions that contribute to the design of future projects, including in-depth exploration of the DTA, comparison of hybrid and exclusively digital models, development of remote crisis management protocols, and analysis of the impact of this modality on communication and resilience in the dyad. Importantly, the fact that this case was collected during the pandemic opened the possibility of exploring the pertinence and effectiveness of brief remote psychoexistencial interventions in palliative care. This possibility should continue to be pursued beyond pandemic scenarios, extending to contexts and populations in which such responses remain essential. By combining technological innovation and humanistic principles, MLT via videoconferencing not only expands access to specialized care but also reaffirms the centrality of the human and relational dimension in palliative care practice.

REFERENCES

Adjei-Boateng, D., & Rph, C. L. I. (2025). Digital Mental Health Interventions for Adolescents and Young People: Evaluating Efficacy and Accessibility. *Cureus, 17*(6). Advance online publication. DOI: 10.7759/cureus.85943 PMID: 40662025

Altaf Dar, M., Maqbool, M., Ara, I., & Zehravi, M. (2023). The intersection of technology and mental health: Enhancing access and care. *International Journal of Adolescent Medicine and Health, 35*(5), 423–428. DOI: 10.1515/ijamh-2023-0113 PMID: 37602724

Argüero-Fonseca, A., Cervantes-Luna, B. S., Martínez-Soto, J., Santos-Ávila, F., Aguirre-Ojed, D. P., Espinosa-Parra, I. M., & Beltrán, I. L. (2021). Telepsicología en la pandemia Covid-19: Una revisión sistemática. *UARICHA, 18*, 1–10.

Arogundade, B., Christine Kalu, O., Olukayode, S., Mayowa Olukayode, S., & Olorunjuwonlo Adebanjo, A. (2024). Digital Mental Health Interventions and Ai in Therapy See Profile Digital Mental Health Interventions and Ai in Therapy. *Article in International Research Journal of Modernization in Engineering Technology and Science*, (September). Advance online publication. DOI: 10.56726/IRJMETS61880

Azcona, M., Ángel Roldán, L., Soria, L., Garzaniti, R., Labaronnie, C., Manzini, F., Maite, L., & del Pilar Bolpe, M. (2022). La telepsicoterapia durante el Covid-19: Repercusiones de la capacitación y del ámbito laboral de las/los terapeutas. *Psicologia Clínica, 34*(1), 169–188. DOI: 10.33208/PC1980-5438v0034n01A08

Bentley, B., O'Connor, M., Williams, A., & Breen, L. J. (2020). Dignity therapy online: Piloting an online psychosocial intervention for people with terminal illness. *Digital Health, 6*, 1–8. DOI: 10.1177/2055207620958527 PMID: 33014409

Brandão, T., Schulz, M. S., Gross, J. J., & Matos, P. M. (2017). The emotion regulation questionnaire in women with cancer: A psychometric evaluation and an item response theory analysis. *Psycho-Oncology, 26*(10), 1647–1653. DOI: 10.1002/pon.4356 PMID: 28010039

Breitbart, W., Gibson, C., Poppito, S. R., & Berg, A. (2004). Psychotherapeutic Interventions at the End of Life: A Focus on Meaning and Spirituality. *Canadian Journal of Psychiatry, 49*(6), 366–372. DOI: 10.1177/070674370404900605 PMID: 15283531

Cardoso, A. R., Remondes-Costa, S., Veiga, E., Almeida, V., Rocha, J., Teixeira, R. J., Macedo, G., & Leite, M. (2023). Meaning of Life Therapy: A Pilot Study of a Novel Psychoexistencial Intervention for Palliative Care in Cancer. *Omega (United States), 0*(0), 1–30. DOI: 10.1177/00302228231209654 PMID: 37884277

Chan, C. L. W., Ho, A. H. Y., Leung, P. P. Y., Chochinov, H. M., Neimeyer, R. A., Pang, S. M. C., & Tse, D. M. W. (2012). The Blessings and the Curses of Filial Piety on Dignity at the End of Life: Lived Experience of Hong Kong Chinese Adult Children Caregivers. *Journal of Ethnic & Cultural Diversity in Social Work, 21*(4), 277–296. DOI: 10.1080/15313204.2012.729177

Chen, M., Gong, J., & Li, Q. (2022). The application of eHealth in cancer survivorship care: A review of web-based dyadic interventions for post-treatment cancer survivors and caregivers. *Asia-Pacific Journal of Oncology Nursing*, *9*(10), 100109. DOI: 10.1016/j.apjon.2022.100109 PMID: 36118622

Chochinov, H. M. (2012). *Dignity TherapyFinal Words for Final Days*. Oxford University Press., DOI: 10.1093/acprof:oso/9780195176216.001.0001

Clark, D. (1999). "Total pain", disciplinary power and the body in the work of Cicely Saunders, 1958-1967. *Social Science & Medicine*, *49*(6), 727–736. DOI: 10.1016/S0277-9536(99)00098-2 PMID: 10459885

Cortiula, F., Pettke, A., Bartoletti, M., Puglisi, F., & Helleday, T. (2020). Managing COVID-19 in the oncology clinic and avoiding the distraction effect. *Annals of Oncology : Official Journal of the European Society for Medical Oncology*, *31*(5), 553–555. DOI: 10.1016/j.annonc.2020.03.286 PMID: 32201224

Crowe, S., Cresswell, K., Robertson, A., Huby, G., Avery, A. S., & Sheikh, A. (2011). The case study approach. *BMC Medical Research Methodology*, *11*(100). PMID: 21707982

D'Alfonso, S., Lederman, R., Bucci, S., & Berry, K. (2020). The Digital Therapeutic Alliance and Human-Computer Interaction. *JMIR Mental Health*, *7*(12), e21895. DOI: 10.2196/21895 PMID: 33372897

Dahley, L., & Sanders, G. F. (2016). Use of a Structured Life Review and Its Impact on Family Interactions. *Activities, Adaptation and Aging*, *40*(1), 53–66. DOI: 10.1080/01924788.2016.1127060

Denys, A., Guiu, B., Chevallier, P., Digklia, A., de Kerviler, E., & de Baere, T. (2020). Interventional oncology at the time of COVID-19 pandemic: Problems and solutions. *Diagnostic and Interventional Imaging*, *101*(6), 347–353. DOI: 10.1016/j.diii.2020.04.005 PMID: 32360351

Dilhani, W. N. S., Mitchell, S., Dale, J., Toor, K., Javaid, M., & MacArtney, J. I. (2024). A mixed-methods systematic review investigating the use of digital health interventions to provide palliative and end-of-life care for patients in low- and middle-income countries. *Palliative Care and Social Practice*, *18*. Advance online publication. DOI: 10.1177/26323524241236965 PMID: 38617095

Donato, S. C. T., Matuoka, J. Y., Yamashita, C. C., & Salvetti, M. de G. (2016). Effects of dignity therapy on terminally ill patients: A systematic review. *Revista da Escola de Enfermagem da USP*, *50*(6), 1014–1024. DOI: 10.1590/s0080-623420160000700019 PMID: 28198968

Finucane, A. M., O'Donnell, H., Lugton, J., Gibson-Watt, T., Swenson, C., & Pagliari, C. (2021). Digital health interventions in palliative care: A systematic meta-review. *NPJ Digital Medicine*, *4*(1). Advance online publication. DOI: 10.1038/s41746-021-00430-7 PMID: 33824407

Fitchett, G., Emanuel, L., Handzo, G., Boyken, L., & Wilkie, D. J. (2015). Care of the human spirit and the role of dignity therapy: A systematic review of dignity therapy research. *BMC Palliative Care*, *14*(1), 8. DOI: 10.1186/s12904-015-0007-1 PMID: 25844066

Goddard, C., Speck, P., Martin, P., & Hall, S. (2013). Dignity Therapy for older people in care homes: A qualitative study of the views of residents and recipients of 'generativity' documents. *Journal of Advanced Nursing*, *69*(1), 122–132. DOI: 10.1111/j.1365-2648.2012.05999.x PMID: 22489609

Grewal, U. S., Terauchi, S., & Beg, M. S. (2020). Telehealth and Palliative Care for Patients With Cancer: Implications of the COVID-19 Pandemic. *JMIR Cancer*, *6*(2), e20288. DOI: 10.2196/20288 PMID: 33049695

Grijó, L., Tojal, C., & Rego, F. (2021). Effects of dignity therapy on palliative patients' family members: A systematic review. *Palliative & Supportive Care*, *19*(5), 605–614. DOI: 10.1017/S147895152100033X PMID: 33818358

Guo, Q., & Jacelon, C. S. (2014). An integrative review of dignity in end-of-life care. *Palliative Medicine*, *28*(7), 931–940. DOI: 10.1177/0269216314528399 PMID: 24685648

Haddouk, L., Schneider, B., Van Daele, T., & Lang, F. (2025). Telepsychology in France Following the COVID-19 Crisis From Changes in Practice to Ethical Considerations. *European Journal of Psychology Open*, *84*(1), 13–19. DOI: 10.1024/2673-8627/a000063

Hall, S., Goddard, C., Speck, P. W., Martin, P., & Higginson, I. J. (2013). "It Makes You Feel That Somebody Is Out There Caring": A Qualitative Study of Intervention and Control Participants' Perceptions of the Benefits of Taking Part in an Evaluation of Dignity Therapy for People With Advanced Cancer. *Journal of Pain and Symptom Management*, *45*(4), 712–725. DOI: 10.1016/j.jpainsymman.2012.03.009 PMID: 22921176

Henry, M., Cohen, S. R., Lee, V., Sauthier, P., Provencher, D., Drouin, P., Gauthier, P., Gotlieb, W., Lau, S., Drummond, N., Gilbert, L., Stanimir, G., Sturgeon, J., Chasen, M., Mitchell, J., Huang, L. N., Ferland, M., & Mayo, N. (2010). The Meaning-Making intervention (MMi) appears to increase meaning in life in advanced ovarian cancer: A randomized controlled pilot study. *Psycho-Oncology*, *19*(12), 1340–1347. DOI: 10.1002/pon.1764 PMID: 20878857

Houmann, L. J., Chochinov, H. M., Kristjanson, L. J., Petersen, M. A., & Groenvold, M. (2014). A prospective evaluation of Dignity Therapy in advanced cancer patients admitted to palliative care. *Palliative Medicine*, *28*(5), 448–458. DOI: 10.1177/0269216313514883 PMID: 24311296

International Association for Hospice and Palliative Care. (n.d.). *Palliative Care Definition*. Retrieved August 11, 2025, from https://iahpc.org/research/consensus-based-definition-of-palliative-care/definition/

Irwin, S. A., Fairman, N., Samsel, C., Hirst, J. M., Webb, J. A., & Trachsel, M. (2021). Psychological and psychiatric aspects of palliative and end-of-life care. In Breitbart, W. (Eds.), *Psycho-Oncology* (4th ed., pp. 589–598). Oxford University Press., DOI: 10.1093/med/9780190097653.003.0074

Jess, M., Timm, H., & Dieperink, K. B. (2019). Video consultations in palliative care: A systematic integrative review. *Palliative Medicine*, *33*(8), 942–958. DOI: 10.1177/0269216319854938 PMID: 31187688

Kaveladze, B., & Schueller, S. M. (2023). A digital therapeutic alliance in digital mental health. In *Digital Therapeutics for Mental Health and Addiction* (pp. 87–98). Elsevier., DOI: 10.1016/B978-0-323-90045-4.00009-5

Keenan, J., Rahman, R., & Hudson, J. (2021). Exploring the acceptance of telehealth within palliative care: A self-determination theory perspective. *Health and Technology*, *11*(3), 575–584. DOI: 10.1007/s12553-021-00535-9

Kim, S. W., Langer, S., Ahern, M., Larkey, L., Todd, M., Martin, D., Weihs, K., & Khera, N. (2023). Hematopoietic Cell Transplantation Patient-Caregiver Dyad Perspectives on Participation in a Digital Storytelling Intervention: A Qualitative Approach. *Transplantation and Cellular Therapy, 29*(8), 520.e1–520.e7. DOI: 10.1016/j.jtct.2023.04.021 PMID: 37137443

Kreitler, S. (2019). Confronting dying and death. In *Psycho-Oncology for the Clinician*. Springer., DOI: 10.1007/978-3-030-06126-5_13

Lederman, R., & D'Alfonso, S. (2021). The Digital Therapeutic Alliance: Prospects and Considerations. *JMIR Mental Health, 8*(7), e31385. DOI: 10.2196/31385 PMID: 34283035

Lee, V., Cohen, S. R., Edgar, L., Lsizner, A. M., & Gagnon, A. J. (2004). Clarifying "meaning" in the context of cancer research: A systematic literature review. *Palliative & Supportive Care, 2*(3), 291–303. DOI: 10.1017/S1478951504040386 PMID: 16594414

Lee, V., Robin Cohen, S., Edgar, L., Laizner, A. M., & Gagnon, A. J. (2006). Meaning-making intervention during breast or colorectal cancer treatment improves self-esteem, optimism, and self-efficacy. *Social Science & Medicine, 62*(12), 3133–3145. DOI: 10.1016/j.socscimed.2005.11.041 PMID: 16413644

Lourenço, M., Gomes, T., Araujo, F., Ventura, F., & Silva, R. (2024). Challenges for palliative care in times of COVID-19: A scoping review. *Frontiers in Public Health, 12*(March). Advance online publication. DOI: 10.3389/fpubh.2024.1330370 PMID: 38596518

McClement, S., Chochinov, H. M., Hack, T., Hassard, T., Kristjanson, L. J., & Harlos, M. (2007). Dignity Therapy: Family Member Perspectives. *Journal of Palliative Medicine, 10*(5), 1076–1082. DOI: 10.1089/jpm.2007.0002 PMID: 17985964

Melo, A. C., Valero, F. F., & Menezes, M. (2013). A Intervenção Psicológica Em Cuidados Paliativos. *Psicologia, Saúde & Doenças, 14*(3), 452–469.

Mirshahi, A., Bakitas, M., Khoshavi, M., Khanipour-Kencha, A., Riahi, S. M., Wells, R., Odom, J. N., Ghiyasvandian, S., & Zakerimoghadam, M. (2024). The impact of an integrated early palliative care telehealth intervention on the quality of life of heart failure patients: A randomized controlled feasibility study. *BMC Palliative Care, 23*(1), 22. DOI: 10.1186/s12904-024-01348-z PMID: 38254058

Mistraletti, G., Gristina, G., Mascarin, S., Iacobone, E., Giubbilo, I., Bonfanti, S., Fiocca, F., Fullin, G., Fuselli, E., Bocci, M. G., Mazzon, D., Giusti, G. D., Galazzi, A., Negro, A., De Iaco, F., Gandolfo, E., Lamiani, G., Del Negro, S., Monti, L., & Petrini, F. (2024). How to communicate with families living in complete isolation. *BMJ Supportive & Palliative Care, 14*(e3), e2954–e2965. DOI: 10.1136/bmjspcare-2020-002633 PMID: 33060189

Nowels, M. A., McDarby, M., Brody, L., Kleiman, E., Henson, S. S., Sweet, C. C., & Kozlov, E. (2024). Predictors of Engagement in Multiple Modalities of Digital Mental Health Treatments: Longitudinal Study. *Journal of Medical Internet Research, 26*. Advance online publication. DOI: 10.2196/48696 PMID: 39509696

Ordem dos Psicólogos Portugueses. (2023). *Documento de Apoio à Prática Profissional: Intervenção Psicológica à Distância, publicado pela Ordem dos Psicólogos Portugueses.*

Payne, S., Tanner, M., & Hughes, S. (2020). Digitisation and the patient–professional relationship in palliative care. *Palliative Medicine*, *34*(4), 441–443. DOI: 10.1177/026921632091150 PMID: 32253996

Perez, J. C. (2025). A look into telepsychology in the Philippines: an exploratory-cross-sectional research. *BMC Health Services Research*, *25*(1), 0–3. https://doi.org/.DOI: 10.1186/s12913-024-12091-9

Phelan, A. L., Katz, R., & Gostin, L. O. (2020). The Novel Coronavirus Originating in Wuhan, China. *Journal of the American Medical Association*, *323*(8), 709. DOI: 10.1001/jama.2020.1097 PMID: 31999307

Richmond, C. (2005). Dame Cicely Saunders. *BMJ (Clinical Research Ed.)*, *331*(7510), 238.

Rodrigues-Ribeiro, J. L., Castro, L., Pinto-Ribeiro, F., & Nunes, R. (2024). Impact of palliative care at end-of-life Covid-19 patients – a small-scale pioneering experience. *BMC Palliative Care*, *23*(1), 1–8. DOI: 10.1186/s12904-024-01368-9 PMID: 38166973

Rojas-Jara, C., Polanco-Carrasco, R., Caycho-Rodríguez, T., Muñoz-Vega, C., Muñoz-Marabolí, M., Luna-Gómez, T., & Muñoz-Torres, T. (2022). Telepsicología para psicoterapeutas: Lecciones aprendidas en tiempos del Covid-19. *Revista Interamericana de Psicología. Interamerican Journal of Psychology*, *56*(2), e1733. DOI: 10.30849/ripijp.v56i2.1733

Rosenfeld, B., Saracino, R., Tobias, K., Masterson, M., Pessin, H., Applebaum, A., Brescia, R., & Breitbart, W. (2017). Adapting Meaning-Centered Psychotherapy for the palliative care setting: Results of a pilot study. *Palliative Medicine*, *31*(2), 140–146. DOI: 10.1177/0269216316651570 PMID: 27435603

Salazar, H., & Duarte, J. (2017). *Intervenção Psicológica em Cuidados Paliativos*. Pactor.

Saldanha, J. (2011). *Fundamentals of Qualitative Research* (1st ed.). Oxford University Press.

Stake, R. E. (2005). Qualitative case studies. In Denzin, N. K., & Lincoln, Y. S. (Eds.), *The Sage handbook of qualitative research* (3rd ed., pp. 443–466). Sage.

Steindal, S. A., Nes, A. A. G., Godskesen, T. E., Holmen, H., Winger, A., Österlind, J., Dihle, A., & Klarare, A. (2023). Advantages and Challenges of Using Telehealth for Home-Based Palliative Care: Systematic Mixed Studies Review. *Journal of Medical Internet Research*, *25*, e43684. DOI: 10.2196/43684 PMID: 36912876

Stoll, J., Müller, J. A., Trachsel, M., Giordano, C., Ambrosiano, I., Graffeo, M. T., Di Caro, A., Gullo, S., Wind, T. R., Rijkeboer, M., Andersson, G., Riper, H., Haddouk, L., Schneider, B., Van Daele, T., Lang, F., Fagundes Machado, L., Paris Feijó, L., & Barcellos Serralta, F. (2020). Ethical Issues in Online Psychotherapy: A Narrative Review. *Frontiers in Psychiatry*, *10*(3), e36529. DOI: 10.4081/ripppo.2022.638 PMID: 32116819

Sutherland, A. E., Stickland, J., & Wee, B. (2020). Can video consultations replace face-to-face interviews? Palliative medicine and the Covid-19 pandemic: Rapid review. *BMJ Supportive & Palliative Care*, *10*(3), 271–275. DOI: 10.1136/bmjspcare-2020-002326 PMID: 32457086

Tajan, N., Devès, M., & Potier, R. (2023). Tele-psychotherapy during the COVID-19 pandemic: A mini-review. *Frontiers in Psychiatry*, *14*(July). Advance online publication. DOI: 10.3389/fpsyt.2023.1060961 PMID: 37476543

Teoli, D., Schoo, C., & Kalish, V. B. (2025). Palliative Care. In *StatPearls*. https://www.ncbi.nlm.nih.gov/pubmed/12231124

Van Goethem, V., Dierickx, S., Matthys, O., Deliens, L., Lapeire, L., Surmont, V., Geboes, K., Renard, V., Grønvold, M., D'Alton, P., Turola, E., Guberti, M., van der Wel, M., Brazil, K., Bristowe, K., Hudson, P., De Vleminck, A., & Cohen, J. (2025). Influence of Digital Competence on Participation and Retention of Patients with Advanced Cancer and Their Family Caregivers in a Randomized Controlled Trial with an e-Health Component: Findings from the DIAdIC Trial. *Telemedicine Journal and e-Health*. Advance online publication. DOI: 10.1089/tmj.2024.0101 PMID: 40331349

van Gurp, J., van Selm, M., Vissers, K., van Leeuwen, E., & Hasselaar, J. (2015). How Outpatient Palliative Care Teleconsultation Facilitates Empathic Patient-Professional Relationships: A Qualitative Study. *PLoS One*, *10*(4), e0124387. DOI: 10.1371/journal.pone.0124387 PMID: 25902263

Vuksanovic, D., Green, H., Morrissey, S., & Smith, S. (2017). Dignity Therapy and Life Review for Palliative Care Patients: A Qualitative Study. *Journal of Pain and Symptom Management*, *54*(4), 530–537.e1. DOI: 10.1016/j.jpainsymman.2017.07.016 PMID: 28716617

WHO. (2020). COVID 19 Public Health Emergency of International Concern (PHEIC) Global Research and Innovation Forum: Towards a Research Roadmap. *Global Research Collaboration for Infectious Disease Preparedness*, 1–10. https://www.who.int/publications/m/item/covid-19-public-health-emergency-of-international-concern-(pheic)-global-research-and-innovation-forum

Wood, M., Walshe, C., & McCullagh, A. (2023). What are the digitally enabled psychosocial interventions delivered by trained practitioners being offered to adults with life-shortening illnesses and palliative care needs and their informal and professional caregivers? A scoping review. *Palliative & Supportive Care*, *21*(4), 727–740. DOI: 10.1017/S1478951523000172 PMID: 36994819

World Health Organization. (2019). *recommendations on digital interventions for health system strengthening*. https://www.who.int/publications/i/item/9789241550505

World Health Organization. (2023).. . *Palliative Care*, *1*(June). https://www.who.int/europe/news-room/fact-sheets/item/palliative-care

Zhang, X., Xiao, H., & Chen, Y. (2017). Effects of life review on mental health and well-being among cancer patients: A systematic review. *International Journal of Nursing Studies*, *74*, 138–148. DOI: 10.1016/j.ijnurstu.2017.06.012 PMID: 28692880

KEY TERMS AND DEFINITIONS

Digital Health: Application of digital technologies in the field of health with the aim of preventing and treating diseases and promoting health and well-being, integrating resources such as telemedicine, e-health, big data, genomics, and artificial intelligence.

Digital Therapeutic Alliance: Alliance between client and therapist in the case of therapy sessions conducted via email, online chat, or videoconferencing.

Dignity: A multidimensional construct that involves recognizing and safeguarding the intrinsic value of the person at the end of life. It implies promoting autonomy, alleviating suffering, and respecting the preferences, values, and sense of identity of the individual, ensuring comprehensive care that preserves their humanity, spirituality, and sense of value until the moment of death.

Life Letter: Final document resulting from the application of the Meaning of Life Therapy is a physical legacy that can be given to family members or significant others, summarizing their life journey and purpose, seeking to convey teachings and guidance to future generations.

Meaning of Life Therapy: brief psychoexistencial intervention, involving a protocol and questions that guide the patients through a process of reflection, (re)signification of the meaning of life, and (re) conciliation with the present and past in order to promote meaning and purpose in life, adaptation to the terminal illness and death, and promotion of dignity and peace.

Palliative care: multidisciplinary approach that aims to respond to the holistic physical, psychosocial and spiritual needs of patients facing a life-threatening illness and/or in end-of-life.

Psychoexistencial Intervention: therapeutic approach that combines psychological and existential perspectives and seek to respond to patient's needs in order to strengthen their sense of identity and continuity, meaning-making, cultivate authenticity and responsibility, focus on meaning and purpose, exploration of personal experiences, providing emotional support.

Videoconferencing: One of the means of communication in digital health, allowing virtual visual contact between communication partners through sound and image (video).

APPENDIX

Table 4. Description of the Category System

Impact of MLT on the Patient (29 REFs)	Positive (29 REFs)	Emotional regulation (7 REFs)	It refers to promoting regulation of the patient's emotions during the intervention process.
		Stimulation of reflection (6 REFs)	It refers to the patient's reflection on life events.
		Communication facilitator (6 REFs)	It refers to the increasing willingness of the patient to communicate.
		Facilitator of the process of disease adaptation	It refers to the adaptation of the patient to the terminal cancer.
		(6 REFs)	It refers to the positive impact of recalling the past and planning for the future.
		Positive balance about the past and the future Encouraging sharing (1 REF)	It refers to increased information shared by the patient during and after the intervention.
Perception of the Impact of MLT on the Patient and his Wife (11 REFs)	Positive (8 REFs)	"It's good to talk..."	It refers to the benefits of communication during the intervention process.
		(4 REFs)	It refers to relational changes in the patient's relationship with his family (from his wife's perspective).
		Relational sphere with the patient's family (3 REFs)	It refers to the patient's increased communication (from his wife's perspective).
	Negative (3 REFs)	Openness to communication (1 REF)	It refers to the wife's uncertainties before the intervention due to its theme.
		Uncertainties regarding the theme of the intervention ("It was difficult...") (2 REFs) It avoids negative emotions (1 REF)	It refers to the wife's avoidance of experiencing negative emotions.
Impact of the Creation of the LL on the Patient (15 REFs)		Structuring (6 REFs)	It refers to the organization of ideas, facilitation of internalization, life review and promotion of comfort.
		Facilitating sharing (4 REFs)	It refers to how sharing of patient´s information was facilitated.
		Relational level (2 REFs)	It refers to the improvement of the relationship.
		Contentment (2 REFs)	It refers to the feeling of satisfaction produced when his wife received the LL.
		Useful for Health Professionals (1 REF)	It refers to how useful the LL was to improve knowledge of Health Professionals.
Impact of Sharing the LL with his Wife (6 REF)		Sharing facilitator (3 REFs)	It refers to more ideas and affection shared.
		Permanent testimony (2 REFs)	It refers to the possibility of keeping the LL permanently (forever).
		Emotional Impact (1 REF)	It refers to the emotions felt when receiving the LL.

continued on following page

Table 4. Continued

Patient´s Recommendation of the Intervention (6 REFs)	Yes (6 REFs)	Universal (2 REFs)	It refers to recommending its implementation on a universal scale.
		Structure facilitator (1 REF)	It refers to the intervention as a stimulus to reflection.
		It promotes acceptance (1 REF)	It refers to communication and writing as a means of facilitating disease adaptation.
		It promotes well-being (1 REF)	It refers to the comfort provided by the intervention.
		It facilitates expression (1 REF)	It refers to the possibility of thinking, rephrasing and correcting the content.
Wife´s Recommendation of the Intervention (5 REFs)	Perhaps (5 REFs)	It varies according to the personality traits (5 REFs)	It refers to recommending the intervention only after knowing the patient's personality (ability to accept/ disease confontration).
Risk Indicators (4 REFs)		Wife's reluctance towards the MLT questions (1 REF)	It refers to the wife's uncertainties before the intervention due to its theme.
		Systematic control (2 REFs)	It refers to the consequences of the methods used by health professionals in the symptomatic control of the terminally ill patient.
		COVID-19 contingency measures (1 REF)	It refers to the rules and restrictions adopted due to the pandemic.
Adaptation Indicators (3 REFs)		“Hearing his voice” (1 REF)	
		Maintenance of interpersonal relationships (2 REFs)	It refers to the LL as a permanent testimony.

About the Contributors

Sónia Remondes-Costa has a degree in Clinical and Counselling Psychology (2001) and a PhD in Clinical and Health Psychology (2012). Postgraduate in Advanced Studies in Health Psychology, Psycho-Oncology and Clinical and Experimental Hypnosis. Since September 2003, she has been an Assistant Professor in the Department of Psychology Education (DEP) at the School of Human and Social Sciences (ECHS) of the University of Trás-os-Montes and Alto Douro (UTAD). Her professional career has included teaching in higher education, primary health care, private social solidarity institutions (IPSSs), and private practice. She started as a Guest Assistant Professor on the degree programme in Curative Psychopedagogy at the Universidade Moderna do Porto (2001-2003). She worked in Primary Health Care at the Alfândega da Fé Health Centre (Bragança District; 2006-2008). She has worked as a clinical psychologist in different IPSS, namely: Francisco António Meireles Foundation (Torre de Moncorvo - Bragança), in the residential care of children and young people at risk and nursing home (2001-2006); 'O Leme' - Association for Psychological Support for Oncological Patients and Families (Torre de Moncorvo - Bragança) (2006-2008); Portuguese League Against Cancer - Northern Regional Centre (Porto) (2009-2011); Laços Prá Vida Association (Vila Real) in collaboration with the Portuguese League Against Cancer - Northern Regional Centre (2010-2012). As well as in different clinics: Psychological and Psychopedagogical Support Centre (2003-2004) - Alfândega da Fé - Bragança; Clínica dos Arcanjos (2004-2008) - Torre de Moncorvo - Bragança). At UTAD, she currently teaches History of Psychology, Group Dynamics, Theoretical Models in Psychology, Therapy Techniques and Behavioural Change, Assessment and Intervention in Health Psychology, Clinical and Health Psychology, Health Psychology, and Oncological Psychology in Psychology (1st and 2nd cycle), Psychomotor Rehabilitation, and Sociocultural Animation degrees. She also supervises internships and theses in the Master's Degree in Psychology, specializing in Clinical and Health Psychology and Educational and Developmental Psychology. She has supervised professional internships for the Portuguese Psychologists' Association since 2012. She is also a guest trainer in the Advanced Specialisation in Psychological Intervention in Bereavement [E-learning], in the Module Bereavement in Childhood and Adolescence: Psychological Intervention and in the Workshop Psychological Intervention in Bereavement: in Childhood and Adolescence [E-learning], at the CRIAP Institute. She is a researcher at CIDESD (Sports, Health and Development Research Centre, UTAD). Her research interests include Health Psychology and Oncological Psychology, specifically Health Promotion (in health and illness); Mind-Body Therapies, such as relaxation, yoga, meditation, and hypnosis, and the development and evaluation of the effectiveness of intervention programs; and Palliative Care, specifically Psycho-Existential Models of Intervention in Palliative Care and Bereavement. She is the author of the book Breast Cancer: pains of Female Suffering from the Experience of the Disease; author and co-author of book chapters in the field of psycho-oncology; author and co-author of national and international scientific articles and present at National and International Congresses in the field of her lines of research.

Jorge Remondes holds a PhD in Communication, in the scientific area of Marketing, from the University of Vigo. He is the coordinator of the 'Digital Marketing & E-Commerce' trilogy. He is the author of the book 'Internal Marketing and Communication - The Impact of using new technologies in SMEs' and co-author of 21 books (technical and scientific). He has published several articles on communication and digital marketing in scientific journals Web of Science and SCOPUS and in technical journals in Portugal and abroad, as well as in the general and specialized press. Founder and Editor-in-chief of the International Journal of Marketing, Communication and New Media, Web of Science Journal. Associate Editor of the scientific journals Management in Review and European Journal of Applied Business and Management. He was a manager for 12 years in national and multinational economic groups and began his academic career in 2005. He has been a business consultant. He is a trainer of business executives in the areas of marketing and sales as well as social media, having totaled more than 13,000 hours of training and consultancy activity. He created the Postgraduate Programme in Digital Content Marketing & Analytics at the Porto Executive Academy (PEA), of which he is Director. He created and coordinated the Postgraduate Programme in Digital Marketing & E-Commerce for 10 years at ISVOUGA Executive Education. He has been a guest lecturer on short courses and seminars at the Universidad de Vigo and the Universidad Europea Miguel de Cervantes. He is the author of the Digitality Podcast, available on Podcasts/Rádio Renascença Multimédia since March 2024. In 2012, he became an Honorary Member of the European High Council of Doctors and Doctor Honoris Causa.

***

Lawal Abdulwahab Olamilekan, with a PhD in Economics from Universiti Brunei Darussalam, is a forward-thinking academic. His research focuses on the intersections of governance, health economics, and sustainable development. He lectures in public health and management at Accord University, Somalia, and has extensive experience mentoring postgraduate and undergraduate students across Africa and Asia. His academic journey is anchored in a deep commitment to evidence-based policy research, with published work in peer-reviewed journals on institutional quality, natural resource governance, and healthcare outcomes. Lawal has presented at several international conferences, and his expertise spans digital health economics, macroeconomic policy, and development evaluation. His vision for the future of healthcare is inspiring, as he is passionate about applying AI and digital tools in academic research and healthcare delivery. He advocates for equitable, data-driven innovations that enhance preventive healthcare systems globally.

Mussa S Abubakari, PhD, is an enthusiastic educational technology researcher and associate researcher with the Dig Connectivity Research Laboratory (DCRLab) in Kampala, Uganda, since 2024. He's an instructor in the Department of Physics and Mathematics at Kondoa Islamic Secondary School, Tanzania. He has a PhD in Educational Technology from Sultan Hassanal Bolkiah Institute of Education, Universiti Brunei Darussalam, and graduated in 2025. Dr. Mussa obtained a Master of Education degree in Electronics and Informatics Engineering at Yogyakarta State University, Indonesia, in July 2021. He obtained his BSc. in Telecommunications Engineering at the University of Dodoma in June 2016. His academic and research interests include educational technology, technology-enhanced learning, technology acceptance, open and distance learning, generative AI, and digital competence, among others. He has over 15 journal articles published in internationally reputable journals, several book chapters, and papers presented at international conferences.

Pedro Amado holds a Ph.D. in Type Design in Digital Information and Communication Platforms from the University of Aveiro (2014), an MFA in Open-Source Type Design and Distribution in Multimedia Art (2007), and a degree in Communication Design (2002) from the Faculty of Fine Arts of the University of Porto (FBAUP). He is currently the director of the Master's in Graphic Design and Editorial Projects (MDGPE), an Associate Professor of Typography (Project) and Typeface Design (Graduate and Undergraduate programs), Web Design, and Research Methodologies (graduate program) at FBAUP. Integrated researcher and member of the board of direction of the i2ADS research institute, was one of the inaugural editors of the i2ADS HUB journal, and is the coordinator member of Ligatures — the Special Interest Group around the exploration of the materiality of language — in the i2ADS Computation Hybrid Practices and Culture Program.

Elmars Baltins, Engineering and economics graduate of Riga Technical University, Elmars Baltins finds his work where the cross-sections of education, research and innovation, business and environment take place. He has been involved with designing and organising entrepreneurial training and business idea valorisation programs for youth, nascent entrepreneurs and inventors in Latvia and across borders. Elmars is interested and keeps developing himself in sustainable and innovative business and education techniques. He is a delegate at the European Commission SME Assembly and a board member of Latvian Inventors Association. He is a co-founder of two innovative companies in Latvia.

Unnathi Bhaktharam holds a B.A. (Honours) in Psychology from O.P. Jindal Global University. Her research interests span adolescent mental health, parenting styles, and the therapeutic role of art and dance in psychological well-being. She has co-authored a study on intimate partner violence (IPV), social capital, and their impact on depression in women, at the St.Johns Hospital, Bengaluru. She also brings substantial research experience from her role as a Research Associate with the UC Berkeley Haas Future Work Lab's India Team, where she served as a key trainer and lead coordinator for their main study. Her broader academic and professional focus lies in applying psychological insights to human behaviour, and aims to be part of the solutions of everyday practical challenges of the underprivileged communities. This is her first co-authored publication.

Maddalena Buonamico, a 2021 Political Science, International Relations, and European Studies graduate from the University "A. Moro" of Bari, deepened her knowledge of European project design through a 2022 Master's course at Venice International University. Joining ALL DIGITAL in March 2022 as an Erasmus+ intern, she focused on European Project Management, participating in project activities, disseminating results, and organizing events. Maddalena also contributed to monitoring EU policy developments, writing project reports, and proposals.

Grażyna Busse, a Master in Pedagogy, specializes in Adult Education and Social Gerontology from the University of Lodz. As a German language teacher and co-founder of the Educational Centre of Intergenerational Integration HIPOKAMP, she organizes events addressing demographic challenges in aging. Grażyna coordinates national and international projects on 'active aging' promoting gerontological knowledge and fostering intergenerational dialogue. Since 2008, she conducts practical courses for seniors in urban and rural areas of the Lodz province. She contributes to curriculum development at the Medical University in Lodz, particularly in the innovative field of study: MANAGED SENIOR CARE. Now, engaged in Nofer Institute of Occupational Medicine in Lodz Poland

Pavlos Carrera, Bachelor's in Social Science from the University of Houston, Texas. Specializing in Intellectual Disabilities, with a focus on Autism, he initially worked as a substitute teacher for Pasadena ISD before joining the management team at IMS R&D. With extensive involvement in European research projects as a project manager and researcher, Pavlos now oversees IMS R&D's European Research and Development projects, managing all aspects of research and financial activity. Additionally, he coordinates activities for IMS private school's Erasmus projects, contributing significant experience and expertise to the organization.

Beatriz Carvalho is a designer, graduated in Interior Design from the School of Arts and Design (ESAD) in Matosinhos. Currently pursuing a Master's degree in Industrial and Product Design at the Faculty of Fine Arts of the University of Porto. Has experience in both Interior and Product Design.

Susanta Das is a seasoned educator with a proven record of teaching and mentoring diverse students, working at multiple institutions, and providing service to the various initiatives of organizations. He received his Ph.D. and M.A. degrees from Western Michigan University (WMU), USA, and M.Sc. degree from Banaras Hindu University (BHU), India all in Physics. He continued his research as a Marie-Curie post-doctoral fellow at Stockholm University, Stockholm, Sweden on beam diagnostics for the DESIREE (Double ElectroStatic Ion Ring ExpEriment) in the project DITANET (Diagnostic Techniques for particle Accelerators – a Marie-Curie initial training NETwork), at the Indian Institute of Science Education and Research-Kolkata, India on high-pressure physics as a Project Scientist-B, and at the University of Electro-Communications, Tokyo, Japan on ion-surface interactions as a Post-doctoral fellow. Throughout his career, Dr. Das worked and collaborated with many researchers, Ph.D., master, and visiting students from different countries. He further visited many countries to discuss research and an international conference participant (UK, Italy, Germany, Greece, Belgium, Bulgaria, Romania, Brazil etc.). He co-authored several research articles in WoS/Scopus indexed international journals, conference proceedings, and scholarly book chapters published by renowned international publishing houses. Beyond his research endeavors, Dr. Das has a storied history of service to academic and administrative committees, exhibiting his commitment to the growth and development of educational institutions. His experience includes tenure at Central University South Bihar, Sri Sri University, and P.K. University before assuming his current role at Ajeenkya DY Patil University. He received the Marie-Curie post-doctoral fellowship in Sweden, Science Academies' Summer Research Fellowship in India, Gwen Frostic Doctoral Fellowship, Department Graduate Research and Creative Scholar Award by WMU, and Leo R. Parpart Doctoral Fellowship by Dept. of Physics, WMU, among many others, throughout his academic journey. At present, Dr. Das continues to delve into cutting-edge fields, with a keen interest in nanotechnology, UN SDGs, and data science. His multifaceted contributions, spanning teaching, research, and administrative leadership, showcase a dedicated professional who is instrumental in advancing the vision and mission of the institutions he serves.

Pooja Dehankar is working as an Assistant Professor at Ajeenkya DY Patil School of Engineering, Savitribai Phule Pune University, Pune. She has completed BE in Computer Engineering from Priyadarshini College of Engineering, Nagpur, and ME in Information Technology from Sinhgad College of Engineering, Pune. She has done Post Graduate Diploma in Advance Computing. She has 15 years of experience in academics. Her areas of interest are Artificial Intelligence, Cyber Security, and Data Mining. She has published papers in Scopus Journals. She actively participates in workshops, faculty development programs, short-term training programs, conferences, and webinars. She is pursuing Ph.D. from Symbiosis Center for Research and Innovation, Symbiosis International (Deemed University).

Jana Gerstmair has been the director of the adult education centre in Schrobenhausen since 2018, where she has actively engaged in various international projects. She holds a degree in business administration, which includes a year of study abroad, and she was raised in a multicultural household. Jana believes that the exchange and collaboration with individuals from diverse backgrounds enrich not only her personal experience but also the learning environment at her centre. She is deeply committed to fostering an inclusive educational community and is grateful for the opportunities to learn from and work with people from different cultures.

Bruno Giesteira, is a Associate Professor with Habilitation at the University of Porto, Faculty of Fine Arts, Design Department, pursuing studies in Human-Centred Design, More-than-Human paradigms, and Embodied Cognition as the ground of knowledge for leveraging the Somaesthetic dimension when mediated by computational interactive artefacts, namely in Health and Wellbeing scopes. Is the Director of the Design Doctoral Program at Fine Arts Faculty of the University of Porto and Postgraduate courses in Interaction Design and Games and Design Technologies for Health. He has extensive experience managing HCI's research teams and has been widely published in his field. Nominated member of the Academic Committee of EUGLOH - European University Alliance for Global Health and selected member of the HFES - Human Factors and Ergonomics Society - Europe Chapter.

Celestino Gonçalves, Adjunct professor of Informatics at School of Technology and Management of Polytechnic of Guarda in Portugal, where he has been teaching courses related to artificial intelligence, machine learning, functional programming and ubiquitous computing to the Computer Science Engineering and Data Science and Artificial Intelligence degrees and to the MSc in Mobile Computing. His research interests are artificial intelligence, pervasive computing and the study of deep learning algorithms for designing ambient intelligence solutions of context-aware and user-centric services.

Filipe Gonçalves, Dietitian/Nutritionist and Physiotherapist, holding a degree in Nutritional Sciences from the Faculty of Nutrition and Food Sciences at the University of Porto, and a degree in Physiotherapy from the School of Health at the Polytechnic Institute of Setúbal. Master's in Cognitive Science from the University of Lisbon and currently pursuing a PhD in Health Sciences at the University of A Coruña. Member of CI-IPOP and the Porto Comprehensive Cancer Centre (IPOP/RISE@CI-IPOP). President of the Board of APELA – Portuguese Association for Amyotrophic Lateral Sclerosis, and founding and active member of ADITGameS – Association for the Development of Technological Innovation and Games in Health. Clinically focused on neuromuscular and oncological diseases, palliative care, nutrition, and metabolism.

João Gregório, Ph.D., in International Health and Development Policies (IHMT, NOVA University of Lisbon). With a background in Pharmaceutical Sciences and Community Pharmacy, he is an Associate Professor and Researcher at CBIOS, Lusófona University. João's research focuses on Health Services, particularly new pharmaceutical services and digital health innovations in primary and specialized care. Actively collaborating internationally, he has published extensively in peer-reviewed journals and contributes as an editorial board member and guest editor for leading journals in health services and pharmacy.

Dilek Gümüş is an assistant professor in the Department of Medical Services and Techniques, First Aid and Emergency Care Program at Bilecik Şeyh Edebali University in Turkey. Her academic interests include innovative nursing practices, postoperative care, nonpharmacological pain management, and the integration of digital health technologies into clinical settings. Gümüş is particularly interested in combining artificial intelligence tools with evidence-based nursing practices to improve patient outcomes.

Mallikharjuna Rao K is an Assistant Professor Gr-I, in the department of Data Science and Artificial Intelligence at International Institute of Information Technology Naya Raipur (IIIT NR), Chhattisgarh, India. Earlier, he worked as Assistant Professor Sr. Grade-1 at VIT-AP University between 2019-2021. He also worked as Associate Professor at SVECW, Bhimavaram, A.P., India between 2018-2019. He served as an Assistant Professor at GITAM University, Visakhapatnam, A.P., India and GRIET Hyderabad between 2007-2011. He received his Ph.D. in Computer Science and Engineering and Master's in Computer Science from Jawaharlal Nehru Technological University Hyderabad (JNTUH) in 2018 and 2010. He obtained his bachelor's degree in Information Science and Technology Engineering from Acharya Nagarjuna University, Andhra Pradesh, India, in 2004. Dr. Rao received a grant of Rs. 6 lakhs from DST, Govt. of India for conducting a national workshop on "Data Science Research". He published more than 15 research papers in various international journals and conferences of repute. He also published 3 Indian patents. Dr. Rao is an editorial member and reviewer of various peer-reviewed journals which are SCI/WOS/SCOPUS indexed like IET Software, IEEE Sensors Journal, CMBBE, IJSAEM, JCS, JSR, IJECE, IJCS, BEEI, IJSER. He also chaired sessions AT various international conferences like IEEE WIECON-ECE 2022, ICCIDE22, TRIBES21, etc. Dr. Rao also served as TPC member and Reviewer in various Springer & IEEE conferences like WCAIC-2023, ICDSA 2023, CVR23, InC4-23, ICCCT23, TENSYMP-22, AIC-22,ICCIS22, etc. He is a life member of CSI and Senior Member of IEEE, IEEE CIS, IEEE CS. His research area includes Artificial Intelligence: Evolutionary Algorithms, Swarm Intelligence, Data Science, Machine Learning, Data Mining, Data privacy, Imbalanced data, and applications of health care and finance.

Gerly Macedo, Graduated in Psychology (Pre-Bologna), with a pre-specialization in clinical and health psychology, from the University of Minho [Portugal] in 2001. I have completed multiple postgraduate degrees (both national and international), primarily in health psychology from 2002 to the present day; most recently, a postgraduate degree in postgraduate degree in occupational health, other such postgarduations ares in Neuropsycology Evaluation and intervention, administrative management in health, in Palliative Care from INSPSIC, Porto [Portugal]); a postgraduate degree in Psycho-Oncology from the Instituto Superior de Estúdios en Psicologia (ISEP), Barcelona [Spain]. i have been working as in clinical and health psychology from 2001 to the present day ate privated and public health institutions as a active member on multidisciplinary teams My professional practice encompasses individuals across their various life cycles, with a special interest in oncology, chronic diseases, and palliative care. I have been responsible for the psychological assessment and intervention (in group or individual settings) of chronic patients, family members, and caregivers who exhibit behavioral complaints and/or significant reactive or adaptive psychological/emotional symptoms that cause distress and/or compromise overall functioning and routine. I have also been a supervisor for undergraduate and graduate internships since 2005, developing several research projects in which I participated as a co-researcher and co-author of book and journal articles, posters, and papers in the areas of interest of health psychology, in collaboration with various public and private educational institutions. Finally, I have experience as an Internal Trainer (at Hospital Senhora da Oliveira since 2001) and External Trainer (at Inspisic in various postgraduate programs and at the University of Minho and CESPU as a Guest Professor in thematic modules since 2003).

Marta B Martins (MBM) is currently a Pharmacist and has recently graduated in Pharmaceutical Sciences (Integrated Master's) from Universidade Lusófona - Centro Universitário de Lisboa, with a dissertation in Nanotechnology and Drug Delivery Systems. Due to her growing interest in research, MBM is the author and co-author of several oral and poster presentations at national and international conferences, with focus on hybrid drug delivery systems. MBM was recently awarded a research grant to join an FCT-funded project entitled "Enhancing Medication Adherence in Portugal: Implementation of Mobili®, an eHealth Medicine Dispensing Solution for Multimorbidity Patients.".

Sandra Martins, Associate Professor of Sport at Universidade Europeia, PhD in Human Kinetics, specialising in Health and Physical Fitness, from the Faculty of Human Kinetics - Universidade de Lisboa, Director of the CIDESD-UEUROPEIA Research Hub at Universidade Europeia. With 21 articles published in WOS indexed journals, 6 books and 10 book chapters, she has participated in 5 funded research projects and her teaching activity has been developed in parallel with academic management positions at Universidade Europeia. Clinical Exercise Physiologist at the Endocrinology and Nutrition Centre of the CUF Tejo Hospital in Lisbon, trainer on the Advanced Training Course in Physical Exercise and Cancer of the Portuguese League Against Cancer (Northern Regional Centre) and AICSO since 2021, member of the ONCOMOVE team and the AIM Cancer Centre team, with 18 years of experience working in multidisciplinary teams in a clinical context in the field of obesity, bariatric surgery, diabetes mellitus and cancer. She also holds positions as Vice-President of the Board of the Portuguese Association of Exercise Physiologists (APFE; 2018-present), Member of the Scientific Council of the National Programme for the Promotion of Physical Activity of the Directorate-General for Health (DGS; 2018-present), Secretary of the Board of the Study Group on Sports Endocrinology and Physical Exercise of the Portuguese Society of Endocrinology, Diabetes and Metabolism (SPEDM; 2025-present), former Vice-President of the Board (2016-2021) and current President of the Supervisory Board of the Portuguese Society for the Study of Obesity (SPEO).

Joana Nogueira completed her Master's degree in Medicine in 2020. In 2021, she began her medical career in Caldas da Rainha and, in 2022, started her residency in Family Medicine in Lisbon. She interrupted her residency in 2024 and has since been working as a physician and researcher at Future Healthcare – Virtual Clinic.

Peter Palvolgyi, a pan-European association, focuses on improving digital skills across Europe and supporting the 42% with insufficient digital skills. It represents 100+ member organizations working with 25,000 digital competence centres, annually training 1.5 million people. Member organizations, including ICT centres, NGOs, universities, and associations, provide non-formal education, internet access, ICT tools, and digital training, certification, and opportunities. ALL DIGITAL supports both general and disadvantaged populations, such as the elderly, unemployed, young people, migrants, and refugees. Fostering knowledge sharing, collaboration, and representing members' interests to the EU, the association plays a crucial role in enhancing digital literacy.

Ana Frade Pina, MD, PhD, is Head of d Health & Care at Future Healthcare, leading Future Healthcare Virtual Clinic. Holds a PhD in Mechanisms of Disease and Regenerative Medicine from NOVA Medical School, an MSc in Information Management and Business Intelligence from NOVA IMS. Certified Professional of Digital Health Transformation by HIMSS, and black-Belt in VBHC. Having clinical and research experience, she integrates medicine, data science, and innovation to advance value-based digital health. She leads projects applying machine learning to chronic disease management and digital health transformation, and has authored numerous peer-reviewed publications in diabetes, artificial intelligence, and dysmetabolism. An active member of national and European medical and technology societies, she serves on the AI Commission of the Portuguese Medical Association. Throughout her career, she has combined clinical practice, academic research, and strategic leadership, committed to delivering evidence-based, technology-driven solutions that create measurable value in healthcare.

Andreia Sofia Pinto de Sousa is a designer, researcher, and lecturer. She holds a PhD in Information and Communication in Digital Platforms from the University of Aveiro and the University of Porto (2017). She is currently an Assistant Professor at Universidade Lusófona – Centro Universitário do Porto, where she teaches communication and interaction design. Her research focuses on the intersection of design, health, and digital technologies, with recent work presented at international conferences such as HCII, DIGICOM, HCist, and IEEE CoG.

Maria Poulain, Cultural Studies MA graduate from the University of Lodz, specializing in cultural geragogy, journalism, and ICT skills for the 55+ generation. A certified coach and social animator, with over 3000 hours of workshops on civic activation for older individuals. Member of the Mobile ICT/ Digital Education Team for 50+, providing services in Lodz and small communes. Since 2015, engaged in educational and advisory roles, coordinating granted projects. As an adviser for the Regional Social Policy Centers in Lodz and Opolskie Voivodeships since 2018, involved in the 'Independent Life' project, developing standards and piloting assisted housing for individuals with neurological diseases and the elderly.

Guido Ragucci, Architect and professor of technology in CPIA Taranto. 38 years old. He graduated from the Bari Polytechnic in the department of Civil Engineering and Architectural Sciences. He studied for one year in University of Fuzhou (China) in Civil Engineering College, specialized in pedestrian bridges.

Diogo Ribeiro is currently in the process of completing a degree in Data Science and Artificial Intelligence at Polytechnic Institute of Guarda and working as an intern at Critical TechWorks in Braga, Portugal.

Liliana Rodrigues is the CEO of the company "More Than Humans – Research and Consultancy for Humans". The company bridges academic research and applied innovation, focusing on product and service design for wellbeing. Its work is grounded in Human-centred Design (HCD) and the More-Than-Human paradigm, embedding the New European Bauhaus (NEB) values of Inclusivity, Sustainability, and Aesthetics.

Marta de Oliveira Rodrigues is a researcher at the University of Trás-os-Montes and Alto Douro (UTAD) and a collaborating member of the Centre for Research and Intervention in Education from the Faculty of Psychology and Educational Sciences of the University of Porto (CIIE - FPCEUP). She holds a Doctorate in Education Sciences (FPCEUP), a degree in Sociology of Organizations from the University of Minho (UMinho), and a master's in Educational Sciences – major in Adult Education by UTAD. She is a member of the research community of practice Youth, Education, Diversity and Innovation (JEDI) of CIIE and External Evaluation Committees of the Agency for Assessment and Accreditation of Higher Education (A3ES), integrating External Evaluation Committees. Her current research interests focus on quality/equity in education, sociology of education, school failure and dropout, academic pathways, digital skills, artificial intelligence, NEET (not in employment, education, or training), formal and non-formal education, and qualitative methodologies.

Biswajit Saha has more than 23 years of academic experience which includes teaching at both under graduate and post graduate level of Computer Science and Engineering. He has authored numerous journal and conference publications and contributed book chapters with highly reputed publishing houses. His broader interests include machine learning, health informatics, AI in education, and outcome-based pedagogy.

Eliana Penedos-Santiago is an Assistant Professor of Design and Drawing at the Faculty of Fine Arts of the University of Porto (FBAUP). Integrated researcher and member at ID+ Research Institute for Design, Media and Culture and collaborator of the i2ADS Research Institute in Art, Design and Society, working within the research program for Computation, Hybrid Practices and Culture, a collective of designers, artists, educators and media researchers. She holds substantial experience relating to human-computer interaction in the context of Computational Design (UX, UI, AR, VR), Design Education and Design for Health. Researcher in several funded research projects, is currently the lead researcher on the project "Drawing for Social Re-connectivity. Exploring Inclusive, Collaborative and Digital Environments for Patients with Partial to Complete Locked-In Syndrome."

Teresa Santos, Clinical Psychologist, Master in Clinical Psychology and PhD in Health Psychology (ISPA-Instituto Universitário). Psychotherapist in Behavioral, Cognitive and Integrative Therapies. Specialist in Clinical/Health Psychology; Psychotherapy; Educational Psychology; and Community Psychology by the Portuguese Psychologists Order. Certified Psychologist by EFPA (European Federation of Psychologists Associations). Dean of the Faculty of Health Sciences, Psychology Coordinator and Associated Professor at the Universidade Europeia in Lisbon. Integrated researcher at the Research Center in Sports Sciences, Health Sciences and Human Development (CIDESD) in the University of Trás-os-Montes and Alto Douro (Vila Real).

Clara Silveira, Coordinator Professor at the School of Technology and Management (ESTG) of the Polytechnic of Guarda. Teaching activities, since 1991, in the field of "Software Engineering and Information Systems" to the Computer Science Engineering degree, the Data Science and Artificial Intelligence degree, the MSc in Mobile Computing and the MSc in Cybersecurity. She holds a PhD in Electrical and Computer Engineering from the Faculty of Engineering, University of Porto (FEUP); Master in Electrical and Computer Engineering, specializing in Industrial Informatics at FEUP; and completed the Training Program on Public Managemen by INA. Director of the Software Engineering and Information Systems field. She has over eight years of experience leading the ESTG management team. She was a member of the Polytechnic of Guarda Ethical Committee. She is the author of several scientific works published in national and international journals, book chapters and conferences.

Tainá de Souza holds a Bachelor's degree in Biomedical Sciences (University of Aveiro, 2022) and is pursuing a Master's in Public Health at the University of Porto. Her work bridges research and innovation in digital health, with a focus on user-centered design, accessibility, and health equity. At UXVolution, she contributed to the development and evaluation of healthcare solutions, supporting usability assessments, technical documentation and participation in innovation and entrepreneurship initiatives. She is the first author of a study mapping mobile health applications for Mpox in Brazil, which was presented at Fiocruz in Brazil. She is also the co-author of two articles on digital interventions to promote appropriate antibiotic use. Her academic and professional activities are guided by the conviction that health technology should be human-centered, respecting the social and cultural realities of users. Her areas of interest include health technology design, digital inclusion, health literacy, active aging, and digital public policies.

Ricardo Teixeira is a clinical and health psychologist and cognitive-behavioral psychotherapist. Director of REACH - Mental Health Clinic, in Porto (Portugal). Instructor of Mindfulness-Based Cognitive Therapy (MBCT) program. Guest lecturer at universities and postgraduate centers. Researcher at the Center for Research in Neuropsychology and Cognitive-Behavioral Intervention (CINEICC) at the University of Coimbra. PhD in Health Psychology (Psycho-Oncology) from the School of Psychology of the University of Minho. Post-doctorate in Psychology (third generation Cognitive-Behavioral Therapies) by the Department of Education and Psychology at the University of Aveiro. Postgraduate in Health Psychology, in Cognitive-Behavioral Psychotherapies (Advanced Course), in Compassion-Focused Therapy (advanced course), and in Continuing and Palliative Care. Practicum at the Department of Biological Psychology at the Humboldt University of Berlin. Research interests: processes of stress, anxiety, affection and interpersonal regulation of emotions in psychotherapy and in the community.

Paulo Vieira, BSc in Pure Mathematics from the University of Porto, MSc in Mathematics from the University of Lisbon, and PhD in Computer Science with a specialisation in Artificial Intelligence from the University of Salamanca. I am currently the Director of the BSc in Data Science and Artificial Intelligence at the Polytechnic University of Guarda.

Guilherme Vila Maior, User Interface Designer with a background in Communication Design, specialised in Interaction Design and a Master's in Multimedia from the University of Porto. Guilherme has designed interfaces for diverse communities, including academic, cultural, and healthcare projects such as 'Skills For a Next Generation,' CETAPS, and Porto's Planetarium. Passionate about Human-Computer Interaction, he focuses on User-Centered Design and experience enhancement. Outside of work, he sings with Coro Mozart and enjoys volleyball, oil painting, and video production.

Tjaša Vozel holds a MA in English Language Teaching and has seamlessly transitioned from education to project managing. She offers a unique perspective with extensive experience from kindergarten to adult education. Her deep understanding of the Slovenian educational system, coupled with International Baccalaureate (IB) certificates for MYP and DP programmes, positions her as a versatile professional. Tjaša's proficiency extends beyond the classroom, showcasing adept mastery of translation and subtitling. Leveraging her teaching and translation background, she specializes in international initiatives like ERASMUS+ and CERV projects.

Aleksandra Wasilewska, Master's degree in physiotherapy, graduate of the Medical University of Łódź, specialist in the field of Neurological Aquatherapy. From 2017 to 2020, she worked at the Rehabilitation Clinic at the Institute of the Mother of Polish Health Center in Łódź. From 2020, co-founder and president of the management board of 'Płyńmy Razem' Foundation, whose main goal is to promote physical activity, the healthy lifestyle and promoting of various forms of comprehensive rehabilitation and treatment for disabled, sick, and needy individuals. Since 2023, she has been collaborating with the Senior Center at the University of Łódź, organizing movement rehabilitation for groups of older adults.

Giovanni Zuccalá, Graduated from the University of Salento, studying Intercultural Communication and Translation, focusing on English and Turkish. Studied English Literature in Stockholm and in Turkey.

Index

A

B

C

D

E

G

H

I

L

M

N

O

P

Q

R

S

T

U

V

W

X

www.ingramcontent.com/pod-product-compliance
Lightning Source LLC
LaVergne TN
LVHW060254011026
849161LV00011B/2713